Infectious Diseases

Prevention and Treatment in the Nineteenth and Twentieth Centuries

by

Wesley W. Spink, M.D.

*Regents' Professor of Medicine
and Comparative Medicine, Emeritus
University of Minnesota Medical School*

DAWSON

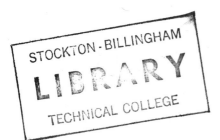
First published 1978

© University of Minnesota 1978

Wm Dawson & Son Ltd, Cannon House
Folkestone, Kent, England

British Library Cataloguing in Publication Data
Spink, Wesley William
    Infectious diseases, prevention and treatment
    in the nineteenth and twentieth centuries.
    1. Epidemics — History   2. Public health — History
    3. Communicable diseases — History
    I. Title
    614.4'09'034   RA649
ISBN 0-7129-0904-4

Printed in the United States of America

To
Dagmar A. Kamprud

Preface

Infectious diseases have been among man's greatest afflictions since ancient times. The full record of the suffering they have dealt in terms of sickness and death would stagger the imagination. Man's endeavor to control infectious diseases also dates back to an early era; real progress was being made by the mid-nineteenth century and is still continuing. The story of this achievement, involving both scientific and institutional developments, is wide-ranging and complex, and often dramatic. This book is an attempt to tell that story for readers in the health sciences and public health, as well as for general readers.

Such a volume is needed because, although advances in the control of infectious diseases have been described in a general way elsewhere, there is still scope for detailed discussion with respect to specific diseases. Medical textbooks have little or nothing to say about the historical aspects of disease. Neither accelerated learning programs nor self-learning projects leave time for such considerations. Yet historical knowledge can be an invaluable asset for individuals involved in health care, if only in deepening their appreciation for the hard-won successes that have been achieved in efforts to maintain healthy populations. One can also gain from the study of past failures a better understanding of what can be done to curtail the spread of infectious diseases. This volume should help provide such information.

. The book is divided into three sections. Section I is introductory; Section II deals in detail with twentieth-century developments in the prevention and treatment of infectious diseases. Section III, which presents the history of specific infections up to the present, comprises most of the text. The extensive bibliography is intended to aid those who may wish to pursue topics further.

Every scientific achievement is built on the efforts of former generations. In the present study Section I is concerned with the origin of concepts of contagion. This section also describes the earliest attempts to control epidemic diseases through quarantine and vaccination. Progress in both these areas was accelerated in the nineteenth century with the most brilliant advance of all in the control of infections, the discovery of the specific microbes that cause them. But even before the knowledge of specificity was acquired, another major achievement was the evolution of the public health movement. I have stressed the development of public health in Great Britain because of its impact on the movement in the United States and on the formation of the United States Public Health Service and of the National Institutes of Health. The success of public health at national levels stimulated cooperation at an international level, first through the League of Nations and later through the World Health Organization.

Section II describes the most dramatic of the achievements in the prevention and treatment of infections, which occurred between 1935 and 1950. These resulted from intensive research on chemotherapy and the development of specific vaccines. I have described the discoveries of sulfonamide and antibiotic therapy in detail because I worked at the time in that field. As one who cared for groups of critically ill patients before the successful introduction of chemotherapy, I could only conclude that the results with the sulfonamides and antibiotics were spectacular. I believe, however, that the greatest good for the greatest number has come through sound public health organization and preventive medicine. Therapy alone has never eradicated any infectious disease.

Section III opens with a discussion of the significance of fever in the interpretation of illness. Ten chapters are then devoted to a historical study of ten groups of infectious diseases. Chapter 12 presents those pandemic diseases still under maritime control — plague, smallpox, yellow fever, leprosy, and cholera. These diseases struck terror among large populations of people in the past, but today through strict quarantine and prophylactic vaccination they are confined to small endemic foci. And it would appear that smallpox will be completely eradicated soon through vaccination. Chapter 14 on respiratory diseases, on the other hand, points out that influenza is a pandemic disease that still cannot be controlled adequately, and the reasons for this deficiency are given. Chapter 13 cites the communicable diseases of childhood that have taken millions of lives in the past, and the prophylactic measures — especially vaccines — through which disability and death have been prevented. This chapter also emphasizes that such precautionary measures must be continued if prevention of these diseases is to be maintained.

The book stresses the fact that although we have the knowledge and the methods for preventing diseases, some infections, such as gonorrhea and syphilis, still afflict millions of people. The most severe challenge remaining among world populations is the control of parasitic diseases, including malaria, leishmaniasis, trypanosomiasis and schistosomiasis, as shown in Chapter 20. Authorities at the World Health Organization have centered attention on this problem. Another major challenge that remains is presented in Chapter 19, which describes virus infections involving the central nervous system, such as encephalitis and hemorrhagic fever, and the slow virus diseases.

I direct further attention to the bibliography. In our pursuit of the references we sought the advice of experienced medical librarians. We have followed their general recommendation of using a format that coincides with the standardized library reference. The complete title has been cited as well as the authors and publication data. English translations of foreign sources have been suggested wherever possible. For the reader interested in a general introduction to historical aspects of infectious diseases, I have added a short annotated list of suggested readings. This is a highly personal selection found in my own collection, one that has been useful to me over the years.

My reasons for writing this book are closely related to my career in infectious diseases, which extends back over fifty years to the time when I was a medical student at Harvard. My interest in the historical aspects of medicine was stimulated initially by my teachers. The surgeon Professor Harvey Cushing aroused this interest through his teaching and through his book *The Life of Sir William Osler*. Dr. Hans Zinsser, professor of bacteriology and immunology, was an incomparable lecturer, introducing each of his lectures with a historical background of the subject. When he told us about the Wassermann reaction for the serological diagnosis of syphilis, he took the time to explain just what Dr. Wassermann originally did in his laboratory. One does not readily forget knowledge acquired in this manner. Dr. Chester Keefer, professor of medicine, was a superb clinician and a medical scholar. He taught me my life-long habit of seeking out historical information about each of the infectious diseases that I saw. Dr. Keefer influenced my academic career more than anyone else. I owe a debt of gratitude to Professor Donald Augustine, who introduced me to clinical research on trichinosis when I was a student. This research was the basis for my first publication on infectious diseases.

I had always wanted to write on the historical aspects of infectious diseases, but circumstances did not permit the sustained time and effort that would be necessary. I had lived and worked through one of the most exciting periods in medical history, dealing with infections before and after the introduction of the sulfonamides, penicillin, and most of the prophylactic vaccines. I was privileged to be associated with enthusiastic graduate students, who contributed much to our knowledge of infectious diseases. As a consultant to United States military authorities and to the World Health Organization I observed and studied infectious diseases in several areas in the world.

When I prepared for mandatory retirement from academic life in 1973, I decided to devote full time to writing this volume. Dagmar Kamprud, who had been my assistant for many years, gladly agreed to join me in the project. She had accumulated my notes and an extensive literature on the subject and had filed them for such a possibility. She typed and edited several drafts of the manuscript and carefully checked the bibliography. Because of her devotion to my work on infectious diseases and because the publication of this book was possible only with her help, I have dedicated this volume to her.

I am grateful to many for the support and advice I have received that allowed me to pursue this project without interruption for five years. A grant from the National Library of Medicine constituted the principal source of financial aid. I appreciate deeply the help of several of my former colleagues in the department of medicine of the Medical School and also the Minnesota Medical Foundation. Dr. N. L. Gault, dean of the medical school, and Professor Glenn Brudvig, director of the Bio-Medical Library, provided us working space in close proximity to collections in that library and in the Owen H. Wangensteen Library of the History of Medicine. The entire library staff was most gracious in their help and advice. John Ervin, Jr., director of the University of Minnesota Press, not only encouraged me to prepare this volume but gave freely of his time for editorial suggestions. I also appreciate the careful editorial assistance of Dorian Kottler and Beverly Kaemmer of the press.

During the preparation of the manuscript I sought the scientific advice of several persons, especially Dr. Abraham I. Braude, University of California Medical School, San Diego; Dr. Craig Howe, former research associate at the University of Minnesota; Dr. Franklin Wallace, professor of zoology, University of Minnesota; and Dr. Martin Kaplan, former director of research, World Health Organization, Geneva, Switzerland, and now director-general of the Pugwash Conferences on Science and World Affairs, Geneva. I am grateful to all these individuals.

The manuscript was written for the most part at home with the help and advice of my wife, Elizabeth, who had long wished that this book could be written — a wish that finally came true.

Wesley W. Spink, M.D.

Minneapolis, Minnesota
February 28, 1978

Table of Contents

LIST OF FIGURES

LIST OF TABLES

SECTION I

Background of the Control and Treatment of Infectious Diseases

CHAPTER 1

Early Concepts of Infection and Methods of Control

The greatest achievement of medical science for human welfare has been the control and management of infectious diseases. This achievement was largely the result of knowledge gained during the second half of the nineteenth century, which came to fruition between 1935 and 1950. The complete history of this knowledge is of course much longer; some concepts of the nature of infectious and epidemic diseases had been formulated over previous centuries on the basis of observation and, in some cases, of experiment. An inquiry into these developments would be very extensive, dating back to early Egyptian and Greek periods. It is possible here to give only a brief sketch of the early background of the control and management of infectious diseases.

Two major achievements contributed to the success in the present century. First, the doctrine of the specificity of each of many infectious diseases was finally proved by the identification of the causative microorganism for each. The Greeks, as recorded in the "Hippocratic Corpus" (Heracleitus, 1931; Hippocrates, 1939), had described the clinical entities of erysipelas, mumps, and puerperal fever, but the causes were left to speculation. Arabic physicians differentiated measles from syphilis (Rhazes, translation 1847 and 1939). The presence of endemic plague was detected by the swollen lymph nodes in the pubic region ("buboes"). But the causes of all infectious diseases remained unknown until the modern period. With the advances of bacteriology and immunology the accurate diagnosis of individual cases was followed by specific methods of treatment.

The second major development was the public health movement, aimed at the control and prevention of epidemic diseases. The early objective of this movement was to protect a healthy population either directly or indirectly from sick and dying people, particularly those suffering from epidemic disease. The earliest attempts to achieve this separation were based on the concept of the contagiousness of disease — the spread of disease from person to person. Contagion became particularly apparent in the seventeenth century with the migration of large numbers of people across Europe, ship travel to American colonies, and exportation of slaves from Africa to Europe and to the Americas. Contagion was abetted by the concentrations of people in the large industrial cities of Europe, in which individuals were crowded together in inadequate living quarters and worked under intolerable conditions.

Another element of the public health movement was the growing knowledge that infections were spread by impure water, unclean air, improper sewage disposal, and poor personal hygiene. Thus social reform toward better living and working conditions, together with sanitary engineering aimed at environmental "nuisances," gave rise to a vigorous and lasting public health movement. (As will be pointed out later, the spread of cholera in the nineteenth century was a specific and powerful stimulus toward implementing the concepts of public health.)

The dual themes, then, of the specific cause of each of the infectious diseases and their management and prevention provide the discussion that follows throughout this book, particularly in the historical survey of each of the infectious diseases in Section III.

The concept of contagion, or the direct spread of disease through contact, appears to have existed during the very early period of human history. The old Hebrew leaders, for example, may have had such a concept in their references to leprosy as recorded in the Book of Leviticus, Chapters XII and XIV. The year 1530 marked a clear departure from the vague thinking of the past regarding contagion and the specificity of disease, with the work of the Veronese physician Girolamo Fracastoro (1930). He had wide clinical experience with epidemic diseases such as plague, typhus, syphilis, measles, and foot-and-mouth disease of cattle) His descriptions of these diseases clearly indicate that he considered them to be specific) Fracastoro's description of syphilis is contained in the greatest of medical poems, "The Sinister Shepherd" (Fracastoro, 1934. See p. 307).

Fracastoro's major contribution was his concept of contagion. He stated that diseases could be communicated by direct contact, by indirect contact through fomites (contaminated bedding, garments, etc.), and from a distance through the air) The causative agents were *seminaria contagium*, or seeds (germs, as translated by others). These small particles could not be seen, but he surmised that they were colloidal, viscous bodies that could endure in the air or on objects for a considerable period. They had some power of resistance to environmental factors, but were inactivated by extremes of heat or cold. Within the body the seeds underwent metabolic changes essential for survival and the production of disease) Fracastoro clarified the meaning of the medieval *miasma* (pollution) as a cause of infection)

The concepts of Fracastoro excited wide interest at the time, but attracted little attention after that until the period when studies were made with the microscope, principally by Anthony van Leeuwenhoek (Dobell, 1932). He communicated his microscopic observations from Delft in a series of over three hundred scientific letters to the Royal Society of London. One of his most famous letters, No. 39, dated September 17, 1683, contained illustrations of bodies observed in scrapings from human teeth, which in a later period could be interpreted as a motile bacillus, micrococcus, leptothrix, and a spirochoete. These were the first bacteria ever seen and described. Leeuwenhoek's published observations made little impact on medical science at the time. Two hundred years were to elapse before the kind of microorganisms he saw were associated with the germ theory of disease.

The confused thinking of physicians on the specificity of infections during the seventeenth century is demonstrated by Thomas Sydenham, perhaps the most influential physician in England. He believed each disease had a natural course of its own. "It is necessary that all diseases be reduced to definite and certain *species* . . . with the same care which we see exhibited by botanists in their phytologies [species]" (Sydenham, 1848, Vol. I, p. 13). He produced detailed descriptions of smallpox, continued and remittent fevers, pneumonia, rheumatism, erysipelas, quinsy, and St. Vitus dance.

Sydenham was persuaded by Robert Boyle to make a systematic study of epidemics in London from 1661 to 1686. His attempted classification shows the confusion of the times over the true nature of infectious diseases in relation to the causes and modes of transmission. (His theory of "epidemic constitutions" (*genius epidemicus*) stated that cosmic and atmospheric factors affect contagious diseases so that they originate from miasms of the earth and have long evolutionary variations and seasonal differences) Thus an epidemic of plague could be preceded and succeeded by a series of other subepidemic diseases whose constitutions were being changed by natural causes such as weather, atmospheric conditions, dryness, wetness, cold, and heat) Geography and meteorological conditions had significant roles in the genesis of epidemics.

The English physician Richard Mead in the eighteenth century advanced the concept of contagion substantially. He stated (1720, p. 2), "Contagion is propagated by three Causes, the Air; Diseased Persons; and Goods transported from infected Places." Mead maintained that it was not the air per se but that which was thrown off by diseased persons that carried contagion. Similarly goods could be contaminated by diseased persons and infect humans.

In the same period Benjamin Marten published a treatise describing his concepts of the mode of transmission and the cause of phthisis. He stated that animalcules residing in tuberculous victims traversed through the air to susceptible persons.

It may be therefore very likely, that by an habitual lying in the same Bed with a Consumptive Patient, constantly Eating and Drinking with him, or by very frequently conversing so nearly, as to draw in part the Breath he emits from his Lungs, a Consumption may be caught by a sound Person; for it may be reasonable to suppose that if the Blood and Juices of such distemper'd People, be charg'd with vast quantities of *Animalcula*, as I have conjectur'd, then their profuse Sweats, and their Breath also, may be likewise charg'd with them, or their Ova or Eggs, which by that means may possibly be convey'd into the Bodies of those who lie, or are most conversant with them (Marten, 1720, p. 79).

Another physician who echoed the specificity of diseases as propounded by Fracastoro was Thomas Fuller (1730). He looked upon contagious diseases as specific entities. "The particles which constitute the material and efficient Cause of the Small-Pox, Measles and other venomous Fevers are of specific and peculiar kinds; and as essentially different kinds are from one another. And since it is most certain that no Effect can be produced but by its own proper cause, I am hard to believe that the Small-Pox or Measles can be produc'd by such Things as have no matter of affinity with them; such are Fevers of any other Sort" (Fuller, 1730, Part I, p. 95). He then stated that plague cannot produce smallpox, nor smallpox cause measles or chickenpox. Neither can a hen produce a duck, or a wolf a sheep. And consequently one condition cannot protect against another. Fuller did not state that the causes of infections are living organisms, but he did delineate the specificity of infections.

Long before the specific causes of epidemic diseases were discovered, efforts had been made to control them through quarantine. This was especially true in the case of plague, the most destructive of all pandemic diseases. The "Black Death" devastated Europe between 1346 and 1350. The population of Europe at that time was estimated to be 105 million; 25 million died of the disease. It was reported to Pope Clement in Avignon that throughout the East, exclusive of China, 23,840,000 persons died (Hecker, 1844).

The most significant early attempt to apply quarantine to protect a population and its commercial enterprise against plague was organized in 1374 in Venice (Simpson, 1905). That city was at its height as a mercantile power. Ships and overland caravans were arriving from around the known world, especially from the East. The Council decided that no ships coming from areas of plague could enter the port or discharge its goods. The vessels were to remain outside for forty (quarantos) days before admission of either cargo or people, because it was believed that during that period the crisis would have subsided. By 1504 the Council of three nobles in Venice had the power of life or death if the regulations were broken. Families with plague were incarcerated in lazarettos for forty days. By 1383 Marseilles had similar quarantine regulations. So progressive were the people at this time that Bills of Health were first introduced in Italy during the plague in 1527.

Epidemics of plague, with their threat to life and commerce, brought about an advanced state of public health activity in Italy during the fifteenth and sixteenth centuries. Between 1361 and 1528 the disease had invaded Venice on twenty-two occasions, and at times had reduced the population by 20 percent (Pullan, 1971). Because plague had raged during the summer of 1485, a permanent magistracy in charge of public health was set up in 1486 — the Provveditori alla Sanità. Not only was quarantine enforced for shipping, but large numbers of vagrants and beggars had to be controlled, since plague was associated with famine and typhus, and the numbers of migrating vagrants increased during periods of such afflictions. By 1528 hospitals for the poor and vagrants were founded and supported by local taxes. Bills of Mortality were also established for plague and typhus. By 1575–1577, at a time when 30 percent of the population had died of plague, poor relief was inaugurated and was supported by taxation.

Carlo Cippola (1973) has described the course of plague and its control in the community of Prato, near Florence in Tuscany, during the epidemic of 1630. A recovered manuscript, prepared originally by Cristofano di Giulio Ceffini, one of the health officers, was his source of information. Prato was a prosperous walled city of six thousand inhabitants. The visitations of plague, recognized as a contagious disease, were vigorously controlled through a board of eight health officers, one of whom was Cristofano. His manuscript detailed the Bills of Mortality and also the methods for controlling plague. All houses with plague victims were quarantined for 22 days, and a local convent was used to house those with the disease for a minimum of 40 days. This combined effort was supported by community taxation. Infected houses were also fumigated with sulphur and perfumes, and objects used by the deceased were either burned or removed from the premises. Trade was also stopped. Cristofano did emphasize the difficulties in carrying out these stern orders.

The experiences with plague during the Renaissance were severe, but out of them came valuable information for the future. The measures for controlling plague at the time contributed to the basic pattern for the public health prophylactic programs of the nineteenth century when the specific identity of the causes of infectious diseases became known.

Another severe pandemic infection was smallpox, which had seriously afflicted Europe and the American colonies in the early eighteenth century. Quarantine measures, largely unsuccessful, had been applied in an effort to control the disease. It had been recognized that a person who had recovered from smallpox did not suffer a second attack. This led to the early practice of *inoculation* as a prophylactic in which material was removed from a smallpox pustule and introduced into the skin of an individual who had never had the disease. This procedure usually resulted in only a localized reaction in the recipient, but conferred protection against smallpox. *Inoculation* must be differentiated from *vaccination*, later introduced by Edward Jenner.

The practice of inoculation entered England from the Far East early in the eighteenth century, mostly through the efforts of Lady Mary Wortley Montagu, wife of the British ambassador to Turkey (Creighton, 1894a, Vol. 2, p. 493). Her own children had been inoculated; because of her social standing and influence, members of the royal family of George I were also inoculated. The royal approval of inoculation resulted in acceptance of the practice by the leading physicians of Great Britain. Its introduction into the American colonies was due principally to the Rev. Cotton Mather[1] of Boston, who maintained an interest in the progress of science in England through the *Philosophical Transactions*. The Rev. Mather persuaded his physician-friend, Dr. Zabdiel Boylston, to try out the procedure. But inoculation was not without its hazards. It caused fatal smallpox in some individuals and was the source of further epidemics. In order to circumvent some of the problems, inoculation hospitals were set up with rigid quarantine. But this procedure was expensive and limited in scope.[2]

Quarantine and inoculation failed to control smallpox toward the end of the eighteenth century. About this time the general practitioner and pupil of John Hunter, Dr. Edward Jenner, proposed the use of cowpox material (*variolae vaccinae*) for protection against smallpox (Jenner, 1798). His thesis was based upon gossip that he had heard among the farm folk in the area of Gloucestershire, where he practiced. Milk cows periodically had a pustular eruption of the teats known as cowpox. Milkmaids, in the process of milking these cows, contracted pustular lesions on their hands, which was followed by lasting protection against smallpox. Jenner believed (incorrectly) that the active agent of cowpox resided in horses having a disease called "the grease."[3] He stated that the farriers who dressed these equine lesions carried the contagious particles on their hands to the bovine teats in the act of milking cows. Furthermore he heard that the farriers often contracted the pustular disease on their hands as a result of contact with "the grease" of horses.

Jenner's publication was seriously flawed scientifically, principally because of the paucity of observations on humans, the dependence upon hearsay evidence for epidemiological data, and the erroneous conclusion relating cowpox etiologically to equine "grease." Severe criticism of Jenner's work has continued for over a hundred and fifty years in Great Britain (Creighton, 1889; Crookshank, 1889; Greenwood, 1936; Razzell, 1977). Nevertheless he did stimulate others in the continued use of prophylactic vaccine, although it is doubtful that the material in such vaccine was the true cowpox virus.[4]

Until the nineteenth century there were but few specific procedures for controlling infectious diseases, such as vaccination for smallpox and partially effective quarantine measures. But there was a progressive, if slow, growth of public health concepts and methods for maintaining good health, particularly among military personnel. Roman leaders were especially cognizant of these principles in binding together their extensive empire through proper drainage of lands for adequate roads required for the movement of troops, through the acquisition of sources of uncontaminated water conveyed in aqueducts, and by an effective means of sewage disposal. Personal hygiene and cleanliness were emphasized.

Later military leaders who emphasized the maintenance of good health in their personnel included Sir John Pringle, surgeon-general of the British Army from 1742 to 1758. During the Austrian wars of succession (1740–1748) he was a military observer, and it was there that he originated the concept of the Red Cross. He laid down "the true principles of military sanitation, especially in regard to the ventilation of hospital wards. . . . ships, jails, barracks and mines. Pringle was also a pioneer of the antiseptic idea; gave a good description of typhus fever; showed that jail fever and hospital fever are one and the same [typhus]; correlated the different forms of dysentery, and named influenza" (Garrison, 1922a, p. 373). His book, *Observa-*

tions on Diseases of the Army (Pringle, 1810), the first American edition of which included notes by Benjamin Rush, had a vast influence in Washington's colonial army.

The Scottish physician James Lind, a member of the Royal British Navy, is best known for his controlled clinical investigations on the prevention of scurvy with fresh citrus fruits carried out on board ship (Lind, 1757b). The volume was dedicated to Lord Anson, who had circumnavigated the globe and had lost 75 percent of his men because of the disease. Lind also wrote one of the first works on tropical medicine (1771), pointing out that geography and weather in some parts of the world determine the presence or absence of certain diseases. He first described the "guinea worm," and commented on yellow fever in the West Indies. He contributed to English naval hygiene, recommending measures for improved ventilation, cleanliness, and food (Lind, 1757a).

In England and elsewhere in Europe there was also an urgent need for prison reform, the inmates often receiving little better care than animals. John Howard, an English Quaker and philanthropist, did much to enlighten his own and other nations, in regard to the abominable conditions not only of prisons but also of hospitals. He toured institutions and lazarettos all through Europe, noting carefully the good as well as the bad ones, and then made recommendations for improvement (Howard, 1791; 1792).

In Germany Johann Peter Frank was a prominent figure in the early development of the concept of public health. He looked upon the states' ruler as the father of all his subjects and believed that with appropriate legislation a healthy population could be protected "from womb to tomb." Frank contended, "At present the authorities give themselves more trouble and spend more money in one week in fruitless attempts to apply remedies than would be necessary if effort and money were expended *to prevent evils through wise ordinances*" (quoted in Baumgartner and Ramsey, 1934, p. 69).

Concepts of contagion and of causes and methods of control developed slowly. Treatment of individual patients was also severely handicapped for centuries because of the lack of this basic knowledge. Through shrewd empirical observations a few specific drugs became available. Opium was widely used in febrile conditions, especially in the eighteenth century in the form of "Dover's powders"

(Dover, 1732). For helminthic infections oil of Chenopodium, or "American oil of wormwood," was probably known to the Aztecs, and Aspidium, or male fern, was used by the Greeks. Ipecacuanha root, used by Indians of South America for dysentery, was later shown to contain the alkaloid emetine, which was particularly effective in amoebic dysentery. Quinine, introduced in the seventeenth century from South America, proved to be highly effective in the treatment of malaria. The history of quinine is discussed in conjunction with the management of malaria in Section III, Chapter 20.

Except for a few such drugs there was little specific therapy available for the febrile patient until the twentieth century. This was due to the fact that the causes of infection were poorly understood and the pathogenesis of the diseases was still defined on the basis of the ancient Greek humoral pathology. Illness resulted from an imbalance of humors; the only relief was through bleeding, purging, and cupping. A brief look at the widespread persistence of the ancient practice of bleeding is warranted here because the final blow to this practice, which was not struck until the nineteenth century, was based on a rather simple scientific approach in clinical medicine that has served as a pattern for evaluating modern specific therapy of infectious diseases, including the use of the sulfonamides and antibiotics.

A thousand years after Hippocrates the first medical school and hospital in Europe was loosely organized in Salerno. Before the age of printing a manuscript was copied and widely distributed known as the *Regimen Sanitatis Salernitanum* (1607 and 1922) or *The School of Salernum*, which was a basic source of knowledge for the laity and physicians. This tract emphasized the value of bleeding in health and in disease. Bleeding continued as a common medical procedure in the fourteenth century. Chaucer (1934, p. 13) described "The Physician" in his *Canterbury Tales*, who was well learned in Greek medicine and based his diagnoses on the humoral theory.

Bleeding and purging were introduced into the United States from Europe and were widely used throughout the eighteenth century. During the yellow fever epidemic in Philadelphia in 1793 the most influential physician, Dr. Benjamin Rush, recommended as standard treatment, purging with ten grains of calomel and fifteen of jalap every six hours; removing eight to ten ounces of blood, repeatedly if there was no improvement; and blistering the skin, as stated in the

Federal Gazette (Philadelphia) for September 12, 1793. Bleeding and purging of the first president of the United States, George Washington, for a respiratory infection led to his untimely death (Rothstein, 1972, p. 55).

The practice of bleeding reached its peak in France because of the highly influential physician François Broussais. He recommended the application of as many as ten to fifty leeches to the body. The scarcity of leeches in 1843 led to the importation into France of 41,500,000 leeches, whereas in 1824–1825 two to three million met all the demands (Garrison, 1922a).

Over the centuries there were able physicians who condemned bleeding as worthless and even dangerous. But it remained for the distinguished French clinician Pierre-Charles-Alexandre Louis (1836b) to reveal in careful comparative clinical studies of different types of infection, with his "numerical method" or medical statistics, that bleeding and blistering were without benefit. Louis's observations, method, and conclusions were soon widely accepted. When any therapeutic procedure or drug was introduced into medical practice, controlled investigations on treated and untreated patients were to be carried out with reference to benefits and dangers. These principles for human therapy should be and are advocated today. Another mollifying effect on the harshness of medical treatment, including bleeding and purging, was the introduction of homeopathy (Hahnemann, 1869).

Quantitative methods of evaluation similar to those of Louis were evolved almost simultaneously for investigations of the causes and management of puerperal fever and septic wounds. These latter studies added significant knowledge to the concept of contagion and introduced an understanding and the practice of aseptic surgery. The acquisition of this fundamental knowledge was a major advance in the control and management of infectious diseases.

Puerperal fever was mentioned as a severe complication of pregnancy in the Hippocratic Corpus, but it was not until 1751 that John Burton of Edinburgh suggested the contagiousness of the disease. Dr. Charles White (1773) of Manchester, England stated shortly thereafter that the highest incidence was in crowded hospitals and that women should be delivered and cared for in private quarters, or at least in uncrowded areas. Clean linen, fresh air, and avoidance of attendance by ignorant midwives were also essential. He opposed bleeding as therapy.

An epidemic of puerperal fever that occurred in Aberdeen between December 1789 and March 1792 was described by Dr. Alexander Gordon (1795). He had encountered 48 patients, 28 of whom died, and presented the classical symptoms and findings in each case, believing that the infection was inflammatory in origin and not putrid. He astutely observed that erysipelas and puerperal fever occurred as concomitant epidemics, with the former involving wounds. He wrote (p. 62), "That the cause of this disease was a specific contagion, or infection, I have unquestionable proof."

In 1843 the first issue of *The New England Quarterly Journal of Medicine and Surgery*[5] contained an essay on "The Contagiousness of Puerperal Fever" by Professor Oliver Wendell Holmes (1843) of the Harvard Medical School. His essay was devoid of any scientific clinical observations of his own in the field of obstetrics, but he was acquainted with the pertinent literature, such as cited in the foregoing discussion. Holmes reemphasized that puerperal fever was a contagious disease. A physician who had attended a patient with puerperal fever or with erysipelas, or who had performed an autopsy on such cases, should not approach a healthy obstetrical patient without thoroughly cleansing himself and changing his clothes completely. Holmes also recommended that the physician should inform his assistant and nurses of the necessity for meticulous precautions against transmitting the disease. But his warnings were severely criticized by some (Holmes, 1855).

At the same time Dr. Ignaz Semmelweis (1861, translation 1941) was carrying out in the General Hospital (Allgemeines Krankenhaus) in Vienna from 1844 to 1855 his definitive observations on the contagiousness and prevention of puerperal fever. The Vienna Krankenhaus had two maternity divisions. Division I was for the instruction of students and assistants, under the supervision of the professors, whereas in Division II, where there were no teaching responsibilities, midwives handled the deliveries. Assigned to Division I for four months in 1846, Semmelweis was appalled by the number of deaths from puerperal fever. His first major observation was the higher death rate in Division I as compared to that in the midwives' Division II. Why the difference? He did not think it was due to the popular hypothesis of a change in the atmospheric-cosmic-telluric conditions in Vienna, although he did not believe at this time in the concept of an epidemic or a contagious disease either. Because of the numbers involved, the authorities called it an epidemic disease. They concluded it was due to the "trauma" induced by the many examiners of the women on Division I, and to control this factor the number of examining students was reduced.

In 1846 Semmelweis was relieved of his appointment because of the controversial nature of his beliefs. In 1847 he was reinstated on Division I. During his absence his friend the pathologist Professor Kolletschka had died as a result of pricking his finger with a knife while performing an autopsy on a victim of puerperal fever. The pathological findings in the tissues and organs of Kolletschka were the same as those found in puerperal fever. Semmelweis brooded over this correlation and concluded that "cadaveric particles" were carried from the autopsy rooms directly to the bedside of parturient women and were introduced by the examining fingers. Semmelweis then insisted that every student had to wash his hands with "Chlorina liquida" before examining a patient. He later changed to the chlorinated lime, which was less expensive. When this simple procedure of washing the hands was followed, the incidence of puerperal fever declined dramatically.

Unfortunately Semmelweis was driven from his position in Vienna. In 1850, at the age of 37, he proceeded to the University of Pest, where he became professor of obstetrics. His concepts and practices were detailed in a Hungarian publication in 1858; his classic summing-up was made in 1861 (Semmelweis, 1861, translation 1941). Semmelweis was a very unstable individual emotionally, but this did not obscure his keen insight and brilliance. He was disturbed that his principles were not universally accepted even though he had the backing in Vienna of such eminent physicians as Carl Rokitansky, Joseph Skoda, and Ferdinand von Hebra. Semmelweis contended that puerperal fever was due to an unknown infectious agent, that it was contagious, that it produced a septicemia, and that it could be prevented. He died abruptly in 1865 at the age of 47 from an infection similar to Kolletschka's.

Why did the excellent work of Semmelweis remain unrecognized for so long? One major factor was that he was reluctant to put his observations into writing, and when he did his prose was unclear and repetitious, and his statistical data ill-conceived for publication. Second, he was an abrasive person with few friends in Vienna and many antagonists. If he had had the dignity and restraint of Joseph Lister, and the clarity in writing of Oliver Wendell Holmes, the acceptance of his work might have swept through Europe.

From a chronological viewpoint it is extraordinary that procedures for preventing puerperal fever were discovered before the establishment of the microbial causes of disease by Pasteur and Koch. Furthermore the basic concepts of Semmelweis were essentially those features of aseptic surgery as outlined by Joseph Lister. There is no doubt about the magnitude of Lister's contribution to the control of surgical sepsis. But his work did succeed that of Semmelweis, and Lister did have some knowledge of Pasteur's studies on fermentation and suspended microbes in the atmosphere. He never referred to Semmelweis's observations, although he had read widely and had traveled extensively, and some of Lister's friends were familiar with Semmelweis and his studies.

Lister received an excellent education in the basic sciences of pathology, physiology, and microbiology, and surgical training under Sir John Erichsen at the University Hospital in London. He then became regius professor of surgery at Glasgow (Godlee, 1917). It was there that he did his most important work on aseptic surgery, and where he was challenged by pyemia, erysipelas, and gas gangrene. He was highly influenced by Pasteur's observations on airborne microorganisms, the cause of putrefaction. Lister's basic principles of treatment for and prevention of sepsis were to establish a clean traumatic wound and to use carbolic acid in wound dressings. He even sprayed the operating room with carbolic acid. He later abandoned the carbolic acid and protected wounds from the immediate environment with dressings (Lister, 1867; 1870).

True to Lister's prophecy that his system would take on a "more perfect shape," disinfectants gave way toward the end of the century to aseptic principles, largely through the fundamental work of Koch on disinfectants and sterilization and through the practice of surgeons in Britain and Germany and, in America, of Dr. William Halsted, chief of surgery at the Johns Hopkins Hospital. The evolution of the treatment of wound sepsis has been further documented by Dr.

Owen Wangensteen (1970; Wangensteen, Wangensteen and Klinger, 1973).

It must be emphasized that these early advances in aseptic surgery were aided by the availability of general anesthesia with ether or chloroform. Doctor Henry Bigelow (1846), surgeon at the Massachusetts General Hospital, introduced the discovery of ether by the Boston dentist William Morton, with a simple and dignified story on its use in general surgery in the November 18, 1846 issue of the *Boston Medical and Surgical Journal*. Shortly thereafter the British obstetrician Sir James Simpson (1847) used ether in Great Britain. He later turned to chloroform because it was not inflammable and was less irritating than ether.

An important factor that contributed to the orderliness and cleanliness in the care of all hospital patients and led to the reduction of infection and deaths was the establishment of professional nursing, principally through the untiring efforts of Florence Nightingale (Cook, 1913). Her devoted work for the sick and wounded in the Crimean War attracted the attention of authorities in England and brought about far-reaching changes in both civilian and military hospitals (Nightingale, 1860).

CHAPTER 2

Development of Bacteriology, Immunology, and Virology

Bacteriology

Fracastoro's view, stated in 1530, that diseases could be transmitted through the air by means of seeds or germs, was finally proved more than three hundred years later. This did not happen suddenly; rather it was the culmination of developments in scientific thought and technology in which the participants were many, with Louis Pasteur and Robert Koch providing the final leadership. Their work was closely related to advances in chemistry, biology, physiology, and pathology, especially the cellular pathology of Rudolph Virchow.

One of the most important questions in the development of the germ theory of diseases was that of the origin of minute animals that were known to appear in decaying organic matter. Did they arise spontaneously or from already existing forms of life that were too small to be observed? For centuries the former view was generally held. The doctrine of spontaneous generation had been a part of biological thought from the time of Aristotle. Flies that evolved from grubs found in the dung gathered in heaps by farmers, fleas and lice that grew out of moisture and filth, fish that rose out of sand or mud — all were thought to have arisen spontaneously. The challenging of this belief that living organisms could suddenly come forth, with no living precursors, was one of Pasteur's most important achievements.

Earlier observers had gathered evidence that contradicted spontaneous generation. In 1678 Francesco Redi concluded that meat exposed to the air containing animalcules became putrefied, whereas meat protected from such air did not (Dobell, 1932). In 1718 Louis Joblot demonstrated that hay infusions became contaminated by animalcules in the air, and in 1776 Lazzaro Spallanzani showed that the infusions remained clear when heated (Bulloch, 1938b). Finally three men independently discovered that the fermentation of sugar solutions or wine formed alcohol and carbon dioxide, owing to the growth of yeast cells in the solutions. Furthermore fermentation and putrefaction could be prevented by the exclusion of air, which contained the living particles (Cagniard-Latour, 1838; Kützing, 1837; Schwann, 1837).

The early part of the nineteenth century was the day of the chemist; J. von Liebig, J. Berzelius, and F. Wöhler would not accept the participation of germs in the process of fermentation. They were aware of the forementioned investigations on fermentation, but they concluded that this was purely a chemical reaction in which atmospheric oxygen played an important role. No living agents were implicated. The crux of the controversy was the question, was microbial activity essential for initiating the chemical reactions?

The story of Pasteur's life and of his many contributions to science and medicine has been fully documented, and numerous versions are available (Dubos, 1950; Duclaux, 1920; Pasteur, 1922–1939). Pasteur began his professional life in chemistry, founding the discipline of stereochemistry with his work on crystals. More immediately relevant in the present context, Pasteur demonstrated that microbes (yeast) initiate fermentation. He showed that some microbes (anaerobic) cause fermentation in the absence of oxygen. His work for the wine industry revealed that fermentation by contaminants could be impeded by heating ("pasteurization"), which later proved to be a major contribution to public health and the prevention of infections. The association of specific microbes with specific fermentations was fundamental to Pasteur's later work on the specific microbial causes of diseases.

Despite his efforts, Pasteur's work did not gain general acceptance because of the inability of others to confirm his results. This was due in part to the irregularity of results with heated and unheated hay infusions. The difficulty was surmounted by the English physicist John Tyndall (1882) with two simple experiments. First, he demonstrated that a sharp beam of light could detect particles in the air in an open box, and he also recovered in culture medium the organisms floating in air. In a closed box devoid of air the light beam was not reflected by particles, and such air yielded sterile cultures. Second, he showed that hay infusions contained heat-resistant forms of bacteria (spores), which could be eliminated only by what he termed discontinuous boiling, i.e., boiling the infusion for one minute five times successively. In this fashion of fractional sterilization, the spores of the hay bacillus were destroyed (Tyndall, 1882).

In 1865 Pasteur began investigations on infectious diseases for the first time, working with a disease of silkworms. The infection turned out not to be a single entity, but a dual one — one called *pebrine* of fungal origin and a second named *flacherie*, probably due to a virus (Pasteur, 1870). His final solution for controlling the disease was through the laborious selection by hand of healthy eggs from disease-free moths.

In his studies on anthrax Pasteur confirmed and extended previous observations (Davaine, 1863), as well as those of Robert Koch (Pasteur and Joubert, 1877a; 1877b). He introduced a prophylactic vaccine for the disease (Pasteur, Chamberland, and Roux, 1881). He successfully established a vaccine for the highly lethal disease of chicken cholera due to *Vibrion septique* (Pasteur, 1880). These were the first successful prophylactic vaccines since that of Jenner for smallpox. And finally, he introduced a prophylactic vaccine for rabies (Pasteur, 1881), which was to bring him universal fame and funds for the establishment of a research institute in Paris.

The significance of Pasteur's work on the present discussion was that he strongly combatted the doctrine of spontaneous generation in showing that fermentation, suppuration, and infections were due to living microorganisms. In addition he stimulated the origins of immunology with his discovery of three prophylactic vaccines.

Robert Koch, a contemporary of Pasteur, can be considered the founder of the discipline of bacteriology. He is remembered today for his exquisite research techniques in that field. Koch was greatly influenced as a student by Professor F. G. Jacob Henle of Göttingen.

Henle had postulated in an essay before the work of Pasteur that living organic matter in the air was the cause of infection, and that to prove this experimentally it would be necessary to isolate the particles from diseased tissue in pure form, transmit them to animals reproducing the infection, and then recover the particles again in pure culture (Henle, 1840, translation 1938). Koch, using simple but ingenious techniques, turned his attention to anthrax and proved the etiology according to the hypothesis of Henle (Koch, 1877 translation 1938). He established what is known as Koch's postulates in bacteriology. Koch had conclusively demonstrated for the first time a specific microorganism as the cause of an infectious disease in an animal or human being three hundred years after Fracastoro had published his concepts on contagion.

Probably Koch's most glorious moment was on the evening of March 22, 1882 before the Physiological Society in Berlin when he delivered his elegant paper on the etiology of tuberculosis. He described with clarity the meticulous isolation of the tubercle bacillus from patients, its successful growth in pure culture, the production of the disease in guinea pigs, and the recovery from the animals of a pure culture of the bacillus, again fulfilling his own postulates (Koch, 1882, translation 1938). Paul Ehrlich, in attendance at the meeting, proclaimed the occasion his "greatest scientific event." Soon thereafter Ehrlich devised the acid-fast stain for identifying organisms microscopically.

Finally, in his studies on wound infections established experimentally in animals, Koch isolated each of several species of organisms in pure culture, "certainly the most important single contribution ever made to the science of bacteriology" (Foster, 1970, p. 37). He also introduced sterilization methods for disinfection in the bacteriology laboratory using dry heat induced by super heated steam (Koch, 1886).

The schools of Pasteur and Koch in their respective institutes in Paris and in Berlin continued to recover and to identify new species of microorganisms as the cause of diseases. With this additional knowledge, a group of men centered in these two institutes also developed the basic concepts of immunology over a period of twenty-five years beginning about 1880.

Immunology

The first immunological principles were established in the Pasteur Institute by Elie Metchnikoff and his pupil Jules Bordet. In a series of observations Metchnikoff established the concept of *cellular immunity* — that certain cells of the body attacked, ingested, and killed invading microorganisms, and that the outcome of this struggle between the cells and microbes often determined the death or survival of the invaded host. Bordet, working in Metchnikoff's laboratory, established the concept of *humoral immunity*, in which the blood, with or without its circulating cells, defended the body against invading microorganisms. Although the controversy between cellular and humoral immunity extended for years, most authorities soon realized that both factors played major roles in the defense mechanism of an invaded host.

Metchnikoff, trained as a zoologist in Russia, was interested in marine biology, centering his research on unicellular organisms. Influenced by Charles Darwin, he sought information about the mechanism of survival of certain species. His first major scientific report dealt with such a mechanism in starfish larvae, which have neither blood vessels nor a nervous system. Placing rose thorns into the bodies of the larvae, he noted that mobile cells immediately surrounded the thorn just as in a man who runs a splinter into his finger (Metchnikoff, 1921). Metchnikoff introduced the term "phagocytosis" to describe this phenomenon. He followed this with observations on a species of daphnia that was often infected with a yeast, *Monospora bicuspidata*; once again the daphnia survived after successful destruction of the yeast spores by phagocytosis (Metchnikoff, 1884).

Upon joining the Pasteur Institute Methnikoff delivered a brilliant series of lectures on inflammation, with the aging Pasteur in attendance. His thesis was that the body's main bulwark against infectious agents was the mesodermal wandering cell, which completed destruction of microbes through phagocytosis (Metchnikoff, 1892, translation 1968). Later he wrote another major work on immunology in which he encouraged immunization against infectious diseases, maintaining that the immune substances in the blood originated in the "juices and ferments" of these digestive cells, the phagocytes (Metchnikoff, 1901, translation 1905).

While Metchnikoff emphasized the role of phagocytosis in immunity, others demonstrated that whole blood killed bacteria, such as the anthrax bacillus; but that if the blood were heated, activity was lost (Nuttall, 1888). At the Koch Institute, R. F. J. Pfeiffer (1894) extended these studies and observed that if cholera spirilla organisms were injected into the peritoneal cavity of guinea pigs that had recovered from the infection, the organisms were lysed by the peritoneal fluid (Pfeiffer and Issaeff, 1894). This bacteriolytic action was specific for cholera because other species of bacteria were not killed. This became known as "The Pfeiffer Phenomenon" in immunological literature. Pfeiffer pursued his studies and demonstrated that serum from guinea pigs that had recovered from cholera when injected into normal pigs protected the animals through the lysis of injected organisms. This was the first description of an antibacterial serum that protected against a lethal infection. But Pfeiffer introduced an immunological enigma with his observation that both heated or unheated sera gave the same protection.

Jules Bordet (1895, translation 1909) soon unified the doctrines of cellular phagocytosis and humoral immunity by showing that normal serum had some bacteriolytic activity that was markedly accentuated by a "preventive substance" in immune serum. Bordet believed that the bacteriolytic activity of serum was dependent on the union of two substances in the blood, the preventive substance and a component designated as "alexin" or complement. Heating serum destroyed activity of the latter substance. Bordet concluded that the defense mechanism of the host against microbes depended on both phagocytosis and the bacteriolytic activity of the serum. Bordet's final achievement was his discovery of the serological test, widely used in the diagnosis of infectious diseases, known as the complement-fixation test (Bordet and Gengou, 1901), which was to be so important in the diagnosis of syphilis (Wassermann, Neisser, and Bruck, 1906).

The results of these immunological discoveries were soon expanded by others, including Emil von Behring and Paul Ehrlich. Their work led to the highly successful toxin and antitoxin for the prevention and treatment of diphtheria. This achievement is discussed in Section III, Chapter 13. This also resulted in serotherapy for other infectious diseases.

Karl Landsteiner (1947), in his studies on the specificity of serological reactions, concluded that an animal could produce a very large number of specific antibodies against each of many foreign substances or antigens never before presented to the body. He introduced the concept that the surface molecular formation of antigen fits into the surface of formed antibody as a key fits into a lock. This concept has had considerable impact on modern immunology.

During World War II chemists defined the components of human serum and discovered that most of the specific antibodies for microbes resided in the gamma fraction of globulin, a discovery that had important applications for prophylactic and therapeutic purposes in bacterial and virus diseases. In one of those fortuitous "experiments of nature" a large body of information was obtained about immunoglobulins through the study of the macromolecules secreted by multiple myeloma (Hood, Campbell, and Elgin, 1975). This malignancy, consisting of plasma cells, the globulin-producing cells of the lymphatic system, provided large quantities of homogeneous immunoglobulin for analytical purposes. It was found that although the myeloma plasma cell represented an abnormal proliferation of a single clone of cells producing an immunoglobulin of questionable significance, normal plasma cells produced a wide spectrum of specific immunoglobulins — including IgM, IgG, IgA, IgE, and IgD — with differing biological and structural characteristics. Finally the molecular structure of the immunoglobulins was defined (Edelman, 1970; Edelman et al., 1969; Porter, 1967a; Porter, 1967b), and the nine protein components of complement were described (Müller-Eberhard, 1972).

While the structure and function of the immunoglobulins were being elucidated for humoral immunity, advances were occurring in studies on cellular immunity. An important concept, designated *selective antibody formation*, stated that antigen does not instruct a cell as to what kind of antibody to make but selects a cell or cells already making preformed "natural" antibody that fits the antigenic structure. The antigen calls for the production of this more specific antibody to aid in the body's defense (Jerne, 1955; 1973). F. MacFarlane Burnet (1959) advanced the *clonal selection theory* that the body possesses multiple clones of globulin-producing cells. When the reactive receptor sites of a population of such cells come in contact with the appropriate antigen, the stimulation calls forth the progeny to produce an abundance of specific antibody (Burnet, 1962). Once the body's cells producing specific antibody have been stimulated in this manner, repeated antigenic stimulus calls forth this new class of antibody very quickly without the lag period characteristic of the primary stimulus.

In studies on cellular immunity two classes of lymphocytes were recognized, including plasma cells, on the basis of their anatomical origins and surface characteristics. "B" lymphocytes originate in the bone marrow and display a high density of membrane-incorporated immunoglobulin. These cells bind antigens and are the progenitors of antibody-secreting plasma cells. The other lymphocyte class (T cells) is thymus-dependent and also binds antigen, but immunoglobulin is not readily detectable at the cell surface. Studies of both viral and bacterial infections have delineated the important role that T cells play in the control of infection (Blanden, 1971; Mackaness, 1971).

Virology

The discipline of virology has produced many discoveries that have added to a better understanding of several infectious diseases and to their control, especially through prophylactic vaccines. Although smallpox and rabies were long considered infectious diseases due to an unknown type of poison, which was called "virus," the first experimental evidence that a disease in mammalian vertebrates could be induced by a cell-free preparation originated with studies on foot-and-mouth disease in cattle, as described by the German Commission under F. Loeffler and F. Frosch (1898). At approximately the same time three plant pathologists (Beijerinck, 1942; Ivanowski, 1942; Mayer, 1942), working independently, contributed to the discovery that mosaic tobacco disease is caused by a virus, one that was to become famous in future research on virology.[1]

An early major discovery in virology that escaped the serious attention of investigators for several years was the observation that filtrable agents from human fecal contents invaded and lysed enteric bacteria (D'Herelle, 1918; Twort, 1915). These bacterial parasites were called "bacteriophage." Subsequently it was learned that there was a variety of phage viruses, each having an affinity for a specific bacterial species (Groman, 1961). The property of bacterial lysogenesis was to produce far-reaching investigations on the pathogenesis of infectious diseases and in the studies of epidemics of staphylococcus infections and typhoid fever. Bacteriophage formed the basis of many of the studies by individuals in the famous "phage" group under Max Delbrück, director of the Cold Spring Harbor Laboratory of Quantitative Biology. Several of the group were awarded a Nobel Prize for their contributions to molecular biology (Cairns, Stent, and Watson, 1966).

Pioneering studies at the Rockefeller Institute for Medical Research described a sarcoma in chicken muscle, presumably due to a virus (Rous, 1911). When a cell-free filtrate of the tumor was injected into normal chickens, a tumor was reproduced at the site of inoculation. Later the tumor was successfully implanted into the developing chick embryo (Murphy and Rous, 1912).

Another early work on virus reproduction was carried out in the Rockefeller Institute when a pure culture of vaccinia virus was obtained following inoculation of the virus into the testicles of intact rabbits (Noguchi, 1915). Other investigators cultivated vaccinia virus and herpes virus in excised testicular fragments of rabbits (Parker and Nye, 1925a; 1925b). Except for further *in vitro* growth studies of vaccinia virus without cultures of tissues (Maitland and Maitland, 1928), utilization of these methods was then delayed for several years.

Many important discoveries are either overlooked or neglected for a long time before they are recognized or "rediscovered." As noted above, J. B. Murphy and P. Rous reproduced a chicken tumor in embryos with cell-free extracts of the sarcoma in 1912. This should have suggested that filtrable viruses could be reproduced in this manner, but it was not until A. M. Woodruff and E. W. Goodpasture (1931) grew fowl-pox virus in the embryo that others pursued this technique. The influenza virus was propagated in the chick embryo, which led to the production of vaccines (Beveridge and Burnet, 1946; Burnet, 1935). Other intact animals were employed for the isolation and growth of viruses such as the intracerebral injection of infected tissues into mice (Theiler, 1930), a technique later utilized for the isolation of yellow fever virus.

Further progress in virology depended on the isolation and production of sufficient quantities of specific viruses for research and for possible prophylactic vaccines. Two technological advances aided in this quest, one the ultracentrifuge (Svedberg, 1937; Svedberg, Boestad, and Eriksson-Quensel, 1934), and the other the electron microscope (Burton and Kohl, 1942). Self-replication of viruses, unlike that of bacteria, requires living cells. Therefore efforts were directed toward tissue culture techniques as explored by H. B. Maitland and M. C. Maitland (1928). Doctor John Enders and his group at the Children's Medical Center in Boston succeeded in growing poliomyelitis virus in cell cultures of various human embryonic tissues (Enders, Weller, and Robbins, 1949), following which the viruses of rubeola and measles were isolated and grown (Enders and Peebles, 1954; Enders et al., 1957; Weller and Neva, 1962). These and similar studies quickly led to the large-scale production of prophylactic vaccines, a major triumph in the control of epidemic diseases of childhood.

The therapy of virus diseases has not been fruitful. Except for prophylactic purposes, antisera have been of no value. Modern research has concentrated on chemotherapy, with limited success.

Exciting and complex research programs have centered on the role of viruses in the etiology of cancer. Although specific viruses have been identified in the causes of malignancy, including leukemia, in lower animals and in subhuman primates, such solid data are still lacking for human forms of cancer.

CHAPTER 3

The Evolution of Public Health
at National and International Levels

The nineteenth century was a time of rapidly changing social conditions. One of the results was the necessity for improving and refining public health measures. Large numbers of people had migrated from Europe to Great Britain and to the United States, settling in urban communities. The cholera epidemic of 1831–1832 made goverment authorities keenly aware of the magnitude of the health problem.

In response to this situation, organized activities were developed to correct some of the social maladjustments that contributed to poor health and epidemic diseases.(A primary objective was to control crowd diseases due to infections.) This was approached through public health procedures at local, national, and international levels in conjunction with the sciences of microbiology and immunology and with epidemiology. In the present discussion the development of public health in Great Britain is considered because it served as a pattern for that in the United States, leading ultimately to the formation of the World Health Organization.

Public Health in Great Britain

A major contribution of Great Britain to public health was the use of statistical methods in dealing with crowd diseases. Vital statistics had its origin in the Bills of Mortality, which were established throughout England under Henry VIII and continued under Elizabeth I. The accumulation of data on births, deaths, and disease was carried out at the parish level. This system was advanced in the seventeenth century by John Graunt, who had been stimulated by his contemporary Sir William Petty, a physician trained in mathematics and interested in statistics. Graunt was a businessman who was attracted to politics and to the Bills of Mortality. He analyzed the weekly data between 1625 and 1665 (Graunt, 1665). He was particularly concerned with the incidence of deaths due to plague. He provided summaries of deaths and the causes from every parish within London and from some outside the city.

Problems relating to the health of the population were handled at the parish level from the time of Queen Elizabeth I until the nineteenth century. Of particular concern during this period was the care of the poor. Unfortunately, however, this was the responsibility of a totally disorganized and often corrupt administration of over 15,000 local groups without communication among them. Approximately one-fifth of the national income was being expended on the poor, and yet little was being done to alleviate the intolerable living and working conditions that contributed to poor health and illness. The basic question facing the nation was, should public monies be expended to eradicate the "nuisances" causing poor health, or should expenditures be strictly for the care of the ill? The "nuisances" included abominable methods for sewage disposal, filthy and inadequate dwellings, scarcity of clothing, outrageous working conditions, occupational diseases, contaminated water supplies, child labor, and malnutrition. Social reformers, sanitationists, and many physicians, believing that illness and the "nuisances" resided on the same side of the coin, demanded that the social evils contributing to poor health be eliminated through government intervention.

There was a tradition already established in Britain for such action as a result of John Pringle's efforts in the Royal Army (1810), James

Lind's recommendations for the Royal Navy (1757a), and John Howard's work in prison and hospital reform (1792). But it was partly the
horror incited by the cholera epidemic that culminated in action by
Parliament. A review of the Poor Laws was made in 1832; a law in
1834 delegated the responsibilities for carrying out the necessary
changes to the local governments. Poor Law Commissioners were
appointed to direct the central office, and Edwin Chadwick was appointed secretary to the commissioners. It was in this capacity that
he executed his sanitary report of 1842, one of the greatest in the
annals of public health (Great Britain Poor Law Commissioners,
1842 and 1965). Because of the influence of his report on the subsequent direction of public health, a brief summary of Chadwick's
life and methods of work, and of his report, is in order.

Chadwick's life spanned the nineteenth century between 1800 and
1890. He elected to study law, and following a custom of the day, he
supported himself as a newspaper reporter. As he roamed through
London he learned of the fevers, the vices and crimes, the filthy
slums, and the workhouses. In the prisons and in the courts he saw
the inadequacies of justice. He became a member of a "radical"
group. He met two young physicians, Dr. Neil Arnott and Dr.
Thomas Southwood Smith, with whom he became close friends.
Chadwick learned about medical schools and their curriculae, and
about hospitals. He visited the "fever dens" of London. He passed
more and more of his time with the circle of "radicals," especially
with the political economists Jeremy Bentham and John Stuart Mill.
He became increasingly interested in the health of the people and
the need for social and political reform.

If parliamentary reform measures were even to be considered, it
was essential that the Poor Law Commissioners supply specific information about the undesirable features of social conditions in Britain. Chadwick, through his own experiences and with his pragmatic
political philosophy, was qualified to acquire the needed facts. He
communicated with the network of physicians throughout England,
Wales, and Scotland, many of whom were associated with the work
of the Poor Law Commissioners. They supplied him with specific
examples of poor sanitation and of degrading working and living
conditions. Chadwick, himself a keen observer, traveled widely
throughout Britain gathering information. He was indebted to Dr.

Neil Arnott and to James Phillips Kay of Manchester for their report on the causes of fever and its relationship to disease, which appeared as a supplement in the Fourth Annual Report of the Great Britain Poor Law Commissioners (1838). He was particularly aided by Dr. Southwood Smith, who as a physician to the London Fever Hospital analyzed epidemic disease in the districts of the metropolis that could be removed by sanitary regulations (Great Britain Poor Law Commissioners, 1838, 1839).

Chadwick's own report, completed after three years of work, comprised 457 closely printed pages with tables and charts (Great Britain Poor Law Commissioners, 1842 and 1965). The report included a careful analysis of the causes of death in 1838 and 1839 under four categories, which included 42 counties in England and two in Wales. Similar information was not available for Scotland, but Chadwick did ascertain that the "mortality from fever" in Glasgow, Edinburgh, and Dundee was greater than in the most crowded towns in England. A condensed version of Chadwick's analysis is shown in Table 1. This information was inadequate from the viewpoint of modern vital statistics. The total morbidity figures were not given, so that the true incidence of the diseases was not revealed, and there was no distribution of the death rate according to age, sex, and occupation. Nevertheless Chadwick's information did show that consumption was the leading cause of death, followed by the fevers of typhus and scarlatina. His study of the distribution of these primary diseases also pinpointed the more troubled localities.

The main body of Chadwick's report gave a vivid picture of the unsanitary conditions existing in England and in Wales, as well as in Edinburgh. His investigators concentrated in detail on the totally inadequate system of sewage disposal with its resultant filth and squalor. The sources of drinking water were a threat to health. Living conditions in the large industrial towns were often undesirable. As cited by Chadwick, several witnesses, including certain clergymen, blamed the poverty and the poor health of the afflicted people on a lack of moral fiber and intemperance, and they were often joined in this conclusion by members of an inept medical profession.

Chadwick's recommendations for reform were based on the principle that better health and less sickness could be obtained through sanitary engineering. This meant improved methods of sewage dis-

Table 1. Number of Deaths for 1838 and 1839

Year	Epidemic, Endemic, and Contagious Diseases				Diseases of Respiratory Organs			Diseases of Brain Nerves and Senses	Diseases of Degenerative Organs	Total Deaths from Four Preceding Causes	Proportion of Deaths in Every 1000 of 1841 Population	
	Fever: Typhus Scarlatina	Small-pox	Measles	Whooping Cough	Con-sumption	Pneu-monia	All Other Classes				From All Preceding Causes	From All Causes of Mortality
1838	24,577	16,268	6,514	9,107	59,025	17,999	13,799	49,704	19,306	216,299	14	22
1839	25,991	9,131	10,937	8,165	59,559	18,151	12,855	49,215	20,767	214,771	14	21

Source: Excerpted from Great Britain Poor Law Commissioners, 1842, table on page 2.

posal and better supplies of water, which could best be attained through public administration. To insure the public against waste and poor workmanship he advised that "securities should be taken that all new local public works are devised and conducted by responsible officers qualified by the possession of the science and skill of civil engineers" (Great Britain Poor Law Commissioners, 1842, p. 371).

Chadwick's report instigated the Royal Commission on Enquiry; this type of investigation was to continue in the interests of public health. The Factory Act of 1847 was passed to regulate the hours and working conditions of women and children. Largely as the result of Chadwick's effort, public health in Great Britain was reorganized, with enduring success. The Act for Promoting Public Health, passed by Parliament on August 31, 1848, was to prove as important in preventive medicine as did the bacteriological contributions to medical science. The General Board of Health, operating through the treasury department with a core of inspectors on a national scale, was not a remote bureaucratic organization that merely handed out decrees from London for the improvement of health. Rather, inspectors were to travel throughout the country to examine sewage, drainage, water supplies, burial grounds, paving of streets, and lighting. The basis of the board's success was the institution of local boards of health with members elected at the local levels of cities, towns, and boroughs. These boards in turn would appoint their own medical officers. The central commissioners of public works were to cooperate with the local health boards. The outstanding feature of this approach was the regulations and supervisions that evolved out of local needs. This important factor was to contribute to the subsequent success of the public health movement in the United States.

In the rapidly changing and expanding public health affairs in Britain, Chadwick was dismissed because of his harshness with people, but he continued to exert his influence on Parliament. In 1836 The Births and Deaths Registrations Act was passed and a director-general appointed. Dr. William Farr, through the influence of Chadwick, was appointed secretary and served from 1841 through 1879. He was a superb statistician; his annual letters to the director-general on the causes of death were a valuable contribution for those concerned with the health of the nation through appropriate legislation.

He was largely responsible for the census. Farr's biography and some of his annual letters were published by the Sanitary Institute of Great Britain (Farr, 1885).

[A contemporary of Chadwick and Farr was John Simon,]who was trained as a surgeon and pathologist and became the medical officer for the city of London from 1848 to 1858. He then served as medical officer under the Privy Council from 1858 to 1872. Simon has been called "the greatest name in the history of Public Health" (Frazer, 1950). As a scientist and consulting surgeon at St. Thomas Hospital, he wrote and spoke with authority. He was a president of the Royal College of Surgeons. As a respected member of the medical community, he bridged the gap between the sanitary engineers and the practitioners in combined ventures that had to be cooperative if the preventive measures were to have any degree of success.] Thus Simon's approach differed from the more abrasive one of Chadwick.

During Simon's combined tenure in London and on the national scene from 1848 to 1872 infectious diseases commanded much of his effort, and he wrote extensively on this subject. One out of every three deaths in England was due to an infectious disease, with tuberculosis responsible for the greatest number of deaths (Lambert, 1963). Other major causes of death were scarlet fever, diphtheria, dysentery of infants and children, typhoid, typhus, cholera, smallpox, and puerperal fever. During Simon's tenure not much could be done specifically for these diseases, since their etiological causes were not known. But he recognized the value of the studies of William Budd on typhoid (1856a, b) and of John Snow on cholera (1853 and 1855, reproduced in 1936).]

[Simon continually stressed the sanitary requirements of the nation, including the importance of clean drinking water.] He emphasized time and time again the national need for smallpox vaccination and worked on administrative procedures in carrying out the prevention of smallpox. In reading through Simon's reports (1887; Great Britain Local Government Board, 1859–1870) one gains a deep appreciation of the breadth of his knowledge, the clarity of his writing, and the soundness of his recommendations. Simon made the public aware of the major health problems of the country. Because of his efforts a public health organization on a national scale was in operation. It was to be a sound foundation for the expansion of the National Health System in the following century.

Public Health in the United States

While the public health movement in England benefited from the efforts of Chadwick, Farr, and Simon, public health in the United States was fortunate in the talents of Lemuel Shattuck. Born in Massachusetts in 1793, he was an itinerant school teacher, a merchant in Concord, Massachusetts, and a book dealer in Boston. As a result of genealogical studies which he undertook in Concord, Shattuck became interested in statistics. He helped to organize the American Statistical Association in 1839 and was active in the registration legislation of 1842 in Massachusetts, which required the recording of all births, marriages, and deaths. He successfully generated a community census for Boston in 1845, the first to be carried out in the United States, and he was instrumental in a more advanced type of federal census that was made in 1850. His greatest achievement came while he was chairman of a board of three commissioners appointed to carry out a sanitary survey of the state of Massachusetts and to produce recommendations for rectifying the deficiencies. The result, generally recognized as the work of Shattuck, is known as the "Shattuck Report" (Massachusetts-Sanitary Commission of, 1850, reprint 1948). It is one of the greatest documents in the history of public health.

This report reviews the history of the sanitary movement on a worldwide basis. The main thrust resides in 50 recommendations, the first 36 on "State and Municipal Measures" and 14 on "Social and Personal Measures" (see Appendix I). In reading these recommendations more than a century after their publication one is struck by their soundness and moderate moral tone, with respect not only to the aims of public health but also to preventive medicine and personal hygiene. It is remarkable that the report was written largely by a layman who knew little of scientific medicine at the time and nothing about the germ theory of disease. The report is a great credit to Shattuck and his two fellow commissioners, Nathaniel Banks, Jr. and Jehiel Abbott.

Massachusetts accepted the Sanitary Report but was not prepared to implement its recommendations (Rosenkrantz, 1972). The 1850s were a period of political instability, with many leaders embroiled in the antislavery movement. The Civil War and the postwar problems added to the deferment of public health concerns. But Massachusetts did organize the first state board of health in the United States in 1869, with Dr. Henry Pickering Bowditch as chairman. A graduate of Harvard, he had trained for two years under Dr. P. Ch. A. Louis in Paris along with his friends Dr. James Jackson, Jr. and Dr. Oliver Wendell Holmes.

[The activation of public health measures was a slow process.]In the first annual report of the board to the legislature, Bowditch proclaimed that "State Medicine" had at long last been established in the Commonwealth and that it was to be concerned with not only the physical needs of man, but with intellectual and moral qualities as well (Massachusetts State Board of Health, 1870). And in the report of 1874 Bowditch again emphasized the importance of physical fitness and a clean environment, as well as the great need for physicians to recognize preventive medicine along with curative medicine (Massachusetts State Board of Health, 1874). These reports reflect the cautious and moral approaches that prevailed just before a more scientific attitude toward disease became firmly established in medical practice and thought toward the end of the century.

The need to protect the health of the public in New York City, America's largest community, also stirred members of the local medical profession and leading citizens during the post-Civil War era (Duffy, 1968). The health administration was entangled in political corruption; even the most obvious means of correcting the threats to health were ignored. There was an urgent need for an independent metropolitan health board. Filth, inadequate housing, poor sewage disposal, and offensive trades and industries were some of the maladjustments of society.[There were epidemics of smallpox, scarlet fever, measles, diphtheria, malaria, tuberculosis, typhoid, and cholera, and occasional visitations of yellow fever.]The stirring documentary report on the corrupt and poorly administered health organization written by Dr. Stephen Smith (1911) for *The New York Times* on March 13, 1865 did much to incite the citizens. The New York State legislature responded to this and other pressures by passing the New York Health Law of 1866, and thereby a strong and independent board of health came into being.

[Simultaneously other states and communities found it necessary to set up administrative boards in the interests of the health of the pub-

lic. In Providence, Rhode Island, under the leadership of Dr. Charles
V. Chapin, the first municipal public health laboratory was opened in
1888 (Cassedy, 1962). His influence was to extend into the twentieth
century; for years he was considered the most outstanding authority
on municipal health in the United States (Chapin, 1910; 1916; 1921).

Public health continued to gain momentum. By 1900 all but eight of
the states had state boards of health, and by 1907 this was accomplished for all states (Ferrell et al., 1929). The founding of the American Public Health Association in 1873 with Stephen Smith as president was to provide an open national forum for a continuing attack on
public health problems. This association, which still continues with a
membership of many thousands, had as its announced purpose in its
constitution a voluntary organization for "the advancement of sanitary science and the promotion of organizations and measures for the
practical application of public hygiene" (American Public Health Association, 1875, p. xiii). It is fortunate that the movements of public
health and preventive medicine became firmly established before the
science of bacteriology brought forth the discoveries on the etiology
and epidemiology of epidemic diseases. The organization of public
health facilities on a local, national, and international scale provided
the operational base for the application of scientific principles in the
control and prevention of infectious diseases.

In summing up the purpose and goals of public health early in the
twentieth century, Professor Charles-Edward Winslow of Yale contended that public health is a social activity, "the science and the art
of preventing disease, prolonging life, and promoting physical health
and efficiency through organized community efforts for the sanitation
of the environment, the control of community infections, the education of the individual in principles of personal hygiene, the organization of medical and nursing service for the early diagnosis and preventive treatment of disease, and the development of the social ma-
chinery which will ensure to every individual in the community a
standard of living adequate for the maintenance of health" (1920, p.
30). ·

United States Public Health Service

Through various agencies, supported by congressional appropri-
ations, the United States has made major contributions to the control

of infectious diseases. This accomplishment has been achieved primarily through the United States Public Health Service, and later through the National Institutes of Health (Furman, 1973; Williams, 1951). The United States Public Health Service (USPHS) had its origin in 1798 when the marine hospitals were established by congressional action for the relief of sick and disabled seamen. The first of the hospitals was opened in Boston in 1803 with Dr. Benjamin Waterhouse physician-in-charge. He first introduced interns and residents into hospitals in the United States. Until 1870 the hospitals were administered within the Treasury Department, but the service became inefficient and lacked strong leadership. Agitated by threats of epidemic cholera, the service was reorganized in 1872, when Dr. J. W. Woodworth became the first supervising surgeon of the United States Marine Hospital Service, a title that was changed to supervising surgeon general in 1902.

Doctor Woodworth made the following recommendations in 1876: (1) Rules were to be established for quarantining foreign vessels. (2) Consular officers in foreign ports were to inform the United States government of sanitary conditions in their area. (3) These officers were to issue weekly reports. (4) National quarantine was to be enforced by the Marine Hospital Service. (5) The origins and causes of epidemics were to be investigated, especially those of cholera and yellow fever (Woodworth, 1875).

A modest but momentous development occurred in 1887 with the establishment of a bacteriological laboratory under the direction of Dr. John Kinyoun at the Marine Hospital, Staten Island, New York. Doctor Kinyoun had received training with Dr. Robert Koch. The primary mission of the laboratory was research on cholera and other infectious diseases. Known first as the Laboratory of Hygiene, the name was changed to the Hygienic Laboratory in 1891, when it was moved to Washington, D.C. Dr. Milton Rosenau succeeded Dr. Kinyoun as director in 1899. For several years the Hygienic Laboratory was concerned mostly with the control of biologicals, and the basic interests were the infectious diseases. Under the direction of Dr. Rosenau the early work was of excellent quality. As examples, Bulletin No. 10 constituted the famous report on hookworm (Stiles, 1903); Bulletin No. 14 was on "Spotted Fever (Tick-Fever) of the Rocky Mountains. A New Disease" (Anderson, 1903); and Bulletin No. 8

was an outline of the "Laboratory Course in Pathology and Bacteriology" (Rosenau, 1902). This course trained public health officers for one year, preparing them for the scientific diagnosis of plague, cholera, diphtheria, tetanus, tuberculosis, typhoid fever, anthrax, malaria, and other infectious diseases. The officers were also encouraged to carry on original investigations themselves.

The Hygienic Laboratory was a part of the United States Marine Hospital Service until 1902, when the name was changed to the Public Health and Marine Hospital Service. The USPHS was organized in 1912 when the Marine Hospital Service was changed to the Public Health Service and the research program, under Dr. Joseph Goldberger, was extended beyond communicable diseases to such studies as pellagra. After World War I many significant changes took place. Doctor Hugh Smith Cumming was appointed surgeon general of the USPHS in 1920, and in 1921 the Rocky Mountain Spotted Fever Laboratory was established in Hamilton, Montana. It was during this period that the National Institute of Health was organized.

National Institutes of Health

In 1930 the name of the Hygienic Laboratory was changed by Congress to the National Institute of Health (NIH), and an extensive reorganization of the federal health services began. The Rocky Mountain Spotted Fever Laboratory was designated as a field station in the USPHS and in 1937 became a part of NIH. Another special research laboratory of the service involving cancer investigations at the Harvard Medical School was inaugurated in 1922 and developed into the National Cancer Institute in 1937. Just before World War II activities of NIH shifted to Bethesda, Maryland with further reorganization and with the building of new administration and research buildings. During the war NIH was still a part of the USPHS, but it was given bureau status within the Public Health Service.

Shortly after World War II the creation of a research grants office of NIH was the outcome of the transfer of funds in 1946 from the Office of Scientific Research and Development (OSRD) to the Public Health Service. This was the beginning of the extramural research grants and fellowship awards, so ably conceived by Dr. Rolla E. Dyer, the director of NIH. The Clinical Center of NIH was opened for patients in

1953. In the same year the USPHS became a part of the new Department of Health, Education and Welfare (DHEW). With the appearance of new institutes involving different categories of diseases and the expansion of intramural and extramural research, the name of *National Institute of Health* had given way to *The National Institutes of Health* in 1948, and by 1968, through continuing reorganization of the government's health activities, NIH had become an independent operating agency within the Department of Health, Education and Welfare (DHEW). The director became responsible to a member of the United States president's cabinet, the secretary of DHEW.

The general mission of NIH has been summarized as follows (United States Department of Health, Education and Welfare-National Institutes of Health, 1976, p. viii):

An agency of the Department of Health, Education and Welfare, the NIH is . . . the focal point for Federal biomedical research and support of research. . . . the NIH conducts biomedical research in its own laboratories; provides grants to nonprofit organizations and institutions for research and for medical education, including improvement or construction of library facilities, buildings, equipment and other resources; provides grants for the training of research investigators and supports biomedical communications through programs and activities of the National Library of Medicine. The NIH reservation is situated on 306.4 acres in Bethesda, Md., a suburb of the District of Columbia. On these campus-like grounds, NIH maintains hundreds of laboratories containing complex and highly sophisticated research equipment, a 516-bed research hospital known as the Clinical Center, and the National Library of Medicine.

As of 1977 all of the major activities of DHEW supported by the federal government are headed by a department head with cabinet status, who is directly responsible to the president of the United States. The magnitude of this enterprise is revealed in the federal budget of 1978 that President Carter submitted to the Congress. The total federal budget was 440 billion dollars, of which 159.4 million was programmed for DHEW. Over 90 percent of the DHEW budget was principally for financing programs for the poor and elderly. The support money designated for NIH, as a federal agency, was approximately 2.5 billion dollars.

The great surge in medical knowledge after World War II was

mainly a result of the basic and clinical research supported by NIH. The NIH training programs for health personnel accelerated the improvement and excellence of medical education, and in turn, better medical care. In the field of infectious diseases the most outstanding accomplishments were in molecular biology, especially in immunology, which led to a more comprehensive understanding of the pathogenesis and management of these diseases. Progress in virology led to the production of more and more effective prophylactic vaccines.

NIH comprises twelve institutes as follows:

(1) National Cancer Institute
(2) National Heart and Lung Institute
(3) National Library of Medicine
(4) National Institute on Aging
(5) National Institute of Allergy and Infectious Diseases
(6) National Institute of Arthritis, Metabolism, and Digestive Diseases
(7) National Institute of Child Health and Human Development
(8) National Institute of Dental Research
(9) National Institute of Environmental Health Services
(10) National Institute of General Medicine
(11) National Institute of Neurological and Communicative Disorders and Stroke
(12) National Eye Institute

The amount of money apportioned to each institute is determined by Congress. In distributing funds for extramural research and for training programs, each of the institutes has competent advisory groups. The peer review system has been one of the outstanding features of the NIH grant system. Although the grants and programs for the study of infectious diseases and allergies and for immunology are centered in the National Institute of Allergy and Infectious Diseases (NIAD), many of the grant requests arise in other institutes because the disciplines of NIAD are utilized in the resolution of many diverse problems of health such as cancer, arthritis, neurological disorders, dental caries, and ocular diseases.

A fortunate development for the control of infectious diseases occurred in the federal government after World War II. These changes were due to the unusual foresight of a group of men in the USPHS.[1] In their vision, intramural and extramural basic biomedical research and the training of personnel would be centered at NIH in Bethesda, and the practical methods and procedures for controlling the infectious diseases at a national level would be located at Atlanta, Georgia. The Communicable Disease Center was the first single public health agency to coordinate this purpose.

The genesis of CDC occurred three months after the Japanese attacked Pearl Harbor, when an emergency war agency was established in Atlanta for the control of malaria. The agency was to be directed especially at the eradication of anopheline mosquitoes. It was called the Office of Malarial Control in War Areas (MCWA). Malaria was endemic in the southeastern states, and because of the year-round favorable weather conditions, the area was selected for military concentrations and for war industries. Malaria was a serious hazard. To facilitate their objectives MCWA activated a multidisciplined staff with five divisions: medical, engineering, entomology, training, and administration. MCWA operated under the Bureau of State Services of the Public Health Service headed by Dr. Joseph W. Mountain.

The success of MCWA in controlling malaria was due to the cooperation of efficient teams in working with several different organizations. Doctor Mountain was supported by Dr. Rolla Eugene Dyer, director of the single existing NIH at Bethesda, and by Dr. Thomas Parran, surgeon-general of the USPHS. Basic to the success of MCWA was the fact that their trained teams acted only in an advisory capacity upon request by the individual states. The eradication work was performed by each state with its own personnel and with the financial aid of its own legislature. This was to be a paramount feature of the future international work of WHO. MCWA also cooperated with NIH, the Tennessee Valley Authority, the United States Department of Agriculture, and various medical centers. The activities of MCWA were extended to an attack against typhus, also endemic in the area, and against typhoid and certain tropical diseases. The agency was highly active in insect and rodent control.

Communicable Disease Center

After World War II Surgeon-General Thomas Parran in 1946 changed the name of MCWA to the Communicable Disease Center. The Veterinary Public Health Division was established in 1947 for problems relating to the zoonoses. The venereal disease and tuberculosis programs of the USPHS were centered at CDC. Basic administrative and functional features of MCWA operated in the evolution of CDC. Strong cooperative relationships continued between the center and the departments of health of the states, especially with reference to communicable and epidemic infectious diseases. Laboratory techniques were evaluated and standardized. Vaccine production was monitored for uniformity. A significant development was the strengthening of the epidemiological division: a system was organized so that data on epidemic diseases could be acquired quickly and then disseminated. Trained epidemiological personnel were available for consultation in any troubled area. In 1951 the Epidemiological Intelligence Service was established so that personnel ("disease detectives") could proceed immediately to any trouble spot in the United States or elsewhere in the world. In 1961 the *Morbidity and Mortality Weekly Reports* on the status of communicable diseases and other infections were widely distributed upon request. In 1968 CDC was changed administratively to a bureau in the USPHS.

The continued attack on infectious diseases was aided by CDC through the establishment in Atlanta of eight branches in the laboratory division, including bacteriology, mycology, parasitology, virology, and rickettsiae. Personnel in these areas did research, assimilated laboratory information for the epidemiological division, acted in an advisory capacity for health departments throughout the country, and organized training programs in Atlanta for health personnel.

CDC has directed extensive programs carried out at local levels for the control of communicable diseases with federal funds, such as immunization for poliomyelitis, diphtheria, whooping cough, tetanus, measles, and rubella. These included the initial field trials for Salk vaccine. In cooperation with WHO, CDC gathered information on new variants of influenza A and participated in international programs for the eradication of smallpox.

The personnel of CDC have been challenged by serious epidemiological problems related to epidemic infectious diseases, as reflected in the sequence of events involved in an epidemic in 1976 of what has been called "Legionnaires' disease of Philadelphia." A second challenge on a national scale was the National Influenza Immunization Program for the same year.[2] The workers and the facilities were severely strained in efforts to resolve all the problems and to maintain relationships with health officials throughout the nation. Public interest in both episodes had given way to alarm, and it was necessary to inform the media periodically on progress being made. One can only commend the center for its excellent work.

Let us first of all consider a summary of the known facts about Legionnaires' disease. On August 6, 1976 CDC issued a brief report on an epidemic of respiratory disease involving 152 persons who had attended a convention of the American Legion Department of Pennsylvania between July 25 and July 31 (Center for Disease Control, 1976c). The illness was characterized by an acute onset of fever, chills, headache, and malaise, followed by a dry cough and myalgia. A state of shock hastened death in those with a high fever and extensive pneumonia. All victims were hospitalized and 22 died, primarily because of pneumonia. The Legionnaires and their families occupied three or four hotels, but most of the cases apparently occurred in only one of them. There was also evidence that the illness had afflicted some nonconventioneers.

Officials of the Philadelphia and Pennsylvania State Departments of Health immediately began investigations with the Bureaus of Epidemiology and the Laboratories of CDC. This relationship was expanded and the work intensified with the passage of time. Mystery surrounded the epidemic at first; interest centered on the environmental factors within one hotel. Was the malady of noninfectious environmental origin, or was a new infectious agent responsible? After intensive work a special report from CDC indicated that an unknown type of bacteria had been isolated from lung tissues through inoculation of chicken embryos and then passed successfully to guinea pigs (Center for Disease Control, 1977b). This result enabled serological tests to be carried out. Because CDC had a serum bank collected from previous epidemics it was revealed on the basis of these tests that a similar outbreak had occurred in a hospital in Washington, D.C. involving 94 cases and 16 deaths. Further serological investigations demonstrated that an epidemic had occurred in Pontiac, Michigan in 1968 with 144 cases and no deaths (Center for Disease Control, 1977c). By March 25, 1977 cultures of the causative bacteria had been successfully grown on artificial media and found sensitive to the antibiotic erythromycin (Center for Disease Control,

1977a). Later it was found that inoculated guinea pigs were protected against a lethal outcome by the administration of erythromycin. A final analysis of the Philadelphia epidemic showed a total of 180 cases with 29 deaths.

Most significant findings based upon serological tests of victims in past epidemics were that Legionnaires' disease was not a new disease and that *after* the Philadelphia epidemic the organism was isolated in a patient in Michigan. By July 1977 a total of 19 new cases had been scientifically proved in 11 different states. Therefore "the disease was neither new nor localized" (Center for Disease Control, 1977d, p. 224).[3]

The plan for the National Influenza Immunization of 1976 constituted the first attempt by a government to finance the production and administration of a prophylactic vaccine. It was a major decision for any government to offer protection against illness by such a procedure, and the decision was reached after serious consultation with many knowledgeable groups. Only the highlights of the available information on the purpose and results of the implementation of the plan can be presented here.

Influenza remains the last pandemic disease for which no completely satisfactory prevention is available. The reason is that the influenza virus is not stable antigenically. About every decade, influenza A, the principal responsible virus, changes antigenically so that a previous exposure or vaccination is without effect immunologically. Even under the best of circumstances the production and testing of a new vaccine takes four to five months. It is obvious that the sudden appearance of a new influenza variant among a susceptible population will cause disease before an appropriate vaccine can be produced, distributed, and administered. But the events of 1976 indicated that a propitious time had arrived when a national program for immunization could be undertaken.

In February 1976 an outbreak of a new variant appeared in military personnel at Fort Dix, New Jersey. It was of great significance in that the strain possessed the antigenic components of the "swine" influenza virus of 1918. The outbreak at Fort Dix was the first transmission of a human-to-human "swine" variant since 1920, and it was called "A/New Jersey/76." The time appeared appropriate to initiate the production of a vaccine with this strain, particularly since there was a vulnerable population under 50 years of age. The virus had appeared late in the respiratory season and there would be enough time to produce and test a vaccine for the following season, which would begin in late 1976. Congress would appropriate 135 million dollars for such a program. The responsibility for the program would fall mainly on CDC for cooperation with the manufacturers in the production, and then for cooperation with the state boards of health for distribution and administration. After many difficulties, the program was instituted by October 1976.

Over 40 million vaccinations were given by February 1977, but by then the program had to be severely curtailed, largely because of the appearance of the complicating Guillain-Barré syndrome, which is of unknown etiology and causes ascending paralysis. There were 843 cases of Guillain-Barré syndrome, 427 occurring in vaccinates and 386 in those not vaccinated. Thirty deaths were distributed equally between the two groups. Another frustrating factor for the public, aside from the dangers attached to any vaccination program, was the failure of a major epidemic of "swine" influenza to materialize in 1977. The public appeared disillusioned and fearful, an additional reason for discontinuing the program. Nevertheless the effort proved that a nationwide program could be implemented for producing, distributing, and administering a vaccine and for evaluating results. That an epidemic did not occur was fortunate. The vaccine proved to be potent and reasonably safe. Finally the program and administrative policy of CDC for protecting the health of the public continued as valuable assets in a national program.

International Public Health

Attempts to control infectious diseases at the international level date back to the introduction of quarantine methods in the fifteenth century (see Section I, Chapter 1). Measures included the application of disinfectants to objects and merchandise being transported into or out of epidemic areas. Instituted at Venice, this practice continued for over five hundred years. International agreements for enforcement of such efforts were unsuccessful, however, until more knowledge had been acquired about the causes and means of transmission of epidemic diseases.

Diplomats and public health authorities of several nations were stirred into action in the nineteenth century by epidemics of cholera. Although knowledge of the nature of cholera was incomplete, the French recognized the urgency of controlling the disease. Through their leadership a series of international sanitary conferences were inaugurated in Paris in 1851 (Howard-Jones, 1975). Between 1851 and 1903 eleven conferences were held, attended by delegates from the leading nations of Europe and in due time from the United States. After 1903 only three additional conferences were held, one in 1912, one in 1926, and one in 1938. Cholera was the principal subject for discussion, but plague and yellow fever were also considered. A summary of fourteen conferences is given in Table 2 (Howard-Jones, 1975). It was not until the seventh conference meeting in 1892, 41 years after the first conference, that the first international treaty on public health was formulated and accepted, which was concerned with cholera and the control of westbound shipping from the East.

The formative period for the International Sanitary Conferences ended with the eleventh, held in Paris in 1903. The preceding year delegates of the American States meeting in Mexico had formulated the world's first *international health organization*, known as the International Sanitary Bureau — later as the Pan American Sanitary Bureau — with offices in Washington. It was agreed that a permanent international health office should be organized. As a result the Office International d'Hygiène publique was established in 1907, with headquarters in Paris.

The twelfth International Sanitary Conference in 1911 was the last one before World War I; no further conferences were held until 1926. The fourteenth and last conference in 1938 was notable because scientific advances in understanding infectious diseases were considered to a greater extent than before. There was a consensus that cholera could be prevented through vaccination. Conference members agreed on some control measures and stipulated that any country should give notice of the *first confirmed* cases of cholera, plague, or yellow fever.

The Office International d'Hygiène publique was a significant advance in international affairs. Popularly known as the "Office," the organization had an elected Permanent Committee, an executive staff, and a president. Such a continuous operative group gave stabil-

Table 2. Summary of International Sanitary Conferences

Conference No.	Place and Dates	No. of Countries	Accomplishment
1	Paris July 23, 1851–Jan. 19, 1852	11 European and Turkey	Cholera, plague, and yellow fever discussed. No conclusions.
2	Paris April 9, 1859–Aug. 30, 1859	Same minus 2 Sicilies	Discoveries of Pacini and Snow largely ignored. No definitive conclusions.
3	Constantinople Feb. 13, 1866–Sept. 26, 1866	16 (USA refused invitation)	Agreed India "home" of cholera. Pettenkofer's concepts overshadowed Pacini and Snow. Printed Proceedings 1130 pages.*
4	Vienna July 1, 1874–Aug. 1, 1874	21 (Pettenkofer German delegate)	Unanimous agreement drinking water could cause disease. Anticontagionist views prevailed.
5	Washington, D.C. January 5, 1881–Mar. 1, 1881	26	Finlay of Spain announced basic principles of epidemiology of yellow fever.
6	Rome May 20, 1885–June 13, 1885	28 (Dr. G. M. Sternberg USA delegate)	Koch delegate — no recognition of his discovery of *Cholera vibrios*.
7	Venice Jan. 5, 1892–Jan. 31, 1892	14	*First International Treaty relating to health protection governing westbound shipping from East.*
8	Dresden Mar. 11, 1893–April 15, 1893	19 (Koch — German delegate)	Pettenkofer experiment on self swallowing *Cholera vibrios* — October 7, 1892. Agreed on notification system of cholera; regulations accepted for ships.
9†	Paris Feb. 7, 1894–Apr. 3, 1894	16 including USA	Sanitary regulations for Mecca pilgrimage. (1893 — severe cholera epidemic).

No.	Place and Date	Participants	Notes
10	Venice Feb. 16, 1897–Mar. 19, 1897	20 including USA	Concerned exclusively with plague. Agreed on bacterial etiology — but no concept of insect transmission.
11**	Paris Oct. 10, 1903–Dec. 3, 1903	23 (Gen. Gorgas USA delegate)	Plans for establishment of permanent international health office in Paris. Yellow fever American problem. Regulation — destroying rats on ships.
12	Paris Nov. 7, 1911–Jan. 17, 1912	41 including China and Siam and 16 countries from the Americas	Discussions of cholera, plague, yellow fever; no basic decisions; importance of carrier state in cholera stressed.
13	Paris May 10, 1926–June 21, 1926	50 sovereign states (almost equally divided between Europe and the rest of the world)	Accepted cholera preventable through vaccination. Yellow fever caused by *Leptospira icteroides* (Noguchi's error). Notification of *first confirmed* case of cholera, plague, yellow fever — and *epidemics* of smallpox and typhus.
14	Paris Oct. 28, 1938–Oct. 31, 1938	50 countries	Egypt given sole responsibility for international quarantine functions previously administered by the internationally composed Egyptian Quarantine Board.

Source: Abstracted with permission of the publisher from N. Howard-Jones, *The Scientific Background of the International Sanitary Conferences 1851–1938*, World Health Organization, Geneva, 1975.

*Very rare — only one copy available in North America (University of Michigan).

†In September 1894, 8th International Congress on Hygiene and Demography held in Budapest. Nongovernmental organization. Opinion on nature of cholera still divided. Yersin and Kitasato submitted reports in absentia of discovery of plague bacillus.

**In 1902, establishment of first international health organization — International Sanitary Bureau in Washington, later the Pan American Sanitary Bureau. In 1907, establishment of Office International d'Hygiene publique.

ity to international health activities, particularly during World War I, and between 1919 and 1939 in cooperation with the Health Organization of the League of Nations. The United States was not a member of the league, but it was a major contributing member of the "Office."

The Paris "Office" supplied information for the International Health Conferences on a variety of subjects, such as epidemic notification, sanitary problems relating to air travel, the problem of venereal diseases in sailors, biological standardization of antidiphtheritic serum, opium and narcotic activities, and a long list of epidemic infectious diseases. When World War I ended in 1918 it had become more apparent that the preservation and protection of health was an international responsibility. Therefore, in the formulation of the League of Nations, organized in 1920 for the purpose of pursuing world peace, Article 23(f) of the Covenant stated that the league was "To endeavour to take steps in matters of international concern for the prevention and control of disease" (quoted in Goodman, 1971, p. 108). The structure of the organization was almost as simple as the stated purpose. Headquarters were in Geneva. During the formative period the Epidemics Commission was set up, principally because of the onslaught of epidemic typhus in eastern Europe and along the borders of Poland and the USSR. The chief body was the Health Committee that met twice yearly to outline the health program. The advisory council was the Permanent Committee of the Office International d'Hygiène publique, which met twice yearly in Paris and appointed some of the members of the Health Committee. The administration's health section, located in Geneva, carried out the program recommended by the Health Committee. With the aid of the Singapore Far Eastern Bureau all epidemiological and technical information was gathered in Geneva and dispersed in published bulletins. Ten annual volumes of the *Bulletin of the Health Organization* were published, and also the *Chronicle of the Health Organization*, *Weekly Epidemiological Record*, and the annual and monthly *Epidemiological Report*.

Perhaps the most outstanding health work of the league was embodied in the efforts of commissions or expert committees probing and advising on different health problems in various parts of the world. This excellent achievement is summarized in the last published *Bulletin of the Health Organization*, Volume XI (League of Nations, 1945). It is apparent that international public health was concerned with more than quarantine measures and a few diseases. Studies were carried out in depth on cancer, leprosy, rabies, dysentery, typhus, typhoid, leishmaniasis, tuberculosis, venereal disease, and malaria. Public health methods, education, and sanitation focused on the needs of developing countries, including the Nationalist Republic of China. Standardization of antibacterial sera was also undertaken.

Although the United States was not a member of the League of Nations, some of the country's outstanding authorities did serve on the Health Committee. The Rockefeller Foundation, chartered in 1913, provided generous financial support for the league's activities. Before and after World War I the foundation also had an important role in aiding international health objectives, such as the control of hookworm disease, malaria, and yellow fever. Education in the medical sciences and nursing was supported in this country and abroad. After 1929 the foundation extended its support to the natural sciences, agriculture, the social sciences, and the humanities. The Rockefeller Institute for Medical Research, founded in 1901, made important contributions leading to the control and treatment of infectious diseases (Corner, 1964). The league also received the cooperation of the Red Cross Organization. World War II closed in on the health activities of the league, but out of the ensuing chaos and destruction a more successful attempt at international health grew up on the foundations of the previous endeavors.

International health activities have successfully bridged the gap between nations during times of war and peace. Professor Hans Zinsser, sanitary commissioner of the health section of the League of Nations and an authority on typhus, visited Russia in 1923. He described the spirit of humanitarianism that prevailed during World War I as follows (1935, p. 293):

It is a curious and heartening fact that international coöperation in the prevention of epidemics placidly continues, however hostile or competitive other relationships may become. At the present moment, — while the world is an armed camp of suspicion and hatred, and nations are doing their best, by hook and crook, to push each other out of the world markets, to foment revolutions and steal each other's political and military secrets, — organized government agencies are exchanging information concerning epidemic diseases; sanitarians, bacteriologists, epidemiologists, and health administrators are coöperating, consulting each other, and freely interchanging views, materials, and methods, from Russia to South America, from Scandinavia to the tropics. It is perhaps not generally known that for several years, during the most turbulent period of the Russian Revolution, the only official relationship which existed between that unfortunate country and the rest of Europe consisted in the interchange of information bearing on the prevention of epidemic disease, arranged in coöperation by the Health Commission of the League of Nations and the Soviet government.

During World War II, on November 9, 1943, 43 allied and associated nations signed an agreement in Washington, D.C. to form the United Nations Relief and Rehabilitation Administration (UNRRA). The total expended budget for health over three years, the life of UNRRA, was to be 168 million dollars (Goodman, 1971). The stated purpose of UNRRA was "to provide for the liberated populations aid and relief from their suffering, food, clothing, and shelter, *aid in the prevention of pestilence and in the recovery in the health of people*, and for preparations and arrangements for the return of prisoners and exiles to their homes, and for assistance in the resumption of the urgently needed agricultural and industrial production and the restoration of essential services" (quoted in Goodman, 1971, p. 140). Doctor W. A. Sawyer (1947), the former director of the International Health Division of the Rockefeller Foundation, was instrumental in the direction of the health activities.

Effort was concentrated on the prevention of epidemic diseases. A major assault was made on typhus with means not available immediately after World War I. A total of 3,393 tons of DDT was supplied to eleven nations, and also anti-typhus vaccine. Steps were taken to prevent the spread of cholera. Diphtheria was combatted with toxoid and antitoxin, and DDT was also available to eradicate the mosquito that causes malaria, especially in Greece. Other work was undertaken for tuberculosis and for venereal diseases. Large amounts of medical supplies and considerable numbers of medical and technological personnel were essential to carry out these assignments. This was the largest international health program ever undertaken.

The objectives of a world organization to extend the work of the League of Nations were worked out during the bleakest days of World War II. The charter of the United Nations had its origin in the

Moscow Declaration of 1943 and in the Conference of Dumbarton Oaks (Washington) in 1944, and was adopted in San Francisco in April–June 1945 at the United Nations Conference on International Organization. Plans for health were overlooked at this charter meeting, but the Brazilian and Chinese delegates quickly corrected this deficiency by suggesting a health establishment within the organization. After three years of extensive preparations the World Health Organization (WHO) was established on September 1, 1948.

The preamble of the constitution of WHO, expressing the principles of the organization, is presented in nine forceful sentences (see Appendix II), in which the social concepts of health are emphasized. A high standard of health and freedom from disease for every individual are the responsibility of government. Chapter I, Article I, of the WHO constitution states the objective in one sentence (World Health Organization, 1947, p. 29): "The objective of the World Health Organization (hereinafter called the Organization) shall be the attainment by all peoples of the highest possible level of health." Membership is open to all states, and members of the UN can achieve membership in WHO by accepting the WHO constitution. The organization is operated through the World Health Assembly, the executive board, and the secretariat, and assignments are carried out through committees and conferences. Geneva was quickly designated the headquarters. Because health needs vary in different parts of the world, the concept of regional organizations was accepted and subsequently six organizations were created, including the Pan American Sanitary Bureau to represent the Americas. Budgetary matters originate with the director-general and the executive board, with final action taken by the assembly.

The basic philosophy of WHO is to advise and inform countries about national public health problems. Such aid can be requested by both member and nonmember nations. From the beginning WHO emphasized that the work should be carried out by the country's own administrative medical and technical personnel. Fellowships are provided for the training of such personnel. Since WHO was to be the only comprehensive international organization dealing with problems of public health, cooperation from the onset with other related agencies has been essential, and the list of agencies is formidable.

In order to disseminate information upon request, precise data on specific subjects have been acquired and distributed through technical publications containing the necessary information gathered by experts with committee or panel appointments. Additional help has been provided by WHO consultants working in field operations. The *WHO Technical Report Series* is available in over five hundred monographs in several different languages. Further information has been published in the *Bulletin of the World Health Organization*, the *WHO Chronicle*, and *Public Health Papers*. These have been supplemented by the *World Health Statistics Report* and the *Weekly Epidemiological Record*. All of these educational activities are supported by competent personnel at Geneva and in the regional offices. Good library facilities are also available. The depth of the different phases of WHO is reflected in the *Catalogue of Publications* from 1947-1973 (World Health Organization, 1974e). Two monographs present a comprehensive review of WHO activities, one for the decade 1948–1957 (World Health Organization, 1958b) and the other for the decade 1958–1967 (World Health Organization, 1968b). Dr. M. G. Candau of Brazil, the director-general of WHO for twenty years, wrote an informative preface on the objectives and the accomplishments of WHO for each of these volumes.

The immediate emphasis of WHO on the control of infectious diseases is recorded in the priority of activities accepted at the first meeting of the assembly in 1948 as follows: (1) Malaria, maternal and child health, tuberculosis, venereal disease, nutrition, and sanitation. (2) Public health administration. (3) Parasitic diseases. (4) Virus infections. (5) Mental disease. The budget to carry out the various enterprises was approximately five million dollars.

Malaria has caused more illness and disability in the world than any other infectious disease, and the most ambitious WHO program against infectious diseases pertained to malaria eradication. In 1955 the Eighth World Health Assembly decided to implement a program for the purpose of eradicating malaria throughout the world (World Health Organization, 1968b, p. 159). This was a costly undertaking largely because the areas affected by malaria were economically unable to share the expenses to any degree. WHO cooperated mostly in an advisory manner in carrying out the eradication. By 1966 100 million people, or 60 percent of the population, of malarious areas were freed from the disease.

But the optimistic plan to eradicate malaria throughout the world soon had to be revised. There was a reappearance of malaria in certain countries in 1975 with two million cases in India and tens of millions occurring annually in Africa, south of the Sahara, where control efforts were minimal. This resurgence is attributed to a combination of the development of insecticide resistance and the increased costs of control, which the governments could not support.

The organization was also actively concerned with the pandemic diseases. In 1968, the International Health Regulations included plague, cholera, yellow fever, smallpox, typhus, and relapsing fever. By 1971 these regulations involved only plague, cholera, yellow fever, and smallpox (World Health Organization, 1971a). The most serious continuous threat to world health was smallpox. In 1958 the Eleventh WHO Assembly voted to embark upon a vast eradication program against smallpox through vaccination. By 1968 the disease was confined to three endemic areas in the world: in South America in Brazil, Argentina, and Colombia; in all countries of Africa south of the Sahara; and in Asia in Afghanistan, India, Indonesia, Nepal, and Pakistan. By 1976 only one country, Ethiopia, reported the presence of smallpox, although very likely other remote pockets of disease can be anticipated. But there is continuing optimism that with an intensive vaccination program smallpox should be eradicated from the world by 1980, if not before.

In many areas of the world parasitic diseases other than malaria afflict millions of people. In tropical and subtropical regions these infections offer the greatest challenge to public health authorities and to WHO. Illustrative of the enormity of the problem is the accompanying tabulation, which was compiled from information for the

Parasitic Diseases	No. of Persons Infected (in millions)
Schistosomiasis	200
Filariasis	190
Hookworm	450
Onchocerciasis	50
Ascariasis	650
Chagas' disease	7

year 1968 (World Health Organization, 1968b, p. 175). A recent evaluation shows the figures to be little changed.

Despite the fact that there are means and therapy available to control such diseases, desperate social and economic factors have tended to hinder progress. The insect-borne diseases of schistosomiasis, onchocerciasis, and filariasis afflict millions of people in the developing countries. The continuous spread of these diseases, and the discovery of new diseases such as arbovirus infections, are often due to a disturbance in ecology, such as the building of man-made lakes, where the vectors of disease can propagate. As in the eradication of malaria, vector control is essential if these diseases are to be eliminated.

WHO activities have also engaged major efforts against virus diseases. Influenza is not one of the diseases subject to international quarantine, but this virus infection remains as the last of the great pandemics that continues to menace civilization at frequent intervals. Prophylactic vaccines, as mentioned above, have been only partially successful because of antigenic shifts of the Type A virus. This challenge is being met by WHO in a worldwide surveillance of influenza virus strains in 93 influenza centers. Recovered organisms are supplied to the World Influenza Center and the Influenza Center for the Americas located in the Center for Disease Control in Atlanta. In this manner new variants of the virus can be speedily detected and steps taken to prepare suitable vaccine.

Hepatitis research on Type B virus is being coordinated in 29 laboratories in 25 countries in tropical and temperate climates studying the prevalence of the antigen by age, sex, and socioeconomic conditions. Attention is being focused on poliomyelitis. Oral vaccines have successfully controlled the disease in the developed nations, but poliomyelitis is increasing in many tropical nations. There remains an urgent need to expand the use of vaccines in these endemic areas. A major threat throughout the world is posed by a growing list of diseases caused by arboviruses. These viruses along with dengue are the cause of epidemic hemorrhagic fever. There is a need for extensive epidemiological studies that will establish the specific etiology and the vectors responsible for the transmission of this group of diseases. WHO is engaged in these efforts.

The most feared animal disease transmissible to man is rabies, and for this reason WHO has expended considerable effort and money on its control. On a worldwide basis, in 1973 more than one million persons received prophylactic vaccine as a result of bites by suspected rabid animals.

Since there are at least 150 diseases of animals transmissible to man, the zoonoses have received continuing attention in cooperation with the United Nations Food and Animal Organization (FAO). Major efforts have been directed at brucellosis, leptospirosis, echinococcus disease, and toxoplasmosis.

Tuberculosis and leprosy are two significant infections under continuous observation by WHO officials and advisors. It is conservatively estimated that there are 10 to 20 million active cases of tuberculosis in the world, three-fourths of which are in the developing countries. Two to three million cases appear each year, with one to two million deaths. Fortunately, decreasing rates are being encountered due to chemotherapy, vaccination (BCG vaccine), and national tuberculosis programs. It is estimated that there are eleven million people with leprosy in the world, four million of whom are disabled. Ten thousand new cases are reported annually from 29 countries and territories. The disease is most prevalent in South America, Africa, Burma, and the South Pacific area. Sulfones have proved effective therapeutically.

At the Eleventh WHO Assembly Meeting held in Minneapolis in 1958, a significant action called for "a special study of the role of WHO in research and of ways in which the Organization might assist more adequately in stimulating and co-ordinating research and developing research personnel" (World Health Organization, 1958a, p. 236). As a part of this objective an advisory committee on medical research was activated. The objectives of the program were the support of national research, provisions of services for research, training of research workers, and improvement of communication among scientists. Doctor Martin Kaplan, the director of the WHO Office of Science and Technology, who has been with the organization almost since its inception, recently reviewed the research objectives and pointed out that "the main health problem of underdeveloped areas is that of infectious diseases, either endemic or epidemic" (Kaplan, M., 1973, p. 1032). The urgent need is to introduce sophisticated technology, equipment, buildings, and personnel into those areas in order to study and investigate the *local* problems.

Infectious diseases still afflict millions of people throughout the world, especially in the developing countries. History is being repeated. Infectious diseases have been controlled among the advanced

countries because of the application of scientific knowledge and because of courageous steps to correct, if not completely eliminate,
socioeconomic "nuisances" that have contributed to disease and poor
health. In the developing nations, poverty, malnutrition, inadequate
housing, and poor sanitation often persist. WHO authorities have not
only aided with new scientific techniques, prophylactic vaccines, and
modern therapy in the control of infections, but have also demonstrated at local levels that crowd diseases, or epidemics, depend upon
elimination of the "nuisances."

SECTION II

The Development of Prophylaxis and Therapy for Infectious Diseases in the Twentieth Century

CHAPTER 4

The Pre-Sulfonamide Era

The establishment of the specific microbial causes of diseases in the nineteenth century rapidly led to specific methods for preventing and treating infections. Prophylactic vaccines were developed for protection against epidemic diseases. Specific antisera became available, followed by the era of the sulfonamides and antibiotics. Chemotherapy was extended to the control of epidemic diseases through chemical insecticides that destroyed insect vectors of diseases.

Microbial Preparations

About one hundred years after Jenner introduced cowpox vaccine for smallpox, Pasteur and his associates initiated the modern era of prophylactic vaccination for fowl cholera, anthrax, swine erysipelas, and rabies, using viable organisms with attenuated virulence. The first heat-killed bacterial suspension was used shortly thereafter in the United States by Daniel Salmon and Theobald Smith for swine plague. Although the scientific basis for vaccination was first firmly established in the Pasteur Institute, continuity of this research did not engage serious attention in Paris. Interest arose in England with the work of Dr. Almroth Wright, who was one of the chief scientific spokesmen for vaccination during the first decade of the twentieth century.

Wright, starting out his career in the British army, was concerned

61

with typhoid fever as a major health problem in the troops. He knew of the work of the bacteriologist W. M. W. Haffkine, who at the time was not only investigating the efficacy of vaccine in cholera, but had started his long pursuit of a vaccine for plague (Haffkine, 1897). Wright was intrigued by Haffkine's suggestion that "the method of vaccination which has proved so effectual in combating cholera epidemics in India might, *mutatis mutandis*, be applied to the prophylaxis of typhoid fever" (Wright and Semple, 1897, p. 256). Wright was largely responsible for the immunization of over a hundred thousand individuals against typhoid fever, using various vaccine preparations. Evaluating results in military populations is difficult, but Hans Zinsser (1927) concluded that Wright's vaccination programs were reasonably successful.

In spite of his interest in morbidity and mortality rates, Wright simply could not master vital statistics, so essential in evaluating a vaccine. His most recognized immunological contribution was the quantitative measurement of the acquired immunity of the individual after receiving vaccine inoculations. He originated and centered his attention on the opsonic index.[1] This is a quantitative enumeration of the number of typhoid bacilli engulfed by the individual's circulating leukocytes. Opsonin, as an immune body, occurs in the blood serum, where it sensitizes the leukocytes to phagocytize and kill invading microorganisms.

Wright and his associates also carried out an extensive immunization program among South African miners with pneumococcus vaccine; but because the preparations lacked specificity, the results were doubtful (Wright et al., 1914). F. S. Lister (1917) in later studies among South African miners did establish immunity against the prevalent pneumococcal infections when he used type-specific pneumococcal vaccines, a result subsequently confirmed in the United States.

Wright (1908) achieved international recognition for his work on vaccination, as shown by his being invited to present a Harvey Lecture in New York. This lecture was essentially an exposition of the value of the opsonic index as a guide to inoculation. Wright also raised some pertinent questions about vaccination in general, especially with reference to its widespread uncritical use. His questions concerned the selection of strains of organisms for vaccine preparation, and the problem of whether attenuated living organisms or heat or chemically killed bacteria should be used for inoculation. What dose of organisms should be inoculated, and how many doses should be given? What about the therapeutic use of vaccines for acute and chronic cases of sepsis? How should one manage chronic localized infections occurring in the sinuses, skin, and lungs?

The early programs of vaccination centered on typhoid fever, cholera, and plague. After fifty years of research, however, such programs yielded only modest success, protection against these diseases waning within a relatively short period of time. Early emphasis was placed on bacterial vaccines, but the most lasting successes were obtained with bacterial toxins. Diphtheria toxin-antitoxin mixtures offered excellent protection against the disease. Similar immunity was established for tetanus, especially when the relatively nontoxic preparations of toxoid were used.

As one surveys the vast literature on immunization one is impressed by the effectiveness of vaccination as developed by Pasteur, and by the clarity of the descriptions of cellular and humoral immune responses contributed by Bordet, Ehrlich, Metchnikoff, and others. But a confused state of thinking often afflicted medical practitioners, particularly when *prophylactic* preparations were administered *therapeutically* for acute and chronic infections, and even for some noninfectious diseases. The basic principles laid down by the pioneers in vaccination were distorted and at times ignored. The selection of appropriate cultures for vaccine production was often superficial, careful evaluation of the administered doses was lacking, and controversy flared over the proper anatomical sites for administering the vaccines. This confusion in clinical medicine persisted during the first quarter of the twentieth century.

World War I provoked epidemic diseases among military and civilian populations, and typhoid fever offered a proving ground to test the value of prophylactic vaccine against typhoid fever. During this period Professor Frederick P. Gay (1918) carried out an extensive survey of typhoid vaccination in the military personnel of several nations including England, France, Russia, Italy, Japan, and the United States. He expressed little doubt that vaccination did protect against typhoid, but he admitted that the results were difficult to interpret because water and food supplies were also controlled. Typhoid vaccine was employed intravenously for the treatment of typhoid fever (Wiltshire and MacGillycuddy, 1915). Even Gay concluded (1918, p. 239), "We regard, then, the intravenous vaccine treatment of typhoid fever as the most effective type of therapy hitherto devised to combat this disease." Even though Wright appeared to be a firm advocate of employing specific vaccines prophylactically for infectious diseases and measured the immune response carefully with his opsonic index, in summing up his experience after World War I he too leaned toward the use of vaccines for therapeutic purposes, even citing Pasteur as an authority. In addressing the Royal Society of Medicine on February 25, 1919 Wright (1919, p. 489) stated that Pasteur "pointed out, in connexion with immunisation against rabies, that a vaccine might legitimately come into application in the incubation period. That was the beginning of therapeutic immunisation." Pasteur never lived to see this thesis proved. As will be discussed shortly, Wright also compromised on the value of strict specificity for prophylactic vaccines.[2]

After World War I a vast array of bacterial vaccines and other preparations such as filtrates and extracts were utilized for prophylactic and therapeutic purposes (Dudgeon, 1927). Many of the vaccines originated from superficially selected cultures of organisms, and most preparations were inactivated by heat or chemicals. Alexander Besredka (1927), working with Metchnikoff, suggested the use of sensitized living cultures in vaccines, i.e., bacteria that had been exposed to immune serum. He also advocated the administration of the vaccine at those body sites that provided the portal of entry of the natural infection — skin, oral mucous membrane, etc. Large lots of prepared (stock) vaccine became available and were widely used for the treatment of many chronic suppurative diseases, such as staphylococcal skin and bone lesions, gonorrhea, streptococcal sepsis, and even for asthma and bronchitis. Autogenous vaccines, which were prepared from organisms isolated from the lesions of the patient, were also used for chronic suppurative conditions. Unfortunately carefully controlled clinical studies were lacking, and scientific evaluation was not carried out. A popular form of prophylactic vaccination for the common cold and other respiratory diseases was the use of polyvalent vaccines made up of heat-killed species of bacteria frequently encountered in the nasal and pharyngeal flora of normal individuals, but the enthusiasm for such preparations gradually waned because of their ineffectiveness.

The introduction of microbial products for prophylactic and therapeutic purposes occasionally had serious consequences, sometimes resulting in death. As discussed elsewhere, this happened with yellow fever vaccine (Section III, Chapter 12), poliomyelitis vaccine (Section III, Chapter 13), and BCG vaccine for tuberculosis (Section III, Chapter 14). One of the early disasters resulted from the use of Robert Koch's (1890) tuberculin. This material is a glycerinated extract of tubercle bacilli and is widely used as a skin test for detecting active or latent tuberculosis. Koch observed that a guinea pig with tuberculosis was highly sensitive to inoculated tuberculin. At the site of inoculation necrosis of the tissue occurred; necrosis of tuberculous lesions also took place. Koch reasoned that tuberculin administered to patients would induce necrosis in the lesions and that the tubercle bacilli would die in the necrotic sites. Some patients highly sensitive to tuberculin died of anaphylactic shock following an injection of it, and viable tubercle bacilli were also widely dispersed from the necrotic lesions into healthy tissue. Nevertheless tuberculin continued to be used therapeutically for a number of years.

After 1940 three major factors limited and stabilized the use of prophylactic vaccines in medical practice. The first was the introduction of the sulfonamides and antibiotics. The second was the discovery of methods for isolating and growing viruses in tissue cultures, which yielded sufficient amounts of organisms for use in specific vaccines. Another contributing stabilizing development was the enforcement of strict biological standards at national and international levels, the latter eventually through the World Health Organization.

At least twenty specific prophylactic preparations of microbial orgin were available by 1970 for human use. The most effective bacterial preparations were diphtheria and tetanus toxoids. Other bacterial vaccines included those for pertussis, typhoid, cholera, plague, tuberculosis, shigellosis, pneumococcal infections, and meningococcal diseases. The most outstanding progress was made with virus vaccines for yellow fever, poliomyelitis, rubeola, rubella, rabies, and influenza.

Serotherapy

The evolution of serotherapy coincided with the development of the vaccines. Dependent on the principles of immunology, the basic problems were complex. Briefly, the early controversies centered on humoral and cellular immunity as defense mechanisms against infections. Some bacteria were killed by exposure to fresh serum alone (humoral immunity). This involved complement, a labile serum factor, which acted in conjunction with bacteriolysin. Certain species of organisms, such as *Cholera vibrio* and typhoid bacilli, were lysed in this manner by serum. On the other hand, some bacteria resisted the action of fresh immune serum, but in the presence of leukocytes, serum aided the killing effect of the leukocytes through phagocytosis, which occurred with gram-positive organisms such as pneumococci, streptococci, and staphylococci (cellular immunity). In addition toxins of diphtheria and tetanus stimulated the cellular production of antitoxins, which circulated freely in the blood and neutralized the toxins. Diphtheria antitoxin, which is discussed in Section III, Chapter 13, was the first successful serum for human use.

Most antisera used for therapeutic purposes until 1940 were obtained by immunizing horses with bacteria. During World War II human serum was fractionated, and the globulin fraction containing concentrated antibodies came into use for prophylactic and therapeutic purposes. Although equine antiserum was highly successful in the therapy of diphtheria, serious problems were encountered because some patients acquired hypersensitivity to this "foreign" protein, expressed as delayed serum sickness or — less often — as the immediate type of anaphylactic reaction. The latter form of hypersensitivity to horse serum produced vascular collapse minutes after injection, with an occasional fatal outcome. The more common delayed type, or serum sickness, appeared seven to ten days after the introduction of the serum and caused chills, fever, diaphoresis, skin rashes, edema, and painful joints. This reaction was incapacitating and could last for several days or even weeks. The potential danger to a patient with serum sickness was that the subsequent injection of a small amount of horse serum, months or years after recovery, could induce acute anaphylaxis and even death. The nature of serum sickness was defined in 1905 (Pirquet and Schick, 1951).

Ten years after diphtheria antitoxin had been introduced the subject of serotherapy was reviewed (Park, 1906). Doctor William H. Park was widely respected for his work on diphtheria in New York City. He stated that the use of specific antisera was of doubtful value in tetanus. Likewise specific antisera were of little or no value in a considerable group of other bacterial diseases. He discussed, at length, serum sickness, which occurred in about 20 percent of the patients receiving serum. He pointed out that bacterial antibody was found in the globulin fraction. This suggested that antibody could be concentrated in smaller amounts of serum, which would reduce the incidence and severity of serum sickness.

Although extensive investigations were carried out on serotherapy over a period of fifty years from 1890 to 1940, consistent encouraging results occurred in relatively few diseases. *Antitoxic* sera continued to have outstanding success in the management of diphtheria, but it was of little or no benefit in suppurative diseases, including scarlet fever, staphylococcal infections, shigellosis, and gas gangrene. Antitoxin proved to be of definite benefit in some types of botulism if administered during the early stages of the disease.

Antibacterial sera were beneficial in some of the common types of pneumococcal lobar pneumonia, as discussed in Section III, Chapter 14. Antimeningococcal serum was used extensively in meningitis, but the results were controversial (Section III, Chapter 16). Specific antiserum for *Hemophilus influenzae* meningitis in young children was of value, especially when combined with a sulfonamide, and later with an antibiotic (Section III, Chapter 16). Preparations of antibacterial sera for pertussis and for plague were of doubtful benefit.

After 1940 human antiviral gamma globulin became a useful adjunct for prophylactic programs in measles, rubella, and mumps. Gamma globulin was widely employed as a prophylactic against viral hepatitis. Antirabies serum was beneficial in the early management of patients bitten about the face by rabid animals. Antiserum became available for herpes zoster infection. And finally, human immune globulin was helpful in patients with infections who had congenital or acquired immune deficiencies.

The evolution of microbiology and immunology after 1900 resulted in a relatively small number of prophylactic and therapeutic agents for infectious diseases. Even so, the impact upon the reduced morbidity and mortality rates in the general population was dramatic. This is particularly applicable to diphtheria, tetanus, yellow fever, poliomyelitis, smallpox, rubeola, rubella, and pertussis. Less outstanding have been the results in animal rabies, typhoid fever, meningococcal disease, tuberculosis, plague, and cholera. Serotherapy has had a smaller but still significant role in the management of infectious diseases. A major impact was produced by chemotherapy between 1940 and 1970.

Bier's Hyperaemia

The trials, errors, and successes of microbiology and immunology as applied to medical practice have been briefly discussed. As usual, the enthusiasm of clinicians in the application of the new knowledge gave rise to some aberrations in everyday practice. Sound scientific principles yielded to philosophical discussion and rationalization in efforts to control infectious diseases. An interesting concept of combatting inflammatory diseases of infectious and noninfectious origin that excited the interest of European and American practitioners during the early twentieth century was the practice of hyperaemia (Bier, 1909). Professor August Bier was a Berlin surgeon who extended the teleological concept that nature has a purpose for that which happens to man in health and in disease, and maintained (1909, p. 1) "that fever, inflammation, suppuration, diaphoresis, expectoration, and diarrhoea, serve to remove from the body 'noxious and impure matter.' " Bier proposed a simple procedure to bring this removal about for a wide variety of suppurative and nonsuppurative inflammatory conditions by means of active and congestive hyperaemia. Hyperaemia was accomplished by bringing more blood to the affected areas with artificial heat, and congestive hyperaemia was produced on the venous side of the circulation by applying bandages to an extremity, thus impeding the flow of blood. In a section on the bactericidal effect of hyperaemia Bier maintained that he was supporting nature by bringing leukocytes and antibodies to the site of tissue injury.

Bier's approach to therapy was like putting modern clothes on the ancient concept of the imbalance of the body humors in disease processes. But the American translator of the sixth German edition of Bier's work was euphoric in his introductory remarks (1909, Preface, p. x): "Bier's work has stirred the minds of able surgeons as no other problem since the discovery of the circulation of the blood, the introduction of antisepsis, and the employment of antitoxin." Even after interest in Bier's application of his methods to a multitude of diseases subsided, his concepts of induced hyperaemia for the treatment of inflammation persisted. They took the form of artificially induced fever, hot fomentations to inflamed tissues, and the use of blistering preparations on the skin.

Nonspecific Protein Therapy

The principle of specificity — that specific vaccines should be used for prophylactic purposes — became more and more difficult to follow, especially when vaccines were used therapeutically. The issue was further clouded by "serum sickness," which often accompanied serotherapy. Clinicians became increasingly convinced that the nonspecific febrile reactions that followed the use of vaccines and serum in the treatment of acute and chronic infections benefited patients. In addition quantitative immunological methods were few and crude, and poorly understood. There was a considerable lag in the evolution of knowledge about serological reactions until Dr. Karl Landsteiner's classic description appeared in 1933 (Landsteiner, 1947). Even as recently as 1962, an authoritative textbook on vaccines and sera stated (Parish and Cannon, 1962, p. 3), "Although many benefits have already been derived from the administration of sera and prophylactics, still greater benefits might result from a better understanding of the non-specific physiological factors which control the phenomena of parasitism."

It is interesting to review Wright's changing attitude toward the specificity of vaccines. In commenting on experience with vaccines for plague, typhoid fever, and pneumonia, he stated (1915, p. 632) that there is a "probability that these vaccines give some protection against diseases other than the particular disease which the inoculation is designed to ward off." Later on (1919, p. 489) he assumed a firmer attitude: "we should discard the confident dogmatic belief; that immunisation must be strictly specific."

Probably because of the improvement patients experienced after serum reactions, chemists became interested in possible substances or changes in the patients' sera that caused these benefits. In exploring this aspect, J. W. Jobling and W. Petersen (1916) injected rabbits intravenously with kaolin, bacteria, protein split products, and trypsin.

They maintained that this was followed by a mobilization of protease in the animals' sera. Jobling and Petersen reasoned that the toxicity of infections was due to protein split products and that these were hydrolyzed by protease to nontoxic forms. They later joined a group in Chicago to carry out extensive clinical studies on nonspecific protein therapy. At the Cook County Hospital good results in arthritis were recorded with typhoid vaccine and the proteose solution of Jobling and Petersen (Miller and Lusk, 1916). Normal horse serum administered intravenously, which provoked systemic reaction, was as beneficial in patients with localized gonococcal infection as was specific antigonococcal serum (Smith, 1916).

The acme of nonspecific protein therapy and its beneficial results was reached with the appearance of a monograph on the subject (Petersen, 1922). A wide variety of substances were used to produce the shock mechanism in many different diseases. Petersen did not minimize the benefits of "specific antigen-antibody balance," but he emphasized the role of bacterial intoxication and the enzymatic degradation of the toxic products. The practice of nonspecific therapy with colloidal agents, vaccines, and other products continued even after the introduction of the sulfonamides and antibiotics. In some forms of chronic inflammatory disease the febrile reactions were associated with improvement, as attested by patients and clinicians.

Focal Infections

At the annual meeting of the American Medical Association in 1914 two presentations attracted considerable attention and were to influence medical practice in the following decade or two. The first was by Dr. Frank Billings, a prominent Chicago physician associated with Rush Medical College and Presbyterian Hospital. Billings (1914) was the chief proponent of the concept of localized infections as a cause of many diseases such as infectious endocarditis, arthritis deformans, rheumatic fever, acute and chronic nephritis, chronic myocarditis, exophthalmic goiter, cholecystitis, peptic ulcer, and diabetes. The primary foci were chiefly in the oropharynx and included chronic infections of the teeth, tonsils, mastoids, and sinuses. The secondary foci, often arising through the bloodstream from a primary focus, included lymph nodes, appendix, gallbladder, prostate, uterus, and kidneys.

The second presentation was by Dr. E. C. Rosenow (1914), a bacteriologist associated with Dr. Billings in his studies and later an experimental microbiologist at the Mayo Clinic. Rosenow discussed the new bacteriology of focal infections in which streptococci, pneumococci, and staphylococci were prominent. He developed the concept of the transmutability of the streptococcus-pneumococcus group, which was to engage his attention for many years.

The pathogenesis and treatment of focal infections was later presented in detail (Billings, 1921). Professor Wilder Tileston (1928) of Yale University described the subject in the leading American textbook of medicine. A two-volume treatise on mouth infections described their relation to systemic diseases (MacNevin and Vaughan, 1930).

The medical profession widely accepted the concept that focal infections caused a multitude of systemic complaints in patients having arthritis, neuralgias, nephritis, ocular inflammation, and general debility and weakness. The physicians' challenge was to locate the focus of infection and then eradicate it through surgical procedures. Autogenous vaccines were supportive measures, but preferably they should be used after surgical extirpation of the focus. As a result, teeth were extracted, tonsils excised, sinuses scraped, and gallbladders removed. Fortunately this surgical practice of treating ill-defined diseases gradually subsided. It is highly doubtful that such surgical procedures benefited the majority of patients. Controlled studies were lacking, even in those conditions due to microbial disease, such as gonococcal arthritis. The pathogenesis of many of the diseases for which a focus of infection was deemed responsible continued as a challenging problem, however.

When one surveys the contemporary status of medical practice in the control and management of infectious diseases, it may be difficult to understand the ill-defined procedures of nonspecific protein therapy, autogenous vaccines, induced hyperaemia, and surgical extirpation of foci of infection for systemic diseases that continued up to the mid-twentieth century. In the light of present-day knowledge one may be tempted to criticize such practices severely. But many afflictions of man, including metabolic and degenerative diseases, still baffle the physician. Some of the practices of today will give way to more definitive treatment with the accumulation of basic knowledge on the pathogenesis of disease.

CHAPTER 5

Chemotherapy and the Sulfonamides

Modern chemotherapy originated in the rapid development of organic chemistry in Germany in the nineteenth century. Chemotherapy owes much to Paul Ehrlich, who is recognized as one of the foremost medical scientists of his generation (Dolman, 1971). Martha Marquardt (1951), his faithful secretary, has written a warm biography, and Sir Henry Dale (1960) has written a brief but excellent summary of his scientific career.

Ehrlich was a chemist and a physician. He was related through his mother to the pathologist Carl Weigert. Ehrlich resembled Metchnikoff in personal traits, being highly imaginative and excitable and enthusiastically dedicated to science. He was a wanderer in pursuit of a good medical education, finally graduating with a medical degree from Leipzig University. It was the anatomist Wilhelm von Waldeyer at Strasbourg who first inspired the young Ehrlich to use aniline dyes for histological preparations, and no scientist ever applied organic dyes to medical science more widely and successfully. Settling later in Berlin, he became interested in a basic problem that he was to pursue all of his life — the interpretation and clarification of chemical affinities in biological processes.

Ehrlich's scientific career can be divided roughly into three phases. The first, which will not be discussed in this volume, includes his studies in hematology and the identification of stained leukocytes. The second phase involves his basic studies on immunology, among them the introduction of quantitative methods in the production of antiserum and the description of his "side chain theory." This has been presented in Section III, Chapter 13 in conjunction with diphtheria antiserum. The third, his most widely known effort, was concerned with chemotherapy and culminated in the discovery of salvarsan for the treatment of syphilis.

When Ehrlich was engaged in his immunological research he was already laying the foundation for his investigations on chemotherapy (Dale, 1960). His first work in this field stemmed from his observations in 1891 demonstrating that methylene blue was lethal *in vitro* for malaria parasites. Then with his colleague P. Guttman in the Moabit Hospital in Berlin, he injected the relatively nontoxic methylene blue into two patients with malaria. Marked improvement occurred within a few days (Guttman and Ehrlich, 1891 translation, 1960). The scientists concluded that further investigations were necessary and suggested that the dye could be possibly used in conjunction with quinine. At this point Ehrlich departed from chemotherapy and became interested in the immunological factors underlying the successful use of diphtheria antitoxin. Beginning in 1904, however, he successfully used leishmaniasis infections in rodents as an experimental model for evaluating dyes of the benzopurpurin series, such as trypan red. He also discovered the *in vitro* phenomenon of acquired parasitic resistance to chemicals.

The greatness of Ehrlich's imaginative genius is displayed in his Nobel Prize lecture, delivered in 1908 (Ehrlich, 1960). In this dissertation he emphasized that future developments in the biological and medical sciences would come from studies on the cell and its chemical processes.

Ehrlich's Nobel Prize address ended with the three famous words: *therapia sterilans magna* (great sterile therapy). He was looking for that agent, "the magic bullet," which following one injection would eliminate not only the microbes of syphilis, but all other pathogens. He thought he had achieved this with his introduction of arsphenamine for syphilis in 1909 and neoarsphenamine in 1912 (Ehrlich and Hata, 1910, translation 1960). This form of treatment was used universally. At the Boston City Hospital in the early 1930s, where I was on the staff, we treated a considerable number of patients having all forms of syphilis with neoarsphenamine and bismuth. These unfortunate victims returned weekly, and then monthly, for a minimum of two years to receive their injections. They often experienced serious toxic drug reactions and were not always cured of the disease. The arsenicals were most effective in acute, or primary, syphilis, and as a result these patients were less contagious. This type of therapy continued until the advent of penicillin therapy in 1943.

Ehrlich's basic contributions to chemotherapy were remarkable. First, he demonstrated experimentally that chemicals would actually kill microbes without serious injury to the host's tissues. Second, he made the fundamental observation that even when chemicals did not kill invading microorganisms, they often destroyed their ability to reproduce, which called forth his second dictum, *therapia sterilisans* (sterile therapy). And third, he demonstrated that organisms could become resistant to the antimicrobial action of chemicals.

At the beginning of the century other chemists were prepared to join Ehrlich in the search for synthetic therapeutic agents for infectious diseases. The chemical industry, especially in Germany at that time, sought out the best minds and supported basic research. One of the drugs that excited the curiosity of several investigators was quinine, which had been first produced as an extract of cinchona bark and found to be effective in the treatment of malaria. But several alkaloids were present in the extract besides quinine, including quinidine and cinchonine. A major achievement had been made in 1820 by French chemists when they first isolated quinine in pure form (Pelletier and Caventou, 1820). Quinine has probably saved more lives than any other drug, inasmuch as malaria has been the most important disease in the world. In a spasmodic type of continuing research, the cinchona alkaloids were investigated for antimicrobial properties. One synthetic agent derived from the cinchona alkaloids was optochin or ethylhydrocupreine. At first, following the report of J. Morgenroth and R. Levy (1911), people believed that optochin would prove valuable in the treatment of pneumococcal pneumonia; but the drug had serious toxic side effects, producing optic atrophy and blindness.

Quinine was such an important drug that plantations were established in the Far East for growing the trees. A few colonial powers held a monopoly on the source of the drug. Following World War I

Germany was stripped of her colonies and did not have her own source of quinine. Accordingly an intensive screening program for synthetic antimalarials was undertaken, directed by Professor W. Schulemann at the Bayer-Meister-Lucius Laboratories under the auspices of the I. G. Farbenindustrie at Elberfeld. Over twelve thousand compounds were systematically prepared and screened, beginning with the basic dye methylene blue and chemically related compounds. W. Schulemann (1932) gave a detailed presentation of the synthesis of the antimalarial agent pamaquine or plasmochin (plasmoquine), which had been patented as early as 1924 (Coggeshall and Craige, 1949).

A second and more important compound resulting from the research of H. Mauss and F. Mietzsch (1933) in the same German laboratories was quinacrine, the alkyl amino derivative of acridine, which was chemically related to plasmoquine and was known as atebrin or atabrine. Although the chemical formula was announced in 1933, all the steps in synthesis were not divulged, a serious handicap to the chemical industry in other countries when at the outbreak of World War II the source of quinine in the South Pacific was cut off by Japanese military forces. Atabrine proved to be moderately toxic, but it was an effective drug and a worthy substitute for quinine.

It is not the purpose here to present the list of antimalarial drugs that evolved in the modern era of chemotherapy. The control and treatment of malaria is discussed in Section III, Chapter 20. Mention should be made, however, of one drug that was used extensively and that resulted directly from the war effort in the United States. The Board for the Coordination of Malarial Studies under the Office of Scientific Research and Development (OSRD) in the United States was responsible for the introduction of chloroquine diphosphate (Aralen) (Coggeshall and Craige, 1949). This proved to be an excellent suppressive agent that could be administered orally once a week.

DDT,[1] a powerful insecticide, was discovered in 1943. This discovery, like that of chloroquine, resulted from cooperative studies between OSRD and the chemical industry in the United States (Coggeshall and Craige, 1949). By 1944 DDT was being incorporated into sprays used in killing mosquitoes in Southeast Asia and hence became an important factor in the control of malaria and typhus.

Sulfonamides

The introduction of the sulfonamides for the therapy of infectious diseases yielded dramatic results and stimulated further scientific work. Within the following decade the whole field of antibiotic therapy was opened up. The impact of the sulfonamides was particularly exciting for those of us who had had our medical training in infectious diseases and had assumed our professional responsibilities during the decade 1927–1937, a period just before the advent of sulfonamide therapy. The contrast that came about in the management of infectious diseases marked one of those great progressive epochs in medical practice.

Again, the evolution of the basic and applied investigations on the sulfonamides was an outgrowth of research in organic chemistry, particularly in Germany. This pursuit was a continuance of Ehrlich's principles in chemotherapy. As one traces this evolution one readily detects the cooperative contributions of the private chemical industries and the academic investigators. Unfortunately this successful cooperative effort carried with it the scramble for priorities in patent rights, as will be pointed out shortly in the discussion of prontosil. On the other hand, one also detects the humanitarian endeavors of scientists of all categories to share their findings internationally with other scientists through formal meetings, printed communications, and personal contacts.

In every scientific revolution there are previous discoveries that contribute to the final achievement. Such was the case in the development of sulfonamides. Paul Gelmo (1908) first synthesized sulfanilamide while doing basic research in organic chemistry on aniline dyes at the Technischen Hochschule in Vienna. Gelmo's report probably occasioned little attention at that time and apparently was overlooked by Dr. Phillip Eisenberg (1913), who as an assistant to Professor Richard Pfeiffer, director of the Hygiene Institute at Breslau, performed a massive screening study on organic dyes, referring to Ehrlich's work with trypanosomes. In the course of his research Eisenberg observed that the dye 2:4-diamino azobenzene ("Chrysoidine") was bacteriostatic *in vitro*. As will be discussed shortly, this dye, when conjugated with Gelmo's product, sulfanilamide, formed "prontosil."

Another major, but isolated, investigation was reported by chemists at the Rockefeller Institute in New York. They were interested in the cinchona alkaloids as potential antimicrobial agents. During their investigations they noted the work of Gelmo, and they too synthesized sulfanilamide. In turn they conjugated sulfanilamide with hydrocupreine. Intending to follow up in their important work, they wrote (Heidelberger and Jacobs, 1919, p. 2132), "Many of the substances described in this paper were highly bactericidal *in vitro*, a property which will be discussed in the appropriate place by our colleague, Dr. Martha Wolstein." But no report ensued. Why not? I could find no published reason. The same question was to be asked of Alexander Fleming when he failed to evaluate penicillin as an antibacterial drug in mice, although he had used that animal species for toxicity studies of the antibiotic.

In putting together the story of the development of the sulfonamides, attention must be centered on the German dye-trust known as the I. G. Farbenindustrie. At approximately the same time that Gelmo completed his synthesis of sulfanilamide in 1908, the Association of German Chemists was meeting at Jena, with Carl Duisberg of the Bayer (Chemical) Works as president (Silverman, 1943). He united all of the German dye industry into one great organization. During the meeting Professor Heinrich Hoerlein, a chemist of the University of Jena, was chosen as the head of the medical division of the newly organized I. G. Farbenindustrie. In 1927 Hoerlein selected Professor Gerhard Domagk, a pathologist, bacteriologist, and clinician, as his assistant and as director of the experimental-pathological laboratory. Within a few years Domagk was to prove that the sulfonamide preparation known as prontosil was a highly effective antibacterial drug.

Figure 1 is a reproduction of a table from the classic paper by Domagk (1935) under the heading "Streptococcus Experiment." The work was done during the Christmas week of 1932. Three groups of mice of the same strain were used. Group 1 (#201–#206) and Group 3 (#315–#322) were untreated control animals that received a lethal injection of streptococci, and all 14 animals died. Group 2 (#303–#314), receiving a similar injection of streptococci, was given one oral dose of prontosil an hour and a half later. All 14 of the treated animals survived. It was the perfect experiment in that there was a

Streptokokkenversuch vom 20. XII. 1932

infiziert mit 1:1000 verdünnter Eibouillonkultur, 0,3 ccm i. p; behandelt 1½ Stunde nach der Infektion

Nr.	Gewicht	Präparat Nr.	%	Dosis	Art der Behdlg.	21. XII.	22. XII.	23. XII.	24. XII.	25. XII.	26. XII.	27. XII.	28. XII.
201	14 g					m	kr.	kr.	†				
202	14 g					m	†						
203	14 g	Anfangskontrollen				m	†						
204	17 g					m	†						
205	19 g					m	†						
206	14 g					m	m	†					
303	18 g	Prontosil	0,01%	0,2	per os	m	m	m	m	m	m	m	m
304	19 g			0,2		m	m	m	m	m	m	m	m
305	18 g			1,0		m	m	m	m	m	m	m	m
306	14 g			1,0		m	m	m	m	m	m	m	m
307	16 g		0,1 %	0,2		m	m	m	m	m	m	m	m
308	15 g			0,2		m	m	m	m	m	m	m	m
309	17 g			1,0		m	m	m	m	m	m	m	m
310	17 g			1,0		m	m	m	m	m	m	m	m
311	14 g		1,0 %	0,2		m	m	m	m	m	m	m	m
312	17 g			0,2		m	m	m	m	m	m	m	m
313	18 g			1,0		m	m	m	m	m	m	m	m
314	14 g			1,0		m	m	m	m	m	m	m	m
315	18 g					m	kr.	†					
316	16 g					m	†						
317	15 g					m	†						
318	14 g					m	†						
319	15 g	Endkontrollen				m	†						
320	14 g					m	†						
321	15 g					m	†						
322	17 g					m	†						

m = munter, kr. = krank, † = tot

Figure 1. "Streptococcus Experiment," table of results of Dr. Gerhard Domagk's classic experiments with prontosil. Reproduced with permission of Georg Thieme Verlag, Herdweg 63, D-7 Stuttgart N. Germany from Gerhard Domagk, "Ein Beitrag zur Chemotherapie der Bakteriellen Infektionen," *Deutsche Medizinische Wochenschrift* 61:250, 1935 (table on p. 251).

100 percent mortality in the untreated animals and 100 percent survival in the treated, an experiment that was verified by other studies, including our own. Furthermore the study proved that in the doses used, prontosil was nontoxic. The experiment is of further historical interest because the same experiment model was used by the Oxford group in proving the therapeutic efficacy of penicillin (Chain et al., 1940).

Why was there such an interval between the time of the completion of the experiment in 1932 and its publication in 1935? In the intervening three years the first patient treated with prontosil was an infant (Foerster, 1933). The drug was particularly effective in streptococcal infections (Klee and Römer, 1935; Schreus, 1935). Patent proceedings on the drug had been started as early as 1930, but publication of the details for manufacturing the chemical were delayed until 1935. A very likely major factor in the delay was that the German investigators did not fully understand the pharmacological or biological activity of prontosil, since it was not bactericidal for streptococci *in vitro*. Domagk was awarded the Nobel Prize for his work in 1939, but the Nazi regime prevented him from accepting it. In 1947 a medal and diploma were presented to him in Stockholm, but he did not receive the monetary award.

Apparently no application of the chemotherapeutic properties of these chemicals was seriously considered before World War I. The only German research on the potential chemotherapeutic value of aniline dyes was recorded by Eisenberg's work in Breslau in 1913, as pointed out above. As noted earlier, the primary attention of the medical group in the I. G. Farbenindustrie after World War I was devoted to the synthesis of atabrine by Mauss and Mietzsch (1933). According to H. Hoerlein (1937), Dr. F. Mietzsch had completed work on atabrine and with another organic chemist, J. Klarer, had developed prontosil as early as 1932.

By 1935 there was no doubt that prontosil was an effective therapeutic agent, at least for streptococcal infections. But a certain degree of anguish unsettled Hoerlein and his business associates at the I. G. Farbenindustrie in their attempt to patent prontosil. Although German and English patents had been obtained for prontosil, such a patent did not apply to France because by law medicinal products could not be patented in that country. In addition the pharmacology and biological activity of prontosil were not wholly understood. The drug was inactive against streptococci in the test tube, but it was effective in experimental animals and in human patients. These factors did not escape the attention of the alert Dr. Ernest Fourneau, director of chemistry in the Pasteur Institute in Paris, and his associate Constantin Levaditi. They were intensely interested in chemotherapy.

The French investigators were anxious to receive prontosil from Hoerlein, and a conference was held involving Hoerlein, Fourneau, and representatives of the large chemical industry of France, Rhône-Poulanc. The Germans wished to make a binding business agreement in supplying prontosil to France, but their efforts were to no avail. Within a brief period the nationalistic French investigators synthesized their own prontosil and called it "Rubiazol" (Gley and Girard, 1936). Levaditi and A. Vaisman (1935) quickly confirmed Domagk's observation with the product. But the key work on the sulfonamides was in France and was reported by the Tréfouëls, Nitti, and Bovet (1935), also working in Fourneau's laboratory. Referring to the work of M. Heidelberger and W. A. Jacobs (1919), in which sulfanilamide was coupled with hydrocupreine, they postulated — and speedily proved — that the active antibacterial principle of prontosil was sulfanilamide. In other words, in the test tube prontosil was inactive against bacteria, but in the body sulfanilamide was split off from prontosil by enzymatic action and was free to act on bacteria.

This brilliant accomplishment of the French investigators presented sulfanilamide to the world without the infringement of any patent rights. Gelmo had synthesized and patented sulfanilamide in 1908, but this patent was no longer valid. Hence a relatively nontoxic major drug could be manufactured easily and marketed at a modest price.

In the meantime, following Domagk's paper and Hoerlein's London lecture, the English also became interested in prontosil. Sir Henry Dale obtained a supply from the I. G. Farbenindustrie in 1935 for a therapeutic trial under the auspices of the Medical Research Council. This was successfully carried out by Colebrook and Kenny (1936) in patients with puerperal sepsis. At the same time a very significant research program was undertaken in the Wellcome Laboratories by G. A. H. Buttle, W. H. Gray, and D. Stephenson (1936). They reported that orally administered p-aminobenzene sulphonamide (sulfanilamide) protected mice not only against strep-tococci, but also against meningococci.[2] Sulfanilamide was not effec-tive, however, against staphylococcal or pneumococcal infections. Both English groups evaluated not only prontosil, which could only be administered orally, but also the German preparation of soluble sodium prontosil (neoprontosil), which could be given parenterally.

It is remarkable that within a year after Domagk's report, experi-mental and clinical work on prontosil and sulfanilamide had been carried out in three European centers. Why did interest lag behind in the United States? The important observations of Heidelberger and Jacobs published in 1919 on the potential antibacterial value of sul-fanilamide and its azo compounds had occasioned no excitement. The general lack of interest was probably related to the fact that experi-mental medical research and clinical investigations in the United States were only slowly acquiring sophistication and competence after the Flexner report on medical education and its shortcomings. Furthermore serotherapy was still engaging the attention of many investigators.

This lag in America is revealed in a personal experience of my own. In 1934–1935 I was carrying out experimental and clinical studies on streptococcal infections at the Thorndike Memorial Laboratory of the Boston City Hospital with Dr. Chester Keefer. Without any available specific therapy the management of patients with these diseases was discouraging. The intellectual and scientific climates were excellent at that institution, and there was always an exchange of ideas among the various investigators. One day a young physician from Holland, working on problems of nutrition, told me that interesting work with a red dye was going on in Germany with streptococcal infections. Why didn't I look into it? This suggestion of a potential antistrep-tococcal agent intrigued me, but I was discouraged from making any further inquiries because a red dye had been extensively tried in recent years in the United States and proved to be without much value. I was referred to the reports on a particular chemical, the sodium salt of dibromoxymercury fluorescin — 26 percent mercury, also known as "mercurochrome," which had been introduced in 1919 by the well-known urologist at Johns Hopkins, Dr. Hugh Young, as a germicide for urinary tract sepsis (Young, White, and Swartz, 1919). An extensive review of the pertinent data in the literature revealed that the chemical was of questionable value (Davis, 1926). After reading this review and heeding the advice given to me, I found that my interest in the new German "red dye" was temporarily suspended.

But American interest in chemotherapy was soon to be aroused. The International Congress of Microbiology was held in London during the summer of 1936. Dr. L. Colebrook of London presented his results on the therapy of puerperal sepsis with prontosil. In attendance at the meeting was Dr. Perrin Long of Johns Hopkins Medical School. He had also received training at the Thorndike Memorial Laboratory and the Boston City Hospital and had gone on to Johns Hopkins as professor of preventive medicine. He was interested in streptococcal sepsis and along with his associate, Eleanor Bliss, a bacteriologist, was a major influence in the introduction of the new bacterial chemotherapy into America. Utilizing sulfanilamide supplied by two chemical firms in the United States, DuPont de Nemours and Winthrop Chemical, Long and Bliss confirmed the experimental work of the English investigators and treated nineteen patients. Their initial report on January 2, 1937 was the beginning of the new era of chemotherapy for bacterial infections in the United States (Long and Bliss, 1937). A monograph by these individuals became a key reference on the subject (Long and Bliss, 1939). They were fortunate in working at Johns Hopkins because Professor Eli Kennerly Marshall, Jr., chairman of the department of pharmacology, and his staff rapidly worked out valuable chemical methods for quantitating concentrations of sulfanilamide in the tissues and body fluids (Marshall, 1939; Marshall, Emerson, and Cutting, 1937).

Shortly after initiating his own studies, Dr. Long aided Dr. Chester Keefer and myself in obtaining supplies of sulfanilamide for investigations on streptococcal and gonococcal sepsis. In our clinical studies with sulfanilamide we confirmed the successful results of others in both types of illness. The findings were particularly gratifying in patients with suppurative gonococcal arthritis. Shortly thereafter, on August 1, 1937, I assumed a position in the department of medicine at the University of Minnesota Hospitals in charge of infectious diseases. I practically carried sulfanilamide from Boston to Minneapolis in my back pocket. Clinical investigations on sulfonamide therapy were made on a large selection of patients during the early stages of evaluation. By 1941 observations had been carried out in over a thousand patients; these results and those of others were incorporated within a monograph on the subject (Spink, 1941b).

A series of new chemotherapeutic agents appeared. They were developed by private enterprise, and the competition for profits was keen. For the most part this progress augured well for human health, but occasionally tragedy followed the introduction of a new drug. One instance occurred in the United States in 1937 with a preparation of sulfanilamide. Sulfanilamide was originally marketed as an oral product in tablet form. Later an effort was made to supply a liquid preparation, which some individuals preferred and which would be more convenient for administering to children. Such a preparation was hastily placed on the open market and called "Elixir of Sulfanilamide-Massengill." During September and October 1937, 76 persons were fatally poisoned by this "Elixir." A prompt investigation carried out by the Food and Drug Administration of the United States Department of Agriculture and by representatives of the American Medical Association revealed that it contained "a 10 per cent solution of sulfanilamide in about 72 per cent diethylene glycol, together with some coloring and flavoring agents" (Geiling and Cannon, 1938, p. 919). Diethylene glycol was quite toxic for the kidneys and liver, as demonstrated in the human material and in experimental animals. This agent was chosen because sulfanilamide was not soluble in water or alcohol.[3] As a result of this tragedy more stringent federal laws were imposed upon the pharmaceutical industry before new drugs were made available for human use.

By 1938, after extensive clinical observations, it became apparent that sulfanilamide had definite advantages, as well as several disadvantages, in the treatment of infectious diseases. Prontosil and neoprontosil had been quickly abandoned in favor of the active principle, sulfanilamide. Sulfanilamide was a tremendous advance in the therapy of streptococcal infections due to Group A hemolytic streptococci, gonorrhea, and meningococcal meningitis, and in the therapy of some urinary tract infections. But the antimicrobial spectrum of sulfanilamide was relatively narrow. The drug had many toxic side effects, some of them serious. A solution for these deficiencies could probably be resolved in part by synthesizing and evaluating other sulfonamide derivatives.

The first of these, sulfapyridine, simply had a pyridine ring added to the SO_2NH_2 moiety of sulfanilamide (Figure 2). The drug was first synthesized and patented by the British pharmaceutical firm, Messrs. May and Baker, and was known as M. & B. 693, or "Dagenon." Sulfapyridine did not replace sulfanilamide but did contribute to an expansion of the sulfonamide antimicrobial spectrum. Sulfanilamide was not effective against pneumococcal infections, but Lionel Whitby (1938) made the pertinent observation that sulfapyridine protected mice against lethal pneumococcal infections. This was an important advance, because in the following year clinical investigations demonstrated that sulfapyridine was effective, not only for pneumococcal pneumonia, but for the highly lethal pneumococcal meningitis (Pepper et al., 1939). At that time we had treated 22 patients with pneumococcal infections at the University of Minnesota hospitals, 14 of whom recovered. We approached our evaluation cautiously, using a combination of specific antipneumococcal serum, when available, and sulfapyridine. But sulfapyridine was relatively insoluble and erratically absorbed from the gastrointestinal tract. Renal complications from precipitated sulfapyridine crystals were also encountered.

In the pursuit of further sulfonamide derivatives, two major syntheses were made, sulfathiazole and sulfadiazine. Sulfapyridine had extended antimicrobial therapy to include pneumococcal diseases, but there was still the need for an antistaphylococcal agent and possibly agents less toxic for the other diseases. Sulfathiazole was synthesized and reported on by two different groups in 1939 (Fosbinder and Walter, 1939; Lott and Bergeim, 1939). Preliminary experimental data indicated that this sulfonamide might be effective against staphylococcal sepsis, and even our own clinical investigations appeared promising (Spink and Hansen, 1940; Spink, Hansen, and Paine, 1941). Sulfathiazole did not extend the antimicrobial spectrum as anticipated, however, and the drug produced a significant increase in the incidence of hypersensitivity reactions.

The year 1940 was a momentous one. Sulfadiazine was introduced, and it practically displaced sulfanilamide, sulfapyridine, and sulfathiazole. On the world front, France had surrendered to the German army, and Great Britain was engaged in combat with the Nazi Air Force. It was the year that the Oxford group under Howard Florey published their first paper on the therapeutic value of penicillin (Chain et al., 1940). Penicillin was to make a dramatic entrance into the

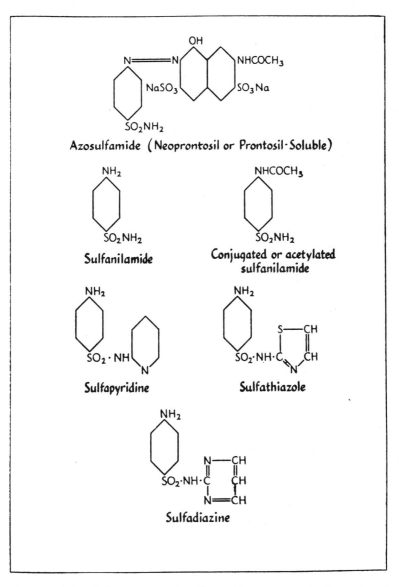

Figure 2. Chemical structure of sulfonamide compounds. Reproduced with permission of Year Book Medical Publishers from W. W. Spink, *Sulfanilamide and Related Compounds in General Practice.* Copyright © 1941 by Year Book Medical Publishers, Inc., Chicago (Figure 1, p. 17).

management of infections and sepsis during World War II. By 1942 the general use of the sulfonamides in medical practice would gradually abate.

The sulfonamide era lasted from 1937 to 1942. During those five years clinical investigations revealed two primary deficiencies of these drugs. First, although sulfadiazine was better tolerated by patients than any of the other drugs and its antimicrobial activity was as effective, the incidence of toxic reactions, such as gastrointestinal intolerance, dermatological reactions, drug fever, blood dyscrasias, and renal complications, was distressing. Some of these reactions were also instances of acquired hypersensitivity to the drugs, in which cases the subsequent use of any of the sulfonamide compounds was excluded.

The second disadvantage of the sulfonamides was the appearance and dissemination of sulfonamide-resistant microbes. The drugs had been particularly effective in streptococcal and gonococcal diseases, but sulfonamide-resistant strains of Group A hemolytic streptococci and gonococci appeared to a serious extent among the civilian and military populations by 1944. Sulfonamide-resistant strains of meningococci were also encountered. The recruitment of millions from civilian life without the benefit of chemotherapy for streptococcal sepsis, gonococcal disease, and meningococcal meningitis would be a threat to the health of military personnel. Resistance acquired for one sulfonamide applied to all of the sulfonamides. Fortunately, as will be described shortly, penicillin became available.

The appearance of sulfonamide-resistant bacteria was a disturbing biological phenomenon. It had been known that the drugs were not effective in the presence of purulent material such as abscesses, and inhibitory activity had been demonstrated experimentally and clinically. The mechanism for the development of sulfonamide resistance was greatly clarified by the observations of D. D. Woods (1940), who attributed the inhibitory effect on the sulfonamides to the presence of the chemically related compound, para-aminobenzoic acid (PABA), an essential metabolite of some bacteria. Certain species of bacteria produced PABA, which competed with the sulfonamides for a position in the metabolic enzyme system of the bacteria. This mechanism of resistance was confirmed in our laboratory in studies with sulfonamide-resistant staphylococci (Spink and Jermsta, 1941; Spink et al., 1944). The struggle of the parasites for survival has been replicated with other microbes and drugs, and was to be demonstrated a decade later in the appearance of penicillin-resistant strains of staphylococci. The Commission on Hemolytic Streptococcal Infections of the United States Army found Group A streptococcal isolates from Army personnel resistant to sulfadiazine in 1944 (Rantz et al., 1946).

Antimicrobial drugs are sometimes used in combinations. The purpose of using two agents is twofold. First, when each of two drugs is destructive for a microbe, each may strike at different metabolic pathways of the organism. In this manner a combination of drugs can have more of a killing effect than the use of either drug alone. The optimal synergistic reaction of the two drugs is dependent upon the proper ratio of the amount of each drug that is present. The second reason for favoring therapeutic combinations is to prevent the appearance of drug-resistant organisms, which occurs at times when a single drug is administered. This biological phenomenon of resistance is not eliminated, but the incidence is reduced in microbial populations. Combinations of drugs have been used particularly for malaria, tuberculosis, and urinary tract infections.

One of the major developments in drug combinations was that of the diaminopyridine drug trimethoprim, first introduced as an antimalarial agent, and the sulfonamide sulfamethoxazole, used primarily for urinary bacterial infections. The antimalarial activity of trimethoprim proved to be less advantageous than its antibacterial effects (Weinstein, 1975b). But the combination of trimethoprim and sulfamethoxazole has been investigated extensively in different bacterial diseases with promising results, especially for infections caused by gram-negative bacteria (Finland and Kass, 1973; Garrod, James, and Lewis, 1969).

During the decade 1935–1945 the sulfonamides provided a remarkable advance in the control and management of infectious diseases. The drugs were particularly advantageous for three major diseases: hemolytic streptococcal infections; gonorrhea and its complications; pneumococcal pneumonia and meningitis; and meningococcal infections. They were also of benefit in selected instances of urinary tract infections. The drugs were of some prophylactic value, as in rheumatic fever, a sequela of streptococcal disease. Limited as prophylactic and therapeutic agents, the sulfonamides were succeeded by the antibiotics, which widened the control of such infections as tuberculosis, staphylococcal sepsis, syphilis, rickettsial diseases, and infections due to gram-negative bacteria. Other chemotherapeutic agents became available for fungal diseases and for parasitic infections. Although chemotherapy was not available for virus diseases, a great advance was made in the prevention of these infections with vaccines. Serotherapy became limited to the treatment of those major diseases produced by exotoxins, such as diphtheria and botulism.

CHAPTER 6

Penicillin and the Cephalosporins

Shortly after the introduction of sulfonamide therapy into medicine, civilization was embroiled in World War II. It would not appear to have been an auspicious time to pursue such revolutionary investigations further. But human imagination and industry sometimes rise to great heights during times of catastrophe. Even under the difficult circumstances of war, much progress was made in therapy for infectious diseases. This came about, not so much through the further synthesis and evaluation of chemicals as through a concern with some old microbiological concepts — those of "antibiosis." The term designates a form of microbial antagonism that occurs during the exposure of bacteria to chemical substances produced by other microbes. Selman Waksman (1945) coined the term "antibiotics" for these chemicals.

Howard Florey has presented an excellent historical review of antibiosis up to the introduction of streptomycin (Florey et al., 1949, Vol. I). His acerbic writing is probably too critical of some of the past efforts of research in this field, but he does write with authority. Florey, like others, selected Pasteur and J. Joubert (1877a) as having presented the first scientific evidence for microbial antagonism, when they observed that the growth of the anthrax bacillus in urine was impeded by the presence of other "common organisms." They even surmised that such bacterial antagonism occurred in animal tissues.

The present survey of the development of modern antibiotic therapy will center on the efforts of three groups of investigators: the research of the soil microbiologists, especially that of Selman Waksman and his student René Dubos; the work of Alexander Fleming; and the results of Howard Florey and his Oxford group. The basic work on the potentials of antibiotic therapy had been accomplished shortly after 1940. "Antibiotic research then received a great impetus when it was discovered at Oxford in 1940 that penicillin belonged to that rare class of drug, the systemic chemotherapeutic agents. This clearly distinguished penicillin from all antibiotics which had been investigated previously. And as the drug was relatively soon introduced into the clinic and achieved widespread success there, most antibiotic work since that date has had as its object the discovery and isolation of many of the hundreds of naturally occurring antibacterial substances, in the hope of finding others endowed with useful therapeutic properties" (Florey et al., 1949, p. 72, Vol. I).

René Dubos was one of the pioneers in research on antibiotics. He was born in France, where he obtained his early education followed by graduate studies in the United States at Rutgers University under the guidance of Dr. Selman Waksman. On March 21, 1940 Dubos presented a Harvey Lecture in New York on "Utilization of Selective Microbial Agents in the Study of Biological Problems," in which he presented his studies on the specific destruction of microorganisms by bacterial enzymes (Dubos, 1940).

The virulence and the type specificity of the pneumococcus is due to a capsular polysaccharide. In the 1930s Dubos, for the first time, isolated enzymes from soil bacilli that "depolymerized" or hydrolyzed the polysaccharides of different types of pneumococci and rendered the organisms nonvirulent, although they continued to multiply. In addition the administration of these enzymes protected highly susceptible mice from lethal pneumococcal infections (Dubos, 1940).

Continuing this approach, Dubos searched for soil bacilli by placing suspensions of viable streptococci, staphylococci, and pneumococci in soil mixtures. In this manner he selected *Bacillus brevis*, which produced a soluble substance that not only killed gram-positive organisms but also protected experimentally infected animals (Dubos,

1939). The material was not effective against gram-negative organisms, however. The preparation, first known as "Gramicidin," was later shown to contain two crystalline substances, gramicidin and tyrocidine, and the mixture became known as "tyrothricin" (Hotchkiss and Dubos, 1940). Tyrothricin was too toxic for systemic therapy and was used primarily for local application.

In summarizing the research of Dubos, Florey stated (Florey et al., 1949, p. 422), "This work and its continuation had the outstanding merit of considering the subject from many points of view — bacteriological, biochemical, biological, and eventually clinical. This was in sharp contrast to all previous work, much of which was adequate on the bacteriological side but suffered from extreme limitation in chemical and other investigations, if indeed these were attempted."

Penicillin

The discovery of penicillin is a major advance in the history of medicine. Having participated in the initial clinical investigations on penicillin under the auspices of the National Research Council (US) and having followed the sequence of events in the succeeding thirty years, I still consider penicillin the grandfather of all antibiotics, and along with the semisynthetic penicillins, the major achievement in antimicrobial therapy.

The key figure in the discovery of penicillin is Alexander Fleming. He was born into a large family on an isolated Scottish farm in 1881. He was shy and reserved, and he loved nature — qualities that probably directed him into a biological science. A good student, he matriculated at London University and received his medical training at St. Mary's Medical School and Hospital. He later joined the faculty of London University as professor of microbiology. He conducted research in a small laboratory in the inoculation department of St. Mary's Hospital, which was under the direction of Sir Almroth Wright from 1908 to 1945.

Because Fleming's observations have often been referred to as a "chance finding," the full import of his previous work, which prepared his mind for the "chance observation," is often overlooked. Fleming's experience under Wright during World War I deeply influenced his future experimental work. A center for the study of war wounds was established at St. Mary's Hospital in London under Wright's direction, with a group of brilliant young assistants that included Fleming and Dr. Leonard Colebrook. Meticulous bacteriological studies were carried out on wounded soldiers transferred to London from the battle fields of France (Douglas, Fleming, and Colebrook, 1920). Fleming pointed out (1919, p. 100) that there were "two schools in the treatment of wounds: the *physiological school*, which concentrated their efforts in aiding the natural protective agencies of the body against infection, and the *antiseptic school*, which aimed at killing the microbes in the wound with some chemical agent."

Wright had propounded the physiological approach; his report with Fleming and Colebrook (Wright, Fleming, and Colebrook, 1918) is a masterpiece of clarity. The host's own defense mechanism is sufficient in the healing of a *clean* surgical or traumatic wound, provided that primary closure eliminates any empty spaces in the tissues. In a severe attack on the antiseptic school Fleming stated later (1924, p. 171), "Many experiments have indicated that the chemical antiseptics in common use, in addition to combining with the bacterial protoplasm and so producing death of the bacterium, will also enter into combination with other albuminous matter and are, in fact, general protoplasmic poisons." His experiments severely indicted carbolic acid and Dakin's solution (sodium hypochlorite), the latter having been used widely during World War I for irrigating septic wounds (Dakin et al., 1917). There could be no doubt that Fleming, as a result of his war experiences, would continue his search for the ideal antiseptic agent for local and systemic use.

Fleming believed that local or systemic therapy for sepsis should be in accord with physiological principles; i.e., an antiseptic should destroy invading microbes without harming the tissues. He represented that lone, thoughtful, and precise investigator whose laboratory efforts were devoid of the hustle and bustle of the "team effort." His studies did not arouse any immediate acclaim, but they did form the basis of the greatest accomplishment in therapy for infectious diseases. His laboratory was incredibly small, his equipment sparse, and his techniques simple. His idol was Pasteur, whose work he praised (Fleming, 1947).

Fleming's scientific output was not large, but his two major discoveries were to influence the Oxford team led by Florey. Between 1922 and 1932 Fleming published a series of ten papers on his discovery of the antibacterial agent lysozyme. His first report in 1922, presented to the Royal Society of London and introduced by Sir Almroth Wright, states (Fleming, 1922, p. 306), "In this communication I wish to draw attention to a substance present in the tissues and secretions of the body, which is capable of rapidly dissolving bacteria. As this substance has properties akin to those of ferments I have called it a 'Lysozyme.' "

It is not clear why Fleming performed these important investigations. He did point out in this first report that a widely-held view was that the function of tears, saliva, and sputum, as far as infections are concerned, was a mechanical one, that of washing away the microbes from the body. This was a view expressed by Metchnikoff, as mentioned by Fleming. However, he proved that these secretions can destroy microbes through their lytic activity.

In his excellent biography of Fleming, André Maurois (1959) has detailed the story of lysozyme. Fleming, suffering from a common cold, placed a small portion of his own nasal secretion on an agar plate upon which he had seeded a culture of bacteria. A clear zone surrounded the growing bacteria. The organisms adjacent to the nasal mucus had been lyzed. He then found the same activity using human tears. Maurois, quoting Dr. V. D. Allison, a young man who aided Fleming with some of the experiments, wrote (1959, p. 110), "For the next five weeks, my tears and his were our main supply of material for experiment. Many were the lemons we had to buy to produce all those tears! We used to cut a small piece of lemonpeel and squeeze it into our eyes, looking into the mirror of the microscope. Then, with a Pasteur pipette, the point of which had been rounded in a flame, we collected the tears which we proceeded to put into a test-tube. In this way I often collected as much as $\frac{1}{4}$–$\frac{1}{2}$ c.c. of tears for our experiments." The organism most easily lysed was *Micrococcus lysodeikticus*,[1] so named by Fleming.

Fleming's tenth and final paper on lysozyme was the presidential address to the Section of Pathology of the Royal Society of Medicine in 1932. He said (1932, p. 71), "My contribution to the subject — apart from the name — has been an elucidation of the properties of the lytic element, a description of its wide distribution in nature, and some estimate of its importance in immunity." Lysozyme was demonstrated in mucus, tears, and egg white. Interestingly enough, one of the references cited by Fleming in this paper was that of Florey (1930), who had been attracted to Fleming's work. Florey's communication was to play an important part in his eventual work on penicillin with his coworker at Oxford, the biochemist E. B. Chain.

A contributing factor in Fleming's approach to the discovery of penicillin was his invitation from the British Medical Research Council to prepare a section on the staphylococcus for a multivolume system on bacteriology (Fleming, 1929b). His 17-page paper was well documented and written in his characteristically concise and clear manner. The same year he published his first communication on penicillin, containing the basic information on this antibacterial agent, along with illustrations and tables, all within 12 pages (Fleming, 1929a).

A careful reading of this publication leads one to appreciate the great contribution that Fleming made. His introductory sentences state (p. 226), "While working with staphylococcus variants a number of culture-plates were set aside on the laboratory bench and examined from time to time. In the examinations these plates were necessarily exposed to the air and they became contaminated with various micro-organisms. It was noticed that around a large colony of a contaminating mould the staphylococcus colonies became transparent and were obviously undergoing lysis." This statement is accompanied by a now well-known photograph of this phenomenon. Fleming grew the mold in broth and then studied the characteristics of the penicillin in the broth filtrate free of organisms. He emphasized the following points: (1) The action of penicillin was considerable against pyogenic cocci (streptococcus, staphylococcus, pneumococcus, and gonococcus). (2) It was nontoxic to animals in large doses. (3) It did not interfere with leucocytic function. (4) It might be an efficient antiseptic for application to, or injection into, areas infected with penicillin-sensitive microbes. Like Fleming's work on lysozyme, this report on penicillin was also to influence the penicillin research of Chain and Florey.

Fleming was 48 years old when he published his findings on

penicillin. Although he lived to be 74, no further significant scientific work came from his laboratory. He was not a chemist; the only attempts to produce penicillin in sufficient quantities for further investigations were made by Professor Harold Raistrick of the London University School of Tropical Medicine and Hygiene. But the chemistry involved was unusual, and the penicillin was unstable in the extraction process. It remained for the Chain-Florey Oxford team to solve the problem of penicillin production.

One fundamental question remains unanswered in relation to Fleming's interest in penicillin. He had demonstrated its marked bacteriolytic property for pyogenic microbes, and he had shown it to be nontoxic when injected into animals. Why did he not proceed one step further and test the therapeutic action of penicillin in mice inoculated with cocci, as the Florey team were to report later? There is no clear answer. R. Hare (1970) has added interesting details on Fleming's historic work with penicillin.

Although Fleming's scientific work had gained only limited recognition by the time he reached middle age, following the brilliant achievements of the Oxford team his fame grew. Having passed many hours with him in London and with him and his wife in our home in Minneapolis, I observed that he was a warm modest person without any driving ambition for adulation.

In a moment of self-assessment Fleming told me that he derived the greatest sense of achievement from his discovery of lysozyme, the nontoxic antibacterial material. The concepts involved and the simple laboratory techniques for studying this enzyme prepared him for the subsequent discovery and investigation of penicillin.

Historians of science have repeatedly emphasized that revolutionary advances are made by individuals whose achievements light the way for the discoveries of others. Thus in the field of chemotherapy for microbial diseases, revolutionary changes were induced by Ehrlich, Domagk, Fleming, and Florey. Ehrlich introduced chemotherapy for infectious diseases with his discovery of Salvarsan for syphilis. But this drug, as well as related arsenicals, were too toxic for continued use, and the therapeutic effects were limited. Domagk's discovery of prontosil and the subsequent development of the sulfonamides by others widened the attack on microorganisms, but the toxicity of the drugs and the appearance of sulfonamide-resistant organisms proved to be severe handicaps in therapy. The outstanding features of the discovery of penicillin by Fleming, and of its subsequent purification and production by Florey and his associates, were the relatively low-grade toxicity of the drug and its successful application to many serious types of infectious diseases. Their investigations opened up the discovery of a series of new antibiotics for infections that did not yield to penicillin therapy.

Professor Howard Florey's own imagination and scientific ability were captured by the two major discoveries of Fleming, that of lysozyme and that of penicillin. Florey's competence was reflected in his relentless drive to select other men of competence and, under the hardships of war, to present penicillin as a therapeutic agent that would save millions of lives.

Florey was born in Australia in 1898, where he obtained his collegiate training in medicine. He was later a Rhodes Scholar at Oxford. Greatly influenced in physiology and biochemistry by Sir Charles Sherrington and Sir Frederick Gowland Hopkins, he chose experimental pathology as his career and eventually became head of the Sir William Dunn School of Pathology at Oxford from 1935 to 1962. His early training also included a Rockefeller Travelling Fellowship for one year with Professor A. N. Richards, chairman of the department of pharmacology at the University of Pennsylvania, thus forming a relationship with Dr. Richards that was to be most helpful in his subsequent development of penicillin production. His wife, Ethel, was an Australian schoolmate and was a physician and clinical investigator. She participated in the early clinical evaluation of penicillin.

Florey was not of the classical school of pathology interested only in the histology of changes in the tissues due to disease, but he related these alterations with the disciplines of physiology and chemistry. One of Florey's early interests in research was the action of lysozyme, first described by Fleming. Florey was interested in the function of mucus in the gastrointestinal tract, which contained lysozyme. He postulated that its presence in duodenal secretions might be related to natural immunity and to the genesis of duodenal ulcers. Studying the lysozyme contents of the tissues in a number of mammals, including man, he could find no alternative function of lysozyme other than antibacterial (Florey, 1930; Goldsworthy and Florey, 1930).

The year 1935 was a fateful one for Florey and for the future of penicillin. He was appointed chairman of pathology at Oxford; and realizing the importance of biochemistry in experimental pathology, he selected for his staff the young enzyme chemist Ernst Chain through the recommendation of Sir Frederick Gowland Hopkins. Educated in Berlin, Chain left his country because of Hitler and studied snake venom under Hopkins at Oxford. He was successful in his work with venom. In his own words (Chain, 1971, p. 295), "For the first time, the mode of action of a natural toxin of protein nature could be explained in biochemical terms as that of an enzyme acting on a component of vital importance in the respiratory chain."

Florey encouraged Chain to study the bacteriolytic action of lysozyme on bacteria. Together with a Rhodes Scholar from America, L. A. Epstein, Chain succeeded in demonstrating that lysozyme was an enzyme that hydrolyzed the polysaccharide of the cell wall of *Micrococcus lysodeikticus*, an action that paralleled that of tyrothricin on the cytoplasmic membrane of the pneumococcus (Epstein and Chain, 1940). After discussing the matter further with Florey and surveying the literature on other bacteriolytic agents, Epstein and Chain selected Fleming's penicillin for study. As Chain has emphasized (Epstein and Chain, 1940), although this work was started as World War II began, it was undertaken not as part of the war effort but as a purely scientific investigation.

The work at Oxford on penicillin is one of the great episodes in scientific medicine. Preparations for war brought about an acute shortage of funds for basic research, and the bombing of London by Nazi airmen hampered cooperative industrial efforts for the production of penicillin. The story of this research has been related by Florey et al. (1949, Vol. II) and by Chain (1971). All through the penicillin investigations at Oxford, beginning in 1939, there was a dreadful lack of financial support. At the beginning Florey and Chain aroused the interest of Dr. Warren Weaver, director of the Division of National Sciences of the Rockefeller Foundation, who awarded them a research grant of $5,000 for five years! Probably no equivalent award ever produced more useful results for humanity.

Chain was joined in his research efforts by Dr. N. G. Heatley. They succeeded in growing the mold *Penicillium notatum* and extracting enough penicillin for Florey to direct initial pharmacological and biological studies. By August 24, 1940 a communication of two pages in *The Lancet* by seven authors described penicillin as a "chemotherapeutic agent" (Chain et al., 1940). The report included a table that simulated Domagk's results with prontosil in 1935. Just one year later on August 16, 1941 the Oxford team published a second paper describing in detail the production of penicillin on a large scale in the laboratory and the first therapeutic trials in human patients (Abraham et al., 1941). This report demonstrated quite clearly that penicillin was not toxic for man and was effective in staphylococcal infections. Shortly thereafter, with penicillin prepared at Columbia University and also at the Mayo Clinic, the clinical results were corroborated in America (Herrell, Heilman, and Williams, 1942; Hobby, Meyer, and Chaffee, 1942).

At this time progress in this important work appeared to be temporarily halted. London was being fire-bombed by German airmen, and the necessary financial aid for large-scale production was not available. Once again Florey turned to Dr. Warren Weaver for aid. He was urged to present his case in person in the United States. In July 1941, accompanied by Dr. Heatley, Florey proceeded to Washington to see Dr. Ross Harrison, president of the National Academy of Sciences, who advised him in turn to see Dr. Charles Thom, America's outstanding mycologist, in the Bureau of Plant Industry of the Department of Agriculture at Beltsville, Maryland. Dr. Thom wisely sent Florey and Heatley on to the Northern Regional Research Laboratory of the Agriculture Department in Peoria, Illinois. The climax of the visit to the United States for Florey really came on July 14, 1941 in Peoria when he first met with Dr. Robert Coghill, director of the Fermentation Division, who suggested producing penicillin from the mold with corn-steep liquor in large, deep fermentation tanks. Events moved quickly. Heatley stayed at Peoria to work out the necessary large-scale techniques and then went on to Merck & Company, Incorporated at Rahway, New Jersey. According to Florey, Merck, E. R. Squibb & Sons, and Chas. Pfizer & Company were the first major pharmaceutical firms in the country to undertake the task of producing penicillin in this way.

An investment of millions of dollars from private enterprise was available for the undertaking, but this was still insufficient. Penicillin production was recognized as a wartime effort, and support for research directed toward that end had been established by President Franklin Roosevelt in the Office of Scientific Research and Development with Dr. Vannevar Bush, the president of Massachusetts Institute of Technology, as director. This office also guided and supported the research on the atomic bomb. Doctor A. N. Richards, with whom Florey had worked for a year at the University of Pennsylvania, was the director of medical research. Soon the penicillin project shared top priority for federal funds with the atomic bomb. Thus the United States government and the pharmaceutical industry, aided by academic scientists, pooled their financial resources and scientific talent to produce penicillin (Coghill and Koch, 1945). Following his visit to Peoria in August 1941, Florey journeyed on to the Mayo Clinic and thence to Minneapolis for a visit with us at the University of Minnesota.

By early 1942 penicillin production was under way in the United States. It was decided that the initial supplies should be stock-piled for the Armed Forces, as the United States was now at war. Further clinical evaluation was essential; toward that end Dr. Richards formed the Committee on Chemotherapeutic and Other Agents of the National Research Council, with Dr. Chester Keefer as chairman. The committee in turn allotted penicillin to designated clinical investigators throughout the country in order to acquire information as quickly as possible on types of infection that would be encountered in the military population. Because of our ongoing investigations on staphylococcal disease at the University of Minnesota Hospitals, we were asked to evaluate penicillin principally in that form of sepsis.

On July 11, 1942 the first patient was treated at the University of Minnesota Hospitals, a child desperately ill with staphylococcal bacteremia and localized inflammatory lesions. Her recovery was dramatic. In the next several months we treated two hundred patients, including some with suppurative conditions such as meningitis, pneumonia, and sulfonamide-resistant cases of gonorrhea and

gonococcal pyo-arthritis (Spink and Hall, 1945). There was no question that penicillin was a superior therapeutic agent in many forms of
sepsis. Serious toxic reactions were uncommon.

By 1943 the Keefer committee reported on five hundred cases
treated in the United States (Keefer et al., 1943). The two Floreys,
Ethel and Howard, provided the first significant clinical paper from
England at the same time (Florey and Florey, 1943). Major Champ
Lyons, a bacteriologist and surgeon in the United States Army Medi-
cal Corps, reported on an extensive group of septic cases treated in
the United States Army under the auspices of the Surgeon General
(Lyons, 1943). And in 1944 a special supplement of the *British Journal
of Surgery* detailed the extensive use of penicillin in the British Army,
for which program Florey was a principal adviser (*Penicillin* Special
Issue, 1944). By 1945 the work of the Keefer committee had ended.
The results of this remarkable cooperative investigation in the United
States were presented in a summary of ten thousand treated cases
(Anderson and Keefer, 1948).

The final team effort of Florey's Oxford group was the publication
in 1949 of two large volumes on antibiotics, with a detailed discussion
and documentation of all phases of penicillin (Florey et al., 1949, Vols.
I and II). A third volume on the clinical results, especially with penicillin, was the sole work of M. Ethel Florey (1952). Fleming, Chain, and
Howard Florey had shared the Nobel Prize in 1945. Fleming's scientific work had ended. Chain was still occupied with enzyme chemistry and future penicillins. It is apparent that he and Florey came to a
parting of the ways, perhaps because of Chain's failure to obtain
adequate fermentation equipment in the laboratory at Oxford. As-
sured of his needs in Italy, he accepted a position as professor of
biochemistry and scientific director of a research center in chemical
microbiology at the Superior Institute of Health in Rome. In 1961 he
became professor of biochemistry at the Imperial College of Science
and Technology in London.

Florey continued at Oxford with his work in experimental pathology, studying particularly the vascular endothelium and the
genesis of atherosclerosis, and engaging in teaching. With his colleagues at the Sir William Dunn School of Pathology, he published a
volume of lectures on general pathology (Florey, 1954).

I first met Florey in 1941, and I was with him a second time in 1947 at the centennial meeting of the American Medical Association. I was chairman of a general session on antibiotic therapy, to which Florey had been invited as a foreign participant. In his remarks to over two thousand persons in the assembly he stated that he did not think that the appearance of penicillin-resistant strains of staphylococcus in clinical medicine constituted much of a problem. This disturbed some members of the panel who thought otherwise. As no one wished to offend an invited guest, nothing further was said at the time. However, as at many other scientific meetings, a quiet conversation on the Atlantic City Boardwalk clarified many issues. During a long walk I presented the evidence of several investigators to him, showing that penicillin-resistant staphylococci did pose a serious threat; he concurred, and we parted amicably.

Subsequently, on a visit to Oxford in 1955, I was alone with both Floreys. On that occasion Howard Florey bemoaned the fact that he had not taken out a patent for penicillin. He was always in search of funds to support research at Oxford, making certain that the investigators were given an adequate salary and desirable equipment. He subsequently gave vent to his feelings publicly in a talk in the United States in 1958. He stated (1959, p. 20), "I have had great extension of my experiences as the result of penicillin. I have seen much of the world and have many friends. There is only one serious regret that I have about the whole affair. That is, that I did not, on the behalf of my colleagues and the laboratory, patent the processes by which penicillin was extracted."

Ethel Florey visited the United States alone in 1956 and included Minneapolis in her journey, staying for several days and seeing at first hand in our laboratories the many strains of penicillin-resistant staphylococci isolated from patients. She needed no convincing on our part that it represented a serious problem in medicine, especially in hospitals. Ethel Florey was a good clinical investigator, but she was hampered in her courageous work by physical disability and deafness. She died in 1966, just a few days before her fortieth wedding anniversary.

From 1960 to 1965 Howard Florey occupied one of the greatest positions in science as president of the Royal Society of London. In

1962 he resigned from his Oxford professorship, having served for thirty years, to become provost of Queen's College at Oxford. He became a life peer in 1965. He later visited Australia and assumed an important part in developing graduate education in that country.

Florey died in 1968 at age 70. He had had progressive angina pectoris for 18 years. As he knew, he was living with a "time bomb" in his chest (Bickel, 1972). Florey was a distinguished scientist, educator, and administrator. An informative account of his life and review of his published works has been offered in an obituary of him by Dr. E. P. Abraham, one of his Oxford associates, who wrote (1971, p. 293): "He proved to be a man of vision, with an energy, persistence and obvious integrity which enabled him to put good ideas into effect."

At the end of World War II penicillin became available for general use. It was relatively nontoxic and inexpensive. It continued to be effective for many infections, especially for streptococcal sepsis, pneumococcal diseases, and gonorrhea and syphilis. For those individuals who had acquired penicillin hypersensitivity, other effective drugs became available. The one serious threat to human life that blocked the successful administration of penicillin was the appearance of penicillin-resistant strains of staphylococci.

Within a decade the widespread dissemination of penicillin-resistant strains of staphylococci resulted in epidemic disease, especially in hospitals. As a result the search by the pharmaceutical industry for antistaphylococcal drugs was intensified. There was considerable apprehension that other strains of bacteria susceptible to penicillin would eventually develop resistance. Resistance of staphylococci to penicillin was due to the production of penicillinase by these strains, an enzyme that hydrolyzed the β-lactam bond of the β-lactam-thiazolidine ring in the nucleus of penicillin, rendering penicillin ineffective. The development of semisynthetic penicillins that circumvented penicillinase activity constituted another major advance in antibiotic therapy. This progress also resulted in the discovery of penicillins effective against gram-negative organisms (Braude, 1976).

It was obvious that the problem of staphylococcal penicillinase would attract the enzyme chemists. Chain, having left Oxford for Rome, stated (1971, p. 311): "It should be possible to change the affinity of the penicillin molecule to this enzyme (penicillinase) if it could be chemically modified so that penicillins with either very high or very low affinity could be produced." A team of research workers from the Beecham Research Laboratories in England joined Chain in Rome in 1955. Meanwhile a fermentation pilot plant was being constructed in England to pursue this problem.

Although the chemical structure of penicillin had become known, it was too difficult and costly to produce penicillin synthetically. By 1959 it was established that the nucleus of penicillin was 6-aminopenicillanic acid or 6-APA, which was isolated in a pure state. This meant that 6-APA could be produced by fermentation methods, and then thousands of penicillins could be synthesized — or, more accurately, semisynthesized — through the free amino group of 6-APA. Chain must have been jubilant over this discovery when he wrote (1971, p. 312), "We found ourselves, in fact, in a very similar situation in which the Trefouëls, Bovet and Nitti found themselves in 1935 when they recognized that the active principle of prontosil was sulphanilamide." Within a short time semisynthetic penicillins became available for staphylococcal sepsis in which the hydrolyzing action of penicillinase did not result in inactivation of the drugs.

A second method of producing semisynthetic penicillins involved the addition of an amidase to the fermentation process. This enzyme, when added to the culture medium, stripped the side chain from penicillin and made possible the addition of precursor side chains to the penicillin nucleus. The basic discovery was made in the Beecham Laboratories. Three groups of semisynthetic penicillins could then be prepared for clinical use: (1) acid-resistant penicillins (alpha-phenoxyalkyl derivatives) with the same activity of penicillin G which could be administered orally, such as phenethicillin, propicillin, and phenbenicillin; (2) penicillinase-resistant penicillins, including methicillin, oxacillin, cloxacillin, diphenicillin, and nafcillin — all but methicillin being absorbed orally; and (3) those possessing greater activity against some gram-negative organisms, such as ampicillin, amoxicillin, and carbenicillin (Klein and Finland, 1963).

Cephalosporins

The discovery of the cephalosporins was a major achievement for antibiotic therapy. Although similar to penicillin chemically, the basic nucleus of the cephalosporins differed enough so that new semisynthetic drugs could be developed, thus widening the attack on pathogenic microbes and resisting the hydrolizing action of penicillinase.

The investigations of the cephalosporins revealed again Florey's competence in selecting individuals for basic and applied research. On April 25, 1955 he addressed the annual session of The American College of Physicians on the subject of "Antibiotic Products of a Versatile Fungus" (Florey, 1955). Many of us learned for the first time of a challenging adventure with some major new antibiotics, similar to penicillin but differing in biological activity. In July 1948 Florey had received a letter from Dr. Blyth Brook, who had been in Sardinia during World War II. Brook called attention to a fungus isolated by Professor G. Brotzu, rector of the University of Cagliari, who during the war searched the sewage outfall on the Sardinian coast for microorganisms that, like penicillin, produced a substance having antimicrobial properties. He recovered the fungus *Cephalosporium acremonium* and reported his finding in an obscure Sardinian journal in 1948, stating that the fungus produced a filtrate that inhibited the growth of gram-negative and gram-positive organisms (Brotzu, 1948). A subculture was received at Oxford, and Florey's two colleagues on the "penicillin team" quickly confirmed Brotzu's observations. The chemist E. P. Abraham was to commit himself to this project for several years.

The initial research was carried out at Oxford and by the Antibiotics Research Station of the British Medical Research Council. Eventually other individuals and investigators from two pharmaceutical companies participated, Glaxo Laboratories, Limited in England and Eli Lilly and Company in the United States. The investigations were complicated because the fungus produced at least six antibiotics, three of which were identified. Cephalosporin P_1 was a steroid; Cephalosporin N was called penicillin N; and the third was named Cephalosporin C. Beginning in 1953 work was concentrated on the third antibiotic, which was not destroyed by penicillinase and which was active against gram-negative organisms as well. The chemical structure of Cephalosporin C was defined by E. P. Abraham and G. G. F. Newton (1961). These investigations were aided by Dr. Dorothy Hodgkin, using X-ray crystallography (Hodgkin and Maslen, 1961). She was subsequently awarded a Nobel Prize in chemistry.

A key discovery related to the nucleus of Cephalosporin C. The nucleus of penicillin, the production of which led to the semisynthetic penicillins, was a thiazolidine-β-lactam ring known as 6-aminopenicillanic acid (6-APA). The nucleus of Cephalosporin C was found to be 7-aminocephalosporanic acid, which is a dihydrothiazine-β-lactam ring (Loder, Newton, and Abraham, 1961). This distinction between the nuclei was responsible for the different biological activities of Cephalosporin C and penicillin. The 7-ACA β-lactam ring was not hydrolyzed by penicillinase, in contrast to that of 6-APA. The difficult problem of producing 7-ACA was finally resolved in the Lilly Research Laboratories (Morin et al., 1962).

A conference held in 1967 at Oxford summed up the pertinent information on cephaloridine, including the therapeutic results in patients (Beeson, 1967). The antibiotic was effective in gram-positive bacterial diseases, such as staphylococcal sepsis due to penicillinase-producing staphylococci, Group A streptococcal disease, and pneumococcal infections. But equally important, it was active against gram-negative bacilli, including salmonellae, *Proteus mirabilis*, *E. coli*, paracolon, *H. influenzae*, and *Klebsiella-Aerobacter*.

Two derivatives of cephalosporin became available commercially. The first included the N-acylderivatives of 7-aminocephalosporonic acid containing the dihydrothiazine-β-lactam ring, known as cephalonidine. Although it was inactivated by penicillinase, this antibiotic had the same antibacterial spectrum as the second derivation. It was administered parenterally and marketed as Loridine (USA) and Cephorin (Great Britain).

The second derivative could be administered orally and was known as cephaloglycine dihydrate (Kafocin). It was advocated for urinary tract infections due to *E. coli*, *Klebsiella-Aerobacter*, staphylococci, *Proteus* sp., and enterococci. Cephalexin monohydrate (Keflex), also prepared for oral administration, was recommended for urinary tract infections and for infections due to streptococci and pneumococci. The most widely used parenteral preparation in this group was a sodium preparation of cephalothrin (Keflin) with a wide antibacterial spectrum for gram-positive and gram-negative organisms.

The toxicity of the cephalosporin preparations simulates that of penicillin, except that they may also cause renal dysfunction. This is reversible if recognized early. There is some cross reaction in the hypersensitivity induced by penicillin and cephalosporin. Therefore patients reacting undesirably to penicillin should not receive cephalosporins.

L. Weinstein and K. Kaplan (1970) provided a helpful pharmacological and clinical review on the status of the cephalosporins. In an informative and extensive volume edited by E. H. Flynn on the chemistry and biology of the cephalosporins and penicillins by several authorities, E. P. Abraham and B. Loder wrote (Flynn, 1972, p. 11),

Eight years elapsed between the isolation of *Cephalosporium sp.* in Sardinia and the discovery of cephalosporin C in Oxford. . . . A further 7 years passed before the isolation of high-yielding mutant strains of the organism and the discovery of a novel method for obtaining the nucleus of the molecule allowed the potentialities of the new ring system of the latter to be adequately explored. During the latter period the difficulties to be overcome appeared at times to be so formidable that it would not have been surprising if the project had been abandoned. Its final success must be attributed to a combination of scientific ability, technical expertise, and willingness to take calculated risks in the pharmaceutical companies that were mainly involved.

The scientific effort that was poured into the elucidation and production of cephalosporin antibiotics for human use constituted a brilliant accomplishment in antibiotic research. Such an achievement was possible only in the mid-twentieth century because it involved the sophisticated techniques of nuclear-magnetic-resonance, mass spectrometry, X-ray crystallography, and vapor phase and thin-layer chromatography, combined with the talents of physical chemists, synthetic organic chemists, enzyme chemists, microbiologists, and geneticists. A statement by Thomas S. Kuhn (1962, p. 26) is applicable: "From Tycho Brahe to E. O. Lawrence, some scientists have acquired great reputations, not from any novelty of their discoveries, but from the precision, reliability, and scope of the methods they developed for the redetermination of a previously known sort of fact."

What would the two chemists Pasteur and Ehrlich have said about this accomplishment with cephalosporin? They would, I think, have been surprised but not overawed. What about Fleming and his mentor Sir Almroth Wright? The achievement probably would have been beyond their comprehension, and very likely they would have asked if the end products harmed human tissues. And what of Sir Howard Florey? He would very likely have smiled and said that ideas come from individuals but scientific accomplishments frequently depend upon "the team effort." He probably would not have been surprised at the accomplishment, but rather would have expected it — provided there was adequate financial backing!

CHAPTER 7

Streptomycin

Tuberculosis was one of the most common infectious diseases until the early twentieth century, causing chronic ill health with a significant mortality rate. Robert Koch isolated tubercle bacilli from human lesions, grew the organisms on a medium containing blood serum, and reproduced the disease in guinea pigs (Koch, 1882, translation 1938). Doctor Edward Livingston Trudeau, himself a victim of serious chronic tuberculosis who established the first tuberculosis sanatorium in the United States at Saranac, New York in 1884, wrote (1916, p. 174), "If I could learn to grow the tubercle bacillus outside of the body and produce tuberculosis at will with it in guinea-pigs, the next step would be to find something that would kill the germ in the living animal. If an inoculated guinea-pig could be cured, then in all probability this great burden of sickness could be lifted from the human race." The prophetic hope of Trudeau was finally fulfilled by the vigorous work of the soil microbiologist Selman Waksman.

Waksman, the only child of Ukrainian parents, migrated to the United States in 1910 at 22 years of age and settled for the rest of his long life at New Brunswick, New Jersey, which is the site of Rutgers University and of the New Jersey Agricultural Experiment Station. He chose this location largely because of relatives who had settled there and who would aid him in his early years. Waksman plunged into the discipline of soil microbiology at Rutgers after graduate training at the

University of California at Berkeley. His financial status, like that of so many intelligent immigrants, was in a precarious state for many years (Waksman, 1954). But this did not impede him in his drive to become an outstanding soil microbiologist. For years he was interested in the formation of humus, which emerges in soil through the action of microorganisms on organic material. His first publication in 1916 was on the actinomyces in soil, a species that was to engage his research activity for many years and that finally would yield streptomycin from *Streptomyces griseus*. He identified this actinomycete as early as 1915.

Waksman did not become actively interested in antibiotics until 1940. He cites discussions he had about that time on the subject with his former graduate student Dr. René Dubos (Waksman, 1954). He also maintained a close working relationship with scientists at the Merck pharmaceutical organization in nearby Rahway. Waksman was alert to the success of the sulfonamides; it is likely that the early efforts with penicillin impressed him. He isolated and purified actinomycin in 1940 and streptothricin in 1942. These antibiotics were antibacterial but too toxic for systemic use.

The discovery of streptomycin was reported in 1944 by Waksman with his graduate student A. Schatz as the senior author (Schatz, Bugie, and Waksman, 1944).[1] This research resulted from a carefully planned approach of studying microbial antagonism in soil impregnated with tubercle bacilli. Almost simultaneously a second paper with Schatz described the *in vitro* action of streptomycin against *Mycobacterium tuberculosis* (Schatz and Waksman, 1944).

Waksman quickly realized that an experimental animal model was necessary to evaluate the effect of streptomycin upon the tubercle bacillus. He turned to the Mayo Foundation in Rochester, Minnesota, where an excellent experimental animal model for therapeutic research on tuberculosis had been established in the Institute of Experimental Medicine by Doctors William Feldman and H. Corwin Hinshaw. Doctor Feldman was a veterinarian in the Institute and was interested in comparative pathology. He had written a superb monograph on avian tuberculosis (Feldman, 1938). Doctor Hinshaw was an internist at the Mayo Clinic and an authority in pulmonary disease. These investigators had done pioneering work in 1942 in the chemotherapy of experimental tuberculosis with the sulfone compounds promin and promizole before streptomycin was known (Feldman, Hinshaw, and Mann, 1944; Feldman, Hinshaw, and Moses, 1942). They were prepared to investigate streptomycin for Waksman.

Feldman and Hinshaw (1945) published an outline of the guinea pig model for evaluating chemotherapy in tuberculosis, accompanied by an excellent illustration that other investigators could and did follow (Figures 3 and 4).[2] These Mayo investigators showed that streptomycin was effective in the tuberculous guinea pig. In 1945 they reported on the use of the antibiotic in human tuberculosis (Feldman, Hinshaw, and Mann, 1945; Hinshaw and Feldman, 1945).

In 1949 Waksman edited a volume on streptomycin. In the opening sentence of the preface he stated (1949, p. v), "Probably no other drug in the history of medical science has had such a phenomenal rise as

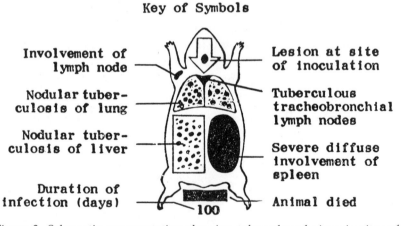

Figure 3. Schematic representation showing tuberculous lesions in sites of predilection of an experimentally infected guinea pig. Reproduced with permission of American Review of Respiratory Diseases, National Tuberculosis Society, New York, New York and of H. Corwin Hinshaw, Sr., M.D. from W. H. Feldman and H. C. Hinshaw, "Chemotherapeutic Testing in Experimental Tuberculosis," *American Review of Tuberculosis* 51:582, 1945 (Figure 1, p. 586).

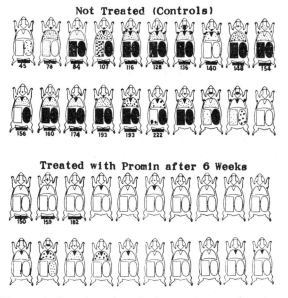

Figure 4. Results of typical experiment showing amounts and situations of tuberculous changes in two groups of guinea pigs consisting of 20 animals each. Reproduced with permission of American Review of Respiratory Diseases, National Tuberculosis Society, New York, New York and of H. Corwin Hinshaw, Sr., M.D. from W. H. Feldman and H. C. Hinshaw, "Chemotherapeutic Testing in Experimental Tuberculosis," *American Review of Tuberculosis* 51:582, 1945 (Figure 2, p. 586).

streptomycin." He listed 1,171 references in the literature on streptomycin from 1944–1948 (Waksman, 1948). Why this phenomenal success? Several factors contributed. For one thing, Waksman was shrewd and energetic in directing his research goals. Furthermore it is known that in his antibiotic program he was assisted by almost fifty graduate students and visiting investigators. He had the benefit of the varied experiences of investigators in the sulfonamide and penicillin programs. He shared the scientific and financial assistance of Merck & Company. And finally, the experience with penicillin during World War II, in which industry, government, and university groups had joined in the evaluation of the antibiotic, was speedily applied to streptomycin. Unlike the case of penicillin, the work on streptomycin came during a time of peace. The Committee on Chemotherapy of the National Research Council under the chairmanship of Dr. Chester S. Keefer, and the Streptomycin Producers Industry Advisory Committee of the Civilian Production Administration, rapidly evaluated the drug with qualified investigators. In rendering his final report Keefer wrote (Keefer and Hewitt, 1948, p. v), "It is truly remarkable that so much information concerning a new therapeutic agent could be accumulated within three years of the announcement of its discovery." In the first report of the committee in 1946, a thousand cases had been evaluated, and in the final report of 1948, three thousand cases were tabulated (Keefer et al., 1946; Keefer and Hewitt, 1948).

Although streptomycin was effective in the acute forms of the disease, there still remained the question of the final outcome and the possibilities of relapse. Perhaps the most outstanding example of a cooperative, long-term evaluation of chemotherapy was the United States Veterans Administration's medical studies on tuberculosis. As a result of these investigations the advantages of streptomycin were summarized, as well as some major disadvantages, which will be discussed shortly.

Other diseases responding favorably to streptomycin therapy included plague, tularemia, and meningitis (Waksman, 1949). Suppurative meningitis due to *Hemophilus influenzae* was the most common form of meningitis in infants under twelve months of age. The mortality rate was 90 percent, and those who recovered often had serious neurological sequelae. While Type B *H. influenzae* antiserum appeared to have some beneficial effect, real progress was made when serum therapy was combined with the administration of sulfadiazine — 68 of 87 patients recovered following such treatment (Alexander, 1944). Further progress was obtained when serum, sulfadiazine, and streptomycin were combined (Alexander and Leidy, 1947). Streptomycin therapy alone was inadequate and was associated with the appearance of streptomycin-resistant organisms. A comprehensive clinical review of streptomycin and dihydrostreptomycin was prepared by Weinstein and Ehrenkranz (1958) after a decade of use.

For several years in our laboratory we carried out studies on the therapy of experimental brucellosis using several animal species, principally mice and guinea pigs. We screened the sulfonamides and penicillin, both experimentally and clinically, and had found these agents to be ineffective. We observed that streptomycin-sensitive strains of brucellae became rapidly resistant when exposed *in vitro* to streptomycin (Yow and Spink, 1949). When we used the chick embryo technique, however, streptomycin plus sulfadiazine had a synergistic and protective effect against lethal doses of brucellae (Shaffer and Spink, 1948). The administration of a combination of streptomycin and sulfadiazine provided the first effective, though not entirely satisfactory, treatment for the disease (Spink, Hall, Shaffer, and Braude, 1948).

Within five years the disadvantages and dangers of streptomycin therapy became manifest. As early as 1946 streptomycin-resistant tubercle bacilli were isolated as a result of treatment, becoming more apparent in a few years (Youmans et al., 1946). The appearance of resistant strains was directly related to the *duration* of therapy, which had to be prolonged because of the chronic nature of tuberculosis. The dissemination of these resistant strains among the susceptible general population was feared.

Streptomycin-resistant bacteria appeared not only with tuberculosis, but also with other treated infections. We demonstrated the appearance of highly resistant strains of brucellae following treatment, and also the development of a streptomycin-dependent brucella strain occurring in a human under treatment (Hall and Spink, 1947; Yow and Spink, 1949). C. P. Miller and M. Bohnhoff (1946; 1947) observed similar streptomycin variants of meningococci, and streptomycin-resistant strains of gonococci. A rapid development of streptomycin resistance appeared in other gram-negative bacterial infections.

The toxic reactions from streptomycin were also alarming, particularly those affecting the eighth nerve. Severe tinnitus, vomiting, and deafness were common and were mostly related to the dose of the drug. Drug fever and skin eruptions were also encountered. The introduction of dihydrostreptomycin did not mitigate these dangers.

When streptomycin was combined with p-amino-benzoic acid, a synergistic therapeutic effect in tuberculosis was observed. This was fortunate because the amounts of streptomycin could be reduced, and simultaneously the appearance of streptomycin-resistant strains of tubercle bacilli and the otological complications became less common.

Isoniazid (INH)

Although streptomycin was hailed as the first successful therapeutic agent for the disease, there was an urgent need for a drug that could be administered orally and that was less toxic. Within a decade streptomycin was largely replaced by an effective oral preparation related to the vitamin nicotinic acid. The discovery of isonicotinyl hydrazine, or isoniazid (INH), is another dramatic story in medical research.

Apparently the first public announcement in the United States about the possible use of nicotinamide in tuberculosis was contained in a brief chemical news summary on "Synthetic Tuberculostats Show Promise" (Fox, 1951), involving a research project carried out by H. Herbert Fox of the research laboratories of Hoffman-La Roche in New Jersey and André Gerard of the French Laboratories of Chemotherapy. Later Fox amplified this report in a historical summary on "The Chemical Attack on Tuberculosis" at the New York Academy of Sciences on April 3, 1953 (Fox, 1953). Three potential groups of synthetic chemical compounds for therapy in tuberculosis had been studied since 1940. The first group were the sulfones, which had been investigated in experimentally-infected animal models by Feldman and Hinshaw at the Mayo Clinic. The second were the thiosemicarbazones, and the third group were the pyridine carboxylic acid derivatives, of which the parent compound was nicotinamide and was first studied by the French in 1945. This French work was largely overlooked in the United States, but Fox, noting the interdependence of vitamin and tuberculostatic activities, had synthesized the most active derivative, isonicotinylhydrazine (INH).

The first successful demonstration of the activity of INH was carried out in 1951 in experimental tuberculosis of mice by Grunberg and Schnitzer (1952) of the Chemotherapy Laboratories of Hoffman-La Roche in New Jersey, and was quickly confirmed by W. Steenken and E. Wolinsky (1952) of the Trudeau Laboratory in New York. Simultaneously at Sea View Hospital in New York, patients with tuberculosis were treated with INH for the first time. The significant results in over a hundred patients were reported in January, 1952 by E. H. Robitzek, I. J. Selikoff, and G. G. Ornstein (1952). In fact this report constituted the entire January issue of *The Quarterly Bulletin of Sea View Hospital*. Investigations were extended by others in which pa-

tients with miliary and meningeal tuberculosis were treated successfully with INH (McDermott et al., 1952).

Success with INH therapy in tuberculosis continued. One valuable
characteristic of the drug was that it penetrated the cell to a site where
the tubercle bacilli were located. No other antimicrobial drug
employed for systemic use acted intracellularly in this manner against
microorganisms. Except for one serious side effect INH was relatively
nontoxic. In some patients the drug did cause peripheral neuropathy,
which could be prevented by the simultaneous administration of
pyridoxine (Vitamin B_6). The modern chemotherapy of tuberculosis
has been reviewed by R. S. Mitchell and J. C. Bell (1958).

Although streptomycin had a meteoric rise from 1952 for the
therapy of tuberculosis and other infectious diseases, by 1965 it has
also had a precipitous decline. Nevertheless streptomycin was the
first successful chemotherapeutic agent for tuberculosis and for some
other major diseases. Doctor Waksman was awarded the Nobel Prize
in 1952 for this contribution. Neomycin was also discovered in his
laboratory, but this agent, which was highly active against gram-
negative organisms, proved too toxic for systemic use (Waksman,
1958).

CHAPTER 8

The Tetracyclines

The pattern of large pharmaceutical companies during and after World War II in the search for new antibiotics was continued in the development of the tetracycline drugs in the United States. Lederle Laboratories in Pearl River, New York and Parke, Davis & Company in Detroit, Michigan initiated research independently in 1939 on the isolation of antibiotics (Dowling, 1959). Chas. Pfizer & Company in Brooklyn, New York shared in the production of penicillin during World War II. The Pfizer research staff also undertook a search for new antibiotics in the soil, although it is not entirely clear when this work started. The search for new antibiotics by private industry required considerable financial risk, greater than that demanded for penicillin production, which had been subsidized by the United States Government as a wartime project. Therefore clearcut therapeutic objectives were necessary in the planning of new projects if the research was to be carried out by private industry alone.

The limitations of streptomycin had become obvious. One gloomy aspect crept into the successful story of penicillin: the threat of widespread dissemination of penicillin-resistant strains of staphylococci, as discussed in Section III, Chapter 16. Would there be a repetition of the sulfonamide experience, and would additional penicillin-resistant species of bacteria appear? Furthermore there was definitely a need for other chemotherapeutic agents for rickettsial diseases, such as

116

epidemic and endemic typhus and Rocky Mountain spotted fever, for typhoid fever, and for the various types of infections caused by gram-negative bacteria.

Chlortetracycline

The research at Lederle Laboratories was under the general direction of Dr. Weed Malcolm. His unusually competent team for basic and experimental research and clinical evaluation contributed to the striking success of chlortetracycline (aureomycin). The research followed the discovery by Professor Benjamin Dugger, who had retired from the department of botany at the University of Wisconsin in 1943, and the following year, at the age of 72, had joined the staff at Lederle supervising the examination of soils for potential antibiotics. On September 4, 1945 he isolated an organism from a sample of soil received from a timothy field on the University of Missouri campus. The organism, later called *Streptomyces aureofaciens* and designated A-377, was the source of the new antibiotic. Chlortetracycline was first isolated in 1945; the first experimental animal studies were made in 1946; crystalline material was prepared for biological research, and the first patients were treated in 1948.

The clinical evaluation of chlortetracycline took the form of what Dowling (1959) has called "a frontal attack" by a group of university investigators. Progress was so rapid that a symposium on "Aureomycin — A New Antibiotic" was held at the New York Academy of Sciences on July 21, 1948. The results published on November 30th of the same year embraced the basic pharmacology and the clinical findings in pneumococcal diseases, streptococcal infections, gonorrhea, meningitis, typhoid fever, bacillary dysentery, typhus, Rocky Mountain spotted fever, Q fever, lymphogranuloma venereum, and other diseases (Williams, 1948). The antibiotic was approved for medical use by the Food and Drug Administration October 20, 1948, and the first "broad-spectrum" antibiotic was marketed on December 1, 1948.

Our interest at the University of Minnesota in exploring the potential value of chlortetracycline was stimulated through a visit to us in March, 1948 by Dr. Y. Subba Row, director of research at Lederle Laboratories, who had been my instructor in biochemistry at Harvard Medical School. As a result of our discussions we embarked upon two investigations with the antibiotic. First, we were interested in its therapeutic potential in brucellosis. No clinical data were available at the time. Second, one of the major unsolved therapeutic problems in infectious diseases related to urinary tract infections and sepsis due to a variety of gram-negative organisms, such as *Escherichia coli*, *Aerobacter aerogenes*, *Klebsiella pneumoniae*, *Pseudomonas aeruginosa*, and the *Proteus* species. We were impressed by the increasing incidence of bacteremia caused by these microorganisms, with and without accompanying urinary tract infections, and the associated circulatory collapse (septic shock). The problem of shock was to engage our attention over the following decade.

As a result of many experimental studies in our laboratories on the possible application of antibiotics to the therapy of brucellosis, the National Research Council (US) and the government of Mexico encouraged an investigation on the possibilities of a combination of streptomycin and sulfadiazine in patients with brucellosis at the Mexico General Hospital in Mexico City. This was undertaken in the summer of 1948 with Dr. A. I. Braude and Dr. M. Ruiz Castaneda and his Mexican group.

Clinical studies with streptomycin and sulfadiazine had to be abandoned, however, because of a high incidence of the otitic side effects of streptomycin. Also the patients complained bitterly about the pain accompanying the intramuscular injections of the drug. We then turned to an evaluation of chlortetracycline. Like tuberculosis, brucellosis is a disease of intracellular parasitism, the brucellae remaining viable in the tissues for a long time, even though there are no overt signs of disease (Spink, 1952b). Although chlortetracycline was bacteriostatic for brucellae *in vitro*, intracellular organisms were protected against the activity of the drug, and also against the bactericidal action of serum (Magoffin and Spink, 1951; Shaffer, Kucera, and Spink, 1953b). Chick embryos were protected by chlortetracycline against lethal infection (Magoffin, Anderson, and Spink, 1949). Using mice as the experimental model, we found that the infected animals were also protected with chlortetracycline against a lethal outcome, but very prolonged administration of the drug did not eradicate the organisms from the tissues (Braude and Spink 1950; Shaffer, Kucera, and Spink, 1953a; Spink and Bradley, 1960). This was the status of our knowledge — much of it unpublished — when the first patients with brucellosis were treated with chlortetracycline in July, 1948. Twenty-four were given an oral preparation. The challenge to any therapeutic agent was severe because many of the patients had been ill for months with persistent bacteremia. But the results far exceeded our expectations (Spink, Braude, Castaneda, and Goytia, 1948). The drug was administered for 11 days. All of the patients recovered, but a relapse in two patients required a second course of therapy. In three recovered patients bacteremia was present after treatment had been stopped. This experience of an occasional relapse and the presence of bacteremia prompted the recommendation that chlortetracycline in a dose of 2 gm. daily should be continued for not less than 21 days. Chlortetracycline became and remained the drug for the therapy of brucellosis.

One side effect of chlortetracycline in these patients occasioned alarm. Following the initial oral dose of the drug, 12 of the 24 patients had a rise in temperature, tachycardia, and hypotension, indicating impending vascular collapse. This initial reaction was circumvented by reducing the amount of the initial dose, and later by the simultaneous use of adrenocorticotrophic hormone (Spink and Hall, 1952). A similar sequence of cardiovascular events was encountered by others in the treatment of typhoid fever with chloramphenicol and was also prevented by the use of cortisone (Smadel, Ley, and Diercks, 1951; Woodward et al., 1951). Within a year chlortetracycline was used successfully in Minnesota in patients with infections due to *Brucella aborus* (Braude, Hall, and Spink, 1949).

The treatment with chlortetracycline of urinary tract infections and bacteremia due to a variety of gram-negative organisms proved to be a difficult and continuing problem. Usually in chronic infections, because administration of the drug would be associated with the elimination of the bacteremia, a relapse of the urinary tract infection would occur. The antibiotic was beneficial in acute urinary tract infections and in some patients with bacteremia. The results of our experimental and clinical studies and those of others in the management of septic or endotoxin shock have been summarized elsewhere (Spink 1958; 1960; 1962; 1965).

Penicillin-resistant staphylococcal infections posed a serious clinical problem at the time chlortetracycline became available, but this antibiotic proved less effective than other agents for these infections

(Spink, 1951). A great advance, however, was the successful use of chlortetracycline in the treatment of the rickettsioses, including the spotted fever and typhus groups. "Atypical pneumonia" (myco-plasma), thought to be due to a virus, was also favorably controlled by chlortetracycline when therapy was initiated early. Subsequently another advance included the successful therapy of suppurative *Hemophilus influenzae* meningitis (Chandler and Hodes, 1950; Drake et al., 1950).

Oxytetracycline

A drug closely related chemically and therapeutically to chlortetracy-cline, oxytetracycline, was marketed as terramycin in 1950. Ter-ramycin was isolated from a new species of actinomycete, *Strep-tomyces rimosus*, from a sample of soil in the laboratories of Chas. Pfizer & Company, Brooklyn. The first report on this new antibiotic appeared January 27, 1950 (Finlay et al., 1950), and the description of its antimicrobial activity was published in March of the same year (Hobby et al., 1950). The basic studies on the isolated antibiotic were carried out in the Pfizer Research Laboratories and its clinical evalua-tion was completed by a group of investigators in the United States. On June 16 and 17, 1950 a conference on terramycin at the New York Academy of Sciences presented a review of this effort (*Terramycin*, 1950). Doctor Gladys Hobby, who had pioneered penicillin studies with Dr. Martin Dawson at Columbia University, coordinated the clinical studies on terramycin at Pfizer and was able to submit a thousand case reports to Dr. Chester Keefer, chairman of the confer-ence.

The results of this conference and subsequent clinical studies clearly indicated that terramycin and aureomycin had essentially the same antimicrobial activity and caused similar side effects (Lepper, 1956; Musselman, 1956). Both of these agents were a distinct advance in the chemotherapy of infectious diseases because the antimicrobial spectrum was widened; the drugs were available for effective oral administration; the toxicity was not serious in the vast majority of patients; and the development of resistant bacterial strains was not alarming.

Tetracycline

Another major development with chlortetracycline and oxytetracycline occurred in 1952. When the C1 atom of the former and the O atom of the latter were removed, the resultant compound was tetracycline (Dowling, 1955). Tetracycline had the same antimicrobial activity as aureomycin and terramycin, and according to most clinicians provoked fewer side effects than either, especially the gastrointestinal disturbances. According to Dowling (1955), tetracycline was marketed in November, 1953 by Lederle Laboratories. Subsequently the drug was prepared by several other major pharmaceutical firms for commercial purposes, thus practically displacing aureomycin and terramycin.[1]

The successful introduction of the tetracyclines into chemotherapy was a major advance in the management of infectious diseases. At the time they became available penicillin was the principal antibiotic in use, but the tetracyclines added to the effective management of infections. First, the tetracyclines were readily absorbed into the blood when administered orally. Second, these drugs were without serious toxic manifestations. Third, the antimicrobial spectrum responding to drug therapy was enhanced, especially for the rickettsioses, salmonella infections, and a wide range of gram-negative bacterial diseases. Fourth, the appearance of antibiotic-resistant strains of pathogens was not a serious problem. And finally, the expense of the tetracyclines was not excessive considering the serious nature of the diseases that responded to such oral therapy.

CHAPTER 9

Chloramphenicol and Other Antibiotics

The search for antibiotic-producing soil microorganisms continued. An important discovery was made in the Research Laboratories of Parke, Davis & Company in Detroit in cooperation with Professor Paul Burkholder of the botany department at Yale University when a new actinomycete, *Streptomyces rimosus*, was isolated from a sample of soil obtained from a mulched stubble field in Caracas, Venezuela. The antibiotic chloramphenicol (chloromycetin) came from this source. Two brief reports on this discovery appeared in *Science* for October 31, 1947 (Ehrlich et al., 1947; Smadel and Jackson, 1947). The first, from the laboratories of Parke-Davis, described the *in vitro* action of the crystalline material for several species of bacteria, and the second, from the Army Medical Center in Washington, D.C., related to the effectiveness of chloramphenicol on rickettsial infections and psittacosis. Independently, David Gottlieb and his associates (1948) at the University of Illinois isolated an antibiotic identical with chloramphenicol from *Streptomyces griseus* found in compost.

A chemical feature of this antibiotic was the presence of a nitrobenzene moiety that was a derivative of dichloracetic acid. The synthesis of the natural product was reported in 1949, and chloramphenicol became the first completely synthetic antibiotic to be marketed. The antimicrobial activity of the natural and synthetic products were the same (Controulis, Rebstock, and Crooks, Jr., 1949; Smadel, Jackson, Ley, and Lewthwaite, 1949).

In the development of chloramphenicol as a therapeutic agent the early and major work was done under the direction of Dr. Joseph Smadel, chief of the Viral and Rickettsial Diseases Section of the Army Medical Center in Washington. Cooperative clinical studies were carried out in Malaya with Dr. Raymond Lewthwaite, director of the Institute for Medical Research in Kuala Lampur; in Mexico; and with Dr. Theodore Woodward and his group at the University of Maryland Medical School.

Because of this association of investigators two significant advances were made in the chemotherapy of infectious diseases. First, the drug proved to be effective in the rickettsial diseases, such as tsutsugamushi disease (scrub typhus) (Smadel, Woodward, Ley, and Lewthwaite, 1949); in epidemic typhus (Smadel et al., 1948); in murine typhus (Ley, Jr., Woodward, and Smadel, 1950); in Rocky Mountain spotted fever (Pincoffs et al., 1948); and in fièvre boutonneuse (Janbon, Bertrand, and Combier, 1949). The second major advance was the use of the drug in the successful treatment of typhoid fever (Woodward et al., 1948; Smadel, Bailey, and Lewthwaite, 1950). Smadel (1949) reviewed the early work on chloramphenicol.

As chloramphenicol became available to physicians the foregoing results were confirmed, especially in typhoid fever. I observed epidemic typhoid fever in Yugoslavia and in Mexico, and the therapeutic results with the drug in these areas were remarkable, especially when administered early in the course of the disease. The mortality rates were greatly reduced, as were such complications as hemorrhage and perforation of the bowel. I also saw epidemic tsutsugamushi disease in American military personnel in the Pacific areas treated promptly and effectively with chloramphenicol.

Other diseases for which chloramphenicol was found to be effective included *H. influenzae* meningitis and selected cases of urinary tract infections (McCrumb et al., 1951). Although favorable results were obtained in patients with brucellosis, most investigators preferred the less toxic tetracyclines. A comprehensive and well-documented review on chloramphenicol was prepared by Woodward and Wisseman, Jr. (1958).

During the twenty-five years that elapsed after the introduction of penicillin, thousands of potential antibiotics were screened for human therapy. Since there was a continuing need, new agents became available. For a comprehensive review of the newer broad-spectrum penicillins and other antibiotics by a large group of competent clinical investigators, reference is made to the conference held at the New York Academy of Sciences in 1967 (Mann, 1967). This group not only assessed the new drugs but compared their clinical value with the older antibiotics, especially with penicillin G and the tetracyclines.

Erythromycin represents one of the macrolide antibiotics derived from the actinomycete *Streptomyces erythreus* by McGuire and his group (1952). Macrolides contain a lactane ring to which sugars are attached. Related antibiotics include *carbomycin*, *spiramycin*, and *oleandomycin*. Erythromycin has continued to be useful in the therapy of infections due to gram-positive organisms such as streptococci, staphylococci, and pneumococci. The drug is administered orally, causes relatively few toxic reactions, and is particularly advantageous in patients who are sensitive to penicillin. Because of the ease of administration, it has been used widely in small children with respiratory infections.

Kanamycin is derived from a group of antibiotics possessing a wide antibacterial spectrum, including gram-negative organisms and penicillin-resistant staphylococci. It was first reported by Umezawa of the National Institutes of Health in Tokyo in 1957, having been isolated from an actinomycete, *Streptomyces kanamyceticus*, and found in the soil at the Nagama prefecture. In the succeeding year clinical experience permitted a conference on this drug at the New York Academy of Sciences (Finland, 1958). It became obvious that like neomycin and streptomycin, kanamycin produced renal and otological toxic reactions, although it appeared to be of value in selected cases of urinary tract infections. Eight years later a second conference was held at the New York Academy of Sciences, at which M. Finland, in summarizing the proceedings, pointed out that kanamycin was indicated in urinary tract infections, as originally suggested, but that it remained potentially toxic (Mann, 1966). This antibiotic has assumed a position of limited use in medicine.

Gentamicin is another of the antibiotics introduced because of its wide antibacterial spectrum. It was discovered, isolated, studied, and reported as a team effort in 1963, being derived from *Micromonospora purpurea* (Weinstein et al., 1964; Rosselet et al., 1964). The antibiotic, also utilized in urinary tract infections, appears particularly advantageous against those due to *Pseudomonas aeruginosa*. An international symposium on gentamicin in 1968 offered further clinical guidelines for the use of the antibiotic, particularly for infections due to gram-negative bacteria (Finland, 1969).

Finally the rifamycins are an interesting group of antibiotics derived from *Streptomyces mediterranei*. After the basic aromatic ring complex had been defined, several semisynthetic products were produced, of which the most widely investigated has been rifampin. The antibiotic is useful orally, along with isoniazid, in the ambulatory therapy of tuberculosis (Newman et al., 1974). Because it is highly active against *Neisseria meningitis* it is an effective prophylactic for those in contact with cases of meningococcal disease (Weinstein, 1975a).

CHAPTER 10

Antibiotics and Animal Nutrition

The successful application of modern chemo-
therapy to infectious diseases and the preservation of human health
has had a corollary in its beneficial effect on animal health. An unexpected success has been a marked improvement in animal nutrition
and a rapid gain in weight accompanying the ingestion of antibiotics
by apparently healthy animals.

The use of antibiotics in animals with infections has been limited to
local application and systemic administration through oral and parenteral routes. Large-scale systematic administration has been greatly
limited because few existing diseases really require the excessively
large, costly doses of drugs. The control of animal diseases, especially
in large animals, has been successful through the use of prophylactic
vaccines and through the elimination of infected animals. Ornithosis,
however, has been partially controlled in birds and poultry through
the use of tetracyclines in drinking water, as have also enteric diseases to a limited extent. Animals have been treated systematically
with antibiotics for anthrax and leptospirosis. The drugs have been
administered selectively to valuable animals and to small pets.

The antibiotics have been effectively used when applied locally to
infected animals, especially in the management of bovine mastitis,
which is commonly of streptococcal origin. The dipping of poultry
and fish carcasses in solutions containing antibiotics has been

employed as a preservative, and also to prevent the transmission of contaminated foods to humans.

The most outstanding use of antibiotics in animals has been to accelerate growth, resulting in increased amounts of animal protein for human consumption and in the addition of millions of dollars to the income of producers of livestock, poultry, and fish. The initial discovery of the potential nutritional value of antibiotics in animals was made in the college of agriculture at the University of Wisconsin in 1946 (Moore et al., 1946). It was noted that when sulfasuxidine or streptomycin was added to the diet of chicks, an accelerated growth rate resulted.

In 1948 a purely "chance experimental finding" by the Lederle group demonstrated that chlortetracycline produced a similar increase in growth of chicks when added to the feed ration (Harned et al., 1948). In the original Lederle studies on the toxicity of duomycin (chlortetracycline) the drug was fed to chicks, and a distinct increase in growth was noted as compared to the untreated controls. They concluded that the drug had eliminated infection. Even though this concept of the effect of the antibiotic on nutrition remained unproved, there was a gradual increase in the use of antibiotics in animal feed for the purpose of preventing infections, especially enteric diseases. There was also a widespread recognition that animals treated in this manner had an accelerated growth rate. T. H. Jukes (1955) summarized the status of antibiotics and nutrition up to 1955.

By 1955 medicated animal feeds had reached such proportions that public health and regulatory officials were apprehensive that the consumption of antibiotic residues in animal foods might have some deleterious effects on human health. In addition more information was needed on the mechanism by which the antibiotics accelerated the growth rate. Two major conferences were held to summarize the known facts and, if necessary, to propose some regulatory action.

The first symposium took place in Washington, D.C. on October 19–21, 1955 under the auspices of the Agricultural Board and the Agriculture Research Institute of the National Academy of Sciences-National Research Council (1956) on the "Use of Antibiotics in Agriculture." The mode of action of antibiotics in stimulating animal growth was again discussed. Several "modes" were suggested but none with definitive proof. There appeared to be some relationship to the antimicrobial action of the antibiotics. I was involved in this symposium as chairman of the session on the "Public Health Aspects" of antibiotics in animal feeds. No substantial evidence was offered that antibiotic residuals in animal products endangered the health of human beings. There was some anxiety that the continued use of antibiotics would lead to the development and dissemination of antibiotic-resistant microbial strains that would afflict human beings, but there was no indication that this had occurred.

The second symposium was sponsored in 1956 by the United States Department of Health, Education and Welfare and by the Food and Drug Administration. This gathering produced several reports, of which the authoritative paper of Whitehair (1956) is pertinent. He summarized the use of penicillin, the tetracyclines, and bacitracin in animal feeds for chickens, turkeys, swine, and calves (bovine). Most outstanding was the increase in growth rate of healthy swine, amounting to 10–20 percent as compared with control groups. There were no demonstrable effects on carcass quality. The mode of action was not clear. C. K. Whitehair concluded (1956, p. 47), "There is much to support the concept that a more nearly 'normal' growth potential is realized because the antibiotics check unknown subclinical infections." Supporting the concept was the fact that "germ-free" animals did not manifest this growth rate. Solid experimental evidence was still lacking for any definitive answer, however.

Continued monitoring took place on the use of antibiotics in animal feeds. A major summary of the subject occurred in 1969 under the auspices of the National Academy of Sciences (1969), the National Research Council, and federal regulatory agencies. There appeared to be more supporting evidence for the concept that the favorable growth effect of the drugs was due to a suppression of subclinical infections. Although apprehension increased over the dissemination of antibiotic-resistant strains of microbes among healthy animals as a result of long-continued use of the drugs, humans did not appear to be affected, either directly or indirectly.

The use of antibiotics in animal feeds has continued with outstanding success for livestock producers. In summarizing the status of this practice Jukes (1973) has pointed out that no significant evidence has been offered that antibiotic residues in the carcasses of treated animals are deleterious to human health or that resistant strains of microorganisms have been disseminated.

The Relationship of Human Infections and Nutrition

Since it was evident that the antibiotics stabilized the health of animals and accelerated growth in the young, many similar studies were undertaken in human beings, which Jukes has also summarized. Interest centered mainly in the developing countries in which malnutrition and infections undermined the health of children. In analyzing the human data Jukes could report only that the administration of antibiotics suggested an improvement of health in the children, but that there were too many complicating factors — such as malnutrition and recurrent, undefined infections — to allow the drawing of definitive conclusions.

The interrelationship of human nutrition and infection has been the subject of international inquiry, particularly with reference to the less developed countries. A symposium in 1955 concluded (Schneider, 1955, p. 314): "It is now more obvious than ever that there is no clear and simple connection between infection and nutrition. . . . we have made but a beginning." Similarly a conference held a little more than a decade later emphasized the very complex nature of the relationship, especially in those areas of the world where malnutrition and infection are so prevalent (Ciba Foundation Study Group No. 31, 1967). And more recently Professor P. C. C. Garnham, a distinguished parasitologist, stated (1971, p. 98), "In order to live, the parasite has to feed, and the principal reason for its adopting the parasitic form of life is that nutriment becomes immediately available from the body of the host. If the host is starved, the parasite suffers from malnutrition, and in conditions of famine of a human population, the virulence of many infectious diseases diminishes. Malaria epidemics lessen, and poorly nourished people or those in the final stages of cancer cannot easily be infected with *Leishmania donovani*." Garnham concluded with specific instances of other deficiency states that actually protect the host against infection.

Further clinical observations have revealed that some human infections are suppressed during periods of starvation and malnutrition (Murray and Murray, 1977). After starving nomadic people in Africa had received relief feeding, latent infections such as malaria, tuberculosis, and brucellosis were converted into active disease. Such observations should have considerable significance in future studies on the relationship of nutrition to infection.

On the other hand, there is accumulating evidence, both experimental and clinical, that there is a synergistic relationship between malnutrition and infectious diseases, especially in infants and young children. That is, a poor state of nutrition leads to more severe infections, and infection accentuates an already compromised nutritional state. The net result of the combination is that severe malnutrition and infection lead to increased mortality rates (Latham, 1975; Mata, 1975; Scrimshaw, Taylor, and Gordon, 1968).

Clearly, if a susceptible population is to be protected against epidemic diseases, strenuous efforts to improve the nutritional status must be made, along with known methods of controlling infectious diseases, which include the availability of clean water, uncontaminated foods, and proper clothing and shelter. To implement this available knowledge toward better health, vast sums of money are necessary. A change toward improved public health took place after 1936 in many areas in the world, not entirely due to the drugs although certainly they had contributed a major part. The dream of Ehrlich, Fleming, and others had almost been fulfilled. The invading parasites had been brought under control with relatively few *severe* toxic effects for the host. Unfortunately, when a drug or drugs are cheap and effective for so many diseases, they are often used indiscriminately. No known drug is without undesirable side effects, and toxic reactions do occur, some of them lethal.

SECTION III

Evolution of Knowledge of Specific Infectious Diseases

CHAPTER 11

The Interpretation of Fever

Fever has been regarded as the sine quo non of infection since the time of Hippocrates, but the true relationship of fever to infection has been understood only in modern times. For two thousand years fever was looked upon not as a part of the symptom complex of an illness, but as the illness itself expressed in many different ways. Until the specific microbial causes of fever were established, physicians tried to classify febrile states on the basis of clinical and epidemiological observations.

For over a thousand years after Hippocrates fever was detected in the patient by the physician through his sense of touch. The daily course of the febrile states was recorded. Each of the "species" appeared to have a definite pattern and its own "crisis." Precise quantitative measurements of fever with the clinical thermometer were not made until the eighteenth century.

The Clinical Thermometer

As with many scientific discoveries, priority for the quantitative measurement of body heat has been shared by several individuals (Allbutt, 1870; Middleton, 1966, 1971; Mitchell, 1892; Woodhead and Varrier-Jones, 1916). Four individuals have been considered the inventors of the thermometer — two in Italy and two north of the Alps (Middleton, 1966). The evidence does not favor the two northerners, Robert Fludd of London or Antonio Drebbel of Holland. Turning to the southerners, although Galileo probably experimented with temperature measurements with his friend Aagredo, credit for the discovery of the thermometer in 1625 should go to the Paduan Professor Sanctorius, known for his quantitative metabolic studies on insensible perspiration. Utilizing open-type glass thermometers with wine as the fluid, Sanctorius measured human temperatures as depicted in Figure 5. Further progress was made by the "Florentine experimenters," who were members of the Accademia del Cimento, especially Ferdinand II of the Medici family. The Florentine spirit-in-glass thermometers were hermetically sealed and similar in design to those produced later, and first appeared around 1654.

The crucial problem in thermometry for the measurement of heat or cold was the lack of standardized instruments. A craftsman for designing dependable thermometers was essential, and such a person eventually appeared. Daniel Gabriel Fahrenheit of Amsterdam, who was probably influenced by the Dutch astronomer Olaus Roemer, selected quicksilver (mercury) as the fluid for his calibrated sealed thermometers. Like his countryman Antony van Leeuwenhoek, inventor of the microscope, he submitted his discovery in brief summaries for publication in the *Transactions of the Royal Society of London* (Fahrenheit, 1724a, b, c, d, e). Fahrenheit's scale had an interval of 180°, with 32° as the freezing point of water, and 212° as the boiling point. Mercury was the ideal fluid when contained in instruments because it withstood extreme degrees of heat and cold.

Other scales were proposed after Fahrenheit's. The most enduring was the centigrade scale. Credit for the centigrade thermometer has been given to Anders Celsius, professor of astronomy in Uppsala. In contrast to Fahrenheit, Celsius selected an interval of 100° between the freezing and boiling points of water. It is of interest that the botanist Carl Linnaeus, also professor of medicine at Uppsala, was a close friend of Celsius and used thermometry in his greenhouse.

The Dutch instrument makers quickly prepared standardized thermometers for wide distribution. Fahrenheit's instrument was generally accepted, but not in France, where the centigrade thermometers were used. Fahrenheit was a friend of Professor Herman Boerhaave at Leyden, and his clinical thermometer was employed by the latter's pupils Gerard van Swieten and Anton de

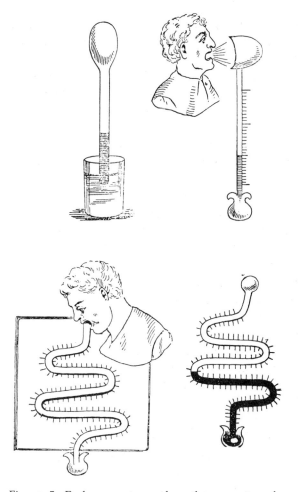

Figure 5. Early open-type glass thermometers for measuring human temperatures. Reproduced from S. Weir Mitchell, "The Early History of Instrumental Precision in Medicine," *Transactions of the Congress of American Physicans and Surgeons* 2:159, 1892 (composite of Figure 2, p. 166, Figure 7, p. 170, Figure 9, p. 172, and Figure 10, p. 173).

Haen. According to Wunderlich, "to de Haen, of Vienna, belongs the honor of having introduced thermometry in the practice and teaching of medicine" (Wunderlich and Seguin, 1871, p. 1).

Perhaps the first scientific investigation on the subject was that carried out by Dr. George Martine (1740). The versatile John Hunter (1778) became interested in body heat, and in a burst of energy measured the temperatures of a wide range of animals, rodents, fish, vegetables, and trees. Always resourceful, Hunter had a Mr. Ramsden produce a mercury thermometer five to seven inches long and 1/6th of an inch thick, with a bulb on the end. The freezing point was marked, and a small ivory scale was used that could slide and retain its position. Also with the aid of Ramsden, Dr. James Currie (1798) of Liverpool advocated the use of the thermometer in clinical medicine, but this suggestion was met with little enthusiasm.

Just as the discovery of the microscope by Leeuwenhoek had to wait two hundred years for its application to medical science, the clinical use of the thermometer did not come about for almost a hundred years. "During the whole of the first four decades of the nineteenth century, . . . the observations made on the temperature of the human body under varying conditions were but scanty" (Woodhead and Varrier-Jones, 1916, p. 175). Perhaps the clinician's reluctance to take precise thermometry seriously was due to the fact that the cause of fever was still unknown; even if measurements were made on humans, what further therapy could be offered the patient? Medicine was greatly benefited by the extensive observation on human thermometry by Professor C. A. Wunderlich of Leipzig, who made literally millions of temperature readings on sick and healthy subjects over a period of seventeen years and in 1871 published his findings on the value of such practice (Wunderlich, 1871). Wunderlich's study coincided with the discoveries of the microbial causes of disease and with scientific investigations on the nature of body heat. Henceforth the recording of the temperature and of the pulse and respiratory rates rapidly became routine in medical practice.

By the mid-nineteenth century measuring the patient's temperature was acceptable practice in Europe and in England. Even in the wilds of Africa, Dr. David Livingstone was determining the temperature of patients, and when he himself contracted the "African fever" (malaria) in 1853 he stated that his temperature varied from 100° to

103° F. (Livingstone, 1857). In American medicine, on the other hand, the use of the thermometer lagged almost incredibly. During the Civil War (1861–1865) the recording of body temperatures was not a routine procedure in the United States Army. Doctor W. W. Keen, professor of surgery at Jefferson Medical College, was a medical officer in the Union Army, and subsequently wrote that no clinical thermometers were available. "Our only means of estimating fever was by touch. It was not until several years after the war . . . that the thermometer became a common instrument. It was then about from ten to twelve inches long, was never used excepting in the axilla, from which it stuck up like a mast, and was often broken by movements of the patient or pressure of the bed-clothes. The first short clinical thermometer, such as we now have, which I ever saw was a gift from my friend, Dr. S. Weir Mitchell,[1] brought from London in 1876" (Keen, 1905, p. 109).

Concepts of Fever

But the most sophisticated techniques for measuring body temperature could be of little benefit medically without some concept of the nature of fever. In early periods physicians merely attempted to classify fevers on the basis of clinical observations. The Greeks described individual cases of representative fevers. In the seventeenth century Sydenham attempted to classify each type of fever in relation to epidemics. Even during the first half of the nineteenth century progress in the clinical understanding of fever was painfully slow. This is revealed in the concepts held by Dr. Thomas Southwood Smith of London. He was recognized as an authority on fever in 1824 when he became physician to the London Fever Hospital. This institution, with a capacity for sixty-two patients, cared for six to seven hundred seriously ill patients a year. Out of this clinical experience came Smith's volume on fever, in which he postulated that it was a genus with several different species (Smith, 1835). Two prominent features of all fever, according to Smith, were a derangement of the nervous system followed by inflammatory localization in an organ or organs. He described the clinical and pathological findings of cases with cerebral, thoracic, and abdominal localization, and "mixed cases." His classification was confusing and his interpretations were opaque.

One of the most influential physicians toward the end of the nineteenth century was Dr. Charles Murchison, who was president of the Edinburgh Royal Society and had succeeded Southwood Smith as senior physician of the London Fever Hospital. In his volume on fevers (1862) Murchison distinguished continued fevers from eruptive fevers, such as those associated with childhood diseases and with smallpox and syphilis, and from intermittent and remittent fevers, such as that accompanying malaria. Murchison believed the continued fevers were not contagious, reasoning that agues and other malarious fevers which had caused the deaths of Cromwell and James I two hundred years earlier had disappeared following the drainage and cultivation of swamps. Plague had subsided in 1666 due to the improved construction of buildings after the great fire.

The first step in fever, according to Murchison, was the entrance of an unknown poison into the blood, followed by a "paralysis" of the nervous system, especially of the vagus and the sympathetic nerves. Here he reflected the influence of the physiologist Claude Bernard. Then a retrograde metamorphosis (metabolism) of the muscles and other tissues occurred, in which no fresh material was assimilated to compensate for the loss, resulting in an increase in fever and loss of weight. Destruction of the tissues was accompanied by an accelerated heart rate. The nonelimination of the products of tissue metamorphosis caused cerebral symptoms and inflammation, leading to a termination of the progress of deterioration at a "definite time in different fevers," the cause of which was unknown. This was termed a crisis, as first described by Hippocrates. The "fever poison" and the products of tissue-metamorphosis were then eliminated. The nervous system resumed normal function, and undue consumption of the tissues was checked. The patient in turn regained weight and strength.

Understanding of fever was furthered in the nineteenth century through the development of experimental calorimetry for the precise measurement of heat production and loss. It had been established clinically and experimentally that excessively high body temperatures followed severance of the cervical cord and traumatic lesions of the brain unrelated to any infection. Also, some persons exposed to unusually high temperatures in their immediate environment would suffer heat stroke and death. The fever was clearly due to a disturbance of the nervous system in the regulation of body heat. One of the most extensive pioneering studies in calorimetry was carried out by Professor H. C. Wood (1881) of the medical faculty of the University of Pennsylvania. Following an incredibly large number of experiments emphasizing the use of the calorimeter for inducing and measuring heat produced and lost in a variety of animals, he corroborated the general belief that fever was due primarily to a disturbance in the central nervous system. However, he still adhered to the belief that fever per se was the cause of the systemic manifestations rather than a symptom of a complex series of metabolic events related to a disturbance in the central nervous system.

Calorimetry continued to advance knowledge on the regulation of body temperature in the twentieth century. The physiologist Professor Eugene DuBois (1948) at Cornell University Medical College summarized the studies in many laboratories, including those of his own and others at the Russell Sage Institute of Pathology. Heating and ventilating engineers supported basic investigations, such as those at the John B. Pierce Laboratory of Hygiene at New Haven (Winslow and Herrington, 1949). Major advances were made during World War II.

But what was the precise relationship between fever and infection? It is difficult to pinpoint the individual or individuals who first clarified this relationship, but no one spoke or wrote more convincingly on the basis of scientific evidence than Dr. William H. Welch, professor of pathology and later dean of the medical school of Johns Hopkins University. After studying basic science in Germany, he returned to the United States and breathed a new spirit of scientific inquiry into medicine. The clarity of his thinking is evident in his Cartwright Lectures on fever (Welch, 1888).

In his introduction Welch stated (p. 365), "The history of opinion regarding fever is in great part the history of medicine itself, for no feature of the great systems of medicine from Hippocrates and Galen to the present century so characterizes these systems as the views held concerning the nature of fever." He based his three lectures on the behavior of heat production, on heat loss, and on the regulating of fever, reviewing the extensive metabolic and physiological studies on heat production and loss carried out in the major laboratories of Europe, especially those in Germany. Welch referred to the important observations of Claude Bernard on the neurogenic regulation of body heat, and concluded that the harmonious regulation of heat production and heat loss resided in the nervous system. After citing the work of others he carried out experiments with indirect calorimetry on rabbits and believed that all of the bodily functions are disturbed by fever.

But the incisive thinking of Welch was projected beyond the physiological responses to fever; he wanted to know the cause of the febrile response, especially in infection. His most outstanding experiment was the intravenous injection of killed typhoid bacilli into rabbits, which not only provoked chills and high temperatures, but also resulted in death. Welch stated that the febrile reaction "depended directly upon affections of the nervous system" (p. 567). He expressed concern over "catheter or urethral fever," but did not know the cause. This problem was to be answered in the succeeding century by the explorations of others. Welch correctly related infection to fever when he concluded that fever was a response to saphrophytic and pathogenic microorganisms and their products.

Progress in understanding the pathogenesis of fever in infectious diseases gained little momentum in the twentieth century until the close of World War II. Most of the studies on heat production and loss were carried out in physiological laboratories, and the experimental model was based on indirect calorimetry. Major advances in knowledge about fever caused by infection were made by Dr. Paul Beeson at Yale and Dr. W. Barry Wood at Johns Hopkins along with their associates (Atkins, 1960). By 1950 a major textbook of medicine contained a substantial section by Beeson on the pathogenesis of fever, including the response to infection. All causes of fever were described under the general heading of "Reaction to Injury" (Beeson, Wintrobe, and Jager, 1950), which besides infections included vascular accidents, neoplasms, hemolytic crises, and trauma. Textbooks of physiology also began to contain formidable discussions of the control of body temperature and the alterations in temperature.

The remaining question was that of the underlying mechanism or mechanisms responsible for fever in infectious diseases. It had been fairly well established in the foregoing studies that pyrogens acted upon the anterior hypothalamus. The problem was clarified by the studies of W. Feldberg (1975), who concluded that microbial pyrogen (endotoxin or lipid A) releases E prostaglandins into the cerebrospinal fluid, causing fever by direct action upon the thermoregulatory area of the hypothalamus. Substantial evidence indicates that antipyretic agents abolish or decrease fever by inhibiting prostaglandin synthesis. The milieu intérieur in the hypothalamus is also governed by calcium ion concentrations.

By the twentieth century fever was interpreted as a nonspecific derangement of bodily heat regulation induced through stimulation of the central nervous system. The most common inciting cause is an infection in which pyrogens are released from the tissues and act upon the hypothalamic region. Other causes of tissue disturbance and inflammation that result in fever are cerebral hemorrhage, cancer and heat stroke. The differential diagnosis of fever, which is a symptom of disease and not the cause, constitutes a frequent challenge to physicians.

CHAPTER 12

Epidemic Diseases
Subject to Maritime Control

Plague [1]

At the beginning of the twentieth century six epidemic diseases were subject to maritime quarantine. These were plague, smallpox, typhus, yellow fever, cholera, and leprosy. The diseases not only caused severe loss of life, but they disrupted the social and economic order of the afflicted communities and states. Plague in particular filled people with fear and terror, stimulating medical historians and others to produce an extensive literature on the subject. Two recent students of plague were Dr. R. Pollitzer (1954), a bacteriologist with the Manchurian Plague Prevention Service who wrote a volume on the subject for the World Health Organization, and Dr. Karl F. Meyer, director of the Hooper Foundation of the University of California in San Francisco, who served in many capacities in the broad field of infectious diseases as a consultant at national and international levels. In the preparation of this section on plague, I obtained information from each of these authorities in personal discussions.

In an unscientific age when epidemics of plague struck whole populations suddenly with high mortality rates, often concurrently with severe climatic changes, droughts, famine, and war, the suffering of the people was looked upon as a visitation from an angry deity. Although the cause and mode of transmission were unknown, contagion must have been suspected, because the first quarantine laws against plague were invoked in the fourteenth century in Italy, and throngs of people left the cities for rural areas.

The cause of plague, *Pasteurella pestis*, was first discovered in 1894 by Dr. Alexandre Yersin (1894) of the Pasteur Institute while working with the Manchurian Plague Commission. Portions of Yersin's historic findings as related in his diary have been recorded by his assistant (Lagrange, 1926). Alexander Rennie (1894) implicated the rat in the transmission of the disease to man, and Mansanori Ogata (1897) described the flea (*Xenopsylla cheopis*) as the vector.

Possessed of these modern scientific facts, we are able to reconstruct the course of plague in the past. During the Middle Ages, rats (*Mus norwegicus* and *M. rattus*) harboring the *X. cheopis* fleas normally fed in the fields and woods, but in times of famine and drought they invaded communities and entered the dwellings of man in search of food. Plague was maintained in endemic form in rats by the passage of infected fleas from rat to rat. Infected rats boarded ships in harbors where plague was prevalent and on arrival in a new land scuttled ashore, entering buildings in their search for food and spreading disease in the process. At the beginning of an epidemic the disease was spread from rats to fleas and thence by fleas to man. After an epidemic was well under way plague was spread directly from man to man through the air because of pneumonia, giving rise to the term "pneumonic plague." In addition viable plague bacilli could become sequestered in the bed clothing and personal belongings of the deceased, providing another reservoir. One of the first visible manifestations of an oncoming epidemic of plague was the appearance of dead rats, victims of the disease, in the buildings and streets of a seaport. In his modern novel relating to plague, Albert Camus wrote (1948, p. 12), "Jean Tarron was gazing down at the convulsions of a rat dying on the step in front of him. He looked up, and his gray eyes remained fixed on the doctor for some moments; then after wishing him a good day, he remarked that it was rather odd, the way all these rats were coming out of their holes to die."

The disease was manifested in humans by an abrupt onset of fever and prominent swelling of lymph glands in the axillae and groin.

Hence the appellation "bubonic plague," the swollen glands being known as "buboes." In a severe case hemorrhagic areas of the skin appeared, which darkened before death; for this reason the disease was known as the "Black Death." When an epidemic of plague intensified, more and more instances of lethal pneumonia were encountered. Because of the expectoration of sputum laden with plague bacilli the immediate environment was contaminated.

A pandemic of historical interest is that of 1346–1350, which spread throughout Europe and was known as the "Black Death." A second invasion of plague had devastating effects in the seventeenth century. The historical aspects of these pandemics and the introduction of quarantine as a method of control are discussed in Section I, Chapter 1.

There are many classical literary writings on plague, some historically accurate, others fictional, and many a combination of both. The Greek historian Thucydides (1954) is often credited — probably inaccurately — with presenting the first description of plague occurring in 432 B.C. in Athens when Pericles was defending the city. It is more likely that he described typhus and possibly typhoid. Perhaps the first description of plague was in the year 320 B.C. as recorded in the first Book of Samuel in the Old Testament of the Bible. The Philistines had captured the Ark of God from the Israelites and brought it to Ashod. And we read (1 Samuel 5:6), "Then the Lord laid a heavy hand upon the people of Ashod; he threw them into distress and plagued them with tumors, and their territory swarmed with rats."

In 1348 A.D. plague wiped out three of every four persons in Florence. It is at this time that Giovanni Boccaccio (1930) set his famous story in a villa at nearby Fiesole to which people had fled for protection. And there, according to Boccaccio (1930, p. vi), "I intend to relate one hundred tales or fables or parables or stories — whichever you choose to call them — as they were told in ten days by a band of seven ladies and three young men during the time of the recent plague."

Daniel Defoe (1908) described the visit of plague in London during the seventeenth century, not as an eyewitness, but from what he had read and heard. Three eyewitnesses of the plague in London did immortalize their observations in their writings. One was the ubiquitous and unbridled Samuel Pepys (1926) in his diary. Pepys was close to the aristocracy of the Court, and he remained in London through-out the epidemic. Thus on July 20, 1665 he wrote (1926, vol. 5, p. 19), "So walked to Redriffe, where I hear the sickness is, and is indeed scattered almost every where, there dying 1089 of the plague this week. My Lady Carteret did this day give me a bottle of plague-water home with me." And on July 25th (p. 24), "This day my Lord Bunder did give me Mr. Grant's (sic) book upon the Bills of Mortality, new printed and enlarged." Pepys examined carefully the Bills of Mortality issued every week as he noted on August 10th (p. 39), "in great trouble to see the Bill this week rise so high, to above 4000 in all, and of them 3,000 of the plague." He concluded his notation for one day (p. 40), "home to draw over anew my will; the town growing so unhealthy, that a man cannot depend upon living two days to an end. So having done something of it, to bed."

A second layman who observed the London plague was the diarist John Evelyn. On September 7, 1665, he wrote (De Beer, 1955, p. 417), "I went all along the Citty and suburbs from *Kent streete* to St. *James's*, a dismal passage and dangerous, to see many Cofines exposed in the streetes and the streete thin of people, the shops shut up, and all in mournefull silence, as not knowing whose turne might be next."

A third eyewitness in London, William Boghurst, was an apothe-cary, or general medical practitioner, who treated up to sixty plague victims daily. He wrote a small tract on the disease and advertised his remedies of water, a lozenge, and an electuary antidote (Boghurst, 1893–1894). He also reviewed the various concoctions of the day gen-erally used in treatment, presented a history of plague, and cited his meticulous clinical observations.

Boghurst did review certain historical aspects of plague and de-scribed the natural history of the disease on the basis of his obser-vations. His treatments were long presentations of concoctions of various chemicals, herbs, portions of animals, seeds, fruits, gums, etc., thus consistent with usual pharmacopoea of the time in medical practice. After an exposition on the causes of plague he concluded with this definition of the disease (p. 19): "The Plague is the perfection of putrefaction, or if you like it better in more words, thus: — The Plague or Pestilence is a most subtle, peculiar, insinuating, venom-ous, deleterious, Exhalation arising from the maturation of the fer-ment of the Foeces of the Earth extracted into the Aire by the heat of the sun, and difflated from place to place by the winds, and most tymes gradually but sometymes immediately aggressing apt bodyes."

The third and last pandemic of plague occurred between 1894 and 1920, originating in the province of Yunnan in China and spreading with fury into India. During the early part of this pandemic valuable scientific information on the cause and epidemiology of plague was acquired in Bombay (India. Plague Advisory Commission, 1906–1917), and in China (Lien-Teh, 1926; Lien-Teh et al., 1936). During this period the bacterial etiology (*Yersinia pestis*) of the disease was discovered and extensive research in animals made possible on the pathology and epidemiology of the disease. The rat was found to be the reservoir for plague and the disease propagated among these rodents by the rat flea (*Xenopsylla cheopis*). Extensive epidemiologic investigations revealed that the disease was naturally transmitted to humans through two pathways. First, the plague bacillus was carried from the rat reservoir to man through the bites of infected rat fleas, resulting in bubonic plague. Second, as the pandemic intensified the serious form of pneumonic human plague occurred, and transmission of the plague bacillus from human to human resulted from airborne transmission. It was these basic findings that contributed to the future prevention and treatment of plague.

The first epidemic of human plague in the United States occurred in 1900 in the port city of San Francisco (Link, 1955). Control measures were hampered initially by the lack of knowledge on the spread of the disease. The rat-flea concept would not be generally accepted until after the work of the Commission for the Investigation of Plague in India in 1905–1916. The second epidemic struck San Francisco in 1907 after a fire had swept the community. There was bitter opposition against federal and state quarantine regulations, but the activities of politicians to thwart this effort were finally overcome by courageous and qualified health officers. Subsequent outbreaks occurred in the ports of Seattle, New Orleans, Los Angeles, Hawaii, and Puerto Rico.

An unusual case of plague that occurred during the 1900 San Francisco epidemic is cited by V. B. Link (1955). Doctor F. G. Novy, a well-known microbiologist at the University of Michigan, was a member of the Plague Commission at the time. Dr. Novy carried back to Ann Arbor a culture of plague bacillus and had a medical student prepare Haffkine's vaccine and serum for him. In the process the student contracted pneumonic plague, from which he recovered. Link concluded by stating (1955, p. 6): "His was the first laboratory infection, the first and only case of plague ever reported in Michigan, the first case in the United States outside of California, the first reported recovery from plague, and the first reported pneumonic plague recovery in the country."

Plague continues to exist in wild rodents (sylvatic plague) in the western states. It is a tribute to the constant efforts of public health authorities at all levels that there were only 523 cases of recognized plague in the United States between 1900 and 1951 (Link, 1955). Although the incidence of the human disease is small, protection has resulted from constant surveillance of the disease in animals and from the application of epidemiological and prophylactic measures when human illness does occur.[2]

A constant surveillance of epizootic plague in wildlife is now maintained in the United States by the Center for Disease Control with headquarters in Fort Collins, Colorado. The first report appeared in July, 1970 (Center for Disease Control, 1970). There is always the threat of urban plague from rat sources, as demonstrated in 1964 when plague transmitted by meadow voles invaded the population of Norway rats near San Francisco. Prompt control measures eliminated this focus. In 1968 a six-year-old girl contracted nonfatal plague in urban Denver. An epizootic of plague was found in tree squirrels (*Sciurus niger*) within the limits of the city. Of 272 dead squirrels, 52 were found to have positive serology for plague, and plague bacilli were isolated from 15 of these (National Communicable Disease Center, 1968). No other mammals were found to be infected. Intensive control measures were carried out against the squirrels, and no further human cases were reported.[3]

Human cases in the western rural areas continue as a menacing problem. The disease has afflicted campers, hunters, and Navajo Indians. From 1908 through 1969 there were 127 cases of human plague with 67 deaths (53 percent), mostly in rural areas, the sources of which were wild animals (Center for Disease Control, 1970). Known reservoirs of the disease were prairie dogs (*Cynomys gunnisoni*), rabbits, fox squirrels, chipmunks, and deer mice. There was a rise in the number of human cases from 1969 through 1973, with 56 cases and 12 deaths (21 percent). The lower mortality rate is attributable to prompt recognition and antibiotic therapy. A review of bubonic plague in the southwestern United States, especially in New Mexico, involved 31 cases in the decade 1960–1969 (Reed et al., 1970).

Plague has not been eradicated as a threat to human health, but the disease has been confined to epizootic areas by constant surveillance through international agreement. No recurrence of pandemic plague has occurred since the third pandemic. The spread of plague from its natural reservoirs has been prevented by breaking the mode of transmission from rodents to humans. Seaports are safely guarded against the debarkation of rats from ships arriving from areas where human plague exists. Ships also have been rat-proofed. Insecticides, including DDT, have been used for destroying the fleas as vectors of the disease. Constant efforts are made to exterminate rats in urban areas, and also to remove the sources of food for the rodents. A continual alert for outbreaks is maintained by the World Health Organization and its expert committee members (World Health Organization Expert Committee on Plague, 1970).

Ever since the discovery of the plague bacillus in 1894 attempts have been made to prepare and use a prophylactic vaccine for humans. Millions of persons over a period of several years were inoculated with vaccines produced from killed cultures with doubtful results. In more recent years live vaccines from attenuated cultures have been investigated, as well as chemical extracts. After more than fifty years of evaluation it is generally agreed that vaccination for plague gives only a short-lived and partial protection against the disease.

In 1939 the white mouse was found to be highly susceptible to plague, and thus provided an experimental animal model for evaluating chemotherapy and serotherapy. Extensive studies were carried out subsequently, especially at the Hooper Foundation, University of California, San Francisco under the direction of Dr. Karl F. Meyer (Meyer et al., 1952). After further evaluation in human cases, streptomycin and tetracycline have proved to be valuable drugs in the treatment of plague, particularly if therapy is initiated early in the illness.

Smallpox (Variola)[4]

In 1815 James Moore, an English surgeon, dedicated a volume on smallpox to his friend Edward Jenner, praising him for his discovery and also tracing the history of smallpox (Moore, 1815). I have described Jenner's contribution of vaccination in Section I, Chapter 1. Moore pointed out that smallpox and measles were known in "remote antiquity in China and Hindoostan," and gradually spread westward. About 910 A.D. measles was differentiated from smallpox by the Arabian physician Rhazes (translation 1847 and 1939). It is difficult to ascertain when smallpox was introduced into Europe, but it is possible that the disease accompanied invaders from the East into the Mediterranean countries as far as Spain. Smallpox is a systemic illness, usually recognized by the skin lesions, the eruption closely resembling that of varicella (chickenpox), measles (rubeola), and syphilis. A distinguishing feature of smallpox is the facial scarring of the skin upon recovery. C. Creighton (1891a; 1894a) confirmed Moore's statements by concluding that smallpox was a relatively uncommon disease in England, and probably in Europe, until the sixteenth century. There is more definite evidence that smallpox existed in epidemic form during the seventeenth century in England and on the continent as a coincidental accompaniment of the plague. This evidence is based on the Bills of Mortality in England, which date from 1629. The disease afflicted all ages and classes. A brother and sister of Charles II, and Queen Mary II, wife of William III, all died of smallpox.

Eventually smallpox was spread to the New World, being introduced into the Caribbean area, and probably into Mexico, by European adventurers during the sixteenth century. During the seventeenth century widespread epidemics occurred in the Indians toward the North. Jesuits from France witnessed the extensive epidemics among Indians in North America and recorded their findings in reports and journals (Stearn and Stearn, 1945). George Catlin (1841), an early student of Indians, lamented over the fate of millions of these people who succumbed to smallpox, warfare, and whiskey.

The introduction of vaccination into the American colonies, especially into Massachusetts, made it increasingly apparent that this was the most effective way to control smallpox. An examination of comparative data between Massachusetts and Minnesota in the twentieth century underscores the importance of vaccination clearly. Massachusetts always had a highly enlightened and well-directed public health program. In 1855 the state made it compulsory for every child attending school to be vaccinated, and by 1872 the law was strictly enforced (White, 1924). In 1904 vaccine was standardized and distributed in the state without a charge. As a result smallpox became and remained a rare disease in Massachusetts. My own medical education extended from 1928 to 1937 in Boston, and during that period I never saw a case of smallpox.

Minnesota also had vigorous leadership in public health, but the independent citizen protected his right to make his own choice regarding vaccination, and Minnesota has never required smallpox vaccination for school children. The result was that a susceptible population awaited the disease. A catastrophe struck Minnesota in 1924 during the pre-Christmas holiday season. A man with variola major, or classic malignant smallpox, had entered the state at its northern boundary from Canada the previous January, causing an epidemic in Duluth, located at the head of Lake Superior. In February sporadic cases began to appear in Minneapolis and St. Paul, with increasing frequency during the following months. By December the published reports of the disease had started a storm of protest in the Twin Cities, due to an undesirable effect of news reports on the Christmas trade in the stores. There ensued a severe attack on the Minnesota Department of Health, and the removal of the director, Dr. A. J. Chesley, was urgently demanded. At that time Professor Benjamin White (1924) of Harvard wrote a small volume on vaccination. He extolled the excellent results from vaccination in Massachusetts and deplored the negligence in Minnesota. A screaming newspaper headline in Minneapolis stated that Dr. White should be sued for libel because he claimed the governor of the state held personal liberty higher than the common good and chose to suffer smallpox rather than to submit to compulsory vaccination. During 1924 and 1925 Minnesota had a total of 4,098 cases of smallpox with 505 deaths, while Massachusetts had only 15 cases and 2 deaths. But the antivaccinationists triumphed, and smallpox was to continue as a serious threat for more than a decade. When I joined the medical faculty of the University of Minnesota in 1937 with the responsibility of teaching infectious diseases, I still had never seen a case of smallpox. After 1937 I had ample opportunity to see patients with smallpox at the Minneapolis General Hospital. Then voluntary vaccination became more widely accepted, and not a single case was reported in the state from 1948 to 1976. The decrease in incidence was probably related to the general acceptance of vaccination.

Although vaccination provided a highly effective means for controlling smallpox, the disease continued to be a serious threat on a worldwide basis. In the twentieth century the appearance of a milder type of illness in many epidemics led to a distinction between the two clinical forms of the disease. The milder form became known as alastrim, or variola minor, and the classic type was called variola major. The milder form is a much less serious disease and carries a low mortality rate. The common appearance of the milder disease is due either to an attenuation in virulence of the virus or to partial immunity in previously vaccinated individuals. The two types are distinct, but both forms have occurred at the same time in severe epidemics.

As recently as 1930 England and Wales recorded twelve thousand cases of smallpox and the United States over forty-eight thousand (Henderson, 1973). Most of these were of the milder type, but elsewhere in Asia, Africa, and South America severe epidemics occurred. In 1959 the World Health Organization agreed on a global eradication program and intensified these efforts in 1967. Remarkable progress has been made largely due to three factors — the use of a potent freeze-dried vaccine, the surveillance of sample populations to detect the performance of vaccination, and mass vaccination programs based upon precise epidemiological data. Doctor Donald Henderson, who has headed the WHO Eradication Program, was so encouraged by the cooperative effort up to 1973 that he was moved to state (1973, p. 499), "It would seem, however, not unreasonable to anticipate that sometime in 1974, a milestone in medical history could be reached, the occurrence of the last case of smallpox."

This was a realistic conclusion since in January 1974 smallpox was endemic in only four countries, Bangladesh, Northern India, Pakistan, and Ethiopia, but the goal had not yet been reached. The disease has still persisted into 1977. In 1973 there was a total of only 132,339 cases in the world reported to WHO. The eradication of a major epidemic disease of human beings would be a public health triumph. "The remarkable progress so far attained is a tribute to what may be achieved by true international co-operation"[5] (Smallpox Editorial, 1974, p. 296).

Yellow Fever

This epidemic disease originated in West Africa (Carter, 1931); it spread to the Americas but never appeared in Asia. The disease was first recognized in Yucatan in 1648, having entered from Africa probably through the slave trade. There is no evidence that yellow fever was present during the visits of Columbus. Epidemics had occurred in the Caribbean islands in 1648 and 1649, and from this area the disease was introduced into the colonies of North America with devastating results. The illness could be mild, but mortality rates up to 85 percent occurred.

The recognized clinical pattern of the recurring epidemics was fever, severe vomiting (often bloody), a yellow skin, and death. Although the main medical problem up to 1793 in the colonies was smallpox, epidemics of yellow fever occurred in New York in 1668, in Boston in 1691–1693, and in Philadelphia and in Charleston, South Carolina in 1699. It is probable that the source of yellow fever was the Barbados, where epidemics appeared in 1647–1648. Recurrent epidemics culminated in a severe form of the disease in Philadelphia in 1793, the terror of which has been vividly described (Powell, 1949). The clinical observations were ably recorded by Benjamin Rush (1794). Many of the colonists held a concept of contagion in the genesis of yellow fever; their main thrust against the disease was that of embargo, particularly against ships arriving from the West Indies. It was the presence of yellow fever in the Barbados that resulted in the first quarantine law of Massachusetts in 1647–1648 (Blake, 1959). On August 19, 1793 Benjamin Rush declared the presence of yellow fever in Philadelphia. Boston immediately enforced strict quarantine by land and sea. In 1794 the citizens of Baltimore and New Haven fell victims, and New York City was severely stricken in 1795. By 1804 yellow fever had moved north to Portsmouth, Newburyport, Providence, and New London.

Because the mode of transmission could not be defined, battle lines were drawn up between the two groups, the contagionists and the anticontagionists, concerning the nature of the disease. This conflict permeated epidemiological thinking during the following century. The contagionists believed that the disease was imported, not indigenous, and that strict quarantine on water fronts was essential. The anticontagionists thought that unusual seasonable atmospheres were responsible and that improved sanitary measures were the proper approach. This epidemiological warfare persisted for decades with respect to yellow fever and to other epidemic diseases as well, with each side contributing to the eventual control of these diseases.

The anticontagionists fostered better public sanitation and improved water supplies. By 1795 Boston was the first city of size to have an aqueduct transmitting clean water. The community also cleared away the putrefying fish and animal refuse from the wharves. Nevertheless yellow fever struck the city in 1798. Through the simultaneous efforts of the contagionists, strict quarantine legislation was brought to bear on the problem.

During the frightful yellow fever epidemic of 1793 in Philadelphia the influential Rush, siding with the anticontagionists, stated that the disease was not imported, but rather that it originated from vegetable putrefaction along the wharves, especially from rotting coffee. On his advice attempts were made to clean up the filth along the wharves. But as the summer wore on the epidemic continued unabated.

Both the physicians and the citizens of Philadelphia were desperate in their search for protection against the infection. A strong garlic breath was recommended. People wore tar ropes around their necks to ward off the disease. They applied vinegar copiously around their houses and held vinegar sponges to their mouths and noses while walking through the streets. Finally, they shot cannon off in the streets and burned gunpowder in their houses.

In such a time of fear and ignorance any authoritative voice could catch the ears of the afflicted. Benjamin Rush was the best known physician at the time and a leading citizen, having signed the Declaration of Independence in 1776. He was besieged on every side for his medical services. The demands for his personal attention were excessive and beyond his ability to fulfill. He widely publicized his therapy of purging and bleeding (Section I, Chapter 1).

Another astute observer of the Philadelphia epidemic of 1793 was

Dr. J. Dévèze (1794), who had had experience with yellow fever in the Caribbean prior to his migration to Philadelphia. During the height of the epidemic it became apparent to the city government that an infirmary for yellow fever was necessary to house the ill, especially the poor, who could not afford medical attention. An old mansion on the edge of the city — Bush Hall — was selected, and Dr. Dévèze was appointed to direct the medical care of the patients. With loyal attendants and devoted assistants he worked under very difficult circumstances. Unfortunately many of the patients were in extremis when they arrived at the institution, and the mortality rate was high. Dévèze believed that yellow fever was not imported, that it was not contagious, but that it was due to a local miasma in the air and was related to the weather. He reasoned that the infection could not be contagious because at Bush Hall it was noted that attendants handling the sick and dying and disposing of soiled clothing and linen did not acquire the disease, an observation confirmed by Walter Reed and his associates a century later. Furthermore patients who were admitted to the infirmary and who were suffering from some other disease did not acquire yellow fever. Dévèze's therapeutic regime was temperate and largely supportive, and he was conservative in bleeding and purging.

Amidst the many professional disputes concerning the causes and treatment of yellow fever in the 1793 epidemic, one very significant contribution by an anonymous writer appeared in the *American Daily Advertiser* on August 29th of that year (Middleton, 1928, p. 440):

As the late rains will produce a great increase of mosquitoes in the city, distressing to the sick, and troublesome to those who are well, I imagine it will be agreeable to the citizens to know that the increase of those poisonous insects may be much diminished by a very simple and cheap mode, which accident discovered. Whoever will take the trouble to examine their rain-water tubs, will find millions of the mosquitoes fishing about the water with great agility, in a state not quite prepared to emerge and fly off: Take up a wine glass full of the water, and it will exhibit them very distinctly. Into this glass pour half a teaspoon full, or less, of any common oil, which will quickly diffuse over the surface, by excluding the air, will destroy the whole brood. Some will survive two or three days but most of them sink to the bottom, or adhere to the oil on the surface within twenty-four hours. A gill of oil poured into a common rain-water cask, will be sufficient:

large cisterns may require more; and where the water is drawn out by a pump or by a cock, the oil will remain undisturbed, and last for a considerable time. Hickory ashes have been tried without effect.

Consider the millions of lives and the human misery that could have been spared if this prophylactic advice could have been followed. A century was to pass before medical science recognized this approach.

All during the eighteenth and nineteenth centuries yellow fever harassed the ports along the Atlantic seaboard and the rivers, especially the Mississippi. New Orleans was afflicted. An epidemic in 1878 practically decimated the city of Memphis (Keating, 1879). The loss of life was great, and the survivors left the community. This epidemic seemed particularly harsh to the people at this time because it followed an economic depression in the country.

When the nineteenth century came to an end the enigma of yellow fever remained. The disease was feared, the cause was unknown, and the mode of spread unclear. And then the solution to the mystery of yellow fever unfolded in a series of brilliant achievements by a small group of courageous and dedicated members of the United States Army Medical Department. Within the first half of the twentieth century the cause of yellow fever was discovered, the epidemiological factors were established, and a successful prophylactic vaccine became available. Toward this end the International Health Division of the Rockefeller Foundation played a significant part (Strode, 1951).

The Spanish-American War in 1898 lasted 118 days, and a frightful toll of human health and life by typhoid fever and yellow fever in American military personnel in Cuba was exacted in this brief campaign, far beyond the lives lost in battle. Fortunately the surgeon-general of the army was a pioneer bacteriologist, Dr. George M. Sternberg. In 1900 General Sternberg dispatched an Army board to Cuba to investigate yellow fever in the American occupying troops. This board consisted of Major Walter Reed, James Carroll, Aristides Agramonte, and Jesse W. Lazear, all physicians. At the same time Major William C. Gorgas, later General Gorgas of Panama Canal fame, was the chief sanitary officer of Havana. It was this small group of men that removed much of the fear that surrounded yellow fever. Reed, whose story has been warmly told by Dr. Howard Kelly (1906), had studied under Dr. William H. Welch at Johns Hopkins. He also was a member of the Typhoid Board (Reed, Vaughan, and Shake-speare, 1900).

When Reed and his men arrived in Cuba they were in possession of a few, but valuable, epidemiological facts relating to yellow fever. They knew that Dr. Josiah Nott of South Carolina had published a report (1848), based on his own observations, on the *probable* trans-mission of yellow fever by small "animalcules." But most important, they were aided by the presence in Havana of the physician Dr. Carlos J. Finlay, who had made careful scientific observations on yellow fever and had concluded that a species of mosquito, *Culex Cubensis (Aedes aegypti)* transmitted the disease (Finlay, 1937). He had cultured the mosquitoes for experimental purposes but had not transmitted the disease. Nevertheless his techniques were helpful to Reed's group. Doctor Henry Carter (1931) of the Public Health Service had established the incubation period of the disease in his studies in Mississippi. And finally, they were considerably influenced by the studies on malaria proving that mosquitoes transmitted that disease.

When the Yellow Fever Board of four members set up their site for experimental studies at Quemados, Cuba on June 25, 1900 they had two well-defined objectives in view, which they attained within a few months. First, they proved that neither the *bacillus icteroides* of Sanerelli nor the *bacillus X* of Sternberg was the cause of yellow fever. Second, they successfully transmitted the disease to nonimmune human volunteers with the mosquito *Aedes aegypti*. (Unfortunately one of the board members, Lazear, died of yellow fever following accidental exposure.) The board proved that the interval between the time when a mosquito ingests blood from a victim with yellow fever and then is able to transmit the disease to another human is 9 to 16 days (Reed et al., 1900). The interval corresponds with the time for the passage of malaria parasites from the stomach to the salivary glands of the mosquito. This simple initial report is a model in scien-tific literature. A second report at the annual meeting of the Associa-tion of American Physicians on April 30, 1901 cited the transmission of the disease to human volunteers by injecting them with blood from yellow fever patients (Reed, Carroll, and Agramonte, 1901). Two commentators at this meeting were General Sternberg and Dr. Welch, both laudatory, with Welch saying of the human volunteers (ibid., p. 71), "These young men, American soldiers, unwilling to accept a cent of pay for their services, submitted themselves for this experimental work, and I think they should be known in the history of the army as well as in medical circles as true heroes." Fortunately no fatalities occurred among the volunteers.

In February 1901 Major Gorgas ordered yellow fever patients to be screened off and mosquitoes to be destroyed. Within three months no yellow fever was recognized in Havana for the first time in 150 years (Garrison, 1922a, p. 752).

After the epidemiology of yellow fever had been clarified, the next step was to prove the etiology, which they thought was a virus, and to produce a successful vaccine. The Rockefeller Foundation played a major role toward this end. Members of the foundation's West African Yellow Fever Commission successfully transmitted the disease in 1928 to the Indian monkey *Macacus rhesus* (Strode, 1951), while others, especially Dr. Max Theiler, established the disease experimentally in white mice, and by 1937 produced a vaccine for human immunization (Theiler, 1930, 1933; Theiler and Smith, 1937).

The epidemiological principles established by Reed and his coworkers indicated that yellow fever was an urban epidemic disease spread from human to human by one species of mosquito, *Aedes aegypti*. But disturbing epidemiological features appeared in the 1920s when it was discovered in rural Central and South America and in parts of Africa that a sylvatic form of yellow fever existed in which monkeys were the natural host, and the vectors included more than one species of mosquitoes. Thus two forms of yellow fever existed, the urban or "house" form and the rural or "jungle" form. Information about the latter type was worked out largely through the efforts of the Rockefeller Foundation (Strode, 1951). In the control of both forms, immunization and the eradication of the mosquito as a vector of the disease were carried out. Mosquitoes were destroyed by eradicating their breeding areas through drainage and the use of insecticides.

Potential hazards have always existed when a new type of viable virus vaccine, even one with attenuated virulence, is employed for human purposes. This has been demonstrated in the use of vaccines for poliomyelitis, for tuberculosis and, in the present discussion, for yellow fever. When the United States was drawn into World War II it was apparent that military personnel would be dispersed to many areas of the world where yellow fever was not only endemic, but occurred in epidemic proportions. Under the auspices of the International Health Division of the Rockefeller Foundation attenuated vaccine was supplied for the immunization of military personnel. The vaccine was suspended with a small amount of normal human serum to prevent the inactivation of the relatively unstable virus, and several million soldiers were immunized with various lots of it. Early in 1942 the largest outbreak of "serum hepatitis" in United States military history occurred in the troops, with many deaths. Viable yellow fever virus in the vaccine was suspected as the cause. Careful epidemiological studies traced the source of serum in the vaccine to a volunteer healthy donor from the staff of the Johns Hopkins University Medical Center (Paul and Gardner, 1960). It was concluded that the initial serum employed for stabilizing the vaccine was obtained from an anicteric and presumed healthy human with viremia. Each injection included 0.04 ml. of serum, enough to induce hepatitis. It is difficult to ascertain the number of cases of hepatitis that ensued and the number of deaths, but it has been stated that twenty-eight thousand cases of jaundice and sixty-four deaths resulted out of 2.5 million United States soldiers inoculated. When a new source of vaccine was used, no further cases occurred.

Leprosy[6]

Leprosy originated in antiquity. Many of the facts surrounding its source and dissemination are shrouded in mythology and folklore (Mackerchar, 1949). Some of the older literature refers to leprosy as "elephantiasis Greco." Leprosy was designated by the Hebrews as *Zaraath* (Kaposi, 1875). The term means scaling of the skin and might have included psoriasis, scabies, leukopathia, and syphilis. In this light all ancient writings that cite the "curing" of leprosy must be interpreted cautiously.

It is possible that reservoirs of leprosy did exist in ancient Egypt and China, and it is likely that the Hebrews fled from Egypt with leprosy in their midst. Reference to leprosy and the advice of the Lord to Moses is found in Leviticus 13:3: "The priest shall examine the sore on the skin; if the hairs on the sore have turned white and it appears to be deeper than the skin, it shall be considered the sore of a malignant skin disease, and the priest, after examination, shall pronounce him ritually unclean." In the New Testament reference to leprosy is made in Luke 16:19, in the parable of the rich man and Lazarus with the sores on the skin; Mark 1:40–45, in the story of Jesus healing lepers; and Matthew 10:8, in the advice of Jesus to the disciples to heal the lepers.

Leprosy is due to *Mycobacterium leprae* (Hansen's bacillus). Like tuberculosis and syphilis, it is a chronic human disease; unlike the other two diseases, it is not highly contagious, but it is dependent on close human association. The incubation period before the appearance of disease can extend over several years. The leprosy bacilli have a peculiar predilection for localization in the cooler areas of the body, including peripheral nervous tissues and the skin, eyes, and naso-oral mucous membranes. Two principal forms of leprosy have been known for centuries. The first displays neurological lesions with anesthesia of the skin, and the second has the features of an inflammatory reaction of the skin and mucous membranes, which is associated with proliferation of the tissues. Hence the arms, hands, legs, and feet have neurological disturbances with crippling and deformities. The inflammatory and proliferating lesions of the skin, eyes, and nasal mucous membranes cause necrosis, hideous disfiguration of the face, and blindness. Because leprosy is visible on the exposed areas of the body, the severe forms made people fearful. Victims were ostracized and segregated from society. In this very action, frequently carried out in a humane way, society — without any knowledge of the contagiousness of leprosy — was protected from the unfortunate victims. The disease was often looked upon as a visitation from God.

Leprosy was known in France as early as the seventh century and in Germany during the eighth. The incidence rose to a peak in the eleventh century and remained so for two hundred years. This was related to the shift in populations involving tens of thousands during the Crusades. In France there were two thousand leper homes during the eleventh century. The St. Lazare Home in Paris became famous. Malmaison, the favorite home of Napoleon, derived its name from a home of lepers during the Middle Ages. During the fifteenth century there were 362 leper houses in Great Britain, 285 of which were in England (Cochrane and Davey, 1964).

Leprosy was introduced into the Sandwich Islands (Hawaii) during the nineteenth century by Chinese coolies. In 1865 the leper colony on the Island of Molokai was established. By 1880 there were two thousand lepers in Hawaii or 5 percent of the population (Thomas, 1947). Between 1865–1899, 5,125 patients were sent to Molokai, while between 1900–1937 there were only two to three thousand cases (Long, 1967). Similarly leprosy abounded in Korea and in the Philippines. The story of Culion, the leper colony in the Philippines, has been related by Perry Burgess (1940).

For reasons not clear leprosy died out in Europe during the fourteenth and fifteenth centuries, having been replaced by the ravages of epidemic syphilis and plague. Leprosy had disappeared in Great Britain by 1798. The entrance of leprosy into the United States coincided with the arrival of Columbus and his adventurers, and with the African slave trade.

Although leprosy gradually disappeared from Europe, a pocket of the disease persisted in Norway for many centuries and eventually led to the introduction of leprosy into the upper Midwest of the United States by Norwegian immigrants. Leprosy had appeared in Bergen as early as 1266 A.D., where a "leper house" from that period still exists. The incidence of leprosy in Norway reached a peak in 1856 with a total of 2,850 cases.Between 1861 and 1865, 1,040 more cases were discovered. But by 1934 there were only 51 (Leonard Wood Memorial Staff, American Leprosy Foundation, 1944).

Leprosy was known in Bergen as "Spédalskhed." The modern era of scientific investigation on leprosy originated mostly in Norway, where Dr. D. C. Danielssen, working in a leprosy hospital, carried out extensive clinical observations with his colleague Wilhelm Boeck (Danielssen and Boeck, 1848). Danielssen believed the disease was hereditary in origin and not contagious. But his pupil Dr. G. Armauer Hansen (1875) concluded that leprosy was contagious. He saw and described the leprosy bacillus for the first time, and along with Dr. O. B. Bull, also of Norway, described the ocular lesions of leprosy (Bull and Hansen, 1873).

The first Norwegian settlers arrived in Minnesota around 1852, and by 1864 physicians in Norway were aware that leprosy had been discovered among the emigrants (Washburn, 1950). The Minnesota State Board of Health, organized in 1872, formed a leprosy committee with a remarkable Norwegian immigrant physician from Christiania as the chairman, Dr. Christian Grönvold. It was he who had recognized leprosy amongst the immigrants, and he took a lively interest in the public health aspects of the problem (Grönvold, 1884). He communicated with the leading scientists of Bergen regarding the disease. Both Dr. Wilhelm Boeck and Dr. G. Armauer Hansen visited Dr. Grönvold in Minnesota and saw the Norwegian settlers with leprosy. The significant contribution of Dr. Grönvold in Minnesota was that he allayed the fears of the people about the spread of leprosy and advocated a sane and humane policy of calm with isolation of active cases. This attitude was in contrast to that in neighboring states, where authorities did little to allay the fear of the people, and the victims remained in abandoned isolation.

I have reviewed the Minnesota cases of leprosy, especially those originating in Norway, noting that there were 16 cases in Minnesota before 1891. Up through 1971 there were 103 cases, but only three had occurred since 1967. Of course, all of these cases did not originate in Norway, some coming from other parts of the world, especially during the twentieth century. At least one case occurred in a child born in Minnesota, whose mother, an immigrant from Norway, had leprosy. The child recovered completely but the mother died in the United States Leprosarium in Carville, Louisiana.

In 1944 there were between fifteen hundred and two thousand cases of leprosy in the United States, the majority of which came from Southern California, Florida, Louisiana, and Texas. In 1944 there were 384 cases at the National Leprosarium in Carville, Louisiana.

Leprosy is still a medical problem on a worldwide scale. According to a WHO report in 1965 there were an estimated 10,786,000 cases distributed throughout Africa, the Americas, Asia, Europe, and Oceania. And in 1973 there were ten thousand new cases reported annually in 29 countries in the Americas (World Health Organization, 1974a).

Contemporary knowledge about leprosy has been documented by R. G. Cochrane and T. Davey (1964) and C. C. Shepard (1971). There have been two outstanding achievements. The first involves the transmission of the disease to lower animals, and the second to treatment. Although *Mycobacterium leprae* have been recognized in tissues since Hansen's discovery, experimental transmission of the disease has been difficult. It had been established that leprosy tends to localize in the cooler areas of the body. Therefore, when infected human tissue was injected into the foot pads of mice, a localized infection occurred at this site in the rodent. More recently, growth of bacilli in the armadillo (*Dasypus novemcinctus* Linn.) has been achieved (Kirchheimer and Storrs, 1971). And equally revealing is the report on the presence of "leprosy-like" disease in armadillos trapped in Louisiana, a state in which human leprosy is indigenous (Walsh et al., 1975). These have been major accomplishments, since therapy can probably be evaluated in laboratory animals and studies on the pathogenesis can be extended.

The second triumph has been in therapy. For years treatment with hydnocarpus (chaulmoogra oil) was the mainstay. Following the observations on use of the sulfones in experimental tuberculosis, these agents were evaluated in human leprosy (Bushby, 1959). The most widely used and successful oral preparation has been dapsone (4, 4'diominodiphenylsulfone, DDS, diphenylsulfone). Side reactions do occur, and treatment must be continued for long periods of time. Other drugs being evaluated are acedapsone, clofazimine, and rifampicin. A possible approach for the lepromatous form of leprosy has been the use of Lawrence's transfer factor or whole lymphocytes obtained from patients sensitive to *Myco. leprae* antigen (Bullock, Fields, and Brandriss, 1972).

Cholera[7]

"Cholera was the classic epidemic disease of the nineteenth century, as plague had been for the fourteenth" (Rosenberg, 1962, p. 1). Although Koch is usually credited with the first recognition of *Vibrio cholerae* as the cause of cholera, he was preceded by the Italian investigator Filippo Pacini, who identified the etiological agent in 1854. As a result the judicial committee of the International Commission on Bacteriological Nomenclature designated the vibrio as "*Vibrio cholerae* Pacini, 1854" (Howard-Jones, 1975). Cholera is one of the enteric diseases, mostly waterborne, and follows the streams and canals on land and ships over seas. The disease strikes an individual suddenly, causing abdominal pain and a profuse diarrhea so severe that patients can quickly enter a stage of shock and die from dehydration and acidosis. The mortality rate of untreated patients may be over fifty per cent. As in any epidemic disease, the spectrum of illness extends from the very mild cases to those having a lethal outcome. Fortunately the disease is not highly contagious but is usually directly related to the numbers of organisms ingested in water or food. And actually, of those infected there are usually more persons who are asymptomatic than those with diarrhea. The carrier state can extend for a relatively long period, but usually does not last beyond a few weeks in the vast majority of those infected. Asymptomatic healthy carriers pose a serious problem in the control of the disease.

Historically the disease was endemic in India and the East Indies until the nineteenth century. The following pandemics pursued the trade routes throughout the world: (1) The first pandemic originated in India in 1817 and lasted until 1823, spreading first by land to China and to Ceylon; thence by sea to Mauritius, East Africa, the Philippines, China and Japan; and finally by land to Iran, Arabia, and Russia. Europe was spared. (2) The second pandemic started in India in 1826, followed a similar course to that of the first, but extended to Moscow, Berlin, Hamburg, and Great Britain and reached Edinburgh in 1832. This epidemic made its way to America in 1832 by way of the Atlantic Ocean, the disease being carried by Irish immigrants. New York City was severely afflicted. (3) The third pandemic, extending from 1840 to 1849, originated in India and caused a million deaths in Europe, including fifty thousand in Great Britain. The disease was introduced into the United States in 1849 through the port of New Orleans and spread throughout the Mississippi Valley. (4) The pandemic of 1863–1866 traveled overland with the pilgrims to Mecca and thence to Europe. Once again the eastern seaboard of the United States was visited in 1866. The last epidemic of cholera in the United States was in 1873. (5) The pandemic of 1884 was brought to Europe through the completed Suez Canal. (6) The pandemic of 1892–1894 also reached Europe via the Suez Canal and was severe in European Russia. The Russian composer Peter Ilich Tschaikowsky died of the disease during this epidemic. (7) The final pandemic involving Europe extended from 1902 to 1910, but intermittent and extensive epidemics of the disease continued after that date in Eastern Europe and the Far East. (8) In 1961 a pandemic of cholera due to the *El Tor* strain of vibrio originated in Southeast Asia, spread to the Celebes, Indochina, the Philippines, India, Pakistan, and the Mediterranean areas of Europe and Africa, lasting until 1974. This train of events in the twentieth century was clearly due to poor sanitation and contaminated drinking water. Only worldwide cooperative health activities, largely through the World Health Organization, prevented an even more catastrophic pandemic. Only one case of cholera due to the *El Tor* strain had been recorded in the United States up to 1974, and that patient was a Texan who had not been out of the country. The source of his infection is still not clear.

Attention has been centered on the epidemics of cholera because the fear of the disease in the mid-nineteenth century did more to stimulate the growth of sanitary reform and public health than any other communicable disease. "Cholera has been described as the sanitarian's best friend" (Napier, 1946a, p. 372) because of its sudden and dramatic appearance and the means at hand to prevent the disease. These features readily attracted immediate attention.

One of the most fascinating stories in medical history involves Dr. John Snow (1853 and 1855, reproduced in 1936), who was a London anesthesiologist and Queen Victoria's obstetrician. During the London epidemic of cholera in 1849, Snow shrewdly noted that the attack rate among Londoners was greatest among those who obtained their water supplies from the Broad Street pump. Working against strong resistance, he finally succeeded in having the handle of this pump removed, and the disease rapidly abated.

During the epidemic of 1854 Snow once again plotted out the areas where the incidence of the disease was highest. Two private companies supplied London with water. Lambeth Company obtained water from the Thames above the entrance of sewage, while Southwork and Vauxhall carried water from a sewage-contaminated area of the river. Snow pointed out that the highest incidence of cholera was among those people who obtained their water from Southwork and Vauxhall. He also revealed that cholera had been reintroduced by ships arriving from the Baltic area and disposing their sewage into the Thames.

Snow stated (p. 2) that cholera "travels along the great tracks of human intercourse, never going faster than people travel and generally much more slowly. In extending to a fresh island or continent, it always appears first at a sea-port. . . . Its exact progress from town to town cannot always be traced; but it has never appeared except where there has been ample opportunity for it to be conveyed by human intercourse."

Doctor John Woodworth, the supervising surgeon of the United States (Merchant) Marine Hospital Service, published a report on the cholera epidemic of 1873 in the United States. His conclusion was (1875, p. 19), "For nothing is more clearly proved by the history of cholera than that epidemics of this dreaded disease can be controlled by *vigorous hygienic measures. The true remedy against cholera is preventive medicine."*

Often in medical history there has been a delay of several years before valuable scientific information has been introduced into medical practice. New ideas are often accepted with reluctance, the opposition being persistent and effective. This course of events is brilliantly analyzed by N. Howard-Jones (1975) in the attempts to control cholera through international agreement. John Snow had clearly defined the mode of transmission of cholera in 1849 and again in 1855, and Pacini had first demonstrated the etiology of the disease in 1854 and repeatedly thereafter. But these scientific facts were either opposed or ignored for many years. It was not until 1892 that the etiology and mode of transmission of cholera was recognized, and the first international treaty for the protection of health, though limited, was consummated.

Why was there such a delay in formulating international regulations for cholera? A major cause was that medical thinking all through the nineteenth century was still divided between the contagionists and anticontagionists. Taking a middle course was the influential German Dr. Max von Pettenkofer, who pioneered successfully in environmental health and hygiene. Von Pettenkofer accepted neither the microbial cause nor the transmission of cholera through vibrios in contaminated drinking water. He practically eliminated typhoid fever in Munich through an improved supply of community drinking water, even though the cause of the disease was unknown.

Von Pettenkofer's concept of the etiology of cholera was bizarre, though convincing for many scientists. He maintained that there were three major factors in its cause and transmission, X, Y, and Z. X, an unknown factor in human feces, was deposited in certain soils containing an unknown Y factor, which was essential to form the unknown causative factor Z. In reality this was practically a return to the medieval concept of contagious diseases.

Von Pettenkofer was so convinced that the vibrio bacillus was not the cause of cholera that he carried out a famous experiment on himself in October 1892 (Howard-Jones, 1975, p. 67): "He swallowed on 7 October (1892) in the presence of witnesses, 1 cm^3 of a broth culture of cholera vibrios prepared from an agar culture provided by Gaffky, after neutralizing his gastric juices with a solution of sodium bicarbonate. He estimated that his 'cholera drink' contained a thousand million vibrios but was not pessimistic about the outcome." Except for borborygmi, some diarrhea, and colic, he continued in good health. But a pure culture of vibrios was found in his watery stools. His disciple R. Emmerich repeated the experiment and passed stools hourly for 43 hours!

But even for those conference delegates who accepted the scientific evidence of the mode and transmission of cholera, there was additional scientific evidence that made an international treaty with regulatory details very difficult to accept, and — more important — to enforce. At the twelfth International Sanitary Conference held in Paris (1911–1912) the president of the conference, Camille Barrère related (ibid., p. 90) "healthy individuals can carry the cholera vibrio for days and even for months and transmit it to their fellows. A healthy person can transmit the disease without being affected himself. This is one of the great discoveries of the last few years. It is rather disconcerting for the authorities responsible for safeguarding the public health."

This scientific fact relating to the healthy carrier of cholera organisms was forgotten and then "rediscovered" fifty years later during the cholera years 1961–1970 (World Health Organization, 1970). Because of the impossibility of identifying healthy carriers of the disease, strict international regulations could not be achieved in 1892. Hence a loose and very limited treaty resulted. The healthy carrier of enteric pathogens still poses a threat in the modern day of international jet travel.

As far as treatment is concerned there are few procedures in medical practice that so dramatically improve the condition of the cholera patient as the administration of fluid. The severe diarrhea, amounting up to 8 to 10 liters of watery stools per 24 hours, quickly and severely dehydrates an individual. An associated vomiting accentuates the problem. As early as 1832 in England physicians recognized the need for infusions of copious amounts of saline solutions (Cholera Editorial, 1832). The specific need is for the salts of sodium and potassium.

In 1964, as a medical consultant for the United States Air Force, I visited an installation in the South Pacific where hundreds of natives with cholera were treated. Even under somewhat primitive conditions the *quantity* of stool was measured, and replacement therapy with hypertonic saline solution was promptly carried out. Cholera struck mostly the debilitated and malnourished of both sexes and all ages. Some patients appeared moribund, but the improvement with adequate fluids was remarkable. No military personnel were afflicted. Immunization with cholera vaccine was helpful, but the maintenance of pure water supplies and careful food preparation were more important, as was the basic good health of the men and women.

In 1973 an epidemic of *El Tor* cholera erupted in Naples, Italy and in the surrounding towns (de Lorenzo et al., 1974). The outbreak provided a clear-cut example of poor sanitation and contaminated food and water as the cause. The primary source was infected mussels, often eaten raw. It is difficult to ascertain the number of cases, but several hundred persons were attacked, and at least a hundred died. The majority of patients were in the older age groups, and most of the deaths occurred in debilitated patients over 50 years of age. Navy frogmen aided in the control of the epidemic through the destruction of the mussel beds in the Bay of Naples.

CHAPTER 13

Communicable Diseases of Childhood

The control of the communicable diseases of childhood is one of the primary medical achievements of the twentieth century. These afflictions include the enteric diseases of infancy as well as rubeola (measles), rubella (German measles), varicella (chickenpox), pertussis (whooping cough), diphtheria, streptococcal diseases, and poliomyelitis. Despite what has been accomplished, many countries throughout the world are still besieged by these illnesses. Certain ones attack both children and adults, such as streptococcal and staphylococcal infections, respiratory diseases, enteric infections, and virus conditions.

There is a spectrum of diseases in which the clinical manifestations are due to bacterial exotoxins that are disseminated systemically. In some instances the toxins alone are responsible for a lethal outcome, as in botulism, tetanus, and some staphylococcal infections. In other instances suppuration is combined with toxemia, as in diphtheria and gas gangrene, but the toxins are the principal causes of death. The term "scarlet fever" is due to the characteristic rash caused by the erythrogenic toxin formed by several strains of Group A hemolytic streptococci. It is the suppuration at localized sites caused by the proliferating organisms that is the most formidable aspect of streptococcal diseases, however, along with the nonsuppurative complications, such as rheumatic fever and nephritis.

Diphtheria

Diphtheria used to be the most common disease of childhood. It is associated with a toxin which is formed in necrotizing inflammatory lesions of the mucosa of the nasopharynx ("false membrane"), frequently extending down to the larynx, bronchi, and bronchioles. The sloughing of the membrane often causes death through suffocation. The exotoxin attacks nerve tissue and the myocardium, causing peripheral paralysis and myocarditis, respectively. At times diphtheria bacilli enter the skin through abrasions, causing a localized ulceration, and the toxin that is formed produces peripheral neuropathy. During World War II it was discovered that focal epidemics of peripheral neuritis among military personnel in tropical zones were due to the localizing of bacilli in traumatized skin, usually of the legs. Recurrent epidemics of diphtheria in the army were often traced to the dissemination of the organisms from the nasopharynx of healthy carriers.

Diphtheria was described as early as the second century A.D. (Rosen, 1958). It was not until the sixteenth century that ulcerated lesions of the pharynx were recorded in epidemic form and the contagiousness of diphtheria was recognized (Loeffler, 1908). All through Europe during the eighteenth century ulcerating throats were commonly encountered. J. Fothergill (1751) described the nasal membranous inflammation and the sloughing pharyngeal membrane that are characteristic of diphtheria.

Diphtheria was widespread in the early American colonies. E. Caulfield (1939) wrote on what was undoubtedly diphtheria: "A True History of the Terrible Epidemic Vulgarly Called the Throat Distemper Which Occurred in His Majesty's New England Colonies Between the Years 1735 and 1740." Beginning in New Hampshire and spreading into Maine, Massachusetts, and Connecticut, the death toll was heavy. Ministers and physicians contributed to the spread of the disease through their visits to afflicted homes, in consequence of which their own families suffered heavily. Evidence of the epidemic can still be seen in the many gravestones of small children in the cemeteries of Massachusetts. There is little question that epidemics of scarlet fever also occurred simultaneously, being differentiated from diphtheria largely on the basis of the rash of scarlet fever. It is likely that diphtheria and scarlet fever spread beyond the confines of New England at this time.

A significant contribution to knowledge of diphtheria was made by Dr. Samuel Bard (1771), professor of medicine at King's College in New York City, who described an epidemic, particularly in children under ten years of age. He cited sixteen cases, with seven deaths. He attended one family with seven children, all of whom were ill, and three died. Autopsy of one revealed the typical diphtheritic membrane extending down through the trachea and bronchi to the lungs. Bard believed that the disease was contagious and that it was spread from person to person through expired air. He concluded that prevention should consist of removing healthy children from contact with the infected. His recommended treatment included calomel, opiates, purges, the bark (quinine), blisters on the throat and neck, snake root, and poultices.

Until the nineteenth century ulcerative pharyngeal diseases, including diphtheria, had not been clearly differentiated from each other. The careful clinical observations of Pierre Bretonneau (1826, translation 1859) during an epidemic of diphtheria in the vicinity of Tours in 1819 defined the disease as a specific clinical entity.[1] The causative microbe was later isolated and described by Friedrich Loeffler (1884). Considerable difficulties had been experienced in differentiating the bacterial species that caused inflammatory membranes of the pharynx. Chains of cocci (streptococci) and bacilli (diphtheria) were often seen together in the membranes. With the use of heated serum and gelatin as a culture medium Loeffler succeeded in growing the diphtheria bacillus in pure culture from the membrane. He inoculated the pharyngeal tissues of guinea pigs, calves, and pigeons with organisms and produced a toxic, lethal disease. Diphtheria bacilli were found only in the mucous membranes and not elsewhere in the body.

Emile Roux, an associate of Pasteur and later director of the Pasteur Institute, joined with Alexandre Yersin and successfully produced crude diphtheria toxin from the bacteria-free filtrate of a culture. They found the toxin lethal for guinea pigs, rabbits, sheep, dogs, and birds, but rats and mice were resistant (Roux and Yersin, 1888–1890).

Emil von Behring had had a long service in the medical department of the German Army. In 1889, at the age of 35, he joined the staff of

Koch's Institute for Hygiene. He had been interested in disinfectants and with S. Kitasato began a series of studies on the possible use of immune serum against bacteria instead of disinfectants. Kitasato (1889) had isolated the microorganisms of tetanus in pure culture. Von Behring and Kitasato (1890) carried out studies with the bacilli of tetanus and diphtheria and their toxins. They recorded that they had inoculated guinea pigs subcutaneously with diphtheria bacilli, and immediately thereafter injected a 1–2 percent solution of iodine trichloride into the same area for each of three days. The guinea pigs given the bacilli and treated with iodine survived, but untreated pigs died. After complete recovery, two of the treated guinea pigs survived a dose of diphtheria bacilli that killed control animals in 36 hours. This observation was to provide the clue for further investigations with the toxins and the production of antitoxins.

Following the basic discoveries of Roux and Yersin, and of von Behring and Kitasato on diphtheria toxin, vigorous efforts were made to produce a more potent antiserum in large quantities. Such efforts were first undertaken at the aniline dye works of Meister, Lucus, and Bruning at Hochst, a suburb of Frankfort. Although von Behring and Roux shared major French prizes for their work on diphtheria, von Behring alone was to receive the first Nobel Award in Medicine.

The history of bacteriology and immunology has often revealed the aid that chemistry has given to these disciplines. It is pertinent here to digress briefly and reemphasize the contributions of German organic chemistry to bacteriology, especially those of Gram and Ehrlich. During the last two decades of the nineteenth century, organic chemistry in Germany yielded hundreds of dyes useful in medical research and in the textile and pharmaceutical industries. With the rapid discoveries of new species of pathogenic bacteria, methods had to be devised for differentiating these microorganisms, since morphological appearances alone were inadequate. The aniline organic dyes were employed for this purpose. Perhaps the most widely used diagnostic procedure in clinical microbiological laboratories today for differentiating strains of bacteria is "Gram's stain," discovered during investigations on the etiology of pneumonia (Gram, 1884). The taxonomy of bacteria was in a confused state at that time (Austrian, 1960). It became apparent that pneumonia was not caused by one species of bacteria alone.

In a successful attempt to differentiate bacterial species in the pulmonary tissues Gram, working in Professor Carl Friedländer's laboratory in Berlin, first applied Ehrlich's aniline-water-gentian violet dye to the tissues and then destained with alcohol. Under these circumstances, some of the bacteria retained the blue stain, while others became decolorised. The latter could then be counterstained with a red dye. In this manner bacteria could be divided into "Gram's positive" (blue) and "Gram's negative" (red) species. This basic methodology and nomenclature still prevail, and each group of bacteria has distinguishing morphological characteristics as well as distinctive biological features.

Ehrlich was born in 1854, the same year as von Behring, and was well acquainted with him and his work on diphtheria antitoxin. Interested in the problem of preparing more potent sera, Ehrlich approached the study of immunology as a chemist and applied quantitative methods. In his initial investigations he used protein toxins of ricin from the seeds of castor oil, and abrin from jequirity seeds (Ehrlich, 1891). By injecting gradually increasing doses of toxin in mice he produced antitoxins of high potency. He found that he could quantitate the amount of toxin neutralized by the immune serum both *in vitro* and *in vivo*. A standardized antitoxin could be prepared with these toxins.

But when Ehrlich turned his attention to the production of diphtheria antitoxin he encountered difficulty. The resolution of the problem, in his own words (1897, translation 1956, p. 123), "required . . . years of painstaking, monotonous work, on account of the complex nature of the toxin solutions," primarily because the toxin and antitoxin were very labile substances. This final, highly technical report constitutes one of the brilliant advances in immunology. Although the potency of diphtheria toxin deteriorated in time, its antigenic property remained, and this changed product Ehrlich called "toxoid." His standard assay of toxin was that amount which when added to one standard unit of antitoxin killed a 250-gram guinea pig within four days. He also recommended the preservation of standardized antitoxin under carefully prescribed circumstances.

In his 1897 report and in his subsequent Croonian Lecture in England (Ehrlich, 1900) Ehrlich discussed his side-chain theory of immunity (Figures 6 and 7). He had to account for the two properties of toxin

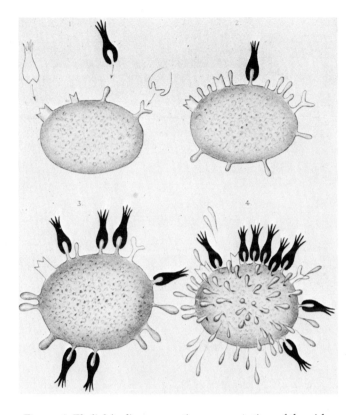

Figure 6. Ehrlich's diagrammatic representation of the side-chain theory. Reproduced with permission of the publisher from P. Ehrlich, "On Immunity with Special Reference to Cell Life," in *The Collected Papers of Paul Ehrlich*, Vol. 2, *Immunology and Cancer Research*, ed. F. Himmelweit, New York: Pergamon Press, 1957 (Plate I between pp. 194 and 195).

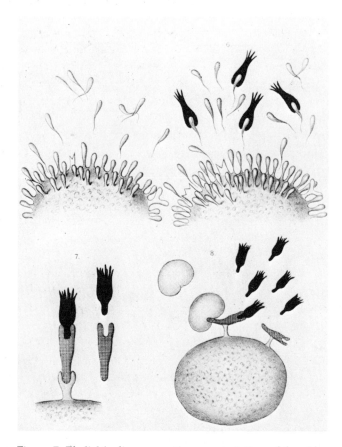

Figure 7. Ehrlich's diagrammatic representation of the side-chain theory. Reproduced with permission of the publisher from P. Ehrlich, "On Immunity with Special Reference to Cell Life," in *The Collected Papers of Paul Ehrlich*, Vol. 2, *Immunology and Cancer Research*, ed. F. Himmelweit, New York: Pergamon Press, 1957 (Plate II between pp. 194 and 195).

— its toxicity and its binding capacity for antitoxin. Being a chemist, he introduced a concept in which the toxin molecule had two different chemical groups, one the *haptophore*, and the other the *toxophore*. In the first stage of toxin activity the haptophore group became anchored to certain "side chains" of the protoplasm of the body cell. This is a "firm and enduring" reaction. As more toxin was formed, the body "became educated" to reproduce more receptors, such as occurred in an inflammatory reaction, and with an abundance of reproduced receptors some were cast off in the blood to become attached to the circulating toxin. This constituted the process of immunization. *"The antitoxines represent nothing more than side chains reproduced in excess during regeneration, and therefore pushed off from the protoplasm, and so coming to exist in a free state"* (Ehrlich, 1900, p. 437, his italics).

The principles worked out by Ehrlich for producing standardized immune serum had a far-reaching effect in biological standardization. His side-chain theory, however, brilliant as it was, did not withstand the passage of time. But potent diphtheria antiserum could be processed, and by 1894 the first specific antiserum was widely used, resulting in marked reductions in the mortality rates of diphtheria.

One of the pioneers in the treatment and control of diphtheria was Dr. William H. Park of New York City. Trained as an otolaryngologist and interested in microbiology, in 1892 he confirmed Loeffler's findings on the role of the diphtheria bacilli in the etiology of diphtheria and the value of pharyngeal cultures in the diagnosis of the disease. The same year Dr. Hermann Biggs of the New York City Board of Health established the first municipal diagnostic laboratory in the United States, and in 1893 Park was asked to head the diphtheria program. Under Park's direction diphtheria antiserum was produced in 1895 and distributed free of charge to indigent patients in New York City. The dramatic impact of diphtheria antitoxin in the reduction of mortality rates by 1908 was reviewed by Park and C. Bolduan (1908) for many principal areas of Europe and for the United States, particularly New York City. In citing statistics they had to include deaths from "croup" as well as diphtheria, since the differential diagnosis was not always readily made with accuracy. (Croup is an inflammation or edema of the larynx in children that causes difficulty in breathing and a harsh, brassy cough. It is associated with a variety of specific infections, including diphtheria, pertussis, and streptococcal disease.) In 1894 in New York City, with a population of 1,809,353, there were 2,870 deaths from diphtheria and croup, or 105 deaths per hundred thousand. In 1896, the year following introduction of the antitoxin, the mortality rate for the first time in a decade fell below 100 per hundred thousand. By 1905, the year after an antitoxin laboratory was established, New York City had a population of 2,390,382 and there were only 860 deaths from diphtheria, or 38 per hundred thousand. Park had also discovered the postconvalescent carrier state in diphtheria and had identified healthy carriers in family contacts. By 1908 B. Schick (1908) had introduced the cutaneous test with toxin as an indication of immunity to diphtheria, and within a few years toxin-antitoxin immunization was advocated (Behring, 1913).

During the ensuing years several advances in knowledge about diphtheria were made. The natural host for *Corynebacterium diphtheriae* is man. The disease is disseminated by the acutely ill patient, and — more significantly — by healthy carriers with nasopharyngeal diphtheria organisms. As a result of extensive studies carried out in Leeds, England, strain differences in the potency of toxin were discovered (Anderson et al., 1933). These strains were classified into three main groups, *gravis*, *mitis*, and *intermedius*. The third is the strain most constantly found, but the gravis provokes the most toxin and hence the most serious epidemics. More refined immunizing preparations and antiserum were developed. Figure 8 shows the decline in diphtheria cases in the United States, primarily as a result of immunization programs.[2]

The major studies on diphtheria carried out in Baltimore by the American epidemiologist Dr. Wade Frost (Frost et al., 1936) were to influence epidemiological work in many other infectious diseases. He clarified the concept that in an infectious disease a pathogen must come in contact with a susceptible host and that the host reaction constitutes the disease that follows. Frost emphasized one further major point: even though such contact does not always result in illness, in these cases it does produce a healthy carrier of the pathogen. He demonstrated graphically that diphtheria is principally a disease of young children. Older children and adults generally escaped diphtheria because in mingling with carriers at early ages, usually in school, they acquired inapparent infections that rendered them im-

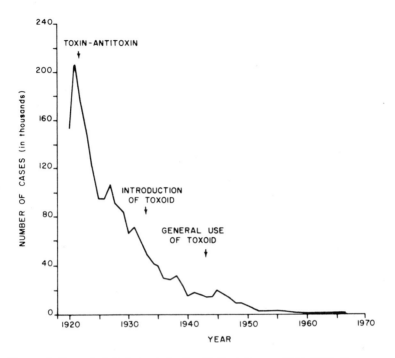

Figure 8. Reported diphtheria in the United States, 1920–1966. Reproduced from Diphtheria Surveillance Report No. 8, 1965–66 Summary, March 1, 1968. Bureau of Disease Prevention and Environmental Control, National Communicable Disease Center, Atlanta, Georgia (Figure 1).

mune. Figure 9 illustrates the age distribution of diphtheria in the United States in 1968. Figure 10 shows the carrier state confined principally to children in the United States.

The most important epidemiological lesson gained in the control of diphtheria is that an inadequately immunized population will invite epidemic diphtheria, as illustrated by what happened in the state of Michigan (Michigan Department of Health, 1945). In 1921 that state had the highest diphtheria mortality rate in the world, but in 1941 it had one of the lowest, the rate declining 98 percent because of an immunization program. Subsequently immunization was neglected, and in 1948 there were over five hundred reported cases. By 1973 there were only 228 reported cases of diphtheria in the United States, 104 of which occurred in the state of Washington. Doctor P. J. Imperato, in the New York City Department of Health, reviewed the pattern of diphtheria in 1972 and concluded (1974b, p. 776): "Diphtheria in New York City today is primarily a disease of nonimmunized children less than 15 years of age who live in low-income areas in the inner city."

The failure to immunize populations often results from a state of complacency. Control programs for diseases are often so effective, and therapy for the occasional case is so successful, that there is not the urgent need to push public health education in order to maintain the control. The unfortunate results of such a philosophy were dem-

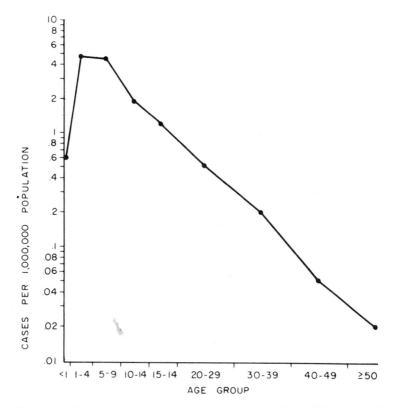

Figure 9. Diphtheria attack rates by age groups, United States, 1968. Reproduced from Diphtheria Surveillance Report No. 10, 1968 Summary, December 31, 1969. Health Services and Mental Health Administration, National Communicable Disease Center, Atlanta, Georgia (Figure 4, p. 4).

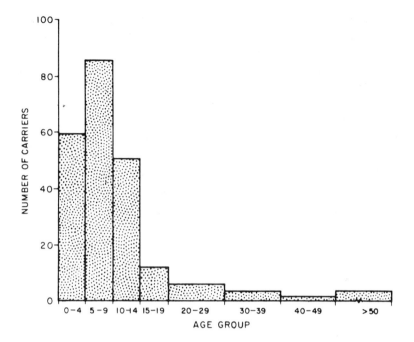

Figure 10. Diphtheria carriers by age group, United States, 1965–1966.
Reproduced from Diphtheria Surveillance Report No. 8, 1965–66
Summary, March 1, 1968, Bureau of Disease Prevention and
Environmental Control, National Communicable Dis-
ease Center, Atlanta, Georgia (Figure 7).

onstrated among American military personnel in World War II.
Diphtheria immunization was not carried out in the inductees at the
beginning of hostilities. From 1942 to 1945 there were 5,724 cases of
diphtheria with 125 deaths, mostly in the European Theater of Operations (McGuinness, 1958). In addition there was a large number of
cases of cutaneous diphtheria ("tropical ulcers"), principally in the
Pacific area, with many instances of peripheral neuritis. In the occupied civilian population of Europe the attack rate was quite high,
particularly in Holland. Beginning in 1946 army personnel were
quickly immunized without any preliminary Schick-testing.

   In the United States the American Academy of Pediatrics (1974) has
recommended that combined absorbed toxoid for tetanus, diphtheria,
and pertussis should be administered to children at age two months

with subsequent doses given at age four months, six months, four to six years and fourteen to sixteen years. Toxoids are prepared by adding formalin to preparations of toxins, which reduces the toxicity but does not alter the immunizing capacity.[3]

Scarlet Fever

In the history of infectious diseases scarlet fever provides a tantalizing story of the difficulties of precise diagnosis and differentiation from other febrile conditions, including those patients with streptococcal sepsis but without the cardinal sign of the scarlatinal skin lesion. Scarlet fever was recognized as a specific disease in the seventeenth and eighteenth centuries because of the characteristic skin rash. A consideration of the present status of scarlet fever as a clinical entity is helpful in interpreting much of the confusion that previously existed in medical practice.

Scarlet fever is due to Group A streptococci, in which several serological types producing the erythrogenic exotoxin cause the characteristic skin eruption in susceptible individuals. Entrance of the streptococcus is usually through the pharynx, sometimes resulting in suppurative pharyngitis, and also through wounds ("surgical scarlet"), or through the uterus in septic abortion and puerperal fever. The rash is only one of the signs of streptococcal sepsis. If a person has an immunity to the toxin due to past exposure, the suppurative lesions will occur without the rash, which is what happens in a large segment of the adult population. Although other streptococcal toxins probably contribute to the severity of the infection, the rash has been overemphasized in the past, and it is very doubtful that the erythrogenic toxin adds significantly to the severity of the disease (Bloomfield and Rantz, 1943).

As a child I was incarcerated for two weeks by the Health Department because I had been sent home from school with a sore throat and a rash. In addition my family was restricted in activity because of a large red placard that was nailed to the front of the house with the black letters "SCARLET FEVER." To be sure, no one ventured near us. At the same time, those of my schoolmates without a rash and with only a mild sore throat, but probably harboring the same offending strain of streptococcus, were allowed back into school after a day or two, or even attended regularly. Such was the confusion in medical practice throughout most of the country for at least the first quarter of the twentieth century. I once attended three people at the same time, each infected with the same strain of type-specific streptococcus. One had suppurative pharyngitis and a rash (scarlet fever); one had suppurative meningitis and no rash; and one had erysipelas. The momentous discovery of the grouping and typing of hemolytic streptococci by F. Griffith (1934) in England and R. C. Lancefield (1933) in the United States did much to clarify the epidemiological dilemma of streptococcal diseases.

The first clear clinical description of scarlet fever was reported by the French physician Armand Trousseau (1861). Hugo Schottmüller (1903) distinguished strains of streptococci by cultural methods in blood agar. Werner Schultz and W. Charlton (1918) observed that convalescent human scarlet fever serum injected into the area of the rash produced a blanching of the skin after a few hours, which proved to be a useful diagnostic test. Simultaneously Gladys and George Dick (1924) at the University of Chicago and A. R. Dochez and Lillian Sherman (1924) at Columbia University demonstrated the erythrogenic toxin in filtrates of streptococcal cultures and produced antitoxin in animals. A brief era of serum therapy for scarlet fever was then introduced. But the introduction of the sulfonamides, and later of penicillin, successfully replaced all other forms of therapy for acute streptococcal diseases. Valuable historical information on scarlet fever has been presented in the reviews of John D. Rolleston (1937) and Arthur Bloomfield (1958e).

Measles [4] (Rubeola) [5]

An authoritative definition of measles is "an acute, highly contagious, ancient viral disease characterized by fever, coryza, conjunctivitis, cough and a specific enanthem (Koplik's spots) followed by a generalized maculopapular eruption, which usually appears on the fourth day of the disease" (Krugman and Ward, 1973b, p. 106).

Recognition of measles as a specific disease is accorded to Rhazes, who in 910 A.D. differentiated it from smallpox (Rhazes, translation 1847 and 1939). Treatment included bleeding "even until fainting comes on." Rhazes intermingled his discussion of measles with his views on smallpox. Between the tenth century of Rhazes and the seventeenth of Sydenham, the Greek humoral theory of the pathogenesis of the disease persisted. Sydenham (1939) also advocated purging and bleeding for treatment.

A new concept concerning the disease, and possibly its prevention, was advanced in the next century. Doctor Francis Home, a Fellow of the Royal College of Physicians, practiced medicine in Edinburgh. Observing an epidemic of measles in 1758, he stated (1759, p. 266), "Considering how destructive this disease is, in some seasons; considering how many die, even in the mildest epidemical constitution; considering how it hurts the lungs and eyes; I thought I should do no small service to mankind, if I could render this disease more mild and safe, in the same way as the Turks have taught us to mitigate the small-pox." But what would he use for inoculation? The persistent doctrine of humoral pathology led him to the source as he wrote (p. 267), "I then applied directly to the magazine of all epidemic diseases, the blood." He probably did transmit the disease in this manner, because he described a febrile eruptive disease in young susceptible children injected with the blood of a patient, although it is not clear whether this procedure resulted in future protection. Nevertheless this was the first attempt to administer prophylactic vaccine for measles, an approach that was successfully applied with attenuated virus two hundred years later. L. Hektoen (1905) transmitted the disease from human to human via blood in 1905, and J. F. Anderson and J. Goldberger (1911) succeeded in passing the disease to the rhesus monkey.

The highly contagious nature of measles and the havoc wrought in a susceptible population have been emphasized in epidemiological studies, one of the outstanding examples in medical history being the 1846 epidemic in the Faroe Islands (Panum, 1939). Peter Panum, a 26-year-old physician just out of medical school, was dispatched by the Danish government in 1846 to the Faroes, an isolated group of islands situated in the mist and fog of the north Atlantic Ocean. No measles had appeared in the seventeen islands since 1781; thus the population of eight thousand inhabitants was highly susceptible to the disease, which was introduced by a cabinet maker who had journeyed from Copenhagen, where he had been exposed to measles. There were six thousand cases with 102 deaths before the epidemic subsided. Panum's observations over a period of five months were not limited to measles; he also described other diseases, as well as the social and cultural life of the people. He encountered no tuberculosis, scarlet fever, or whooping cough, and smallpox had not been seen since 1705. Twenty cases of syphilis over a period of two years were traced to one individual.

The seriousness of measles in a susceptible adult population is reflected in the morbidity and mortality rates of the United States Army. "Apparently no disease was more closely allied to mobilization than was measles" (Michie and Lull, 1928, p. 414). In the Union Army during the Civil War there were 67,763 cases with 4,246 deaths. In World War I there were 96,817 cases with 2,367 deaths in a mobilized force of four million persons. In 1918, out of a civilian population of 100 million there were 529,498 cases. In World War II, however, the United States Army statistics showed only 60,809 cases with but 33 deaths in an army "four times as large and the duration of the war twice as long" (Kneeland, Jr., 1963a, p. 32). The change between World War I and World War II was due to a shift in the civilian population from rural to urban areas between the two wars and to the more widespread exposure of the younger age group to measles because of urbanization.

Perhaps the most unusual epidemic of measles in medical history occurred in Greenland in 1962 (Littauer and Sørensen, 1965). The epidemic was purposely instigated over a large area by health authorities during the warm summer months because medical attention would not be readily available during the severe winter weather. Previous epidemics of measles had occurred in 1951, 1954, 1955, and 1959. It had become apparent that faster means of transportation and travel permitted exposed individuals to arrive in the country during the incubation period of the illness, and before the appearance of symptoms, so that health authorities could not alert communities about the possibilities of an impending epidemic. In 1962 a violent epidemic of influenza broke out in May, with measles appearing in July. The focus was the community of Umanak, where a population of eight hundred was in contact through trade and travel with nine other trading posts and small villages. In order to speed up and terminate the inevitable measles epidemic during warm weather, hundreds of persons over a wide area were artificially infected by exposure to acute cases, with the expectation that there would be a guided epidemic of relatively short duration. These hopes were rewarded with almost twelve thousand cases and a mortality rate of only 0.47 percent. The most common complication was pneumonia. The epidemic extended from July to October, fulfilling the purpose of the experiment. Anti-measles gamma globulin was administered to high-risk individuals.

It was not until World War II that specific prophylaxis and therapy for measles became available. Through a research program at the Harvard Medical School engendered by the war effort, fractionation of human plasma resulted in the isolation of immune gamma globulin (Ordman, Jennings, and Janeway, 1944). Administration of this immune substance produced a milder form of the disease, and at the same time immunity was established against future attacks. In addition measles could be prevented completely after exposure during the initial stage of incubation, but this precluded the acquisition of immunity. A second advance in the therapy of measles was the successful use of the sulfonamides and penicillin for the suppurative complications of pneumonia, otitis media, mastoiditis, and meningitis, usually of streptococcal origin. This reduced the mortality rate and the chronic disability of children.

The development of a measles vaccine was a major step forward in the control of infectious diseases, one that ranks with poliomyelitis vaccine. Both vaccines came out of the laboratory of Dr. John Enders and his group in Boston following the successful large-scale growth of viruses. Enders and T. C. Peebles (1954) first announced the isolation and growth of measles in tissue culture, and by 1960 they had successfully evaluated an attenuated live vaccine in humans (Enders et al., 1960). Fortunately the measles virus was antigenically stable, making the production of vaccine and the control of the disease a continued success. Live attenuated measles vaccine was licensed in the United States in 1963. Before that time there were at least five hundred thousand cases of measles per year with three to four hundred instances of the dreaded encephalitis, an occasional complication of measles. By 1968 only 22,231 cases were reported, and the incidence of encephalitis decreased. Postvaccinal encephalitis was rare.

In modern society reliable medical care for illness is expensive.

Likewise the preservation of good health takes effort and finances. The comparative costs in lives and money have been graphically portrayed for measles in the United States since the introduction of measles vaccine. The decade of 1963–1972 has been summarized by the Center for Disease Control as follows (Center for Disease Control, 1973a, p. 11): "In the 10 years since vaccine licensure. . . . Over 60 million doses of vaccine have been distributed, nearly 24 million cases [of measles] have been prevented, and the economic savings, both from direct medical expenditures and indirect costs from loss of productivity, total nearly 1.3 billion dollars." Additional data gathered by D. J. Sencer and N. W. Axnick are presented in the accompanying tabulation.

Cases averted	23,707,000
Lives saved	2,400
Cases of retardation averted	7,900
Additional years normal and productive life saved by preventing premature death and retardation	709,000
School days saved	78,000,000
Physician visits saved	12,182,000
Hospital days saved	1,352,000

Source: Center for Disease Control, 1973a, p. 11

The results of measles vaccination have indeed been dramatic, but unless persistent efforts are made to continue universal vaccination, the incidence of the disease will rise with the appearance of new generations of nonimmune infants and children. This phenomenon has already been demonstrated. In the United States there were only 25,826 reported cases of measles in 1968, but by 1972 this number had tripled with 75,290 cases. The increase was due to the failure to vaccinate children in certain areas of the country. Alerted to this rise, health authorities once again encouraged vaccination, and in 1973 there were only 26,690 reported cases. The duration of immunity to measles following vaccination is not clearly known (Linnemann, Jr., 1973); it will be necessary to follow groups of children into adult life to answer this question. There is still the necessity to extend the use of measles vaccine throughout the world, not only in the developing countries but in those with advanced technology. As of 1974 measles vaccination had not been widely used in Denmark, for example (Horwitz et al., 1974).

Rubella (German Measles)

Rhazes recognized measles, or rubeola, as early as the tenth century, but the similar but milder rubella was not clearly defined until eight centuries later. The delay was due to a confusion of rubella with measles and with scarlet fever. Rubella was generally known as German measles or *rötheln* [6] until H. Veale (1866) suggested the designation *rubella*, a term that has only gradually attained universal acceptance (Wesselhoeft, 1947).

Until 1940 rubella was regarded as a mild exanthem of adolescents and young adults. A widely used textbook briefly defined and described the disease as follows (Dowd, 1928, p. 285): "Rubella is an acute, highly contagious disease, similar to but quite distinct from measles and scarlet fever. It is characterized by a long incubation period, short invasive stage, benign course, and almost complete freedom from complications." This mild statement is to be compared with a more recent formidable review of the disease (Krugman and Ward, 1973c, p. 236): "Since 1941, a great deal of interest has been focused on this disease because of the association of rubella during pregnancy with an increased incidence of congenital malformations."

Doctor N. McAlister Gregg (1941), an ophthalmologist in Sydney, Australia, published a report in the *Transactions of the Ophthalmological Society of Australia* in which he called attention for the first time to the relationship of rubella to congenital malformations. An epidemic of the disease had swept through Australia. The epidemic coincided with a large number of congenital cataracts in infants that he observed in Sydney. Upon further investigation he gathered additional information about 78 infants from various parts of the country. He described not only cataracts but other congenital malformations such as microcephaly, deafness, congenital heart disease, and mental and growth retardation.

Because Gregg's report appeared in a journal not widely recognized and during World War II, a decade elapsed before the significance of his observations was recognized; but confirmation did take place in other areas of the world, including New York City (Greenberg, Pellitteri, and Barton, 1957) and Sweden (Lundström, 1962). Several thousand infants manifested the rubella syndrome of congenital defects in the 1964 epidemic in the United States, which was studied exhaustively as a scientific and community project in Houston, Texas (Baylor Univ. Rubella Study Group, Houston, Texas 1967). It became apparent from pathological studies that practically every organ in the body could be invaded. The pathology and pathogenesis of the disease have been well summarized by Menser and Reye (1974). Of particular importance is the persistence of live virus in the tissues of children, which can be shed into the environment for many months. This presents a serious problem of strict isolation in nurseries and hospitals against the spread of the disease. The Houston experience demonstrated the necessity for long-term followup of the patients and their families by many different social agencies of the community, and for the dispensing of information and advice to parents and other members of the families.

It had been postulated by A. F. Hess (1914) through transmission studies that rubella was due to a virus. This was proved definitively by Y. Hiro and S. Tasaka (1938) and by K. Habel (1942). In 1962 two groups of investigators simultaneously grew the virus in tissue cultures (Parkman, Buescher, and Artenstein, 1962; Weller and Neva, 1962). Four years later, in 1966, live, attenuated rubella virus vaccine was ready for evaluation, and by 1969 licensure for the general use of vaccine in the United States as a prophylactic against rubella had been granted (Meyer, Jr., Parkman, and Panos, 1966).

The highest incidence of the disease is in older children, adolescents, and young adults, which makes it a real threat in pregnancy. Since immune globulin did not offer the necessary protection *before* pregnancy, reliance for this immune effect depended upon vaccination. In evaluating the vaccine several questions had to be answered. First, how safe was it? Second, would vaccinates disseminate the disease and thus serve as reservoirs for epidemics? Third, who should get the vaccine, and at what age? And fourth, what was the duration of the immunity following vaccination?

These questions were answered in the five years between 1969 and 1974. Up to 50 million doses of the vaccine were administered. The reactions to the vaccine were exceptionally mild. Vaccinates did not transmit the disease to susceptible individuals. It was recommended that children of both sexes, one to twelve years of age, should receive the vaccine. Serological evidence of persistent antibody response persisted up to six years in some of the original vaccinates.

The most challenging problem is that of the young female who has had no history of the disease and in whom pregnancy may be anticipated. No general rules can be laid down except that such individuals must be carefully advised by a physician. It has been recommended that serological evaluations should be carried out on such women, and those having rubella antibody should not require vaccination. Under no circumstances should vaccination be carried out during pregnancy, especially during the first few weeks. In those vaccinated, pregnancy should be avoided for two months after vaccination.

Vaccination programs should reduce the dangers of the complications of congenital rubella in the years ahead, *if such programs are continuously monitored and carried out*. In 1966, the first year of reporting, there were 46,975 cases and 11 of the rubella syndrome. In 1973 there were 27,804 reported cases of rubella in the United States with 35 cases of congenital rubella syndrome. Epidemics appear to occur at six- to nine-year cycles. For this reason, vaccination programs should be constantly offered in the intervening years to susceptible populations.

Varicella [7] (Chickenpox) [8]

Varicella, like scarlet fever illustrates the painfully slow evolution of concepts of the specific nature of a disease and its control. Like measles, it is a highly contagious and common disease of childhood. And yet, unlike measles, varicella received little notice until the sixteenth century, when the disease was differentiated from scarlet fever. Varicella was also differentiated in this period from smallpox by the London physician Dr. William Heberden, Sr. in the initial volume of the *Transactions of the Royal College of Physicians*. He stated (Heberden, 1768, p. 427), "The chicken-pox and swine-pox differ, I believe, only in name; they occasion so little danger or trouble to the patients, that physicians are seldom sent for to them, and have therefore very few opportunities of seeing this distemper. Hence it happens that the name of it is met with in very few books, and hardly any pretend to say a word of its history." Swine-pox is not the same as chickenpox, however. The former is a specific dermal eruption in swine due to a virus that afflicts no other species.

Heberden looked upon varicella as a benign disease. In comparing it with smallpox he wrote (1768, p. 433), "these two distempers are surely totally different from one another, not only on account of their different appearances . . . but because those, who have had the small-pox, are capable of being infected with the chicken-pox; but those, who have once had the chicken-pox are not capable of having it again, though to such, as have never had this distemper, it seems as infectious as the small-pox. I wetted a thred in the most concocted, pus-like liquor of the chicken-pox, which I could find, and after making a slight incision, it was confined upon the arm of one who had formerly had it; the little wound healed up immediately, and showed no signs of any infection." Thus he concluded that a person who had had one attack of chickenpox would not have a second attack, and demonstrated in a simple experiment that the disease could not be transmitted to an "immune" subject.

In reflecting on early medical history I have often wondered why so much emphasis was placed on the differentiation of measles from smallpox beginning with Rhazes in the tenth century, and culminating with Sydenham in the seventeenth. It is more difficult to differentiate a mild case of smallpox from that of varicella, and the "mild" case of smallpox may be easily overlooked or misdiagnosed.

Although varicella is usually a benign disease of childhood, rare but serious and lethal complications include hemorrhagic varicella and encephalitis. It is a severe disease in newborn infants. Suppurative secondary bacterial complications of the respiratory tract are common and potentially dangerous. The disease can also be serious in adults, and varicella pneumonia is common. This specific form of pneumonia was first defined in 1942 (Waring, Neubuerger, and Geever, 1942), and since then many groups of cases have been reported (Knyvett, 1966). The histology of the lung lesions is similar to that described in 1906 for the dermal lesions (Tyzzer, 1906), in which there was a ballooning of epithelial cells with the appearance of multinucleated cells and of intranuclear and cytoplasmic inclusion bodies.

One of the most intriguing aspects of varicella has been its relation to herpes zoster, which is a painful eruption of the skin ("shingles") over the course of peripheral nerves, occurring mostly in those over 50 years of age. Zoster[9] was described by the Greeks and was known as "zona" because of the characteristic distribution of the rash (Downie, 1961). Bókay (1909) stated that varicella had been contracted from cases of herpes zoster; according to A. W. Downie (1961) children developed varicella following inoculation of material from zoster lesions. The histological picture of the two lesions is the same. There has been repeated confirmation of Bókay's observation (Garland, 1943). Zoster is rarely contagious, and it is now postulated that the herpetic inflammation is due to activation of latent varicella virus residing in the sensory nerve ganglia of individuals with a history of having had varicella. Isolation of the varicella-zoster (V-Z) virus in tissue cultures was accomplished in 1953 (Weller, 1953).

In contrast to measles, varicella was of minor concern in the armed forces during World War I and World War II. A previously unexposed and nonimmune population, however, may suffer severely from varicella, as it may from measles. This is illustrated by the epidemic in French Cameroun in 1936 in which there were 1,919 cases with 370 deaths, mostly among adults (Millous, 1936). In the United States there was a total of 182,927 reported cases in 1973.

The highly contagious nature of varicella was recognized long before the etiology was established. Control of the disease depended on strict isolation techniques, especially in institutions and hospitals. But even under the utmost precautions varicella did spread to a susceptible population. No satisfactory vaccine is yet available, but zoster immune globulin (ZIG) can be obtained in the United States from the Center of Disease Control for the protection of high-risk children against varicella and also for selected adults. It is most effective when administered within 72 hours after exposure (Brunell et al., 1969).

There is no specific therapy for varicella. The secondary suppurative infections can be successfully managed with antibiotics, however. This has reduced the period of convalescence and — appreciably — the number of fatalities.

Pertussis [10] (Whooping Cough)

No more vivid description of pertussis has been presented than that of Professor Thomas Watson when he lectured to his students in London during the early nineteenth century as follows (1853b, p. 552):

"The phenomena that characterize hooping-cough are, I say, remarkable. It begins with the symptoms of an ordinary catarrh arising from cold. The child (for it is most especially a disease of children) has coryza, and coughs; and mothers and nurses are aware that the disease commences in this way, and express their apprehensions lest it may *turn* to the hooping-cough. After *this*, the *catarrhal* stage, has lasted eight or ten days, or a fortnight, or sometimes a day or two longer, that kind of cough begins to be heard which is so distinctive. It comes on in paroxysms, in which a number of the *ex*piratory motions belonging to the act of coughing are made in rapid succession, and with much violence, without any intervening inspirations; till the little patient turns black in the face, and seems on the point of being suffocated. Then one long-drawn act of *in*spiration takes place, attended with that peculiar crowing or hooping noise, which denotes that the rima glottidis is partially closed, and which gives the disease its name. As soon as this protracted inspiration has been completed, the series of short expiratory coughs, repeated one immediately after the other till all the air appears to be expelled from the lungs, is renewed; and then a second sonorous back-draught occurs; and this alternation of a number of expiratory coughs, with one shrill inspiration, goes on, until a quantity of glairy mucus is forced up from the lungs, or until the child vomits, or until expectoration and vomiting both take place at once. During the urgency of the paroxysms, the face becomes swelled and red or livid, the eyes start, the little sufferer stamps sometimes with impatience, and generally clings to the person who is nursing him for support, or lays hold of a chair or table, or of whatever object may be near him, to diminish (as it would seem) the shock and jar by which his whole frame is shaken. As soon as expectoration or vomiting have happened, the paroxysm is over. The child may pant a little while, and appear fatigued; but commonly the relief is so complete, that he returns immediately to the amusements, or the occupation, which the fit of coughing had interrupted, and is as gay and lively as if nothing had been the matter with him. When the fit terminates by vomiting, the patient is in general seized immediately after with a craving for food, asks for something to eat, and takes it with some greediness."

Pertussis must have been recognized as a major childhood disease for centuries. The earliest known description was by G. Baillou (1736, translation 1945) in 1578. Another early description of the disease was that of Dr. Robert Watt (1813) of Glasgow. Watt arbitrarily called the disease Chincough, one of the three synonyms in use at the time, the others being hooping cough and, as the Scotch called it, Kinkcough. In addition to his careful clinical descriptions based on thirty years of observation, Watt brought forth two other important facts. First, he described the results of autopsies he had performed on children who had died of the disease, including two of his own. Second, he appended the monthly mortality rates on several diseases over a period of twenty-nine years (1783–1812). Three leading causes of deaths were smallpox, measles, and whooping cough. During that period one half of the children born died before ten years of age! Watt did recognize pertussis as a contagious disease. His therapeutic suggestions were, at best, supportive.

Progress in the control and the treatment of whooping cough was slow. J. Bordet and O. Gengou (1906) first isolated the causative bacteria. Known first as *Haemophilus pertussis*, the organism is now called *Bordetella pertussis*. Initial attempts to produce a suitable prophylactic vaccine were not successful. The disease was highly contagious, and few children escaped infection. It was a frightful illness in very young infants because of the suppurative complications of secondary bacterial pneumonia and otitis media. Convulsions with cyanosis were serious, resulting in organic brain damage in those who recovered. Sporadic pertussis in adults was also a severe disease.

P. H. Leslie and A. D. Gardner (1931) established the four phases in the growth of the pertussis organisms, which proved to be fruitful in the subsequent production of successful vaccines. The vaccination of young children has caused a marked reduction in the incidence of the disease. In the United States there were only 1,759 reported cases in 1973. Antibiotic therapy in the form of erythromycin and ampicillin is also effective when given early in the course of the infection.

Mumps [11] (Epidemic Parotitis)

Mumps was recognized as a distinct clinical entity by the ancients. In *Of the Epidemics*, Book I, Hippocrates (1939, p. 98) described mumps as follows: "Swellings appeared about the ears, in many on either side, and in the greatest number on both sides . . . inflammations with pain seized sometimes one of the testicles, and sometimes both." Mumps was not considered a serious disease, although, as Bloomfield (1958c) has pointed out, a surprisingly large literature has appeared on the subject.

Robert Hamilton (1790), a leading physician of Edinburgh, gave an account of a distemper in England, which the common people "vulgarly" called mumps. He elaborated on the description of Hippocrates and prescribed blistering to one or both sides of the face, presumably to prevent the subsequent testicular swelling. If the brain was threatened with involvement (encephalitis), Hamilton would not hesitate to blister the testicles to prevent this cerebral complication. He made the astute observation that the disease was common among soldiers.

Contrary to measles, varicella, and pertussis, mumps is not a highly contagious disease, rarely afflicting infants. The majority of cases occur between five and ten years of age, and 30 to 40 percent of the cases have inapparent infections. Complications include testicular swelling and encephalitis, usually not succeeded by any residuals. Contrary to popular belief, mumps is rarely a cause of male sterility.

Because mumps is not a highly contagious disease, many children escape infection. Under certain circumstances epidemics of the disease occur among adults, as illustrated by the incidence of mumps among army recruits. During World War I "mumps was of great importance" (Michie, 1928b, p. 451) in the United States Army. "From a standpoint of noneffectiveness [disability], mumps stood third on the list of important diseases . . ." (Michie, 1928b, p. 451). There were 230,356 cases in the Army of four million. During World War II mumps was again the most common of the so-called communicable diseases of childhood in the Army, with a total of 103,055 cases (Kneeland, Jr., 1963b). Of particular concern in the troops was the appearance of orchitis, because it prolonged convalescence and extended the period of disability. In my own experience, in one Army division of ten thousand men we encountered an incidence of orchitis in 35 percent of the cases. There was no effective specific therapy for the parotitis or orchitis.

Mumps can also appear in epidemic form in isolated communities, afflicting both children and adults, as does measles. In 1957 an unusual epidemic occurred among Eskimos on St. Lawrence Island in the Bering Sea (Philip, Reinhard, and Lackman, 1959). There were 363 cases among a "virgin" population of 561, an incidence of 65 percent. Only one death was recorded. A second epidemic was studied in 1965 on St. George Island, also in the Bering Sea (Reed et al., 1967). No mumps had been recorded on the island since 1907. There were 156 cases out of 212 natives, an incidence of 73 percent. The rather high incidence was due to the fact that modern serological methods revealed 37 instances of inapparent infections. In this epidemic the administration of immune gamma globulin did not alter the course of the disease.

Claud D. Johnson and Ernest W. Goodpasture (1934) succeeded in transferring mumps to monkeys via Stensen's duct with a filtrate of saliva from patients. Karl Habel (1945) grew the virus in the chick embryo and in 1946 reported on the preparation of a vaccine (Habel, 1946). The virus was then successfully propagated in tissue culture (Henle and Deinhardt, 1955).

Epidemiological investigations of mumps were enhanced by the development of serological methods for detecting antibodies following recent exposure to the antigen (Enders et al., 1945). J. F. Enders and his associates (1946) demonstrated the acquisition of dermal hypersensitivity in humans to mumps antigen, indicating the presence of resistance to the disease.

A live, attenuated mumps vaccine was licensed for use in the United States in 1969. It is not recommended for use in infants under twelve months of age. The vaccine can be administered effectively alone and does protect against the natural disease. It is also available in combined vaccines for use against measles, rubella, and mumps in children. Immune gamma globulin is of doubtful prophylactic value.

There has been a steady decline in the incidence of mumps in the United States since 1968, when the disease was first reported nationally; there were 152,209 cases reported in 1968 as opposed to 69,612 in 1973. This decrease may be related in part to the use of prophylactic vaccine.

Cytomegalovirus (CMV) Infections

The advances in virology beginning in the 1940s brought forth new knowledge about host-parasite relationships in human disease. Information about CMV infections stemmed not only from new virological techniques but also from the contributions of comparative medicine. The CMV viruses, of which there are two or more serotypes, belong to the herpes-virus group and are antigenically related to varicella-zoster, herpes simplex type 2, and the Epstein-Barr (EBV) virus of infectious mononucleosis. The uniqueness of CMV virus is the widespread distribution in the tissues of man, beginning *in utero* and extending through adult life. The virus may remain latent for years and then explode into a lethal infection. This discussion will emphasize two major clinical features, congenital CMV disease and the acute illness in adults.

Acute congenital or postnatal illness with viremia may be either asymptomatic or severe with many tissues and organs involved. The characteristic histological feature is the ballooning of the cells, as in varicella, with large bodies occurring in the nuclei (CMV) and sometimes in the cytoplasm. These characteristics are present in tissue cultures of fibroblasts — hence the term "cytomegalic."

Ernest Goodpasture and Fritz B. Talbot (1921) reported on lesions in an infant that in some respects simulated those of varicella. They commented extensively on the appearance of the "protozoan-like" cells. Later S. Farber and S. B. Wolbach (1932) contributed a major study on "Intranuclear and Cytoplasmic Inclusions ('Protozoan-Like Bodies') in the Salivary Glands and Other Organs of Infants." They studied autopsy material on 183 infants and found inclusion bodies in the salivary glands of 22 and also throughout other tissues. Further human studies were probably impeded by the lack of techniques for studying the nature of the "protozoan bodies," but important contributions on this problem came from studies on the natural disease in animals.

R. Cole and A. Kuttner (1926) first isolated what they considered to be a filtrable virus from the salivary glands of guinea pigs, a study confirmed by C. H. Andrewes (1930), who also found that the animals with salivary gland disease provided immune serum that neutralized growth of the virus. Margaret Smith (1954) propagated the virus of the salivary glands of the mouse in embryonic mouse tissue and later isolated and grew the mouse virus in tissue cultures of human fibroblasts. She stated (1956, p. 425), "The incidence of intranuclear inclusions in the salivary glands of infants and young children, regardless of the cause of death, has been reported from different geographical areas as 10 to 30% in routine autopsies." Viral isolations from human material were soon recorded by others (Weller et al., 1957).

By 1960 CMV infection was recognized as a serious disease in infants: "congenital CMV infection is probably the most common fetal infection of man" (Krugman and Ward, 1973a, p. 9). The studies were greatly aided by the occurrence of viruria with large cells having inclusion bodies that could be readily detected in stained urine specimens (Fetterman, 1952).

Knowledge of the nature of the disease and of congenital CMV infection was greatly extended by the studies of J. B. Hanshaw and T. H. Weller (1961) at Harvard. They confirmed the viruria in children, especially in those with leukemia, lymphoma, and neoplastic diseases. But more important, they defined the syndrome of congenital inclusion disease in infants, which included jaundice, petechial rash, microcephaly, and psychomotor retardation. The virus has been isolated from the urine of infants for months and years after birth, an unusual phenomenon in human biology. Latent infections are apparently activated in pregnancy, with and without symptoms, producing viremia and infection of the fetus. J. B. Hanshaw (1970) in an extensive review described the extraordinary number of congenital defects arising in 260 infants from birth to twelve months of age.

The acute illness in adults mimics infectious mononucleosis, including the lymphocytosis and atypical lymphocytosis, but without heterophile serological reactions. An infectious mononucleosis-like syndrome following transfusions with fresh blood has been apparent in patients who have had open heart surgery (Kääriäinen, Klemola, and Paloheimo, 1966). Acute and disseminated disease has been activated in patients with immune deficiency states, often induced by chemotherapy for malignancy. The problem of CMV infection has also been encountered in recipients of renal transplants who have been treated with immuno-suppressive agents (Kanich and Craighead, 1966).

The host-parasite relationship in humans, enduring from early life until late adult years, will continue to enlist the interest of epidemiologists, virologists, and clinicians. CMV infections are common and distributed throughout the world. Although animal strains do exist and are antigenically related to the human strains, it is not clear whether the animal reservoir is significant as far as human disease is concerned. Control measures are not available, and there is no specific therapy for the disease. T. H. Weller (1971) has contributed an excellent review of the entire subject.

Poliomyelitis[12]

Many infectious diseases have been recognized as distinct clinical entities for centuries, but it was not until the late nineteenth and early twentieth centuries that epidemic poliomyelitis was defined. Epidemics appeared in the more advanced countries, and few diseases were more feared than poliomyelitis because it attacked healthy, normal children, leaving many with physical disabilities for the rest of their lives. The conquest of poliomyelitis provides a brilliant example of the successful efforts of medical science combined with intelligent public health measures. For the United States and for other afflicted countries the successful control of poliomyelitis was related not only to a unified national effort, but to one that was international in scope through the World Health Organization.

Many of the historical aspects of the disease have been summed up by John Paul (1971), while M. Fishbein, E. M. Salmonsen, and L. Hektoen (1951) have provided 10,367 bibliographic references pertaining to all phases of poliomyelitis. The first dependable description of the disease was recorded by Michael Underwood (1795), who wrote on "Debility of the Lower Extremities" in children. He described what later became known as "infantile paralysis." J. Heine (1840) in Germany and O. Medin (1890) in Sweden first recognized poliomyelitis as a distinct epidemic disease involving the nervous system, and Ivan Wickman (1913) introduced another synonym, "Heine-Medin disease." Wickman's monograph, based mostly on the 1905 Stockholm epidemic, established many of the epidemiological factors, described the histological findings in the central nervous system, and cited the clinical features of the disease.

The first recognized epidemic of poliomyelitis in the United States occurred in Vermont with 183 cases (Caverly, 1896). Major studies were made by Wade Hampton Frost (1913) of the United States Public Health Service in epidemics occurring in Iowa in 1910, in Cincinnati in 1911, and in Batavia, New York in 1912. Frost made two important epidemiological contributions. First, he pointed out the similarities between measles and poliomyelitis, both diseases occurring in epidemic waves and both involving mostly children. In both diseases there was a younger age distribution in urban as compared to rural areas. Second, he stated that a much larger segment of the population was exposed and infected without manifest illness, as compared to those who became ill. Immunological studies carried out later by others were to substantiate this point. Excellent epidemiological studies by the United States Public Health Service were made during the severe epidemic of 1916, which occurred in New York City and the northeastern United States (Lavinder, Freeman, and Frost, 1918). Among the definitive clinical and pathological studies at the same time were those of F. Peabody, G. Draper, and A. R. Dochez (1912) at the Rockefeller Institute for Medical Research.

While the foregoing studies were under way a momentous discovery was announced in Vienna by Karl Landsteiner and Erwin Popper (1909). They had injected the nerve tissue of a fatal human case into monkeys, reproducing flaccid paralysis and typical histological lesions in the spinal cord. No bacteriological cause could be ascertained, and the disease was presumed to be due to a virus, such as that in rabies. This was a most fortuitous experiment since it involved only one human case and two monkeys. The scientists were particularly fortunate in their selection of the species of monkey for transmitting the disease, since subsequent studies with many other different species of laboratory animals failed to transmit the disease. Landsteiner's and Popper's experiment was soon confirmed, and the observations were extended by S. Flexner and P. A. Lewis (1910a) at the Rockefeller Institute. They transmitted the disease from monkey to monkey, and Flexner (1916) later observed that the virus was inactivated by both convalescent monkey and human serum.

By the 1920s several basic facts about poliomyelitis had been discovered. It was an acute febrile disease of virus origin afflicting principally children during the warmer summer months. Man was its only known reservoir. The epidemics followed the pattern of measles, as a highly contagious disease in which the majority of the population were infected but relatively few developed paralysis. No known means for preventing poliomyelitis existed, and no convincing type of specific therapy was available. Once nerve tissue had been attacked and necrosis had occurred, regeneration did not take place, and permanent paralysis resulted, usually involving one or more extremities. The clinical features followed four possible courses: (1) inapparent infection in probably over 90 percent of those infected; (2) vague febrile illness with upper respiratory manifestations, gastro-enteritis, or generalized body pains like "grippe" or "influenza;" (3) nonparalytic poliomyelitis, in which there were many of the clinical and laboratory findings indicating inflammation of the nervous tissue but without succeeding paralysis; (4) paralytic poliomyelitis involving the spinal cord, or bulboencephalitis, in which the higher nerve centers were involved. This last type was accompanied by a high mortality rate. The primary cause of death was respiratory failure with circulatory collapse.

Although most authorities agreed that poliomyelitis was caused by an unknown type of virus, one startling report appeared in 1916 by Dr. E. C. Rosenow and his associates of the Mayo Clinic stating that a specific strain of a filtrable form of streptococcus was the cause, a thesis that Rosenow relentlessly pursued for over thirty years (Rosenow, 1917; 1949; Rosenow, Towne, and Wheeler, 1916). This could not be confirmed, and general interest subsided.

At this stage of knowledge about poliomyelitis, I had an intensive professional experience in the care of afflicted children during the summer of 1933 in the south department of the Boston City Hospital, which was the unit for contagious diseases. During the epidemic we often worked all night, examining as many as a dozen children and performing an equal number of lumbar punctures to establish or to rule out the diagnosis of poliomyelitis. At the time there was little to offer the patients during the acute phase except steps to relieve the intense pain and spasm of the involved muscles of the extremities. Boston was an outstanding center for orthopedic surgery, and the recommendations of this group predominated in the care of the patients, since orthopedic measures and surgery would be necessary after the pain had subsided and paralysis with its deformities had been established. One of these respected surgeons was Dr. Robert W. Lovett (1917), who had had an extensive experience with the disease. He advocated rest in bed during the acute stage and cautioned against massage and manipulation.

It was surprising to observe the severe amount of muscle atrophy and flexure deformity that could occur in a relatively short period when an extremity was kept constantly at rest. This was particularly evident when the pain was relieved by placing an extremity in a plaster cast, as was practiced so often on patients with poliomyelitis or in the management of sepsis of a large joint, such as the knee or hip. The acute phase was often followed by deformity and lifelong partial disability, in spite of corrective surgical procedures carried out after recovery.

More precise knowledge was needed regarding the pathogenesis of poliomyelitis, which would be dependent on isolation and propagation of the virus. As noted, epidemiological studies had suggested similarities between measles and poliomyelitis. Did this mean that poliomyelitis was an airborne type of infection with passage of the virus from the nasopharynx through the lungs into the circulation and final localization in the nervous system? Or was poliomyelitis an enteric disease with transmission of the virus from human to human through the fecal contamination of milk, water, and food? And would this imply that the virus multiplied in the intestinal tract causing a viremia with systemic disease? Subsequent investigations as detailed by J. R. Paul (1971) supported the enteric thesis, but still left incomplete the manner in which the disease was spread from human to human (Anderson, 1947).

Progress in virology depended on the refinement of techniques, and this was well exemplified in the isolation and growth of the poliomyelitis virus. Although the virus had been demonstrated in human tissues as early as 1908, it was not until 1931 that A. Sabin and P. Olitsky (1936) successfully isolated and propagated the virus in pure culture in human nervous tissue. Unfortunately their strain, maintained by repeated transfers in monkeys, became neurotropic and reproduced only in nervous tissue. J. Enders, T. Weller, and F. Robbins (1949) announced the growth in pure culture of the Lansing strain of poliomyelitis virus in extraneurol human embryonic tissues. This finding was to mark the beginning of a successful approach to vaccine prophylaxis. In the meantime an important sequence of events occurred in the search for further knowledge.

The fact that the spinal cord of monkeys contained an abundance of poliomyelitis virus suggested to investigators that they pursue the concept of Pasteur and use the emulsified spinal cord of monkeys for immunization as he did in rabies with rabbit cord. It should be possible, they thought, to "inactivate" the virus with a chemical such as formalin before such a procedure was carried out in humans. Immunization appeared reasonable because monkey convalescent serum neutralized the virus, and recovered monkeys were immune to lethal doses of virus.

In the field of medical sciences there has always been a calculated risk in going from the laboratory with experimental data obtained in test tubes and with lower animals to the human being. This has been particularly true in the use of vaccines since the time of Jenner. The most successful vaccine is a viable product with attenuated virulence. It takes courage and confidence, combined with a respect for human life, to evaluate a new vaccine. If it is successful, deserved honors go to the pioneers, but if the outcome is disastrous, the consequences are severe. In retrospect, the decision to use emulsified monkey spinal cord for immunization was not justified, because precise techniques for evaluating such a step were not available at the time. Two groups did use such preparations. The first trial on humans was with a preparation of monkey cord exposed to formalin, which was considered by some to be inadequate for *complete* inactivation of the virus (Brodie and Park, 1935). The second trial preparation employed during the same period was subjected to more severe chemical treatment (Kolmer, 1935). Medical science was not ready for the continuation of such vaccinating programs, however, particularly after J. P. Leake (1935) of the United States Public Health Service reported that poliomyelitis occurred in a group of children living in an unexposed area where vaccine was being evaluated.

Another approach to the management of poliomyelitis was the administration of antipoliomyelitis convalescent human serum, encouraged by the work of Dr. Simon Flexner at the Rockefeller Institute for Medical Research. A precedence had been established in the very successful use of diphtheria antitoxin. Although there was no evidence that the poliomyelitis virus produced a toxin, Flexner and P. A. Lewis (1910b) had proved that convalescent monkey serum inactivated the virus, and monkeys pretreated with such serum withstood lethal doses of virus despite the fact that there appeared to be no benefit after the onset of paralysis. Extensive trials on humans with human antiserum were carried out over a period of twenty years by competent investigators without benefit. At best the serum appeared useful as a prophylactic in the preparalytic stage.

For many years research on poliomyelitis was thwarted because the natural course of the disease could be studied experimentally only in monkeys. This was always an expensive and arduous undertaking. Doctor Max Theiler (1934; 1937) of the Rockefeller Institute reported on a form of spontaneous encephalomyelitis in mice that stimulated further research on poliomyelitis. Although the causative virus was unrelated to the human virus, the model, called ''mouse poliomyelitis," had considerable possibilities in future viral studies, including poliomyelitis, as M. Theiler (1941) later pointed out. After Theiler's finding Dr. Charles Armstrong of the United States Public Health Service received specimens of human spinal cord obtained from fatal disease by Dr. Max Peet, professor of surgery at the University of Michigan. C. Armstrong (1939b) succeeded in transmitting the virus in this preparation to monkeys and then to the eastern cotton rat (*Sigmodon hispidus hispidus*). This selection of a rodent was due to the fact that such rats were available at the National Institute of Health. This famous strain of poliomyelitis virus later became known as the Lansing (Mich.) Type II strain. Shortly thereafter Armstrong (1939a) was able to adapt the strain to the white mouse. It is indeed fortunate that rodents, especially mice, were readily available by the time Enders and his group were growing virus in tissue culture. Again we have the demonstration of progress in medical research made possible by the availability of new techniques.

Sometimes a new technique can clarify a complex clinical problem, and at other times wide application of refined procedures may add to the complexity. The advent of tissue culture techniques for viruses led to highly successful vaccine preparations for poliomyelitis, but at the same time it revealed that encephalomeningitis, with and without paralysis, was a malady caused by viruses other than that of poliomyelitis. In 1947 Dr. Gilbert Dalldorf, director of the New York State Health Laboratory, studied a group of cases in children at Coxsackie, New York and isolated a new type of virus from the feces of the children with the use of suckling mice for isolation purposes. In this murine model the virus caused a diffuse myositis. Shortly thereafter he was able to report on a spectrum of what became known as related Coxsackie enteric viruses (Dalldorf and Sickles, 1948). Since many different enteric viruses were found in the fecal contents of febrile and normal children a group of viruses also became known as "orphan viruses" or Enteric Cytopathogenic Human Orphan (ECHO). The name was applied because they were viruses in search of known diseases. These are now known as ECHO viruses, and many produce the clinical features of Coxsackie disease.[13]

As far as poliomyelitis was concerned, the discovery of the Coxsackie and the ECHO group of viruses complicated the previous epidemiological statistics of acute poliomyelitis, especially "abortive" poliomyelitis, since it was impossible to differentiate febrile epidemic diseases without the advantage of specific serological and cultural techniques. Adding to this confusion of differential diagnosis in a modern era was the identification of a large number of Arboviruses, so named because these viruses are transmitted to humans by arthropods, especially mosquitoes, and cause encephalitis and encephalomeningitis. It is because of this complex picture that public health diagnostic laboratories at local, national, and international levels became so helpful in clinical medicine.

While startling advances were being made in understanding the specific cause of poliomyelitis, supportive therapy was all that could be offered to the patient during the acute paralytic stage and physiotherapy during the convalescent period. Two therapeutic advancements merit brief discussion, however. The first was the introduction of the respirator, or "iron lung," of Dr. Philip Drinker and his associates (Drinker and McKhann, 1929) at the Harvard School of Public Health. One of the serious features of poliomyelitis occurred in patients with severe respiratory distress due to paralysis of the intercostal muscles and the diaphragm, and in those with involvement of the brain stem. Death was inevitable in many patients unless breathing was assisted mechanically. My first professional experience with the cumbersome early model of the respirator was with that used in the 1930s at the Boston City Hospital. In 1946 I also observed a severe epidemic of poliomyelitis in Minnesota. In a period of four months, 183 cases of bulbar poliomyelitis were admitted to the University of Minnesota Hospitals under the care of Dr. A. B. Baker, chief of neurology. An entire floor of the department was filled with respirators. The patients in these respirators received meticulous and thorough care. Doctor Baker stressed the necessity of maintaining a free air passage; in the more severe cases, respiratory assistance was combined with tracheostomy and the introduction of oxygen through a tube into the trachea. He believed that anoxia and cyanosis could lead to brain damage. This was a distinct advance in treatment, the details of which have been recorded (Baker, 1949).

A second, more dramatic advance was made by the Australian nurse Sister Elizabeth Kenny. In 1940, at the invitation of Dr. Harold Diehl, dean of the University of Minnesota Medical School, she demonstrated her methods of treating patients during the acute paralytic stage of poliomyelitis at the University Hospitals. I was on the committee that shared in the responsibility of having her with us. Doctor Milan Knapp, director of the department of physical medicine, and Dr. John Pohl, an orthopedic surgeon in Minneapolis, were most closely associated with her. She immediately revolutionized treatment through the utilization of wet heat, massage, and early involuntary movement of the muscles. During this acute, painful, and spastic stage, skill and patience were necessary, and Sister Kenny possessed these qualities, except that she had no patience with the orthopedic surgeons! Unfortunately she was not content to teach only her therapeutic approach but asserted, in her own terminology, her opinions on the pathogenesis of the disease; and she brooked no criticism. I was so convinced of the success of her methods, however, after seeing the recovery of patients without deformity as well as the rather early return of the voluntary use of muscles with little or no atrophy, that I could only subscribe to her efforts. They marked a radical departure from the immobilization of extremities with plaster casts observed during the 1930s. Her stormy career has been thoroughly recorded by a capable science writer (Cohn, 1975).

By 1950 it appeared that a vaccine for the prevention of poliomyelitis would be forthcoming. Large amounts of virus could be harvested by the new culture techniques, and — fortunately — only three immunological types of virus were involved. The National Foundation for Infantile Paralysis (NFIP) sponsored research programs, such as that carried out by Dr. Jonas Salk at the University of Pittsburgh. Born in New York City, Salk was a physician who was also trained in biochemistry and virology. He inactivated the virus cultures with formalin, as had been done previously, and successfully carried out preliminary testing in humans (Salk, 1953).

After feverish consultations and meetings attended by American authorities, a field trial with the Salk vaccine was undertaken. The evaluation of the trial was under the direction of Dr. Thomas Francis, Jr. at the University of Michigan. Between March 1954 and June 1954, 1,829,916 American children in 211 areas of 44 states were involved. Some received the vaccine, some a placebo, and some neither. On April 12, 1955 the famous report by Dr. Francis announced in Ann Arbor that the vaccine trial was successful. But within 15 days disaster occurred, with the information that 214 cases of poliomyelitis were associated with the vaccine study, of whom 79 had received the vaccine, the remainder being contacts. There were 11 deaths, mostly due to the Type I (Mahoney) strain present in the vaccine. The source of the incriminated vaccine was the Cutter Laboratories, and the United States Public Health Service quickly terminated any further vaccine emanating from that source. But by 1960 the Salk vaccine had regained its useful position, except that an oral preparation was urgently needed if the vaccine were to be used widely in developing countries.

Intensive investigations with oral forms of attenuated living virus were under way, with the support of the World Health Organization and the United States Public Health Service (U.S. Public Health Service, Report to the Surgeon General, 1964; World Health Organization, Expert Committee on Poliomyelitis, 1958). Pioneers in this effort included Dr. Harold Cox of the Lederle Laboratories, Dr. Hiliary Koprowski in Philadelphia, and Dr. Albert Sabin at the University of Cincinnati. Sabin had been interested in poliomyelitis for many years. He was an accomplished scientist and virologist, and he successfully prepared an effective oral preparation for immunization (Sabin, Hen-

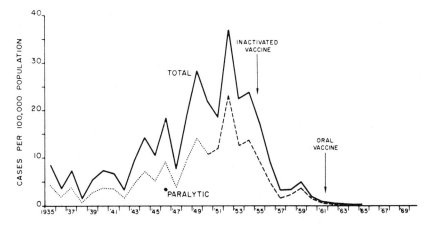

Figure 11. Annual poliomyelitis incidence rates, United States, 1935–1964, and paralytic poliomyelitis cases, United States, 1961–1967. Reproduced with permission of publisher from John R. Paul, *A History of Poliomyelitis*, New Haven: Yale University Press, 1971 (Figure 58, p. 439).

nessen, and Winsser, 1954). It was largely through his energetic efforts at an international level that the oral vaccine preparation received its general acceptance and proved highly successful, a story Sabin told when he received the Lasker Award (Sabin, 1965). In those areas where oral vaccines have been properly used, paralytic poliomyelitis has become a rare disease (Figure 11). The control of poliomyelitis is a great achievement, but the disease has not been completely eradicated. Persistent surveillance and immunization programs are essential.

CHAPTER 14

Respiratory Diseases

The Common Cold (Upper Respiratory Infections)

In a modern industrial society upper respiratory infections cause more disability in otherwise healthy individuals than any other affliction. A pertinent scientific study carried out on twenty-five thousand illnesses in a group of families in Cleveland, Ohio between January 1, 1948 and May 31, 1957 showed that each person in a family of three or more averaged 5.6 respiratory infections per year, which were caused by a wide spectrum of microbes, mostly viruses (Dingle, Badger, and Jordan, Jr., 1964). In this as in many other studies bacteria were not found to be the primary cause of the common cold (Andrewes, 1965; Tyrrell, 1965).

Although man had probably suffered from minor respiratory ailments over the centuries, little prominence was given to discussion of the common cold before the eighteenth century. During the first part of the nineteenth century one of the influential English medical teachers was Thomas Watson (1853a) of London. There were four editions printed of his *Lectures on the Principles and Practice of Physic*. He discoursed on catarrh[1] as an "inflammation of the mucous membrane of the air passages" plaguing the sinuses, nose and trachea. "Not one man in ten thousand passes a winter without having a *cold* of some sort. . . . It does not always or often result, I apprehend, from cold air brought into contact with the membrane itself, in the process of breathing; but from cold, and especially from cold and wet, applied to the external integument" (Watson, 1853a, p. 532). Relief of symptoms, according to Watson, was obtained with opium, a mild purge, hot wine, and rest. The cause was suspected to be exposure to cold and wet, a concept that trailed well into the twentieth century. Watson concluded that catarrh and other epidemics were connected with a state or contamination of the atmosphere.

Almost one hundred years after Watson's recommendation for the treatment of the common cold, Dr. Harold Diehl (1933), director of the student health service and later dean of the medical school at the University of Minnesota, carried out controlled studies on the treatment of this disease among hundreds of students. He concluded that opium given during the acute phase produced the best relief and recommended a combination of codeine sulphate and papavarine.[2]

During the twentieth century scientific interest in the common cold increased as the disability afflicted military personnel in two world wars. Investigations were encouraged within the new discipline of virology. A mammoth review by the Pickett-Thomson Research Laboratory referred to two thousand papers on the subject (Thomson and Thomson, 1932), and Arthur Bloomfield (1958f), a student of respiratory diseases, summarized a group of pertinent studies.

Interest in the possible viral etiology of the common cold was aroused by research at Columbia University (Dochez, Shibley, and Mills, 1930). Colds were produced in human volunteers with cell-free filtrates of human nasal secretions, but attempts to isolate a virus and to transmit the infection to lower animals yielded doubtful results. Some of the most successful research was directed by Dr. C. Andrewes (1965) and his associates, who organized The Common Cold Research Unit at Salisbury, England just before World War II. They employed carefully controlled experimental procedures with human volunteers and dispelled the myth that physiological alterations caused by cold and wet induced common colds. On the other hand, there remained little question that a respiratory infection could be transmitted with the filtered nasal secretions of patients. Perhaps the most outstanding finding of this group and others — summarized by D. A. Tyrrell (1965) — is that the common cold is due to a wide spectrum of viruses. These include the myxovirus group, para-influenza and respiratory syncytial viruses, as well as the influenza viruses A, B and more rarely C; the adenoviruses; the reoviruses; the enteroviruses, including the coxsackieviruses and echoviruses; rhinoviruses; and *Mycoplasma pneumoniae*, to be discussed in conjunction with pneumonia.

With such an array of viruses causing the common cold, the outlook for the control of these respiratory infections with vaccines is gloomy. But there remains hope that drug therapy may prove beneficial. The importance of viral nasopharyngitis is that the inflammatory reaction induced by these organisms supports secondary bacterial infection and contributes to the onset of bacterial pneumonia.

Pneumonia [3]

William Osler's *Practice of Medicine* was the most universally used medical textbook at the beginning of the twentieth century. The introductory chapter discussed typhoid fever, probably the leading cause of the hospitalization of patients with acute illness at that time. Osler's work was subsequently replaced by an American text, edited by Dr. Russell Cecil (1928), to which numerous authors contributed. Cecil's book reflected a change in emphasis on diseases; in its introductory pages typhoid fever was replaced by respiratory infections, including influenza and pneumonia. Typhoid fever had become an uncommon disease, but in many hospitals pneumonia became the leading cause for admission.

Pneumonia is an inflammatory condition of pulmonary tissue caused most commonly by different species of bacteria, but also by viruses and occasionally by chemicals. In the classic clinical sense pneumonia means infection due to pneumococci; pneumococcal lobar pneumonia was graphically and correctly delineated clinically and pathologically by R. Laennec (1819, translation 1823), although the etiology was not established until fifty years later (Fraenkel, 1886; Weichselbaum, 1887b).

Although knowledge on the pathogenesis and management of pneumonia was rapidly acquired during the twentieth century and serotherapy proved successful, as will be discussed shortly, such specific therapy was not yet available during World War I. The impact of influenza during the war is discussed later. The United States Army, with a total strength of slightly over four million, had almost one million cases of influenza; over 99 percent of the deaths due to influenza were caused by pneumonia, including pneumococcal lobar pneumonia, as well as those caused by hemolytic streptococci, *H. influenzae*, and staphylococci. There were at least seventy-six thousand cases of lobar pneumonia, and the most serious complication was empyema (Hall, 1928; Opie et al., 1921).

The 1890s brought the introduction of serotherapy for diphtheria, and it proved to be a lasting triumph. G. Klemperer and F. Klemperer (1891) in Germany investigated antipneumococcal immunity. F. Neufeld (1902) made the important observation that the pneumococcus capsule swelled (the so-called quellen phenomenon) when the organism came into contact with specific antiserum. Another milestone was reached when A. R. Dochez and L. J. Gillespie (1913) discovered three main antigenic types of pneumococci, designated Types I, II, and III, and an ill-defined Type IV group. O. T. Avery (1915) subdivided the groups still further; by 1932 thirty-two types had been described (Cooper et al., 1932). The classification of pneumococci became the basis for the extensive studies on specific serum therapy carried out by the group at the Rockefeller Institute for Medical Research (Avery et al., 1917).

The State Public Health Laboratories of New York and Massachusetts assumed an aggressive policy in developing and dispensing antipneumococcal horse serum. An extensive program with appropriate advisory committees was inaugurated in Massachusetts in 1931 and in New York in 1935. The Massachusetts program was carried out over a five-year period (1931–1935). During this time hundreds of patients were treated at the Boston City Hospital under the able direction of Drs. M. Finland and W. D. Sutliff. As a member of the house staff between 1932 and 1937 I had an extensive experience in treating these patients. It was laborious work, entailing long hours of effort. We had to type the pneumococci in the sputa of the patients by the Neufeld method, and then cautiously administer the type-specific antipneumococcal horse serum intravenously. Serum reactions occurred frequently, sometimes of a serious nature. At a later period, antipneumococcal rabbit serum was used, which caused fewer reactions. Serotherapy was successful, especially in the uncomplicated cases, and the death rate from pneumonia was reduced.

The literature on pneumococcal pneumonia is extensive, but fortunately two monumental volumes summarize the experimental and clinical work (Heffron, 1939; White, 1938). The Massachusetts program of serum treatment was summarized by F. T. Lord and R. Heffron (1938).

Although lobar pneumonia due to pneumococci was the most commonly encountered form of pneumonia during the foregoing period, it must be emphasized that the disease was also frequently caused by other pathogens, including hemolytic streptococci, staphylococci, *Hemophilus influenzae*, and Klebsiellae (Reimann, 1954). In contrast to pneumococcal pneumonia, no successful serotherapy was acquired for these other forms of the disease, except for suppurative meningitis due to *H. influenzae*.

After type-specific antipneumococcal sera had become available the question arose as to whether there was any immunological basis for the development of a prophylactic vaccine. This question did not go unanswered. Invasiveness of the pneumococcus is dependent on the type-specific capsular polysaccharide. Recovery from pneumococcal pneumonia is accompanied by the appearance of serum antibodies for the type-specific capsular polysaccharide, and the acquired immunity endures for as long as a year. It was clearly demonstrated that humans could be protected for one season by a single injection of small quantities of one or more type-specific pneumococcal polysaccharides (MacLeod et al., 1945). Such a prophylactic program was not seriously expanded, however, because of the advent of successful chemotherapy.

Sulfanilamide became available in 1937, and for the first time chemotherapy was effective against streptococcal infections, including pneumonia due to Group A hemolytic streptococci. This success was particularly applicable to the cases of highly lethal streptococcal empyema. But sulfanilamide was without effect in the pneumonias caused by other species of bacteria.

In 1938 an analogue of sulfanilamide, sulfapyridine, was shown to be effective in the treatment of pneumococcal pneumonia (Whitby, 1938). This drug was also beneficial in the treatment of the universally fatal pneumococcal complication, suppurative meningitis. But other bacterial causes of pneumonia were not influenced by sulfapyridine. By 1943 penicillin was shown to be valuable therapeutically for pneumococcal, streptococcal, and staphylococcal pneumonia. In the ensuing quarter of a century other antibiotics were used for a wider spectrum of microorganisms, so that bacterial pneumonia was brought under control but by no means eradicated.

Mycoplasma Pneumonia (Primary Atypical Pneumonia)

While suppurative bacterial pneumonias have a fairly well-defined clinical pattern and the pathological findings are distinctive, there is a group of "atypical pneumonias" in which the differential diagnosis is not easy. In an era when specific drug therapy was readily available, precise differentiation became a major factor for the welfare of the patient, and with modern technological and laboratory aids the distinction could be made.

H. Reimann (1938) called attention to a form of atypical pneumonia that was considered to be viral in origin. Shortly thereafter I saw a number of young adults on the student health service at the University of Minnesota Hospitals with clinical findings similar to those described by Reimann. The features were a gradual onset of malaise, fever and chilly sensations, and severe headaches and body pains, followed by a nonproductive cough. The severity of the symptoms was in marked contrast with the few abnormal physical findings in the chest. The mortality rate was low, and convalescence was often prolonged. Having been hospitalized with this disease myself, I reviewed the subject (Spink, 1943).

As a member of the United States Army Commission on Hemolytic Streptococcal Infections in World War II, I observed many cases of atypical pneumonia in young recruits. No specific treatment was available. The surgeon-general of the Army issued a clinical description of the disease (Commission on Pneumonia, Board for the Investigation and Control of Influenza and other Epidemic Diseases in the United States Army, 1942). Important work on this illness was conducted by the Commission on Acute Respiratory Diseases, Fort Bragg, North Carolina (1945b). Working with healthy human volunteers, this group transmitted the infection to them with bacteria-free nasopharyngeal washings from patients. It was presumed that an unknown virus was the etiological agent. Independently M. D. Eaton, G. Meiklejohn, and W. van Herick (1944) isolated what was considered a virus from patients and successfully transmitted it to cotton rats, hamsters, and chick embryos. Subsequently "Eaton's agent" was found to be a unique genus of the microorganism *Mycoplasma* (Couch, 1973). Other species in this group do infect animals naturally, causing contagious pleuropneumonia in cattle (Nocard and Roux, 1898). Mycoplasmas are not viruses. The organisms grow on artificial media, but unlike bacteria, they do not have a cell wall and hence are not affected by penicillin. If the disease is recognized early, however, the administration of tetracycline is beneficial.

Influenza

Influenza is one of the afflictions that has continued to elude man's efforts to control and limit all pandemics of infectious diseases. According to Charles Creighton (1894b, see p. 304) two origins have been proposed for the term "influenza," the first of Italian derivation meaning influenced by the stars. He accepts the second, originating from humoral pathology, *influsso* or *influxio*, meaning catarrh or defluxion. The terms *la grippe* and *influenza* were often used interchangeably in the medical literature, even until recent times. *La grippe* is the name of an insect that was very common in France prior to an epidemic of influenza that people believed contaminated the atmosphere (Creighton, 1894b).

I remember vividly a double disaster that occurred in 1918 in Duluth, Minnesota. On Saturday, October 12th a forest fire raged around much of the city and destroyed two hundred thousand acres of wooded land. Almost five hundred lives were lost. A bloody sun was high in the sky and wood smoke permeated the atmosphere. Crowds of refugees, having lost all of their possessions, streamed into Duluth and were housed temporarily in every available building, including the National Guard Armory. I was one of the high school volunteers who joined in collecting clothing, bedding, and food for the victims.

The day before, October 11th, the school had been closed because of an epidemic of the "flu." This was the second wave of the pandemic to be discussed shortly. Wherever people were congregated gauze masks were worn. I gathered bedding in a car driven by a young woman, seemingly healthy, but two days later she was dead, a victim of influenza. This terrible pattern swept through the community, killing rich and poor alike, healthy young adults and the aged especially. One of the remarkable features of the epidemic was that some families, including my own, were repeatedly exposed but suffered no ill effects, while near neighbors had visitations of sudden death.[4]

There is scattered, but doubtful, evidence that influenza was recognized as early as the twelfth century. Until the seventeenth century, however, if influenza did occur, plague was so extensive and severe that clear-cut descriptions of influenza at that time are lacking. There appears little doubt that influenza was correctly observed in the eighteenth century by many leading English physicians. Doctor C. H. Stuart-Harris, a contemporary authority on the disease, enjoys quoting the physician Dr. John Huxham, who described an epidemic in and around Plymouth, England in 1743 as follows (Stuart-Harris, 1961, p. 54):

A kind of fever, in general slight, but some times not a little fatal to old men and children who had weak lungs, raged throughout all this country. At once and at the same time, innumerable persons were seized with a wandering kind of shiver and heaviness in the head; presently also came on a pain therein and also in the joints and back; several however, were troubled with universal lassitude. Immediately a very great and acrid defluxion from the eyes, nostrils and fauces, and very often falling upon the lungs, which occasion almost perpetual sneezings, and commonly a violent cough.

And as Stuart-Harris commented (p. 54), "Epidemics come and epidemics go, but the clinical picture of influenza remains remarkably unchanged." T. Thompson, writing on the history of influenza stated (1852, Introduction, p. x), "There is a grandeur in its constancy and immutability superior to the influence of natural habits."

Medical historians have cited the appearance of influenza epidemics in past centuries. Not until the nineteenth century, however, was scientific evidence adequate to substantiate many of their conclusions. This was largely due to the developing disciplines of bacteriology and pathology, and also to the new science of statistics. Influenza does have a constant type of clinical pattern, but it also simulates a number of acute respiratory infections, each due to a different virus.

The initial appearance of epidemic influenza in any area (first wave) is characterized by a febrile disease of sudden onset with generalized body aches, prostration, sore throat, headache, insomnia, and intermittent gastro-intestinal complaints. A prominent feature is a cough with bright red blood in the sputum. Recovery usually takes place in the uncomplicated case within a week or ten days, although convalescence may be prolonged. Secondary pulmonary infections may occur due to a spectrum of bacteria such as staphylococci, streptococci, pneumococci, and *H. influenzae*. In recent years staphylococcal pneumonia has been one of the more severe complications (Wollenman, Jr. and Finland, 1943).

During a large-scale epidemic, or pandemic, such as that of 1918–1919, after a lapse of several weeks a second wave of the disease appears, and in more severe form. Those afflicted during the first wave are immune. In a serious attack of influenza, fever, prostration, and collapse can occur suddenly with the rapid onset of pulmonary manifestations such as cough and copious, bloody sputum. The toxemia is accompanied by respiratory distress and a heliotropic type of cyanosis of the face. Death may occur within a few days after onset. Another form is the onset of a febrile illness that progresses for several days, after which a lethal secondary bacterial pneumonia occurs. One can readily appreciate why the mortality rate is exceptionally high in those with cardiac or pulmonary disease and in the aged.

The pandemic of 1889–1892 was the first time that the rhythm of the first and second waves of influenza was clearly defined. The disciplines of pathology and bacteriology contributed new information, which supplemented the clinical observations of previous generations. Out of this came a controversy concerning the etiology of influenza that was not to be resolved for another half century. R. Pfeiffer (1892) reported that he consistently found a gram-negative bacillus in the pulmonary tissues and exudate of influenza victims. This became known as *Hemophilus influenzae*, or "Pfeiffer's bacillus." It was widely, though not universally, accepted as the cause of influenza.

Although epidemic influenza occurred periodically after 1892, it was not until 1918 during World War I that a pandemic again appeared. The pandemic of 1918–1919 was more widespread, afflicting more people and carrying with it a mortality rate greater than any other epidemic disease since the Black Death of the fourteenth century. It is estimated that throughout the world there were 21,642,283 deaths due to influenza among a population of two billion, or 527 per hundred thousand (Jordan, 1927). There were 548,452 deaths in the United States and 112,329 deaths in England and Wales (Great Britain Ministry of Health, 1920). Starting in the spring of 1918, the first wave of the epidemic spread rapidly to Europe and thence to the United States. The second wave struck with fury in October of 1918. The rapid spread and the severity of the pandemic were marked by the number of cases that appeared simultaneously in Boston and in Bombay. The highest attack rate was in those under fifteen years of age, and the greatest mortality rates were in infants, young adults, and the aged. According to Dr. Hans Zinsser (1922), in India the number of deaths was about five million. In the American Army the total hospital admissions for influenza in 1918 was over six hundred thousand with 23,007 deaths. If to this are added the deaths from pulmonary complications the total number was 39,371.

The origin of this pandemic is subject to controversy. Although Spain was long considered the area of origin and the disease was called "Spanish influenza," there is no substantial evidence to support this. The records of the United States Army indicate clearly that the first group of cases appeared in troops at Fort Riley, Kansas in March 1918. It is possible, though not proved, that this was the original focus of the worldwide expansion of the disease (Kaplan and Webster, 1977).

The pandemic of 1918–1919 stimulated many investigations on the disease during and after the war. In two massive volumes Thomson and Thomson (1933–1934) reviewed the literature on influenza up until 1934. Zinsser (1922), an active observer of the pandemic in the armed forces, had previously reviewed the etiology and epidemiology and reserved his judgement as to whether influenza was due to H. influenzae or to an unknown virus. Among the outstanding advances made during World War I on the nature of influenza were the superb pathological studies, especially those of M. C. Winternitz and his associates (Winternitz, Wason, and McNamara, 1920), and those carried out by the United States Medical Department in the Armed Forces (Callender, 1929). The notable pathological feature was the extensive hyalinization and necrosis of the entire endothelial surfaces from the trachea to the pulmonary parenchyma.

But the most elusive question was that of the precise cause of influenza, the answer to which came from an unusual source. Doctor J. S. Koen was a veterinarian and an inspector for the Bureau of Animal Industry in charge of hog cholera control in Iowa. He made some remarkable observations in the fall of 1918 and winter of 1919 describing the close relationship between an illness in swine and in man, and stated (1919, p. 468),

I have no apologies to offer for my diagnosis of "flu." Last fall and winter we were confronted with a new condition, if not a new disease. I believe I have as much to support this diagnosis in pigs as the physicians have to support a similar diagnosis in man. The similarity of the epidemic among people and the epidemic among pigs was so close, the reports so frequent, that an outbreak in the family would be followed immediately by an outbreak among the hogs, and vice versa, as to present a most striking coincidence if not suggesting a close relation between the two conditions. It looked like "flu," it presented the identical symptoms of "flu," it terminated like "flu," and until proved it was not "flu" I shall stand by that diagnosis.

The search for the etiology of influenza was encouraged by the important investigations of the veterinary medical scientist Dr. Richard Shope (1931; 1944) of the Rockefeller Institute for Medical Research, who demonstrated that a virus was responsible for swine influenza, which acted synergistically with *Hemophilus influenzae suis* in producing the disease.

Shortly thereafter Wilson Smith, C. H. Andrewes, and P. P. Laidlaw (1933) isolated the influenza virus from ferrets that had been inoculated with the nasopharyngeal secretions from human patients. Thereafter growth of the virus was achieved in mice and in chick embryos, and the antigenic relationship between swine influenza virus and human virus was established. This was designated Type A influenza virus. Another type of human influenza virus known as Type B was isolated later (Francis, Jr., 1940). A third, Type C, is found only occasionally.

A significant epidemiological finding was made concerning the occurrence of Type A and B epidemics (Commission on Acute Respiratory Diseases, Fort Bragg, North Carolina, 1946b). Sixteen widespread epidemics of influenza occurring in the United States between 1920 and 1944 were analyzed, and it was determined that influenza A had a cycle of every two to three years, and Type B every four to six years. The sequence of cyclic epidemics in relation to the evaluation of prophylactic vaccines was to provide considerable confusion subsequently.

Following the isolation of the Type A in 1933, the British investigators found an opportunity to test a vaccine in the 1936–1937 epidemic (Stuart-Harris, Andrewes, and Smith, 1938). Although the parenteral administration of formalized vaccine to human volunteers was associated with the appearance of neutralizing antibodies in the sera, its efficacy remained uncertain. Fortunately influenza was not a serious problem in World War II, as it had been in World War I. There was no pandemic, but epidemics did occur in 1940–1941 and in 1943, the latter being the more severe. Field trials of a combined Type A and B vaccine indicated that a more lasting immunity appeared with Type B. The vaccine appeared to offer protection, but further evaluation was necessary.

By 1956 it had been established that viruses causing fowl plague, duck influenza, and equine influenza, as well as swine influenza, were antigenically related to human influenza A (Kaplan and Beveridge, 1972). These important findings had a bearing on investigations relating to the pandemic of 1957–1958, called "Asian flu," which originated in interior China. This strain was antigenically different from those previously isolated, and there was suggestive evidence that there was an animal reservoir for "Asian flu." WHO officials then supported a worldwide survey of domestic animals as possible reservoirs of influenza virus. It was found that swine influenza was present in Czechoslovakia as well as in the United States, and equine influenza was reported from many countries.

In the 1968 pandemic caused by the "Hong Kong" strain, a marked antigenic difference was detected between this newly isolated strain and the previously recognized Asian strains. Furthermore antibodies for the Hong Kong virus were found in the sera of persons in Taiwan, Hungary, Great Britain, and the United States. It is now known that dogs, as well as several species of birds, harbor the virus.

Influenza is the last uncontrolled pandemic infectious disease. Epidemics recur because of the appearance of new antigenic types, especially Type A. Exposure of human populations to previous types through either natural disease or immunization does not result in immunity to these newer types. The basic immunological and epidemiological principles underlying the occurrence of repeated epidemics of influenza can be summarized. The main antigenic and biochemical components of the virus are hemagglutinin and neuramidase found in the genetic composition of RNA, which is present in eight separate single-strand segments. Specific immunity for influenza depends on the development of antibodies against hemagglutinin and neuramidase. Major shifts in the recombination of the RNA genetic material during replication in animal or avian reservoirs can result in a new antigenic type, however. It is predicated that such a mixture of virus particles might invade a susceptible human population, especially very young children, and initiate infection against which no immunity exists. A major shift in the genetic composition of the virus necessitates the production of a new prophylactic vaccine. The biological shifts in the influenza virus are unlike the more stable viruses of the other pandemic diseases, such as smallpox and yellow fever, and the viruses of childhood diseases, such as measles. For this reason standardized vaccine preparations for these diseases are readily available at the very early appearance of recurring epidemics. Intensive research is necessary so that a combination or combinations of influenza vaccine can be prepared and used at the earliest stage of an epidemic caused by a new variant of virus.

The appearance of a human "swine" type of influenza A in 1976 produced alarm and the fear of a repetition of the pandemic of 1918. As a result, for the first time a national immunization program was inaugurated in the United States. This is discussed in Section I, Chapter 3.[5]

Tuberculosis

Epidemics of cholera during the nineteenth century aroused the public and the medical profession more than any other infectious disease. Cholera was a spectacular illness, appearing suddenly, the patients either dying or recovering within a few days. In contrast, tuberculosis was a treacherous, insidious, and debilitating disease that afflicted more people than cholera or any other illness, with death occurring in the majority of cases only after a lingering sickness. Until 1909 tuberculosis was the chief cause of death in the United States (Long, 1961). Around 1850 the mortality rates of tuberculosis in the United States and England approached 25 percent of all deaths.

The magnitude of the problem of tuberculosis over a period of a hundred years is revealed in the statistics of the state of Massachusetts. In the first annual report in 1842, "consumption" caused 22 percent of all deaths. In an analysis of two 40-year periods, however, progressive control of the disease occurred as follows (Chadwick and Pope, 1942, p. 3): "from 1860 through 1899 the rate declined from 444 to 254 for 100,000 population, a drop of 190 points or 43 percent. From 1900 through 1939 the rate declined twice as much, from 253 to 36, a drop of 217 points or 86 percent." The horrible attack rate of tuberculosis that occurred in Massachusetts over a century ago parallels the incidence of the disease in many parts of the world today where proper control measures are lacking. The records of the Minnesota State Department of Health show that the death rate was 108.1 per hundred thousand in 1887, a level that was maintained for the next quarter of a century.

Although tuberculosis alarmed several medical leaders early in the twentieth century, it was not until after World War I that determined efforts were made to control the disease in the developed nations. Several volumes have appeared on the history of tuberculosis (Brown, 1941; Castiglioni, 1933; Cummins, 1949; Flick, 1925; Kayne, 1937; Webb, 1936). Most students of the disease agree, from evidence of lesions in recovered skeletons, that human tuberculosis existed in prehistoric periods. Hippocratic recordings in the section "Of the Epidemics" state (1939, p. 99), "Consumption was the most considerable of the diseases which then prevailed" and malaria proved most fatal in "phthisical persons."[6] Tuberculosis was known "throughout medical and nonmedical writings under a bewildering variety of names. Besides the words 'phthisis,' 'consumption' and 'scrofula,' the expressions 'asthenia,' 'tabes,' 'bronchitis,' 'inflammation of the lungs,' 'hectic fever,' 'gastric fever,' 'lupus,' and many more, referred in most cases to conditions now known to have been caused by tubercle bacilli" (Dubos and Dubos, 1952, p. 10).

The ancient Greeks managed patients with an unusual degree of common sense. "The treatment of tuberculosis . . . was rational and in some respects similar to that which we use at the present day. In the acute stages they treated it as they did pneumonia and pleurisy, with baths, cleaning out of the bowels, liquid diet, rest, and drugs which opened up the secretions and quieted the circulation. In the chronic form they used relative rest, a diet of rich, easily digested food, moderate exercise in some cases, and occasionally change of climate" (Flick, 1925, p. 21).

Although it was not until the latter part of the nineteenth century that *Mycobacterium tuberculosis* was established as the cause of tuberculosis, and that the disease was transmitted from human to human, it is remarkable that some of the earlier physicians possessed a keen insight into the nature of the disease, which they obtained through shrewd clinical observations. Girolamo Fracastoro (1930) stated in the fifteenth century that contagious phthisis was contracted by people living in contact with the disease. Benjamin Marten (1720) wrote an extraordinary treatise in which he postulated the contagiousness of the disease. He believed that animalcules residing in tuberculous victims could find their way through the air to susceptible persons.

It may be therefore very likely, that by an habitual lying in the same Bed with a Consumptive Patient, constantly Eating and Drinking with him, or by very frequently conversing so nearly, as to draw in part the Breath he emits from his Lungs, a Consumption may be caught by a sound Person; for it may be reasonable to suppose that if the Blood and Juices of such distemper'd People, be charg'd with vast quantities of *Animalcula*, as I have conjectur'd, then their profuse Sweats, and their Breath also, may be likewise charg'd with them, or their Ova or Eggs, which by that means may possibly be convey'd into the Bodies of those who lie, or are most conversant with them (Marten, 1720, p. 79).

Basic to the evolution of knowledge about the nature of tuberculosis were the thorough clinical and pathological studies in the nineteenth century by G. L. Bayle (1810, translation 1815). René Laennec (1819, translation 1823) correlated the physical findings in pulmonary tuberculosis with the underlying pathological changes of the lungs, bronchi, and pleura by percussion of the chest wall and auscultation of the breath sounds with the stethoscope.

The most outstanding advance in the history of tuberculosis was the discovery of the etiology of the disease (Koch, 1882, translation 1938). It was not only superb experimental work, but convincing to the medical world. Although the justification for the general admiration of Dr. Robert Koch's clear-cut investigations cannot be denied, priority for demonstrating the infectious nature of tuberculosis rests with the French Army surgeon and academician Jean Antoine Villemin. Over two decades before the celebrated announcement of Koch, Villemin was impressed with the similarities between glanders in the horse and tuberculosis in man. Glanders could be transmitted by inoculation from animal to animal, thus demonstrating the infectious nature of the disease. Villemin inoculated sputum and caseous material from humans with tuberculosis into guinea pigs and rabbits and described disseminated disease in the animals. This showed that tuberculosis too was transmitted from animal to animal through inoculation. Villemin injected rabbits with the tuberculous tissues of cows and concluded that this source of tuberculosis provoked a more virulent disease in rabbits than that obtained from human sources, thus antedating the later discovery by Theobald Smith (Villemin, 1868).

Almost simultaneously with Villemin, Dr. William Budd of typhoid fame had written a note upon the contagious nature of tuberculosis. He put his ideas in writing about 1857, but they were not published until October 12, 1867 in *The Lancet* (Paget, 1867). According to Budd, tuberculosis was a zymotic disease such as typhoid fever, scarlet fever, typhus, and syphilis and was disseminated to susceptible persons, usually under crowded conditions, by specific germs cast off in the tuberculous matter (sputum?) of persons suffering from the disease. Budd cited the unfortunate victims under the crowded circumstances of jails, ships, convents, and harems!

Although Villemin transmitted bovine tuberculosis experimentally to rabbits, the importance of the bovine in the epidemiology of the human disease was not clearly demonstrated until the experiments of Dr. Theobald Smith (1898) thirty years later. Cattle proved to be a major reservoir of the disease, and milk was the source of considerable tuberculosis in humans. The concentration of the disease in cattle was emphasized by the incidence in one of the cleanest herds in Great Britain, that of Queen Victoria. "In 1890, Queen Victoria ordered that the dairy cows on the Home Farm at Windsor be tested with tuberculin. Thirty-five of the forty cows were found to be tuberculin-positive and tuberculous lesions were found in all of them!" (Dubos and Dubos, 1952, p. 260)

One of the great advances in the control of human tuberculosis was the use of tuberculin for skin testing (Mantoux, 1910; Pirquet, 1907). This offered a simple epidemiological tool for ascertaining the incidence of the disease. Finally the introduction of X-ray techniques for chest examinations in the twentieth century provided an additional screening process for large populations in surveys for evidence of pulmonary tuberculosis.

As people were surveyed for the presence of active disease, major epidemiological data were acquired that would aid control programs. An important feature of the natural course of tuberculosis was the age distribution. From birth to one year there was great susceptibility, and the mortality rate was high. The trend receded between five and sixteen years, rose between sixteen and twenty-five years, and then declined again, only to afflict the aged. The majority of children and young adults who became infected, as demonstrated by a positive tuberculin reaction or by roentgenological evidence of a healed pulmonary lesion, usually had inactive disease for the rest of their lives, but during advanced age the disease frequently became reactivated. These age factors were important in preventive programs against the disease.

One of the questions concerning the pathogenesis of tuberculosis related to the natural resistance or susceptibility to the disease on a familial or hereditary basis. Studies in experimental animals supported a genetic relationship, but evidence in human tuberculosis was less clear-cut (Rich, 1944). Nevertheless studies on identical human twins revealed a close relationship for susceptibility in monozygotic partners compared to other control groups (Kallmann and Reisner, 1943). J. B. McDougall, who has studied tuberculosis from a global viewpoint, has concluded (1949, p. 197), "in the case of a slow chronic disease like tuberculosis it may be many generations before the effects of native resistance can be determined."

Likewise there has been considerable confusion concerning the susceptibility of certain ethnic groups or races to tuberculosis. American statistics on tuberculosis correctly emphasize the high morbidity and mortality rates of blacks. But the blacks in slavery suffered little from it (Mays, 1904). They were members of an apparently healthy, well-nourished, and isolated group, relatively free of tuberculosis. Only when they were liberated and gravitated to the large industrial areas with poor housing and crowded living conditions did they fall victims to the disease. The African black did not suffer from tuberculosis until he was exposed to the inroads of civilization. The attack rate was also very high among the newly-arrived Irish immigrants in the slums of New York and Boston. Here again many of these people migrated from isolated rural areas. But the fact that tuberculosis was a prominent cause of death in the poor working class of the Irish cities suggests that the migrants may have brought the disease with them (Ireland, Medical Research Council of, 1954). It was not a unique susceptibility to the disease that resulted in tuberculosis but rather the heavy exposure to tubercle bacilli present in the environment. In summary, as McDougall (1949) has emphasized, since knowledge is incomplete it is well not to be too dogmatic on the susceptibility of racial groups to tuberculosis.

The status of knowledge during the early years of the twentieth century on tuberculosis and the means for controlling the disease can be summarized: (1) The causative microorganism of human and bovine tuberculosis had been isolated and defined. (2) Studies on the pathogenesis of tuberculosis indicated quite clearly that the core of the problem resided in the individual patient with open pulmonary lesions, who disseminated the disease through his sputum either directly or indirectly to susceptible persons. Unpasteurized cows' milk was also a source of disease. (3) The incidence of infection distributed among populations could be determined by the cutaneous tuberculin reaction and with chest X-ray examinations. Such surveys would also serve to detect early disease. (4) Vital statistics on the disease were assembled at local, state, and national levels that would provide ample evidence for the necessity of control. Since political and voluntary monetary support was essential to start and carry through any control program, information on the magnitude of the problem was necessary. (5) Finally isolation of ill patients with open pulmonary lesions under competent medical and nursing supervision was essential. Adequate support would be needed for family dependents. A system of case-finding required a closely coordinated community operation directed by knowledgeable administrators.

Medical leadership was a paramount requisite for initiating such a program. The first tuberculosis dispensary in the world was started in 1887 in Edinburgh by Dr. Robert W. Philip and was one of the foundation stones for the formation of the British National Association for the Prevention of Tuberculosis in 1898. The important feature of this progressive movement was the appearance of an alerted citizenry.

In the United States, New York, Massachusetts, and Pennsylvania were pioneers in antituberculosis efforts, and in each of these areas dedicated individuals were at the center of activities. Doctor Herman Biggs of the New York City Health Department not only participated in the antidiphtheria program, but in 1894 he established the first community diagnostic laboratory for the examination of specimens for tuberculosis (Winslow, 1929). In 1897 institutions and physicians in New York City were required by law to report all active cases of tuberculosis to the health department. In 1903 Dr. Biggs inaugurated the first group of public health nurses employed in the systematic control of tuberculosis, having established the first school for nurses in the United States in 1902. Later he went to Albany to reorganize the New York State Board of Health with Dr. A. B. Wadsworth as the Director of Laboratories. It must be emphasized that this movement represented a statewide thrust at tuberculosis with a core of competent individuals. This pattern was to be repeated in many states and communities throughout the United States.

In Massachusetts, through the efforts of Dr. Vincent Bowditch and his father, Dr. Henry Bowditch, the state established the first public institution for the care of tuberculous patients in 1898. In 1892 Doctor Lawrence Flick almost single-handedly started the program in Pennsylvania when he organized the Pennsylvania Society for Prevention of Tuberculosis, the first such group in the United States. He was largely responsible for establishing the first American institute for tuberculosis research in 1903, the Henry Phipps Institute, later associated with the University of Pennsylvania.

While antituberculosis efforts were centered in national governmental agencies in Great Britain and on the continent of Europe, the movement in the United States was carried out through local and state agencies, and nationally in nongovernmental groups such as the National Tuberculosis Association founded in 1904. This organization had a powerful impact on the fight against tuberculosis through educational efforts, support of public health nursing, and mass surveys of the population for active tuberculosis (Jacobs, 1940). The highly successful Christmas Seal Sale, first directed by the American Red Cross and later by the National Tuberculosis Association, aided antituberculosis work. One of the successful efforts of the association was close cooperation with other agencies and with the communities. Major assistance was given to child health programs in antituberculosis campaigns.

This concerted movement against tuberculosis did bring forth good results through the application of scientific achievements with community participation. The natural course of tuberculosis was that of a dreadfully lingering malady requiring painstaking and sympathetic care. I was always impressed with the patience, attention, and almost evangelical zeal that many physicians displayed in directing their professional training toward the solution of this community problem. Many had themselves remained for years in sanatoria as patients because of tuberculosis they had acquired during their medical training. Numerous professional organizations supported the movement to curb tuberculosis. These included the American Public Health Association, the American Medical Association, and state and community societies. The membership of one of the most distinguished medical organizations in the United States, the American Clinical and Climatological Association, was initially largely concerned with pulmonary tuberculosis. The association, founded in 1884, included some of the foremost academic leaders in the country. It was a period when basic care was rest and rehabilitation carried out in sanatoria in Europe and then in the United States, which were located in quiet country areas with a pleasant climate. Clear air with sunny days were believed to have a salutary recuperative effect on persons with tuberculosis.

It is interesting to note that the state of Minnesota was promoted by the railroads and others as an ideal place for individuals with tuberculosis to live because of its lakes, forests, clean atmosphere, and vigorous climate. Among others, Henry David Thoreau in 1861 and Dr. Edward Livingston Trudeau in 1873 sought aid for their tuberculosis in Minnesota. Ironically, in this fashion tuberculosis was brought to the state and attacked the susceptible population (Myers, 1949).

A major step in the control of tuberculosis was the campaign to eliminate bovine tuberculosis (Myers and Steele, 1969). The Bureau of Animal Industry of the United States Department of Agriculture directed this eradication effort through cooperation with veterinary medical leaders. The program involved a test (tuberculin) and slaughter procedure rather than the simple expedient of isolating diseased cattle. Another important measure was legislative action prohibiting the sale of unpasteurized milk. As in most public health matters in the United States, legislative measures of public concern started at the local and state levels. Efforts to obtain needed legislation in the interest of human health requires persistence, a fact to which I can attest, having participated in the fight for a state law requiring the pasteurization of milk in relation to human brucellosis and its transmission from cattle through unpasteurized milk. In such a process one learns to appreciate the conflict between economic interests and human health as well as the severe pressures placed on legislators.

Bovine tuberculosis as a source of human infection was so successfully controlled that a state of self-satisfaction ensued. With the combination of complacency and a disease that still smoldered, it was not surprising that the worst epidemic in the history of Georgia swept through herds of cattle in that state in 1974 (United States Department of Health, Education and Welfare, 1974). Over 200 head of cattle had positive tuberculin tests and 250 herds in 19 counties were placed under quarantine. Since all the animals involved were registered beef cattle, there was a severe economic loss as well as a threat to human health.

The establishment of sanatoria in Europe was a major advance in the control of tuberculosis. Dr. Edward Livingston Trudeau initiated the sanatorium movement in the United States at Saranac, New York. Furthermore in many areas a patient could be placed in a sanatorium near his home so that frequent visits by family and friends were possible. The availability of institutions for the isolation and proper care of patients not only protected susceptible populations but also intensified the search for unsuspected cases of tuberculosis. This was reflected in a seemingly paradoxical rise in the morbidity statistics for tuberculosis, even though those with the disease were actually receiving improved treatment and the public was being protected.

The value of screening susceptible populations for tuberculosis was observed in a study carried out among the student nurses at the Boston City Hospital between 1932 and 1937 (Badger and Spink, 1937). During the five-year period, 273 nurses were examined periodically. On entrance to training 57.6 percent were tuberculin-positive, while on the completion of training 95 percent were positive. Eight of the nurses developed active pulmonary tuberculosis, seven of whom had had negative tuberculin reactions initially. One of the nurses in the latter group developed a primary pulmonary tuberculosis that progressed rapidly to death. Obviously the main hazard to these nurses was the presence of active cases of tuberculosis on the wards. Observations were made in other hospitals, with similar results.

After World War II the United States Veterans Administration provided isolated care in special units for patients with tuberculosis. One of the most successful cooperative studies on therapy ever carried out was by the Veterans Administration, as discussed in Section III, Chapter 16.

Although care in sanatoria was offered primarily to adults and older children, important advances were also made in controlling the disease in infants and young children. This was achieved by means of the school systems throughout the United States and by special dispensaries in the larger cities. The accomplishments were remarkable, as described by Edith Lincoln (Lincoln and Sewell, 1963) of the Children's Medical Service at Bellevue Hospital in New York City and by Dr. J. A. Myers (1944) for the Minneapolis children at Lymanhurst School.[7] Careful screening and followup of young children and adolescents reduced the mortality rates to very low levels. The effort represents a combined effort of medical leadership, a dedicated visiting nursing service, an enlightened school system, and an educated public.

In the comparative evaluation of any prophylactic or therapeutic agents for tuberculosis it is exceedingly important that the morbidity and mortality statistics be considered in the light of the influence of public health education and procedures developed during the nineteenth century and carried on intensively into the twentieth. The major factor in the control of the disease was the detection and the isolation of the active cases, particularly in the early stages. In areas where such preventive measures were carried out it became difficult to evaluate a prophylactic vaccine such as a BCG (Bacillus Calmette-Guerin) preparation.

Doctor Albert Calmette was the associate director of the Pasteur Institute in Paris during World War I and an authority on the pathogenesis of tuberculosis in animals and in man (Calmette, 1923). Calmette and Camille Guerin (Calmette et al., 1927) reported on a bovine culture of tubercle bacillus that had attained a state of attenuated virulence after repeated *in vitro* subcultures. They proposed human vaccination with this strain for prophylactic purposes, particularly for young children in families with active tuberculosis. For almost fifty years BCG vaccination has been carried out in many areas of the world, with results not always easy to evaluate. A grim tragedy marred the use of the vaccine, as a result of a catastrophe in Lübeck, Germany beginning in 1930 when a total of 72 out of 251 vaccinated infants died. Death was due to tuberculosis. After a thorough investigation a German commission concluded that the vaccine had been contaminated with a virulent strain (Germany: Reichsgesundheitsamte, 1935).

One of the difficulties with BCG vaccine is that hypersensitivity to tuberculin is induced so that inoculated individuals respond to tuberculin with a positive reaction. The tuberculin test is a valuable epidemiological tool, and in an area where a successful control program is under way, as judged by the number of active cases and the number that convert to a positive tuberculin reaction, morbidity statistics are altered by sensitizing individuals with BCG vaccine. Many of us were persuaded that BCG vaccination did not have a place in Minnesota because of the effective program of control already under way before, during, and after World War II. Evidence from England (Pagel et al., 1964) and Scandinavia indicates that vaccination programs in some areas did reduce the incidence of tuberculosis. Vaccination is probably desirable in populations — especially children — in which there is a high incidence of the disease, in selected children within families having active cases, and for students in some medical schools, and for personnel in hospitals (Wilson and Miles, 1964d; see esp. page 1636).

An informative survey of the problem of tuberculosis and its control before the introduction of streptomycin is revealed in the changing status of the disease in New York City between 1900–1950 (Drolet and Lowell, 1952). In the first decade of the century tuberculosis was the leading cause of death in that community. Beginning with the second decade it was third; in the third decade, third; in the fourth and fifth, fifth; and in 1950, seventh. Factors responsible for the decline were improved environmental sanitation, immunization, and nonspecific therapy. There was a shift in the death rates from the younger to the older groups and a marked decrease in the rate for children under fifteen years. The mass of statistical data demonstrated improvement in the control of the disease *before* the advent of specific therapy with streptomycin, indicating quite clearly that other public health measures had been responsible.

The discovery of streptomycin, which has been discussed in Section II, Chapter 7, was one of the primary achievements in the management of tuberculosis. There is little question that the introduction of streptomycin accelerated the control of tuberculosis and decreased the mortality rate. The impact of chemotherapy on the disease in the

Table 3. Deaths from Tuberculosis for Selected Years, 1932–72

Year	Number*	Rate*
1932	78,890	62.9
1942	58,190	43.2
1952	24,861	15.9
1962	9,506	5.1
1972	4,000	1.9

Source: Edwards, 1973, p. 484.
  *Includes estimates for nonreporting areas in 1932 and 1942 and preliminary data in 1972.

United States between 1952 and 1972 has been analyzed by Dr. Phyllis Edwards (1973) of the Center for Disease Control. Streptomycin was introduced for general use around 1950. Therefore the statistical data of Edwards are significant since the incidence and mortality rates for the decades 1932–1952 and 1952–1972 are presented, the former period of twenty years being termed the prechemotherapy years. The comparative death rates and case rates for these two eras are shown in Tables 3 and 4. Edwards commented on the marked drop in death rates for the chemotherapy period of 1952–1972. Referring to the case incidence, she emphasized that chemotherapy at first caused an abrupt decline in the number of cases, but that subsequently the incidence leveled off rather than continuing to decrease.

Edwards reviewed the impact of chemotherapy and what it meant to the patient. She stated (1973, p. 484),

Before chemotherapy the outlook was bleak, especially for the large numbers of patients with advanced cavitary disease at the time of diagnosis. For those who survived, a lifetime of chronic and relapsing disease lay ahead, with long periods of hospitalization. Today the prognosis for complete recovery is virtually 100 per cent. Some patients still need initial hospitalization for a few weeks or months, but many patients may be treated entirely on an ambulatory basis. Relapse or reactivation is so infrequent following effective chemotherapy that followup examinations every year for life are no longer indicated.

The success of the oral antituberculosis drugs has reduced the bed occupancy of sanatoria and general hospitals. Thus not only has this success resulted in the preservation of human life, but it has been an economic gain for the patients and the communities. It is likely that

Table 4. New Active Cases of Tuberculosis for Selected Years, 1932–72

Year	Number*	Rate*
1932	96,500	76.7
1942	92,500	68.7
1952	86,700	55.4
1962	53,315	28.7
1972	33,500	16.1

Source: Edwards, 1973, p. 484.
*Includes estimates for nonreporting areas in 1932 and 1942 and preliminary data in 1972.

tuberculosis can be eliminated as a public health problem in many countries. The major obstacle toward this end is the failure of patients to continue with chemotherapy for a sufficient period of time. The maintenance of therapy must be carefully monitored for every patient.

As tuberculosis has been brought under control, types of chronic pulmonary disease due to atypical mycobacteria have been observed occasionally. Many of these cases have suppurating lesions that respond poorly to chemotherapy. Properly quantitated tuberculin tests yield negative dermal reactions. Although these patients do not carry the epidemiological threat of infections due to the human strains, the individual cases do constitute therapeutic problems.[8]

Comstock (1975), reviewing the modern epidemiology of tuberculosis, has underlined the value of the standardized *quantitative* tuberculin test in detecting rates of infection. Such a procedure will aid in differentiating the cases due to atypical mycobacteria from those caused by *Mycobacterium tuberculosis.* He has also emphasized that the elimination of tuberculosis as a human disease will not occur in the immediate future. The age distribution for active tuberculosis is in the older groups of people who have contracted the disease in younger years. In other words, tuberculosis is an unusual disease in that it has an incubation period of many years.

Finally, when one looks upon the problem of tuberculosis from a global point of view the outlook for effective control of the disease is ominous. Doctor M. Takabe, director of the WHO Division of Communicable Diseases, stated (World Health Organization, 1974d, p. 5), "tuberculosis remains a major health problem in all the developing countries. In some areas of Africa, Asia, and Oceania the reported annual incidence of pulmonary tuberculosis is 250–300 cases per 100,000 inhabitants and the prevalence is usually at least twice as high [World Health Organization, 1974c]. The number of infectious cases of tuberculosis in the world at present is estimated to be in a range of 15–20 million." Also, in some technically advanced countries, although tuberculosis is considered rare, the disease often causes more deaths than all of the other notifiable communicable diseases combined.

Infectious Mononucleosis ("Glandular Fever")

A contemporary definition of infectious mononucleosis is (Niederman, 1974, p. 1063) "an acute and usually benign infectious disease caused by the Epstein-Barr virus (EBV). It occurs most commonly among adolescents and young adults, who have a characteristic clinical picture consisting of fever, pharyngitis, lymphadenopathy, an increase of peripheral lymphocytes with a high proportion of atypical cells, and the development of transient heterophil and persistent EBV antibody responses."

Infectious mononucleosis has excited the interest of many investigators in different basic disciplines. Its unusual feature as a relatively benign virus disease is the marked general reaction of the lymphoid tissue, resulting in hyperplasia and a profuse production of young and atypical lymphocytes, as seen in the peripheral blood. The disease has entered into the speculation and hypotheses relative to the role of viruses in leukemia and other malignancies. Although mononucleosis commonly exists in all parts of the world and has probably been observed for years but not defined, the evolving knowledge of the disease is strictly a product of the twentieth century. In the development of this knowledge advances have resulted from two fortuitous research observations, one describing a diagnostic serological reaction and the other the virus etiology of the disease.

It is often cited that infectious mononucleosis was recognized by Emil Pfeiffer (1889), but from his clinical descriptions — without supporting data — of a febrile disease in children, it is difficult to accept this conclusion. J. P. West (1896) described an unusual epidemic involving 96 children in 43 families in Ohio and called it "glandular fever." The outstanding features were enlarged lymph nodes, and abdominal symptoms and diarrhea in infants and young children. The most frequent complication was nephritis! Only one adult was afflicted. Is it possible that these cases represented "acute infectious lymphocytosis" as described by C. H. Smith (1944)? The first convincing presentation of infectious mononucleosis was that by Thomas Sprunt and Frank Evans (1920) when they described six patients at Johns Hopkins Hospital, in whom the peripheral blood had a marked increase in lymphocytes with pathological forms. Further supporting evidence of a distinct clinical entity was presented at the same time by Warfield Longcope (1922) in New York City.

Infectious mononucleosis is a disease with protean clinical manifestations because the lymphocytic proliferation involves so many tissues and organs. Except in well-defined localized epidemics the correct diagnosis of sporadic cases is often troublesome. For instance, the differential diagnosis of brucellosis and infectious mononucleosis is at times difficult (Spink and Anderson, 1951). The disease may simulate epidemic hepatitis with or without jaundice. In a United States Army hospital in Korea I observed jaundice in many patients with hepatomegaly and splenomegaly that suggested either epidemic hepatitis or infectious mononucleosis. The correct diagnosis of the latter disease was made by supporting laboratory data. In a group of 63 patients, 26 different diseases had been diagnosed initially before hematological and serological evidence yielded the correct diagnosis of infectious mononucleosis (Davidsohn and Walker, 1935).

The confusion surrounding the clinical diagnosis of infectious mononucleosis was diminished by the observation made by J. Paul and P. P. Bunnell (1932) at Yale University when they introduced the heterophile antibody reaction as a serological test. It had been known since 1911 that different antigenic substances could stimulate the formation of antibodies contained in serum that would agglutinate sheep erythrocytes *in vitro*. Intrigued by Davidsohn's observations that heterophile antibodies were present in patients with serum sickness due to horse serum, and because the clinical picture of serum sickness simulated rheumatic fever, the Yale investigators carried out heterophile antibody tests on the sera of patients with rheumatic fever and other diseases. They stated (Paul and Bunnell, 1932, p. 92), "Quite by accident it was discovered that heterophile antibodies . . . were present in a specimen of serum from a patient, ill with infectious mononucleosis, in much higher concentration than has been described in serum disease or in any other clinical condition which we have studied." The specificity of this test was improved by others (Davidsohn and Walker, 1935). Almost simultaneously more precise descriptions of the atypical lymphocytes (Downey-type) in the peripheral blood of patients were made (Downey and Stasney, 1935). As a result definitive epidemiological studies could be pursued.

A second major advance was the discovery of the etiology of infectious mononucleosis, which was established through a series of unusual observations that were unrelated at first. Denis Burkitt (1958), a surgeon at the Mulago Hospital in Kampala, Uganda, reported on a malignant lymphoma of the jaw and abdomen in 38 children seen over a period of seven years. More remarkable, by 1967 he had recorded 127 jaw tumors of which 52 had completely regressed, possibly abetted by chemotherapy (Burkitt, 1967). Known as "Burkitt's lymphoma," this type of tumor was confirmed by observations from other areas. M. A. Epstein, B. G. Achong, and Y. M. Barr (1964), in London, described a herpes virus (EBV) isolated from the tissues of Burkitt's lymphoma, which has also been confirmed.

Gertrude and Werner Henle, working in the virus laboratory of the Children's Hospital of Philadelphia, were interested in the oncogenic role of viruses in malignancy. Their attention was drawn to EBV in Burkitt's lymphoma. They established cell lines of growth for this virus in their laboratory and then proceeded to screen groups of children by serological methods in order to detect the exposure rate to EBV. For a normal control serum they used the blood of a technician in the laboratory (Elaine Hutkin). During the course of her work she developed infectious mononucleosis. While she was convalescing, her blood, which had previously displayed no antibody for EBV, revealed a high persisting titer. A cautious report of the observations appeared in which EBV was implicated in the etiology of infectious mononucleosis (Henle, Henle, and Diehl, 1968). Several convincing communications indicated quite clearly that EBV antibody in high titer appeared in the blood of patients recovering from infectious mononucleosis (Evans, Niederman, and McCollum, 1968; Niederman et al., 1968; 1970). A successful prospective study at Yale was carried out, which gave added impetus to the concept that EBV was etiologically related to infectious mononucleosis (Sawyer et al., 1971). And — very important — EBV was found in oropharyngeal washings from eight days to seventeen months after the onset of infectious mononucleosis, showing that a persistent carrier state existed (Miller, Niederman, and Andrews, 1973). Two serological methods became available for the screening of selected populations, the heterophile antibody reaction and the EBV antibody test.

Serological investigations in different parts of the world indicated that infectious mononucleosis was like poliomyelitis in the age distribution. In those countries with a low socioeconomic basis, younger children were commonly involved, and the disease was mild. In the more developed countries the young children escaped, but a more severe form of the disease appeared in older children and young adults. Important epidemiological data were contributed by college students and military personnel, such as those studied at Yale (Evans and Robinton, 1950; Sawyer et al., 1971), the University of Minnesota (McKinlay, 1935), the University of Michigan (Zarafonetis, 1949), Sweden (Pejme, 1964), and West Point (N.Y.) Military Academy (Hoagland, 1952). The student health service at the University of Minnesota is one of the largest in the country, and hundreds of cases of infectious mononucleosis have been observed and treated at that institution. Little information is available on the problem of infectious mononucleosis in military personnel during World War I. But in World War II, "Infectious mononucleosis was a fairly frequent disease among troops, 13,571 admissions in continental United States and 4,961 abroad" (Gordon, 1958, p. 51).

Further information was gained during and after World War II about the extensive pathology in many tissues and organs, especially in fatal cases (Custer and Smith, 1949). One of the most common and serious complications is an enlarged and fragile spleen that may rupture and cause severe hemorrhage. Recovery has followed only with prompt transfusions of blood and surgical intervention.

Control measures against the disease are not effective, and no prophylactic vaccine is available. No specific therapy has been developed. Adrenocortical hormones are effective in the more severe cases such as those with painful pharyngeal edema, hepatitis with jaundice, neurological involvement, and thrombocytopenic purpura (Bender, 1967). An important symposium on infectious mononucleosis that reviewed contemporary knowledge and projected into the future was held in 1972 (Glade, 1973). Further studies on the disease should help clarify the nature of lympho-proliferative disorders in general.

Psittacosis[9] (Ornithosis)

Although psittacosis is one of the zoonoses, the human disease is primarily a respiratory infection and therefore it is discussed here. It occurs sporadically, and also in epidemic form, often with the manifestations of atypical pneumonia. The etiology was discovered about the same time in Germany (Levinthal, 1930), England (Coles, 1930), and the United States (Lillie, 1930). A. C. Coles had successfully transmitted the disease to mice and recognized the stained organisms in the splenic tissues. He concluded that they had the appearance of rickettsial bodies. Doctor R. D. Lillie, with the United States Public Health Service, studied the tissues of diseased parrots and also those of a fatal human case accidentally infected in the laboratory, and likewise stated that the organisms had the appearance of rickettsiae. He suggested the name *Rickettsia psittaci*. At first the etiology was thought to be bacterial; then a virus was considered; but the agent is now known as a member of the Chlamydia genus, *Chlamydia psittaci*, which genus also includes the causes of trachoma and lymphogranuloma. The organism exists as an intracellular form of specialized bacteria, somewhat like the rickettsias (Moulder, 1964). The important clinical feature of this taxonomical distinction is that Chlamydias are sensitive to the action of antibiotics, and the diseases can be treated successfully, if properly recognized.

The disease is gradual in onset, causing a toxemia and clinical signs much like those of typhoid fever, with splenomegaly and a rash resembling typhoid "rose spots." The principal manifestation is a diffuse infiltrate in the lungs. The disease can be prolonged, and the mortality rate is significant in elderly patients. Some of the patients seen at the University of Minnesota Hospitals (before the present era of antibiotics) had been ill for many days, and hospitalized for several weeks, with the diagnosis long in doubt. Convalescence was exceedingly prolonged.

The disease was not recognized until the latter part of the nineteenth century, when epidemics in Europe were associated with sick parrots. The birds displayed lethargy and a bloody diarrhea, and death often occurred. Psittacosis is highly contagious; the infection is probably airborne with entrance through the respiratory tract, although human-to-human transmission is rare. The first recognized cases in the United States involved a family of three in New Hampshire (Vickery and Richardson, 1904). In 1929–1930 a pandemic of psittacosis appeared suddenly in the Argentine Republic, in the United States, and in European countries. The source of the disease was a large exporting center of parrots in Argentina. The birds had originated in Brazil. There were 117 cases recognized in England with 25 deaths, a mortality rate of 21.36 percent. The excellent experimental, epidemiological, and clinical studies of this English epidemic merit consideration (Sturdee and Scott, 1930), as does the review by S. P. Bedson (1959).

The outbreak in the United States from November 22, 1929 to May 7, 1930 involved 169 cases with 33 deaths occurring in 15 states and the District of Columbia (Armstrong, 1930). In addition there were 16 laboratory infections and two deaths. The ecology of psittacosis was reviewed by Dr. K. F. Meyer (1942), who not only emphasized the role of parrots and canaries in the transmission of the disease, but also called attention to a probable reservoir in pigeons, which was later actually demonstrated (Meyer, Eddie, and Yanamura, 1942).

Following the pandemic of 1929–30 drastic quarantine regulations against the importation of parrots were inaugurated in several countries, including the United States. The parakeet, or "love bird," is particularly susceptible to the disease; interstate shipment of parakeets was strictly prohibited in the United States. It was subsequently found, however, that the parrot family and pigeons were not the only source of the disease, but chickens, turkeys, and ducks were also involved (Meyer, 1958). Birds other than the parakeet were generally not acutely ill with the disease, but they were important healthy carriers of *Chlamydia psittaci*. Psittacosis was recognized as an occupational disease for those raising pigeons and for persons working in plants processing chickens and turkeys (Meyer, 1959).

The introduction of the antibiotic chlortetracycline in 1948 provided not only successful therapy for human patients, as reflected in a marked drop in mortality rates, but also a prophylactic against the disease in parrots and in poultry. When this antibiotic was added to the drinking water of parakeets the disease was curtailed (Meyer and Eddie, 1954–55). It is likely that the addition of antibiotics to animal feed has controlled the disease in other species, a procedure recommended by K. F. Meyer (1959).

Since prophylactic procedures against the avian reservoirs of psittacosis are now available, the restrictions on marketing parakeets have been reduced. The disease has not been completely controlled, but the incidence in humans has been reduced to fewer than about fifty reported cases a year in the United States since 1970.

Trachoma [10]

Although trachoma is not strictly a respiratory infection, the causative organism, *Chlamydia trachomatis*, belongs to the same genus causing psittacosis (*C. psittaci*). Trachoma is a chronic inflammatory infection of the conjunctivae, often associated with secondary invasion by bacteria, resulting in scarring of the cornea and loss of vision. It is still the single most important cause of preventable blindness in the world (World Health Organization, 1971c).

Trachoma is a very ancient disease, probably recognized by the early Egyptians (Boldt, 1904). It was introduced into northern Europe in epidemic form in the nineteenth century. It became known among armies as "Military Ophthalmia," and more widely, as "Egyptian Ophthalmia." The disease is widely disseminated in the Middle East, North Africa, and Northern India. The American Indian was afflicted; such patients were observed at the University of Minnesota in the early days of sulfonamide therapy, which was effective against the secondary bacterial invaders in trachoma. It is estimated that at present there are 20 million persons in the world with blindness due to trachoma (World Health Organization-Expert Committee on Trachoma, 1962).

According to the World Health Organization, persistence of the disease is related to socioeconomic factors such as overcrowding, lack of clean water, unsanitary habits, and an abundant fly population. Because the disease is so prevalent, because it can be prevented, and because antibiotic therapy is effective in the early stages, WHO has expended considerable effort in controlling trachoma (World Health Organization-Director General, 1974; World Health Organization-Expert Committee on Trachoma, 1962). An authoritative contemporary monograph on control and treatment has been prepared by G. Bietti and G. H. Werner (1967).

CHAPTER 15

Enteric Diseases

The enteric diseases have probably disturbed man since his earliest days and were of concern to Moses, as shown by his insistence on appropriate sanitary laws. These diseases are transmitted directly from human to human, or indirectly to man through contaminated food and water and by insect vectors. The diseases, though ancient in origin, still afflict millions of people all over the world. The control of these diseases has been most successful through improved sanitation, public health measures to eliminate contamination of food and water, and — to a lesser extent — the modern achievements of specific vaccines and antibiotics. The major enteric diseases are those grouped under the term salmonellosis. Historically typhoid fever due to *Salmonella typhi* has been the most devastating.

Typhoid Fever [1]

Typhoid fever and typhus were not distinguished from each other until the nineteenth century. (Typhus is discussed in Section III, Chapter 18.) Both were considered diseases of filth, crowding, and unhygienic living conditions. Thomas Willis (1684) may have been the first to recognize typhoid fever; in his "Treatise on Fevers," Chapters IX, X and XI, he dealt with a disease that he called "Putrid Fever," and his clinical observations do suggest typhoid. Chapter XIV of this work indicates that he may have been describing typhus.

240

This early recognition of typhoid by Willis is supported by recent evidence. W. C. Gibson (1970) has related that Christopher Wren assisted Willis by engraving the intestinal lesion of typhoid fever. Wren also made the famous engraving of the "Circle of Willis," which depicts the pathway of the large blood vessels at the base of the brain. Gibson wrote that Wren assisted Willis when he was seeing typhoid patients (1970, p. 336): "One of Wren's signed anatomical drawings, in colour, has been found recently in the Wellcome Institute of the History of Medicine in London, by the Director, Dr. Noël Poynter. It shows a section of small intestine which has been opened to reveal a hemorrhagic ulcer of the type described by Willis in his work on 'Putrid Feaver' as 'little ulcers and exudations and flowing forth of the Blood.' "

The specific identity of typhoid fever was established on the basis of epidemiological, clinical, and pathological findings before the typhoid bacillus was isolated by C. J. Eberth (1880) and more precisely defined by G. Gaffky (1884 translation 1886). Two French clinicians, Pierre-Charles-Alexandre Louis and Pierre Bretonneau, clearly delineated the clinical and pathological features of typhoid and believed that epidemics were due to contagion, although the mode of transmission was not known (Bretonneau, 1829; Louis, 1836a). It was the physician and founder of the Dartmouth Medical School, Nathan Smith (1824), who published the first essay on typhoid fever, and Elisha Bartlett (1842) of Philadelphia, who wrote the first complete book on the disease in English. W. W. Gerhard (1836–1837), also of Philadelphia and a pupil of Louis in Paris, published the first clear-cut distinction between typhoid and typhus.

The transmission of typhoid was presumed to be airborne following these initial studies. William Budd (1856a), a medical practitioner in Bristol, England, suspected the diarrheal discharge of the patients as the source of typhoid, although he was not sure in what manner the disease was distributed. But as a result of careful epidemiological studies suggestive of those of Snow on cholera, Budd (1856b) concluded that typhoid fever was spread through water, milk, and food. He also continued to believe in an aerial route of transmission, however.

Typhoid had a devastating effect among armies during the nineteenth century (Holmes, 1940). In the federal armies of the Civil

War in America a total of 186,216 men died of diseases, principally typhoid fever and malaria, while 44,238 were killed in battle and 49,731 died of wounds. In the Confederate armies there were two hundred thousand deaths, with only one-fourth due to battle casualties. The Spanish-American War was "a military and naval success, a sanitary fiasco" (Holmes, 1940, p. 197). There were 243 battle casualties out of 107,973 men, but typhoid killed 1,580. In the Anglo-Boer War, the Boers killed eight thousand soldiers, and 8,022 died of typhoid. As Dr. Walter Reed and his associates pointed out after the Spanish-American War in one of the most precise epidemiological investigations made on any infectious disease (Reed, Vaughan, and Shakespeare, 1900, p. 214), "Indeed, the history of this disease justifies us in stating that whenever men congregate and live without adequate provision for disposing of their excrement, there and then typhoid will appear." The success in controlling typhoid fever in the massive warfare of the twentieth century attests to the truth of this statement.

Typhoid also struck heavily at the civilian population. At the beginning of the twentieth century mortality tables for the United States revealed the leading causes of death to be tuberculosis, pneumonia, and cancer, with typhoid fever fourth, the leading cause of illness in the large municipal hospitals at that time. In searching out the medical records for the year 1900 at the Boston City Hospital, I found that typhoid was the most common ailment for which patients were admitted to the hospital. As physician-in-chief of the Johns Hopkins Hospital, William Osler, together with the staff at this period, published a series of thirty-five reports on various phases of typhoid (Osler et al., 1891–1900).

But what to do about it? People began to realize in the early part of the twentieth century that a knowledge of sanitary engineering was essential to prevent the spread of diseases, including typhoid. Osler wrote (1901, 4th Ed., p. 40), "In cities the prevalence of typhoid fever is directly proportionate to the inefficiency of the drainage and the water supply." Doctor Milton Rosenau, the first professor of preventive medicine at Harvard Medical School, stated (1913, p. 74), "Every case of typhoid fever means a short circuit between the alvine discharges of one person and the mouth of another."

The development of public health engineering was stimulated by two outstanding leaders. Professor Max von Pettenkofer (1869), a German chemist and physician, is considered the founder of experimental research in hygiene. In 1875 he became director of the world's first institute of hygiene at Munich. His most significant contribution was the virtual elimination of typhoid in Munich through an improved system of handling sewage. He is also widely known for his controversial stand on the epidemiology of cholera (See Section III, Chapter 12).

Professor William T. Sedgwick, a graduate of the Sheffield Scientific School at Yale University, obtained a doctorate in biology at Johns Hopkins University. He was influenced by von Pettenkofer, but unlike him, Sedgwick had accepted the principles of the new bacteriology. He was also interested in environmental sanitation and in 1883 joined the engineering faculty of the Massachusetts Institute of Technology in Cambridge, Massachusetts. In an era before the development of schools of public health he organized a department of biology and public health with research and educational interests in pure water supplies and adequate sewage disposal. The results of this research and the training of graduate students in the new field of public health were his greatest contributions.

Sedgwick worked closely as a consultant with the Massachusetts State Board of Health. In 1913 he organized a school for health officers through Harvard University and the Massachusetts Institute of Technology, which was a forerunner of the Harvard School of Public Health. He also aided in the development of the United States Public Health Service in Washington. His vast experience in sanitary engineering was incorporated into a widely accepted textbook (Sedgwick, 1902). One of his disciples, a consulting engineer, wrote an authoritative text on typhoid fever (Whipple, 1908). Sedgwick was later memorialized as a pioneer in public health (Jordan, Whipple, and Winslow, 1924).

The identification of typhoid fever depended on precise bacteriology and serological procedures. With the advent of bacteriophage typing of typhoid strains in the twentieth century, a useful epidemiological procedure became available in identifying the strain of typhoid bacillus that caused epidemics and even in directing attention to the responsible human carrier. The universally employed epidemiological and diagnostic tool for typhoid has been the serological reaction known as the "Widal agglutination test" (Gruber and Durham, 1896; Widal, 1896). The agglutination reaction is not a specific test in an acutely ill, febrile patient, however, because the typhoid bacillus has common antigens with other enteric organisms. Furthermore typhoid agglutinins can persist in the blood of healthy individuals for long periods following an attack of the disease or after immunization with vaccine.

Typhoid vaccine was introduced by Richard Pfeiffer and Wilhelm Kolle (1896) and by Almroth Wright and David Semple (1897). Over the ensuing half century it was difficult to ascertain the efficiency of killed bacterial vaccines, but during the 1950s carefully controlled studies in Yugoslavia and in British Guiana with acetone-killed and heat-killed phenolized vaccines demonstrated definite and significant protection against the disease (Typhoid Panel, UK Department of Technical Co-operation, 1964; Yugoslav Typhoid Commission, 1964).

A therapeutic achievement of the twentieth century was the introduction of the antibiotic chloramphenicol (Woodward et al., 1948). Therapy with this drug successfully reduced the mortality rate of typhoid fever, especially in children, and prevented complications. In addition a potentially prolonged illness and convalescence were shortened to a febrile illness of a week or two. But chloramphenicol did not prevent the development of a carrier state, nor was it of benefit in the elimination of typhoid bacilli from the intestinal tract of established carriers. Continued clinical experience with this drug and other antibiotics has revealed the appearance of strains of typhoid organisms resistant to chloramphenicol on the basis of transferrable R factor. This poses the possibility of typhoid bacilli showing resistance against several antibiotics and emphasizes the importance of prophylactic procedures for the disease, especially the strict surveillance of food and water for human consumption.

Typhoid fever still continues as a threat even though immunization methods are satisfactory and drug therapy is effective. The main difficulty is that typhoid is strictly a human disease, and infected individuals, whether or not they have been ill, can continue to be carriers and discharge typhoid bacilli in the feces for years. In the vocabulary of public health a carrier is defined as one who continues to discharge typhoid organisms in feces for twelve months or more after having acquired the disease. In most areas of the world sanitation is not adequate and the water supply is unsafe.

The danger posed by a typhoid carrier, especially one who prepares food for others, is dramatically illustrated by the story of the famous "Typhoid Mary," known as the "human culture tube" (Soper, 1919). Mary Mallon was a healthy woman who lived until she was 70 years old. She was a cook, and during her life was known to have infected 54 persons with typhoid, 3 of whom died. She denied ever having had typhoid fever. Her fascinating life history was published in detail in the *Minneapolis Star Journal* for December 11, 1938. Between 1964–1974 only one registered typhoid carrier existed in the state of Minnesota. Between 1914 and 1974 there was a total of 459 carriers, most of whom harbored the organisms in chronically infected gallbladders.

In the United States in 1973 there were only 680 reported cases of typhoid. There were 19 states with a maximum of 5 cases, and 9 not reporting a single case. Improved sanitation and carefully controlled drinking water have been responsible for the decline. Although typhoid fever has been controlled in the more developed countries, epidemics have occurred in these areas under unusual circumstances. Zermatt, Switzerland enjoyed the reputation for years as a center for winter sports, but became a ghost town as a result of a typhoid epidemic in 1963, caused by a contaminated water supply and involving 437 identified cases. Over twenty thousand visitors returned home from Zermatt to European communities and to the United States (Bernard, 1965). Under such circumstances there is always the danger of introducing the disease into distant communities. In 1964 a major epidemic of typhoid fever occurred in Aberdeen, Scotland involving 515 patients, which was traced to a six-pound can of Argentine corned beef (Aberdeen's Typhoid Bacillus, 1973).

An outbreak of typhoid fever occurred in 1970 aboard a ship on a world cruise with a thousand passengers and six hundred crew members (National Communicable Disease Center, 1970). The ship sailed from Southampton, England on December 12, 1969 and stopped at several points, including Madeira (December 20), Bermuda (December 26), Nassau (December 30), Canal Zone (January 2), and Acapulco (January 6). On January 9, 1970 the ship docked at San Pedro, California, and two crewmen were hospitalized for respiratory symptoms and diarrhea. Four additional crew members were hospitalized in San Francisco for the same reasons. *Salmonella typhi* had been isolated from a blood specimen of one of the hospitalized crewmen following the departure from San Francisco for Vancouver, where the ship was quarantined. At least 42 persons were hospitalized in Vancouver, Canada, and 350 passengers were traced in 22 states for investigation.

The largest outbreak of typhoid fever in the United States in twenty years appeared in 1973 in a migrant farm labor camp adjacent to Miami (Center for Disease Control, 1973b). There was a total of 188 patients, and typhoid bacilli were recovered from the blood of 105 (Hoffman et al., 1975). The patients responded satisfactorily to treatment with ampicillin; there were no fatalities. Approximately an additional 150 suspected cases were hospitalized, with the diagnosis confirmed in 63. This was a waterborne epidemic traced to a contaminated well.

Epidemic typhoid fever is still a serious disease in the developing countries, primarily because of poor sanitation and contaminated food and water. The attack rate is high in these areas, but the introduction of chloramphenicol has reduced mortality rates. Modern epidemics of typhoid fever are usually contained within a given area through prompt surveillance and investigations on local, national, and international levels. Public health authorities are quickly alerted so that the epidemics are kept localized and controlled.

Diarrhea[2] and Dysentery[3]

The "bloody flux" was recognized for centuries among military and civilian populations. Acute diarrhea can be a manifestation of a systemic disease, but it is not always infectious in origin. It can be caused by metabolic disturbances, chemical poisoning, and drugs. Acute ulcerative colitis and regional enteritis, diseases for which the etiology has not been established, can simulate dysentery due to microbial causes. Only the more precise diagnostic techniques of microbiology have permitted a definitive classification of acute febrile diarrheal conditions. This in turn has contributed to enlightened epidemiological studies and to the control of these diseases.

Acute diarrhea is a common affliction of travelers. In the jet age one can hop from country to country within a few hours. The drinking water in the vast majority of developing countries is contaminated, and diarrhea will often follow its consumption. Fortunately most cases of diarrhea acquired in this manner are not serious and abate within a few days. Travelers often assume that nothing more complicated than a "change in water," dietary indiscretion, or an excessive intake of alcohol has been the cause of their gastroenteritis. In the case of persistent diarrhea, however, especially when it is accompanied by chills, fever, abdominal pain, and blood in the feces, the condition can be serious. A specific diagnosis can be made only by careful bacteriological examination of the feces. Since proper therapy is available for these enteric afflictions, a physician should be consulted.

Salmonellosis

Salmonellosis embraces a wide spectrum of enteric microorganisms that cause an acute febrile disease with gastroenteritis as the predominant feature. After the ingestion of organisms, usually in food or drink, there is an incubation period of twelve to twenty-four hours, followed by the onset of nausea and vomiting, abdominal pain, and diarrhea. Recovery usually takes place within a few days to a week. In the United States it is estimated that two million human cases of salmonellosis occur annually (Bauer, 1973).

The term Salmonella is derived from the name of the veterinarian Dr. Daniel Salmon, who was the first director of the Bureau of Animal Industry in the United States Department of Agriculture. Doctor Salmon (1886) engaged in research on "swine plague" with Dr. Theobald Smith, a young physician in the department, and isolated an organism from swine now known as *Salmonella choleraesuis*. Their identification of the organisms was correct, but "swine plague" is now called hog cholera and is known to be caused by a virus. The work of Salmon and Smith is important, however, in that *Sal. choleraesuis* was the first of many different strains of animal salmonellae to be isolated. It also causes human dysentery.

Thousands of isolates of different salmonella strains have been derived from a large number of vertebrates, causing a serious problem in taxonomy. Most have been isolated from humans and from fowl; some have been associated with disease, and some have not. As more sophisticated serological methods became available for differentiating bacterial strains, the Kauffmann-White classification, which included over one thousand serotypes, was introduced by the 1930s. Comprehensive reviews of the methods and results of a survey of different strains are available (Edwards, 1962; Van Oye, 1964; Wilson and Miles, 1964c).

Epidemiological factors responsible for the dissemination of salmonella infections involve three major groups of hosts that harbor the organisms (Bauer, 1973). First, *Salmonella typhi* and *paratyphi* utilize humans as the primary host, and the organisms are spread either directly or indirectly (via food and water) from human to human. Second, several species of vertebrates and fowl act as hosts for *Sal. pullorum* and *Sal. gallinarum* in poultry, *Sal. Dublin* in cattle, *Sal. abortus equi* in horses, *Sal. abortus ovis* in sheep, and *Sal. choleraesuis* and *Sal. typhisuis* in swine. Of these, *Dublin* and *choleraesuis* are the important pathogens in human disease, especially *choleraesuis* in children. Third, there is a large group of thirteen hundred distinct serotypes with no particular host preference, attacking both man and animals and causing gastroenteritis. Infection can be disseminated through cat and dog foods with salmonellae being distributed in the feces of the animals. This reservoir is the principal cause of the modern problem of salmonellosis.

Typhoid fever, primarily a human disease, has been controlled through public health efforts and with vaccines and chemotherapy. On the other hand, the complex system of preparing and distributing foods from animal and fowl sources that are easily contaminated has made it difficult to control the other common salmonella infections. No satisfactory vaccines are available. Antibiotic therapy is usually not indicated for patients with these infections because of the short, uncomplicated, natural course in the majority of cases. One therapeutic problem in the more severe cases is the genetic transmission of antibiotic-resistance from *E. coli* to the offending salmonellae. In addition the presence of antibiotics in animal and poultry feeds can lead to the development of such resistance.

Outbreaks of salmonellosis in institutions such as hospitals and other health care centers are a constant threat because of the likelihood of food contamination. The incidence is generally higher in patients who have other debilitating conditions. In 1964 an outbreak due to *Sal. infantis* took place in the University of Minnesota Hospitals, involving nurses, housestaff, and patients, a total of 23 people. The epidemic was traced to the contamination of food in the kitchen by a carrier who had recently convalesced from an intestinal disturbance (Kohler, 1964). In 1970 a similar type of epidemic traced to contaminated food with *Sal. enteritidis* occurred in a Baltimore nursing home for the aged (Farber et al., 1970). At least 104 of 145 patients and 19 of 66 employees became ill, and 25 of the patients died.

One of the most unusual large-scale epidemics of salmonellosis occurred in Riverside, California in 1965 (Collaborative Report, 1971). More than sixteen thousand cases occurred in a population of 133,219; at least 70 patients were hospitalized, and 3 died. The source of the epidemic was a contaminated water supply and the causative agent was *Salmonella typhimurium*, phage type 2. The epidemic was controlled by chlorination of the water supply. An interesting epidemiological finding was the low coliform counts in the water compared to the high salmonellae figures (Boring III, Martin, and Elliott, 1971).

Waterborne epidemics of salmonellosis probably occur more commonly than reported. Attention has been directed to cruise ships in which passengers and crew members have incurred salmonellosis as a result of contaminated water taken on board at ports of call (Center for Disease Control, 1974e).

The control of salmonellosis is largely a public health problem. A continuous national surveillance of the incidence of human cases can often pinpoint unusual local epidemics, and serotyping can elicit the strain and source of the disease. With the widespread distribution of prepared foods for human use, scrupulous hygienic and environmental procedures must be enforced by public health officials to prevent contamination. Public health education is highly effective in alerting a population to the disease.

Shigellosis

Dysentery was a serious problem in Japan during the last decade of the nineteenth century, with the occurrence of ninety thousand cases and twenty thousand deaths. Doctor K. Shiga (1898) isolated a causative bacterium, which was distinct from the other enteric pathogens in man and which became known as *Shigella dysenteriae*. This organism was unusual in that it caused not only dysentery but neurological disturbances due to a neurotoxin elaborated by the bacteria. Subsequent studies by many others established definitive strains closely associated with Shiga's. At present there are four main subgroups, known as A, B, C, and D or *Sh. dysenteriae* (Shiga-Kruse bacillus), *Sh. flexneri* (*Sh. paradysenteriae*), *Sh. boydii* (*Sh. paradysenteriae*), and *Sh. sonnei* (Wilson and Miles, 1964c; see Vol. I, p. 849). Unlike the salmonellae group, shigellae have man as the primary host; like typhoid, shigellosis is spread from human to human either directly or indirectly.

The incidence of shigellosis cases in the United States almost doubled during the years 1968–1973. The rise is probably related to better surveillance and reporting of cases, and possibly to increased travel. Most of the cases were due to *Sh. sonnei* and occurred principally in children.

An epidemic in Minnesota in 1973 due to *Sh. sonnei* involved a total of 996 culturally-proved cases with almost one-half occurring in Minneapolis, and almost one-half of the total in children under ten years of age. In Minneapolis alone, 292 cases were hospitalized, although the epidemic in general was mild. More than 95 percent of the cultures were resistant to ampicillin, tetracycline, and streptomycin. No common source for the epidemic was found.[4]

Vaccines for prophylactic purposes against shigellosis appear promising. Both sulfonamide and antibiotic therapy have been hampered by the appearance of resistant strains — shigella become resistant to several antibiotics simultaneously on the basis of the episomal or R transfer factor, as in other enteric organisms (Farrar, Jr. and Eidson, 1971). Shigellosis remains a major public health problem calling for intense educational campaigns on the importance of careful hygiene and improved sanitation toward the prevention of infections.

Escherichia coli Diarrhea

Although *Escherichia coli* was long considered the cause of the lethal *white scours* of young calves, other organisms — including viruses — are now implicated. But there is no doubt that enteropathic human strains of *E. coli* do cause epidemic diarrhea in young infants and at times in adults. The first definitive serological, clinical, and epidemiological studies were carried out in the children's wards of Leipzig University (Goldschmidt, 1933). This work was later confirmed in London during an epidemic in which there were 21 deaths among 51 children (Bray, 1945). Subsequent reports from Great Britain (Taylor, 1960) and from the United States (Ewing, Tatum, and Davis, 1957) have emphasized the serious nature of *E. coli* dysentery.

Continuing investigations in adults have revealed the presence of two groups of *E. coli*, each producing distinctive clinical courses (DuPont et al., 1971). Clinical studies were carried out in normal human volunteers infected with each of the strains, and experiments

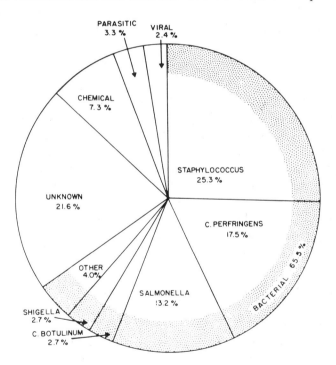

Figure 12. Foodborne disease outbreaks (confirmed and unconfirmed), by causative organism. United States, Annual Summary, 1969. Reproduced from Foodborne Outbreaks, National Communicable Disease Center Annual Summary, 1969. United States Department of Health, Education and Welfare- Public Health Service, Atlanta, Georgia (Figure 2, p. 3).

were performed on rabbit ileal-loops. One group invaded the intestinal wall, causing an inflammatory reaction with blood and mucus in the stools, similar to shigellosis. A second group produced a watery diarrhea, similar to that of cholera, due to an enterotoxin. *Escherichia coli* dysentery is included in that cluster of disorders known as "traveler's diarrhea."

Foodborne Illnesses

The Center for Disease Control issues "Status Reports" on foodborne outbreaks of illness,[5] defined as "disease by ingestion of a pathogenic organism or noxious agent contained in water or a food vehicle" (National Communicable Disease Center, 1969, p. 1). In the 1969 summary for the United States there were 371 such outbreaks. As officials have pointed out, however, there are varying degrees of efficiency in reporting from the individual states. One state may seem to have had a higher incidence than others, but the difference may really be due to more rigid surveillance and prompt reporting.

The important data on the etiology of the 371 foodborne illnesses in 1969 are illustrated in Figure 12. In 46 percent of the outbreaks the causes were not known. Note that 65.5 percent were bacterial in origin, with the staphylococcus the most prominent cause, followed by *Clostridium perfringens*. Salmonella was the third. The staphylococcus is such an ubiquitous organism that food can readily be contaminated unless it is scrupulously prepared and refrigerated. *Clostridium perfringens* is a pathogen of the normal intestinal tract, and contamination of foods is possible through careless food handlers.

Botulism

Botulism[6] is a relatively rare but highly lethal disease due to the spore-bearing anaerobe, *Clostridium botulinum*, which produces a potent neurotoxin. Most human cases are traced to the ingestion of home-canned vegetables. Outbreaks have been associated with contaminated fish (Koenig et al., 1964). *Clostridium botulinum* may also gain entrance to the body through wounds where the toxin is formed and disseminated through the bloodstream. The disease was first recognized and the etiology defined by E. M. P. van Ermengem (1897)

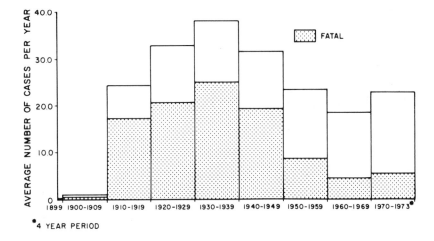

Figure 13. Cases and deaths due to foodborne botulism, 1899–1973. Reproduced from Center for Disease Control: Botulism in the United States,
1899–1973. Handbook for Epidemiologists, Clinicians, and Laboratory Workers, issued June 1974. United States Department of Health, Education and Welfare-Public
Health Service, Atlanta, Georgia (Figure 2,
p. 24).

when several villagers in Belgium at a festival in 1896 contracted
botulism after eating a ham. The disease afflicts animals as well as
man (Roberts, 1959). Tanisieke is botulism in cattle. The sickness in
ducks results from the ingestion of water containing the toxin distributed along shorelines. Mink are also naturally susceptible.

Doctor Karl F. Meyer did much to clarify the epidemiology of
botulism in the United States (Meyer and Eddie, 1965). An excellent
handbook on botulism in the United States from 1899–1973 has been
issued by the Center for Disease Control (1974a). Figure 13 illustrates
the average number of cases in the United States with the mortality
rates during this period. There was an upsurge in the incidence of this
disease during World War I because of an increase in home canning of
vegetables. During 1919–1920 severe epidemic botulism was traced to
deficiencies in the packing of California ripe olives (Young, 1976).
K. F. Meyer (1956a) reviewed the literature on botulism on a worldwide basis for the period 1930–1946 and recorded 5,635 cases with
1,714 deaths, or a mortality rate of 30 percent. Figure 13 shows a

marked rise in the incidence of the disease in the years 1930–1939. This rise was related to the increase in home canning during an era of economic depression, a failure to educate people about the hazards of home processing of foods, and the slow reporting of cases in rural areas prior to this period.

The anaerobe produces six antigenically different exotoxins, Types A, B, and E being the most important in human disease. Shortly after a person ingests contaminated food, the toxin is disseminated through the bloodstream, localizes in the cranial nerves, and produces the symptoms of visual disturbances, difficulty in swallowing, and respiratory distress.

The treatment of botulism requires early diagnosis and supportive therapy in an intensive care hospital unit. Polyvalent and monovalent antitoxic sera are available and should be administered as quickly as possible. Since determination of the precise type of toxin responsible for the illness requires time, polyvalent serum should always be administered. Most epidemics have been caused by the faulty preparation of home-canned foods. Because the toxin is heat-labile, it can be destroyed in food by boiling for ten minutes or by heating at 80° C. for thirty minutes.

Staphylococcal Food Poisoning

The ubiquitous staphylococcus has been considered a probable cause of food poisoning ever since the early days of bacteriology. G. M. Dack (1956) has presented the historical background of the sporadic reports that implicated this organism, the first basic proof that a staphylococcus toxin was the cause of food poisoning having originated from his laboratory at the University of Chicago (Dack et al., 1930). He described the circumstances as follows (1956, p. 115):

In 1929 the role of staphylococci in food poisoning was rediscovered when Dr. W. E. Cary brought to the laboratory two Christmas cakes which had been submitted to him by two of his physician-friends who knew he was interested in food poisoning. These three-layer sponge cakes had a thick cream filling and had been ornately iced and decorated with chopped pistachio nuts and maraschino cherries. They had been baked on December 23 or 24 in a commercial Italian bakery in Chicago and were delivered on the afternoon of the twenty-fourth. The cakes were presumably refrigerated at the bakery but were not kept in ice boxes later. One cake had been served at various times on the twenty-sixth to 5 adults and 3 children and the other at dinner to 3 adults. The 11 individuals who ate the cakes became ill. The victims were from four families, so that other items of food could easily be eliminated. More than half of each cake was available for laboratory study, and work was begun 15 hours after the cakes were first cut.

A filtrate of staphylococci obtained from portions of the cakes produced gastroenteritis in rabbits and in human volunteers.[7] It is now established that certain strains of staphylococci produce enterotoxin. At least five enterotoxins have been identified, although type A is the most common cause of epidemics (Hobbs, 1969).

The epidemiological and clinical pattern of such epidemics is as follows: the contaminated food is usually custard-filled bakery goods. Within six hours of ingestion, nausea, vomiting, abdominal cramps, and diarrhea ensue. Chills and fever are not prominent, and bloody stools rarely occur. Recovery usually takes places within 24 to 48 hours. The illness results from contaminated food that is improperly refrigerated, permitting the reproduction of staphylococci and the formation of enterotoxin, and is rarely lethal.

Viral Hepatitis

Most recognized epidemics of viral hepatitis in the past have resulted from the ingestion of contaminated food or water, and for this reason the disease is discussed under enteric infections. It is also transmitted through inoculation or transfusion of blood or blood products, however. The etiology and pathogenesis of viral hepatitis are complex, but the evolution of knowledge has been rapid, and control of the disease can be anticipated.

Epidemics of jaundice, presumably of virus origin, have occurred periodically in civilian and military populations for centuries. A paradoxical feature is that viral hepatitis has become a disease of modern scientific progress, often resulting from procedures used in the management of other diseases. W. P. Havens Jr., writing on the history of viral hepatitis after World War II, stated (1968, p. 331), "The emergence of viral hepatitis as one of the most important causes of loss of time among U.S. troops during World War II was as unexpected as it was dramatic." In an attempt to foresee the medical conditions that would confront military personnel deployed to various parts of the world during this war, priorities for investigating infectious diseases were influenced by the experiences of World War I. Emphasis was placed on pneumonia, influenza, yellow fever, typhus, malaria, dengue, sandfly fever and venereal infections, "but viral hepatitis received little or no consideration as a potential troublemaker" (Havens, 1968, p. 331). Hepatitis became a major military disease.

The cardinal signs of liver injury are fever and jaundice, which can be caused by many factors, such as toxins, chemicals, malignancy, and blood dyscrasias and may appear during the course of several infectious diseases. Nevertheless there is ample historical evidence that epidemics of fever and jaundice, compatible with contemporary epidemic viral hepatitis, occurred in the past. Present knowledge suggests the existence of at least two types of viral hepatitis. Viral hepatitis A includes catarrhal jaundice, epidemic jaundice, and infectious hepatitis. Viral hepatitis B is also called homologous serum hepatitis, Australia antigen hepatitis, and MS-2 hepatitis.

Since it is now known that type A virus is disseminated in the feces, resulting in the contamination of food and water as in typhoid fever, it is probable that historical accounts of epidemic jaundice related to this type. Viremia in type B, like that of type A, occurs in patients during the acute phase of illness, but unlike type A, may persist in the tissues and blood for months and even for years after apparent recovery from the disease. For this reason type B hepatitis is often associated with transfusions of whole blood and blood products obtained from presumably healthy donors with viremia.

Several accounts of epidemics of probable type A hepatitis occurred in armies throughout Europe during the eighteenth and nineteenth centuries (Paul and Gardner, 1960). According to E. A. Cockayne (1912), probably the first authentic description of epidemic jaundice consistent with type A occurred in Minorca in 1745. Accounts of probable type A hepatitis described 71,691 cases in the white northern troops during the American Civil War between 1861 and 1866 (United States Surgeon-General's Office, 1888). Type A hepatitis was not a medical nuisance among American military personnel in World War I, but the incidence of the disease was considerable in the French and British troops in the Middle East, and in the Dardanelles campaign.

Type A hepatitis attracted the attention of medical investigators during the early years of the twentieth century, particularly of the pathologists and clinicians. Chester Jones and George Minot (1923) in Boston attempted to clarify the pathogenesis of the disease, referring to it as "catarrhal jaundice." They suggested that four basic factors contributed to the pathogenesis: (1) it was an infectious process; (2) there was a disturbance in liver function; (3) bile was excluded from the intestine because of a swelling and obstruction (catarrh) of the bile ducts; and (4) bile was retained in the circulation (jaundice). The authors applied quantitative measurements to the blood and feces to determine the degree of obstruction and described the hematological features of the disease. At the same time George Blumer (1923a) in New Haven reviewed the extensive outbreaks in the United States, doubting the role of food or water in the transmission of the disease but accepting the theory of person-to-person transmission. Arnold Rich (1930) at Johns Hopkins did much to clarify the pathogenesis of jaundice on the basis of the retention and regurgitation of bile.

One of the outstanding contributions to the epidemiology of type A hepatitis was that of an English country practitioner, William Pickles (1939), on the basis of observations made during 1929–1930 and 1935–1936. Studying epidemics of the disease among individuals in various villages, he worked out the incubation period, the clinical course, and the prognosis. His modest and instructive observations, communicated without the advantage of any biochemical data, make pleasurable reading.

About the same time the Copenhagen studies by K. Roholm and P. Iversen (1939) contributed another important advance. They performed 38 aspiration biopsies of the liver on 26 patients with catarrhal jaundice during the acute phase of the disease. This technique, performed on the living subject, was to aid in the future understanding of the histopathology during the progress in studying both types A and B hepatitis. It then became possible to correlate the hepatic pathology with the clinical status of the patient and with abnormal biochemical information. Their report was accompanied by excellent photographic illustrations of the inflamed liver parenchyma.

By 1940 type A hepatitis (catarrhal or epidemic jaundice) had been established as a definite clinical entity, probably caused by a virus. The pathogenesis of the jaundice, based on histopathological studies of the liver, showed hepatic inflammatory disease and stasis of the biliary caniculi. The incubation period was about thirty days. The disease most commonly involved children and young adults. The prognosis was good, and hepatic regeneration restored normal liver function. Remaining enigmas included the precise etiological agent and the modes of transmission.

Interest in type B viral hepatitis (homologous serum hepatitis) increased in 1942 when thousands of military personnel developed hepatitis and jaundice following immunization with the vaccine of yellow fever virus, which out of necessity had been stabilized by the addition of human serum. Unfortunately the serum contained the icterogenic agent. In the United States Army there was a total of 49,233 cases with 84 deaths (Havens, 1968; Paul and Gardner, 1960). Similar results occurred in the armies of allied nations. During the years 1942–1945 there were 182,383 cases of combined types A and B hepatitis in the United States Army with 352 deaths (Havens, 1968; Paul and Gardner, 1960). The catastrophe with yellow fever vaccine sparked many investigations on hepatitis. Type B hepatitis is the more severe form, and epidemics still occur. Scientific papers that should have served as a warning of the possible appearance of epidemic disease on a large scale had appeared prior to World War II.

A. Lürman (1885, translation 1972) probably described the first epidemic of type B hepatitis. He inoculated 1,289 workmen in Bremen, Germany against smallpox with glycerinized human lymph, and 191 of them developed jaundice, while no jaundice appeared in five hundred persons receiving a different source of lymph. He remarked upon the long incubation period of the disease, a characteristic of type B hepatitis. Aside from the inoculated men there were no other cases of jaundice in Bremen at the time.

Many advances in human medicine have come from the observations of abnormal phenomena appearing in species other than man. Equine viral hepatitis was reported by Sir Arnold Theiler (1919), director of veterinary research in South Africa.[8] This was graphically called "staggers" and was associated with acute atrophy of the liver. It was concluded that the disease was due to a virus, and suspensions of virus with and without added immune serum were used for prophylactic purposes. After several thousand horses had been immunized, however, the fatal disease appeared in large numbers in those animals that had received the vaccine *along with immune serum.* In other words, living virus persisted in the "immune serum." It is ironic that a quarter of a century later the same disastrous sequence of events occurred following the immunization of humans with yellow fever vaccine.

Between 1920 and 1940 several clinical reports appeared in which human serum and contaminated inoculating needles were implicated in the genesis of what must have been type B hepatitis. At the Mayo Clinic there were 70 cases of "epidemic infectious jaundice" associated with the treatment of syphilis with arsphenamine between 1916–1920 (Stokes and Ruedemann, Jr., 1920). Hepatotoxicity due to arsphenamine appeared to be ruled out. In a diabetic clinic in Lund, Sweden a nosocomial epidemic of jaundice was observed in 1923 involving 20 patients following injections of insulin (Flaum, Malmros, and Persson, 1926). A most significant report on probable type B hepatitis was made by MacNalty (Great Britain Ministry of Health, 1938) in Great Britain, in which of 82 to 109 children receiving pooled convalescent measles serum, 37 developed jaundice and 7 died.

Two other important communications on type B hepatitis following inoculation with yellow fever vaccine suspended in human serum appeared before World War II. A British report comprising thirty-one hundred persons inoculated between 1932 and 1937 described jaundice in 89 (Findlay and MacCallum, 1938). Fred Soper and H. Smith (1938) in Brazil immunized 795 persons with 17E yellow fever vaccine and hyperimmune serum, and 20 to 30 percent developed jaundice after long incubation periods. Similar observations were recorded by others (Fox et al., 1942). Homologous serum jaundice was recognized by M. L. Trumbull and D. J. Greiner (1951).

It also had become apparent by 1943 that type B hepatitis followed transfusion with whole blood and blood products, especially plasma (Beeson, 1943; Great Britain Ministry of Health, 1943; Morgan and Williamson, 1943). As late as 1938 some experienced investigators still believed that types A and B hepatitis were both due to the same virus (Findlay, MacCallum, and Murgatroyd, 1939; Great Britain Ministry of Health, 1938). But between 1944 and 1946, after studies had been carried out on human volunteers with feces or serum from acute cases, it was concluded that at least two types of virus were involved, causing two forms of hepatitis with distinguishing clinical features (MacCallum and Bauer, 1944; Paul and Gardner, 1960).

Thus by 1960 at least two forms of viral hepatitis had been delineated clinically, one with a sudden febrile onset followed by jaundice and recovery; the second with a longer incubation period and an insidious onset, frequently resulting in a prolonged illness. Occasionally progressive and fatal hepatic necrosis occurred, especially with type B, or biliary cirrhosis resulted in those who recovered. There was no specific treatment for either form. With the aid of more sophisticated biochemical procedures, however, progress had been made in understanding the nature of the diseases, and precise histopathological techniques have defined the amount of hepatic involvement. Preventive procedures included warnings of the dangers of hepatitis from contaminated food and water and of the hazards of accidental or therapeutic inoculation of contaminated human blood. The pressing need was to isolate and define the etiology of each type.

The isolation of viruses responsible for types A and B hepatitis eluded investigators until an unrelated research program uncovered a clue to the etiology of type B hepatitis. Two geneticists, A. C. Allison and B. S. Blumberg (1961), interested in the genetic aspects of cancer, were attracted to concepts of polymorphism in plants. The work of E. B. Ford at Oxford University directed their attention to the same phenomenon in animals and man. According to Ford polymorphism is "the occurrence together in the same habitat of two or more discontinuous forms of a species in such proportions that the rarest of them cannot be maintained merely by recurrent mutation" (Ford 1957, p. 1315). Discussing aberrations of human erythrocytes, Ford selected the example of sickle cell anemia in the African blacks, in whom the heterozygotes are at an advantage compared to the homozygotes. In the homozygotes death occurred early in life, while the heterozygotes carrying the "sickle cell trait" lived to advanced adult life and were protected at the same time against the severe endemic infection of malaria in Africa caused by *Plasmodium falciparum*.

A. C. Allison and B. S. Blumberg (1961) decided to probe genetic disturbances in the proteins of human serum. Such human polymorphism traits had been found in proteins relating to haptoglobin, transferrin, gamma globulin beta-lipo-protein, group-specific substances, cholesterase, and esterase. Using relatively simple immunological techniques, they initially studied the interaction of sera from two groups. One group included "post-transfusion sera," i.e., sera from patients who had had multiple transfusions. The second, "panel sera," contained sera representative of all of the genetically controlled serum protein-types from individuals of different ethnic groups. Their key observation was made on the serum of one male, 64 years of age, who had received 47 units of blood. His serum yielded a strong precipitin reaction with some of the panel sera involving the alpha 2-globulin (Blumberg, 1964). Further investigations emphasized that patients receiving multiple transfusions develop precipitating antibodies against serum beta-lipoproteins (Blumberg, Dray, and Robinson, 1962). These antisera defined "a system of inherited antigenic specificities on the serum low-density beta-lipoproteins. . . . In 1964 an antibody was detected in the serum of a transfused hemophilia patient which was clearly different from the lipoprotein precipitins previously found" (Blumberg, Sutnick, and London, 1968, p. 1566). The antibody of the patient reacted with only one of the antigens present in the sera of the panel of 24, which was from an Australian aborigine. Therefore the antigen was named Australia antigen. Subsequent studies revealed that this reaction rarely occurred with sera in American populations, except in those having acute viral hepatitis, those with leukemia, and patients institutionalized with Down's syndrome.

The possible relationship between Australia antigen and viral hepatitis inspired further investigations. A major result was the discovery that antibody for the Australia antigen was present in many of the sera of patients with type B hepatitis, but not in those with type A. Was Australia antigen in reality the virus that caused homologous type B hepatitis?

The role of Australia antigen in viral hepatitis has received some clarification. Virus-like particles were seen in the sera of hepatitis patients who had positive antibody reactions with Australia antigen (Dane, Cameron, and Briggs, 1970). The particles measured about 42 nanometer (nm.) in size. Smaller particles of 22 nm. and long forms were also found. It was suggested that the 42 nm. particle ("Dane particle") was the complete virus of type B hepatitis. The Australia antigen has proved to be a useful tool in epidemiological and clinical studies. It is used extensively in screening prospective blood donors who may be potential carriers of type B virus.

The second, more direct approach to defining the viral cause of hepatitis came from studies at the Willowbrook State School for re-tarded children in Staten Island, New York. There were 1,153 cases of infectious hepatitis observed between 1953 and 1967, with 5.5 percent having second attacks. The children were three to ten years of age, "incapable of being trained and prone to put everything that they pick up in their mouths" (Krugman, Giles, and Hammond, 1967, p. 365). For these reasons viral hepatitis with more than one cause was anticipated. In initial but carefully controlled studies, sera from acutely ill patients were inoculated into human subjects. For further studies the sera from one patient, Mir, was selected since she had had two attacks of hepatitis, one of a shorter incubation period than the other, suggesting that she had had both types of illness. The serum obtained during the first illness from Mir was labelled MS-1 and that from the second MS-2. The authors concluded that serum MS-1 indi-cated classical infective jaundice (type A), while MS-2 was the result of homologous serum jaundice (type B). They also confirmed that immune globulin greatly reduced the incidence of type A hepatitis and prevented or modified the severity of type B (Krugman, Giles, and Hammond, 1971). Subsequently it was demonstrated that MS-2 correlates with Australia antigen in that no antibody for Australia antigen was demonstrated in the sera from patients with MS-1 infec-tion, whereas antibody appeared regularly in the MS-2 patients (Giles et al., 1969).

Further advances in knowledge of the nature of hepatitis have been rapid through the research of many investigators (Zuckerman, 1972). The results have been monitored and recorded by the National Re-search Council Committee on Viral Hepatitis (1974). An important symposium outlined the basic clinical and laboratory studies that had been carried out up to 1975 (Viral Hepatitis: Symposium, 1976). Type A virus has been successfully identified morphologically and de-scribed as an enterovirus with a RNA core and has been successfully transmitted to marmoset monkeys. Blumberg's type B antigen has been identified morphologically by Dane (Dane particle), with a sur-face antigen ($HB_s Ag$), and a core particle ($HB_c Ag$) having DNA polymerase activity and circular double-stranded DNA. Four sub-types of type B antigen are recognized. Type B virus has been trans-mitted to chimpanzees. A most unusual characteristic of type B as a virus is that active virus particles circulate in the blood in profusion for years in healthy carriers. Collection of these particles has permitted the production of type B vaccine. Neither type has been isolated and grown in tissue cultures. Finally evidence that is still open to question indicates that another virus, type C, is also a cause of hepatitis.[9]

Despite the importance of such discoveries, progress in the prevention and management of hepatitis has been slow. Immune serum globulin is still recommended as a prophylactic, especially for type A hepatitis. Further studies are under way with type B preparations. Rigid, well-established public health measures must be enforced in institutions where exposure to type B infections is most likely, and individual precautions must be carried out for the control of type A infections, the sources of which are food and water. An excellent summary of the procedures for containing hepatitis B disease has been made available (Center for Disease Control, 1976b).

Type A hepatitis is a continuing problem because presumably healthy carriers acting as food handlers are a difficult source of disease to control. In 1974 an epidemic of 107 cases of type A hepatitis occurred in Minneapolis and was traced to a lunch counter where cold sandwiches were served.[10] A sandwich-maker was identified as the source of the epidemic. Over ten thousand injections of immune serum globulin appeared to have modified the severity of the epidemic.

Type B hepatitis is particularly localized in hospitals. It has been emphasized that "hepatitis is the scourge of dialysis and transplantation units. In 1969 there were 150 cases of hepatitis with 16 deaths among 2000 patients on dialysis and 88 cases with one death among the dialysis staffs in Europe" (Kjellstrand et al., 1972, p. 433). J. M. Matsen (1973) pointed out there were 74 cases of hepatitis among the personnel of the University of Minnesota Hospitals between 1968 and 1972, and 65 of the cases were associated with the hemodialysis-transplantation unit or with the clinic laboratories. Most of the cases were type B infections.

Since January 1, 1974 hepatitis has been a specified notifiable disease in the United States under the three headings of hepatitis A, hepatitis B, and hepatitis unspecified. For this reason it is difficult to arrive at definitive national figures, but there is no question that viral hepatitis constitutes a serious public health menace at both national and international levels.

CHAPTER 16

Suppurative Diseases

Little progress was made in the control and treatment of suppurative conditions until the nineteenth century. Before that time there was not much hope for the patient nor aid from the physician in cases of suppuration following surgery or trauma. Acceptance of the germ theory of disease and the concept of contagion contributed to the principles of aseptic surgery as formulated by Semmelweis for puerperal sepsis and by Lister for wound suppuration.

Streptococcal Diseases

Professor Arthur Bloomfield has stated (1958d, p. 135), "So much has been written on every phase of rheumatic fever that the bibliographer is confronted with an almost hopeless task." But rheumatic fever is only one aspect of the complex subject of streptococcal diseases, a subject that has interested me for over forty years. The history of the understanding of these diseases can be divided into four eras. First, the period from Hippocrates to the nineteenth century was one of medical confusion, in which the classification of disease was based largely on clinical observations. The etiology of diseases was unknown, although the concept of contagion gradually became accepted during the eighteenth and nineteenth centuries. Certain characteristic skin eruptions did lead to an early recognition of specific streptococcal entities, such as erysipelas and scarlet fever, but this limited descriptive delineation perpetuated the confusion over the nature of streptococcal diseases into the twentieth century. Treatment was largely supportive and often accompanied by disastrous surgical and obstetrical procedures.

The second era was that from 1850 to 1920, when dramatic progress in the understanding of streptococcal diseases was made through the disciplines of pathology and microbiology. Streptococci were identified, classified, and grown in pure culture, and were assigned as causes of such conditions as erysipelas, scarlet fever, tonsillitis, otitis media, mastoiditis, meningitis, pneumonia and empyema, puerperal fever, endocarditis, and osteomyelitis. Although specific therapy was lacking, the surgical techniques for the management of wounds and of suppuration were greatly advanced during World War I by debridement and drainage. Still the morbidity and mortality rates for streptococcal diseases remained alarmingly high.

The 1920s and 1930s marked several steps forward in the control of these diseases. The classification of streptococci was extended, and the complexity of the biology and chemistry of this family of microorganisms was recognized. Available knowledge during the early years of this era can be gleaned from an examination of Zinsser's (1927) standard *Textbook of Bacteriology*, which was widely used at the time. He wrote about the streptococci (p. 337), *"This broad classification into the haemolyticus and viridans is the practical basis on which bacteriologists at the present time deal with the classification of pathogenic bacteria."* This simple distinction was partially clarified by J. H. Brown (1919), who had recognized *alpha*, *beta*, and *gamma* types of streptococcal hemolytic activity on agar plates, a classification that aided the clinical interpretation of diseases caused by these groups. Most of the suppurative complications were due to the *beta* group of streptococci. The host-parasite relationships were defined by immunological techniques. The surge of investigations on the pathogenic streptococci was emphasized by 1929 in the documentation of over sixteen hundred studies (Thomson and Thomson, 1928–29). By the end of the period the sulfonamides had provided the first definitive therapy for streptococcal diseases, especially those due to *beta* hemolytic streptococci.

During this presulfonamide era from 1928 to 1938, we were confronted by the appalling disability and death from streptococcal sepsis at the Boston City Hospital. In that decade a severe economic depression gripped the nation, and hospital space was taxed with seriously ill "charity cases." The strain on the overworked hospital staff was almost overwhelming and terribly frustrating at times. Although there was no specific therapy, we did learn the natural course of infectious diseases, a valuable preparation for the later evaluation of the sulfonamides and antibiotics. The death rate from streptococcal complications with bacteremia approached 75 percent (Keefer, Ingelfinger, and Spink, 1937). The hospital had large numbers of children with suppurative otitis media and mastoiditis. Recovery from streptococcal meningitis was uncommon. The mortality rate was around 90 percent in patients with streptococcal pneumonia and empyema. And recovery from streptococcal pyoarthritis of the larger joints was invariably followed by ankylosis. Measles was complicated by lethal streptococcal pneumonia. There was a continuing threat of epidemic puerperal sepsis between 1926 and 1933 (Williams, 1936).

The period 1940–1975 included World War II, when Group A hemolytic streptococci were the cause of extensive epidemics of upper respiratory infections — including scarlet fever — and of the nonsuppurative complication of rheumatic fever in the armed forces. A major advance in the prevention and management of streptococcal diseases was provided by penicillin. After World War II the extensive epidemiological data brought together during the conflict were carefully analyzed, and basic investigations were directed toward the nonsuppurative streptococcal complications of rheumatic fever and nephritis. Research was carried out on the chemical and biological properties of the cell structure and of the enzymes of the streptococcal groups, and was summarized in several major symposia (McCarty, 1954; Thomas, 1952; Uhr, 1964; Wannamaker and Matsen, 1972).

Identification, Isolation and Classification of Streptococci

A small book of eighty pages by the general practitioner Dr. Robert Koch (1878, translation 1880) on *Investigations into the Etiology of Traumatic Infective Diseases* appeared in 1878 and "created something of a sensation" (Bulloch, 1938a, p. 149). Koch's twofold monumental contributions were the staining of microorganisms in septic material with aniline dyes, and the use of the microscope for descriptive purposes. But the medical profession was bewildered by his findings. It remained for Alexander Ogston (1881), a surgeon in Aberdeen, Scotland, to clarify Koch's report by employing the latter's techniques in studies on abscesses. Ogston had been greatly impressed by Lister's investigations in Edinburgh. He attacked the mysterious problems of pyemia, septicemia, and other infective processes. He recognized micrococci, often in chains, in human abscesses, although bacilli and spirilla were also present. Pus inoculated into animals established abscesses with the micrococci in evidence. Ogston confirmed Pasteur in describing anaerobic micrococci. He was the first to grow bacteria in abundance in chicken eggs and to produce abscesses in animals by inoculating them with these cultures. He concluded (1881, p. 373), "Suppurating wounds contain micrococci, . . . Listerian dressings prevent micro-organisms from gaining access to wounds. Micrococci in wounds withstand most antiseptic applications. Where no micrococci are present in wounds, no pus is produced; the discharge is serous."

Ogston (1881) designated the micrococci that occurred in chains as *Streptococcus*, and those that appeared like bunches of grapes as *Staphylococcus*. F. J. Rosenbach (1884, translation 1886) clarified the pathogenesis of septic wounds still further, dividing the staphylococcus into the *aureus* and *albus* varieties, and named the micrococci in chains *Streptococcus pyogenes*.

Serological techniques aided greatly in the classification of streptococci and in epidemiological studies. Fred Griffith (1934) described about twenty different types of *beta* hemolytic streptococci and pointed out that there was no specific *Scarlatinae* strain. Rebecca Lancefield (1933) established the basis for the modern differentiation of streptococci by utilizing a carbohydrate fraction of the bacterial cell, with which she produced anticarbohydrate rabbit sera for purposes of identifying strains of streptococci by means of the precipitin test. In this manner she divided 104 of 106 strains into five major groups; Group A strains were found to be the principal human pathogens.

The expansion of this classification during the ensuing twenty years appears in the eighth edition of the authoritative *Bergey's Manual of Determinative Bacteriology* (Buchanan and Gibbons, 1974). Gram-positive cocci from all sources are divided as follows: Family I, *Micrococcaceae*, under which Genus II is *Staphylococcus*; and Family II, *Streptococcaceae*, in which Genus I is *Streptococcus* and Lancefield's

Group A is known as *Streptococcus pyogenes,* twenty-one different species having been recognized. The classification of the *Pneumococcus* is now incorporated under *Streptococcus* as *Streptococcus pneumoniae.* Further clarification on the classification of streptococci can be obtained in the sixth edition of *Topley & Wilson's Principles of Bacteriology, Virology and Immunity* (Wilson and Miles, 1975).

One of the most dramatic achievements of modern medicine is the control and management of streptococcal diseases, brought about largely through the introduction of the sulfonamides followed by penicillin. For this reason certain suppurative diseases and nonsuppurative complications are reviewed here to illustrate this progress and to introduce some remaining problems.

Streptococcal Respiratory Infections

Streptococcal disease was known at the time of Hippocrates; erysipelas was described then. There are many references in the older medical literature to the "ulcerative sore throat," which was undoubtedly confused with diphtheria and exudative pharyngitis (tonsillitis) of streptococcal origin. The latter infection gave rise to many suppurative complications including erysipelas, sinusitis, otitis media, mastoiditis, meningitis, pneumonia (often with empyema), and to bacteremia with metastatic suppurative lesions of various tissues. In contemporary medicine few of these complications are encountered in hospitals.

Serious epidemiological studies on streptococcal upper respiratory infections were hampered before 1933 by the lack of means of differentiating the strains of streptococci present in the nasopharynx, blood, and tissues of healthy and sick individuals. This deficiency was rectified through the use of Lancefield's immunological techniques. It was clearly established that the human oropharynx was a reservoir of the pathogenic strains of Group A hemolytic streptococcus. Up to 5 percent of the healthy population were carriers, a rate that increased appreciably during the colder months. Epidemic streptococcal respiratory disease was usually airborne; but epidemics were also foodborne, especially in military installations (Commission on Acute Respiratory Diseases, Fort Bragg, N.C., 1945a; Purvis, Jr. and Morris, 1946). Similar foodborne epidemics occurred in civilian populations. In 1943 one hundred cases of epidemic "septic" sore throat occurred in a Minnesota village with a population of one thousand. The source was milk from a herd of cattle heavily contaminated with streptococcal mastitis. The herd was attended by similarly infected personnel.

We became aware of the severity of streptococcal respiratory infections soon after the Lancefield technique for typing strains of streptococci was introduced on the IV Medical Service (Harvard) at the Boston City Hospital. Between January 1, 1933 and July 1934, charged with the medical care of the student nurses, we attended 57 hospitalized nurses with streptococcal exudative pharyngitis. Eleven, or almost 20 percent, developed acute rheumatic fever, with one fatality. Several had permanent cardiac valvular damage as a result. This sequence of events also occurred commonly in military personnel in World War II.

At the same time I became concerned with the dermal lesion of *erythema nodosum*, a red, inflammatory, nodular eruption of the lower extremities that occurred principally in young women having a systemic febrile condition. The most widely held interpretation of this condition at the time was that it was a manifestation of tuberculosis; however, an extensive survey showed that it occurred more commonly with streptococcal disease, and also with rheumatic fever (Spink, 1937). It was further established that this eruption appeared in other infectious diseases, and also as a part of a systemic drug reaction.

As World War II approached, knowledge of streptococcal disease had advanced considerably. Bacteriological and immunological techniques had been developed so that epidemiological studies could be carried out. Furthermore, for the first time in medical history, effective systemic chemotherapy with the sulfonamides was available. Streptococcal diseases had not been stressed in the medical history of World War I, but events in World War II soon demonstrated large epidemics of streptococcal respiratory infection in Army and Navy installations in the United States and in Great Britain. Perhaps for security reasons, Army and Air Force camps, and Naval training stations, were established in the Rocky Mountain areas of Colorado, Wyoming, and Idaho. As public health authorities were aware before World War II, this section of the country, as well as New England, had the highest incidence of acute rheumatic fever in the United States among civilian populations. Fortunately few large military installations were established in the New England area. The attack rate of streptococcal disease among new military recruits in the western areas became so severe that special groups were organized to study the cause, prevention, and treatment of this problem. Captain Alvin Coburn had a major role in the epidemiological studies in the United States Navy. The Commission on Hemolytic Streptococcal Infections, of which I was a member, was stationed at Camp Carson, Colorado Springs, Colorado under the Board for the Investigation of Epidemic Diseases, United States Army. During World War II I also had the opportunity to review the excellent work of the United States Army's Commission on Acute Respiratory Infections at Fort Bragg, North Carolina.

Doctor Lowell Rantz (1958), the director of our Streptococcus Commission at Camp Carson, wrote the official United States Army medical report. The principal problem was the high incidence of acute rheumatic fever. From 1942–1943 in the United States Army, largely in the domestic zones, there were at least 26,062 cases of scarlet fever and approximately 150,000 cases of streptococcal respiratory disease. Rheumatic fever is an insidious disease; there were 18,339 cases reported, and the incidence may have been significantly higher. Captain Coburn, summarizing the experience of the United States Navy, stated, "during the four war years at least 1,000,000 personnel contracted a streptococcal infection" (Coburn and Young, 1949, p. 8); and "rheumatic fever ranked third in the loss of man days to disease" (p. 9). It is of interest that although acute glomerular nephritis is an important sequela to streptococcal infection, it did not approach the significant incidence of rheumatic fever.

Fortunately the death rate from streptococcal infections was low, and suppurative complications were markedly reduced because of sulfonamide therapy. On the other hand, a catastrophe occurred midway through the war and was averted only when penicillin became available. It was discovered that several of the most important pathogenic types of Group A streptococci had acquired resistance to the antibacterial action of the sulfonamides. In comparing penicillin to sulfadiazine in the treatment of streptococcal upper respiratory infections, including scarlet fever, we learned that because of the scarcity of penicillin supplies, therapy was discontinued too soon (Spink et al., 1946). Although the patients were remarkably improved after receiving penicillin for 24 to 48 hours, many of them relapsed. This sequence of events was prevented by administering larger amounts of the antibiotic for a week to ten days. We did not appear to alter the course of acute rheumatic fever when penicillin therapy was initiated *after* the onset of this complication (Rantz et al., 1945).

Another major advance in the control of streptococcal infection during and after the war was the use of small amounts of penicillin to prevent upper respiratory disease in selected healthy groups. In large general populations, however, there is no satisfactory approach to prevention.

Erysipelas

Erysipelas, along with other streptococcal diseases, is now rarely observed, but it was a common disease before the introduction of the sulfonamides and penicillin. Erysipelas is a streptococcal invasion of the nose, cheeks, and ears, and is associated with a nasopharyngeal infection (Bloomfield, 1958a). Probably the earliest description of erysipelas was recorded by Hippocrates as follows (1939, p. 126): "Early in spring, along with the prevailing cold, there were many cases of erysipelas, some from a manifest cause, and some not. They were of a malignant nature, and proved fatal to many; many had sore-throat and loss of speech." The first definitive discussion of the disease was that of E. M'Dowel (1835), who considered erysipelas to be contagious. The recommended treatment included bleeding, purging, incision, blistering, leeches, poultices, and mercury — all for a disease that is usually self-limiting. F. Fehleisen (1882, translation 1886) elicited the streptococcal origin of erysipelas.

Doctor Chester Keefer and I made extensive studies on erysipelas during the 1930s at the Boston City Hospital. In the winter months there were two adult isolation wards for the disease, one for males and one for females. In a review of twelve hundred cases from that institution we arrived at two significant conclusions (Keefer and Spink, 1936–37). First, contrary to prevailing medical opinion at the time, erysipelas is not caused by a specific strain of streptococcus, but rather by a number of different Group A strains, including those causing scarlet fever. Second, erysipelas is rarely followed by acute rheumatic fever in children or in adults. It is of interest that acute nephritis but not rheumatic fever is encountered as a sequela of streptococcal skin infections (Wannamaker and Matsen, 1972; see p. 593). Erysipelas is rarely seen in modern hospitals because the initial streptococcal upper respiratory diseases respond so readily to antibiotics such as penicillin or erythromycin.

A severe facial and scalp complication seen in the Boston series of erysipelas was extensive necrosis of the involved skin. This was due to secondary invasion of the lesions by staphylococci that produced a dermonecrotoxin (Stookey et al., 1934). The overall mortality rate of the twelve hundred cases was around 5 percent, usually associated with debilitated conditions and streptococcal bacteremia.

Bacterial Endocarditis

The localization of bacteria on the heart valves, with an ensuing lethal *septicemia* and *pyemia*, remained unrecognized until the nineteenth century. William Kirkes (1852 and 1945) first described the emboli resulting from infectious endocarditis, and Samuel Wilks (1868) detailed the resulting pyemia. In 1869 Winge (1945) implicated bacteria in the valvular vegetations.

William Osler presented the first comprehensive description of bacterial endocarditis in his Gulstonian Lectures before the Royal College of Physicians in London (Osler, 1885). At that time neither the etiology was known nor was any effective therapy advanced, the mortality rate being 100 percent. The most common bacteria in the genesis of bacterial endocarditis proved to be *Streptococcus viridans* (Schottmüller, 1910). Further excellent clinical surveys of the disease were made by George Blumer (1923b) of Yale and by William Thayer (1926) of Johns Hopkins.

As a medical student at Harvard I was introduced to the harsh reality of the lethal nature of bacterial endocarditis when my brilliant classmate Alfred Reinhart learned that he had the disease. I saw him intermittently during the painful weeks of his hopeless illness, and after he died I witnessed the autopsy performed by Professor Soma Weiss. Alfred had meticulously recorded the localization of the emboli in his organs from the vegetations on his heart, which were demonstrated subsequently by Dr. Weiss. Two weeks before he died Alfred gave me a reprint of his scholarly paper on "Evolution of the Clinical Concept of Rheumatic Fever" (Reinhart, 1931). As in his case, bacterial endocarditis usually localizes bacteria of the *viridans* type of streptococcus on cardiac valves previously damaged by rheumatic fever or on a congenitally deformed valve. Alfred had known that he could become a victim of bacterial endocarditis, and he was emotionally prepared. Subsequently I saw and attended several hundred persons with bacterial endocarditis, without a single survivor.

Although many forms of systemic therapy had been attempted in the treatment of bacterial endocarditis, none was successful until penicillin became available. We, among others, had reported our failure with the sulfonamides (Spink and Crago, 1939). Our own struggles with the acute and with the more chronic form of subacute bacterial endocarditis at the University of Minnesota before, during, and after the introduction of the sulfonamides and penicillin, have been recorded (Pankey, 1961).

The therapeutic problem in bacterial endocarditis was that the offending bacteria were enmeshed in the avascular fibrinous vegetations on the cardiac valves. Although penicillin proved to be, and has remained, the most successful therapeutic agent, early investigations proved that the amounts of the drug administered were inadequate. The blood concentrations of the antibiotic were too low. Only when large amounts were infused into the patients for many days did recovery ensue. At present, acute cases caused by the more pathogenic bacteria such as the staphylococcus, gonococcus, and Group A streptococci are much less frequently encountered. This is the result of prompt treatment of the primary diseases that lead to the sustained bacteremia necessary for the establishment of endocarditis. It is difficult to ascertain the mortality rate of the more common instances of bacterial endocarditis caused by the *viridans* form of streptococci, but in our own experience about 75 percent recovered after pencillin therapy, a rate that corresponded roughly with the experience of others (Finland, 1954).

Intermittent bacteremia without ill effects often occurs in many normal individuals following tooth extraction, during surgical procedures, and in acute respiratory infections; but this is a potentially serious threat to individuals with congenital or acquired rheumatic valvular lesions, since the bacteria may localize on these damaged valves. Evaluation of antibiotic prophylaxis against endocarditis under such circumstances has yielded questionable results.

Bacterial endocarditis has not been eliminated as a serious threat to human health. Successful antibiotic therapy for the disease has been one of the major triumphs of medical science, but this is one of many instances in which medical progress has created new challenges. It has now been firmly established in many large hospitals that a changing pattern of bacterial endocarditis has taken place (Finland and Barnes, 1970; Rabinovich, Smith, and January, 1968). The widespread use of antibiotics has resulted in the establishment of infections caused by organisms resistant to the antibacterial action of the drugs. Cases of endocarditis due to resistant strains of staphylococcus, gram-negative organisms, and fungi are being encountered, and therapy is often fruitless.

The remarkable advances of cardiac surgery, in which damaged valves have been successfully replaced by artificial valves, has been associated with the subsequent implantation of antibiotic-resistant organisms on these valves (Sarot, Weber, and Schecter, 1970). In many of these instances systemic drug therapy has failed, and survival has followed only when the infected valves have been removed and replaced with new ones. In addition, when antibiotic therapy has been unsuccessful in those persons whose own valves remain infected, surgical removal of the valves and replacement with artificial valves have led to recovery.

Acute Rheumatic Fever

The modern concept of acute rheumatic fever is an acute febrile respiratory illness due to Group A hemolytic streptococci, which is followed by painful swollen joints and occasionally by Sydenham's chorea, and is associated with an inflammatory reaction of the heart, often resulting in chronic rheumatic heart disease. The disease occurs most commonly in children and young adults. The evolution of this concept was gradual and was associated with considerable controversy.

The first definite advance in the understanding of rheumatic fever was made in the nineteenth century by the French cardiologist Dr. Jean Baptiste Bouillaud. Reviewing his own clinical observations and the scattered information of others, he wrote (1837, Preface, p. iii), "It is, I will venture to say, a discovery of some attention; to wit, the almost constant coincidence, either of endocarditis, or of pericarditis, or endo-pericarditis, with violent articular rheumatism. This fact, which daily observations more and more confirm, is of such vast importance that it constitutes, in some measure, a true revolution in the history of acute articular rheumatism. I am not at all astonished that so many are opposed to it: that is the fate of all new truths of any importance." He considered cold temperatures to be the inciting factor. For treatment he relied principally upon bleeding and quinine for fever.

Further knowledge about the nature of rheumatic fever was attained slowly. Doctor W. B. Cheadle (1889) of London published a monograph comprising his Harveian Lectures, in which he described the clinical features of the disease. His observations seem almost contemporary, except for the absence of the streptococcal etiology. Cheadle presented tonsillitis and chorea as antecedents of the endocarditis. He emphasized that endocarditis could occur without rheumatism and pointed out the subcutaneous rheumatic nodules and the characteristic skin eruptions.

As therapy for rheumatic fever, Cheadle advocated rest and salicylates for therapy. T. Maclagan (1876) had introduced salicin for treatment, which alleviated the pain, toxicity, and fever of the patients. Salicin, a glucoside found in poplars and willows, was changed upon ingestion into salicylate in the body. Immediately thereafter salicylates became the standard treatment for the disease. Over fifty years later some authorities believed that large doses of salicylates would not only alleviate the symptoms of rheumatic fever but would also prevent the development of cardiac lesions. But this conclusion was disproved during World War II.

No specific biological test is available to the clinician for the early detection of endocarditis or myocarditis. The pathologist L. Aschoff (1904, translation 1941), with his assistant S. Tawara, described the characteristic nonsuppurative myocardial nodules of rheumatic fever, which became known as "Aschoff bodies." The precise origin of this inflammatory lesion remains obscure, although such lesions can be reproduced experimentally in lower animals.

After H. Schottmüller's announcement in 1910 that *Str. viridans* was the cause of vegetative bacterial endocarditis, and that it most often invaded a cardiac valve previously damaged by rheumatic fever, the streptococcus was widely considered to be the cause of rheumatic fever. For the next twenty-five years, however, confusion swirled around the concept of the streptococcal origin of the disease. This period has been summarized in a large bibliographic volume (Thomson and Thomson, 1928). At that time the conservative statement by Homer Swift in Russell L. Cecil's standard *Text-book of Medicine* was accepted by most medical authorities (Swift, 1927, p. 77): "Rheumatic fever is a disease of undetermined etiology characterized by fever and a toxic state, and by the presence of the body of small disseminated focal lesions of a proliferative type." After reviewing the theory of the streptococcal origin, Zinsser (1927) concluded that the etiology of rheumatic fever remained unproved. Controversy lingered; students in 1937 were being taught that subacute bacterial endocarditis, rheumatic fever, and rheumatoid arthritis had a common etiology, that of *Str. viridans*. In fact a vaccine prepared from a *viridans* strain was widely employed in the treatment of rheumatoid arthritis.

A considerable part of the controversy stemmed from the knowledge that *Str. viridans* bacteria are omnipresent, existing on the skin and nasopharynx and in the intestinal tract of healthy individuals. It is not unusual for small numbers of these organisms to enter the bloodstream periodically without ill effect, but — paradoxically — it is these bacteria that localize on the valves damaged by rheumatic heart disease, causing bacterial endocarditis.

In spite of such sources of confusion, some progress was being made in the effort to identify the origin of rheumatic fever. Reference has already been made to the accomplishments of Captain Alvin Coburn in the United States Navy in studying the problem of rheumatic fever. As a young clinical investigator in 1931 at Columbia University, he had published a monograph of major importance, *The Factor of Infection in the Rheumatic State*. His significant conclusion read (1931, p. 273),

The observations detailed in this study have led us to the final conclusions that the rheumatic process is a human reaction, which appears in susceptible individuals, and which represents a special type of tissue response to chemical substances arising from disease of the upper respiratory tract. That unrecognized infectious agents may be associated with these upper respiratory diseases is possible; nevertheless the findings in this study justify the conception that Streptococcus hemolyticus is an important factor of infection in the rheumatic state.

Finally S. Lichtman and his associates reported that in a group of nine different diseases, including rheumatic fever and rheumatoid arthritis, "transient" streptococcemia with nonhemolytic organisms occurs frequently. But "these organisms cannot justifiably be considered as the causative agents of these diseases" (Lichtman and Gross, 1932, p. 1094).

Upper respiratory streptococcal diseases, scarlet fever, and rheumatic fever became major medical problems in the armed forces during World War II. By that time it had been clearly established that several different types of Lancefield's Group A hemolytic streptococci caused the majority of upper respiratory infections, and that acute rheumatic fever was a sequela in selected patients of this infection. Scarlet fever resulted from infection by several different types of Group A streptococci that produced an erythrogenic toxin, causing an erythematous rash in individuals lacking immunity to this toxin. Patients infected with these strains, with or without a rash, could develop rheumatic fever. *Streptococcus viridans* was the most common cause of subacute bacterial endocarditis, but there was no evidence that this strain was implicated in the genesis of rheumatic fever or of rheumatoid arthritis.

After more than twenty-five years, millions of doses of penicillin have been administered for streptococcal infections, and there is no evidence that Group A streptococcal types have acquired resistance to the drug. The antibiotic continues as an effective prophylactic and therapeutic agent. Continuous prophylactic doses of penicillin administered to people from childhood well into adult age will prevent recurrent attacks of rheumatic fever, and penicillin therapy will prevent the onset of an initial attack of rheumatic fever in those given the drug early in the course of a streptococcal respiratory disease, including scarlet fever.

Acute Glomerular Nephritis

One hundred and fifty years ago the physician Dr. Richard Bright published a book on the clinical course and morbid anatomy of a series of medical cases he had seen at Guy's Hospital, London (Bright, 1827). In one group of cases he described generalized anasarca, or dropsy, associated with chronic renal disease and "albuminous urine." For the first time chronic glomerulonephritis was delineated as the primary cause of congestive heart failure and death. His descriptions were accompanied by excellent hand-colored engravings of the kidneys studied postmortem. A few years later he presented his observations on the natural history of nephritis.

Since Bright's time it has become recognized that chronic glomerulonephritis represents a "melange" of different diseases that cause a chronic vascular inflammation of the kidneys. The acute form does occur during the course of several infectious diseases, those of streptococcal origin being a major cause.

Rheumatic fever and glomerulonephritis are both nonsuppurative complications of Group A streptococcal infections, but by no means do both diseases occur simultaneously in patients. Investigations were undertaken to analyze the biological reasons for this difference, and it was clearly demonstrated that certain strains of Group A hemolytic streptococci did cause acute nephritis, especially types 12, 4, and 49 (Rammelkamp, Jr., Weaver, and Dingle, 1952; Seegal and Earle, Jr., 1941). As a result of this knowledge, whenever a cluster of persons within a family or an institution develop a streptococcal infection with nephritis, prophylactic procedures with penicillin are usually instituted immediately for the contacts. Although we encountered large numbers of acute rheumatic fever in our experience with the Hemolytic Streptococcus Commission during World War II, we saw relatively few cases of acute glomerular nephritis, probably because the predominant types of Group A streptococcal strains were types 17 and 19.

Staphylococcal Diseases

The sulfonamides were of dubious value in the treatment of staphylococcal diseases, and the initial successful results with penicillin were thwarted within a few years by the development of penicillin-resistant strains of staphylococci. The early therapeutic triumphs over the staphylococcus and the subsequent sharp reversal presented a challenge to medical science.

In the introductory statement on streptococcal diseases reference was made to the complex nature of streptococcal organisms, as suggested by the nineteen-page description of the family *Streptococcaceae* in *Bergey's Manual of Determinative Bacteriology* (eighth edition) (R. E. Buchanan and N. E. Gibbons, 1974). This is to be contrasted with the six pages given over to the *Staphylococcus*. The general literature on the staphylococcus was also, until the late 1950s, considerably less than that for the streptococcus (Wilson and Miles, 1964a). Alexander Fleming (1929b), in an authoritative discussion on the staphylococcus, developed the subject in twenty-five pages. Thousands of scientific papers, on the other hand, have been devoted to the streptococcus and the diseases of scarlet fever, erysipelas, puerperal fever, rheumatic fever, and nephritis. But a sudden interest in the staphylococcus was manifested in Professor S. D. Elek's (1959) definitive monograph of 767 pages, which included over four thousand references. This burst of investigations and publications on the staphylococcus was largely due to the problem of managing and controlling penicillin-resistant staphylococcal diseases.

Classification of Staphylococci

The recognition of the genus *Staphylococcus* evolved into a very simple classification of only three species — *S. aureus*, *S. epidermis* and *S. saprophyticus* (Ogston, 1881; Rosenbach, 1884, translation 1886). The present discussion centers on the pathogenic species *S. aureus*, which reproduces on agar as orange, yellow, or white colonies. A simple but reliable procedure for identifying pathogenic strains is the coagulation of rabbit plasma by staphylococcus cultures. Pathogens produce different toxins, two of which are of major significance clinically. The alpha-toxin is lethal, dermatonecrotic, hemolytic, and leucocidal, and damages platelets. The enzyme enterotoxin is discussed under "Staphylococcal Food Poisoning" (see Section III, Chapter 15).

Epidemiology of Staphylococcal Disease

The natural reservoir for pathogenic strains includes man and several species of animals. Most important in the maintenance of staphylococci and spread of infection is the human nasal carrier, particularly significant in a hospital environment. In studies of healthy hospital personnel at the University of Minnesota, coagulase-positive strains were cultured from the nasopharynx of almost 40 percent, an incidence in accord with other studies (Wise, Cranny, and Spink, 1956). Similar strains can be cultured from the hands of up to 20 percent of healthy individuals, which accounts for the frequent contamination of wounds by staphylococci. Vigorous and prolonged scrubbing of the hands with soap and water, followed by the application of an antiseptic, will not completely remove these carrier strains; even after these procedures staphylococci can be cultured from the perspiration contained within the rubber gloves of surgeons.

Another source of epidemic disease, especially in hospitals, is patients with suppurating wounds and abscesses. Undoubtedly such patients were a major cause of suppurative disease and death in pre-Listerian days.

Staphylococcal Sepsis — Prepenicillin Era

It became apparent between the two world wars that staphylococcal sepsis was a serious problem. Interest was stimulated in 1928 following the Bundaberg tragedy in Queensland, Australia when twelve children died shortly after receiving inoculations of a diphtheria toxin-antitoxin preparation that had been contaminated by *S. aureus* (Kellaway, MacCallum, and Terbutt, 1928). The deaths were due to a strain that produced the highly lethal alpha-toxin. Shortly after this report I investigated the toxin of the "Bundaberg" strain and observed that rabbits died within a few minutes after the intravenous injection of the toxin. Its lethal quality was dramatized for me when I attended a desperately ill patient who had contaminated a small abrasion on her hand with a culture producing this toxin. Without any evidence of suppuration, locally or systemically, she died fifty-two hours later (Spink, 1941c).

The severity of staphylococcal sepsis has been emphasized in several investigations. One of the best prepenicillin clincal reports reviewed the outcome of 122 cases of bacteremia seen over a period of seven years in Boston (Skinner and Keefer, 1941). Most significant was the fact that only 22 of these patients recovered, yielding a mortality rate of 81.97 percent. The authors stated (1941, p. 871), "Treatment was unsatisfactory. The best results were obtained by the drainage of an abscess, when possible, and by blood transfusions." The most common portals of entry were the skin, the respiratory tract, and primary osteomyelitis. Having seen and attended many of the patients cited in the above report, I experienced the same problems at the University of Minnesota from 1937 until 1942, a period just before the introduction of penicillin.

The most disabling and serious staphylococcal infection in the pre-penicillin era was osteomyelitis, especially of the long bones. My interest in this complication extended over the decade 1932–1942. Every large civilian general hospital struggled with the management and care of these patients. They had intermittent febrile attacks and continuing drainage of purulent material, and they underwent multiple surgical procedures, a course that often endured for years. Beginning in 1937 I devoted half a day a week with one of my surgical colleagues to seeing up to a dozen hospitalized patients with osteomyelitis. Management of these patients followed the principles of rest, immobilization of the extremity with plaster casts, and surgical drainage (Orr, 1927; Trueta, 1943). Irrigations with antiseptic solutions were employed spasmodically but were of no more value than sterile saline solution.

The use of maggots or the larvae of certain species of flies for therapeutic purposes in the putrefaction of chronic osetomyelitis had been commented on favorably as early as the seventeenth century. It was not until after World War I, however, that W. S. Baer (1931) proposed a standardized technique for implanting maggots into such areas. Improvement was believed to be due to unknown chemical factors brought about by the parasites, such as the change of the exudate from an acid to an alkaline state. The procedure gave rise to undesirable psychological factors, and its extended use was abandoned because other more acceptable therapeutic methods became available. A comprehensive historical review of osteomyelitis prior to the introduction of penicillin was written by A. O. Wilensky (1934).

The pattern of staphylococcal diseases prior to the sulfonamide-penicillin era at the University of Minnesota Hospitals can be readily summarized. The mortality rate of staphylococcal bacteremia approximated 80 percent. For reasons not clearly understood, the mortality rate of bacteremia in patients with chronic osteomyelitis was around

35 percent. Patients with bacteremia frequently developed acute staphylococcal endocarditis, with a mortality rate approaching 100 percent. Staphylococcal pneumonia was a severe and lethal complication, especially when associated with influenza in patients over 40 years of age. Patients with suppurative staphylococcal meningitis rarely recovered.

Sulfonamide preparations became available for basic and clinical investigations in 1937, and we carried out extensive studies with the drugs over a five-year period until 1942. Each of the sulfonamides, including sulfanilamide, sulfapyridine, sulfathiazole, and sulfadiazine, was evaluated both in the laboratory against staphylococci and in the clinics. It was quickly confirmed that staphylococci were resistant *in vitro* to the bacteriostatic action of sulfanilamide in the presence of peptone (Spink, 1939a). Likewise pathogenic staphylococci were resistant to the bactericidal action of human blood both in patients and in normal controls (Spink and Paine, 1940; Spink and Vivino, 1942). In other words, the patient with a chronic staphylococcal infection did not develop evidence of humoral immunity. The ineffectiveness of sulfonamides against the staphylococcus, especially in the presence of peptone or purulent material, was clarified by D. D. Woods (1940), who showed that p-aminobenzoic acid (PAB) inhibited the antibacterial action of the drugs. Our initial enthusiasm for the potential benefits from sulfonamide therapy in severe sepsis was later tempered by the reports of others and by our own subsequent observations (Spink, Hansen, and Paine, 1941). In short, after five years of extensive investigations we concluded that the sulfonamides were not the therapeutic solution for staphylococcal sepsis. In spite of our frustration and disappointment, our efforts did have one important value: we were prepared in the laboratory and hospital to evaluate penicillin when that drug became available.

Staphylococcal Sepsis — Penicillin Era

Sparse supplies of penicillin were supplied to Dr. Wendell H. Hall and myself for evaluation at the University of Minnesota in 1942.[1] We were requested to evaluate the antibiotic in staphylococcal sepsis. The first patient treated on July 10, 1942 was a young girl with acute osteomyelitis, staphylococcal pneumonia, and bacteremia. The pediatric service held out little hope for her recovery. The strain of staphylococcus isolated from her bloodstream was highly sensitive *in vitro* to penicillin. Although this patient presented a severe challenge to any therapeutic agent, she recovered, and over thirty years later she is a healthy housewife and mother.

Our experience after two years with penicillin therapy for patients with staphylococcal bacteremia revealed that the former mortality rate of 80 percent had been reduced to 35 percent (Spink and Hall, 1945). As other results were channelled into the combined statistics of the National Research Council Committee, the overall mortality rate in the United States of treated cases was 37 percent (Keefer et al., 1943)!

Shortly after our early experience I visited a large United States military hospital devoted principally to the treatment of staphylococcal sepsis, especially osteomyelitis. Penicillin had become available in adequate amounts, and the debilitated patients presented a challenge for the antibiotic. They had survived the early onslaught of the Japanese in the South Pacific and had been airlifted to the United States. They suffered from a combination of diseases such as malaria, hepatitis, dysentery, and malnutrition, with osteomyelitis following battle wounds. The recovery of these patients was due to several procedures, including rest and surgical drainage of the wounds. They were also given whole blood transfusions, an adequate diet, and large amounts of penicillin administered parenterally and locally.

From all of the allied military fronts, continuing success with penicillin in staphylococcal sepsis was recorded and later extended into civilian life (Lyons, 1943; *Penicillin* Special Issue, 1944). It appeared that this type of suppuration would no longer be a major medical problem, but ominous evidence of penicillin-resistant strains of staphylococcus appeared after increased use in the civilian population.

C. H. Rammelkamp and T. Maxon (1942) isolated penicillin-resistant strains of staphylococci from human subjects, an observation later confirmed in our clinic (Spink, Ferris, and Vivino, 1944). It became apparent that wherever penicillin was widely used, especially in hospitals, epidemics due to resistant staphylococci could break out. A primary question in resolving the problem of penicillin resistance was that of the nature of this bacterial resistance. Information was also needed about the magnitude of the epidemics due to penicillin-resistant staphylococci, on the mode of spread of the disease, and on methods of control.

In approaching the problem of penicillin-resistant staphylococci we were mindful that the bacteriostatic action of the antibiotic was on the cell wall of the coccus. Penicillin interfered with bacterial growth by preventing the synthesis of constituents of the wall in rapidly multiplying organisms, information that was to be the focal point of studies on the nature of penicillin resistance.

An early communication by the Oxford group was "An Enzyme from Bacteria Able to Destroy Penicillin" (Abraham and Chain, 1940). This note appeared before a human case had been treated. The enzyme was isolated from extracts of gram-negative resistant organisms, and from *Micrococcus lysodeikticus* but not from staphylococci. The enzyme was called penicillinase, but its precise significance was not clear. W. Kirby (1944) extracted an inhibitor for penicillin from penicillin-resistant strains of staphylococci, an achievement confirmed in our laboratory (Spink and Ferris, 1945a). We also demonstrated that the degree of resistance was quantitatively related to the amount of inactivator present (Spink and Ferris, 1945b). Unlike sulfonamide resistance, in which resistant strains could be established permanently by growing cultures in the presence of the drug, this was only a temporary *in vitro* phenomenon when penicillin was used (Spink, Hall, and Ferris, 1945). In the absence of penicillin these strains reverted to a state of penicillin sensitivity. Penicillin inhibitors could not be extracted from staphylococci with this temporary form of resistance. M. Pollock (1962) established that the inhibitor was an adaptive enzyme, penicillinase, occurring in *naturally resistant* strains of staphylococci, and that its inactivating power was due to the opening of the beta-lactam ring of the penicillin molecule by the enzyme with the formation of penicilloic acid.

In summary, the increasing failure of penicillin in the management of staphylococcal sepsis after five years of use was due to an innate property of some strains of staphylococci. Within the population of a given strain a few organisms are naturally resistant to the bacteriolytic action of penicillin because of the enzyme penicillinase. With the increased use of penicillin these penicillinase-producing strains were selected out by the penicillin and permitted to reproduce. Such strains were particularly abundant in hospitals where penicillin had been extensively used, and it is for this reason that hospital epidemics of staphylococcal sepsis appeared (Spink and Ferris, 1947).

The two decades that followed the successful introduction of penicillin for staphylococcal disease were associated with increasing frustration in all parts of the world because of penicillin resistance. Reports from Australia (Rountree and Thomson, 1949), Great Britain (Barber and Dutton, 1958), and Denmark (Jessen et al., 1969) emphasized widespread hospital epidemics of infections due to penicillin-resistant strains. Advisory groups at state, national, and international levels, including the World Health Organization, reviewed epidemiological surveys and made recommendations for the control of these epidemics (Great Britain Ministry of Health, 1959; Nahmias and Eickhoff, 1961; New York State Department of Health Joint Committee on Staphylococcal Infections, 1958; United States Department of Health, Education and Welfare, 1958; World Health Organization Expert Committee on Streptococcal and Staphylococcal Infections, 1968). And, most important, the pharmaceutical industry was stimulated into an intensive search for drugs that could be successfully used in place of penicillin.

Epidemiological studies were undertaken at the University of Minnesota Hospitals. It was quickly learned that the problem of penicillin-resistant staphylococci arose within the hospital (nosocomial infections) rather than having been introduced by entering patients. The reservoirs of these strains resided in patients, and in the nasopharynges and on the skin of hospital personnel. There was a rise in mortality rate from staphylococcal bacteremia, approaching that of prepenicillin days, and from serious cross-infections of traumatic and surgical wounds transmitted by healthy hospital carriers or from other patients with sepsis. Osteomyelitis was encountered more commonly, and lethal staphylococcal endocarditis appeared more frequently. Of added significance, there was an increased incidence of penicillin-resistant strains being isolated from all sources in the laboratory.

We at the University of Minnesota Hospitals had attended national symposia relating to the problem, read the reports and recommendations of others for control, and observed the trend in our own institution. We decided to review the epidemiological factors responsible

for the increase in sepsis in our hospital and to make recommendations to the staff for control measures. The entire staff and administration of the hospital agreed on this; an epidemiological team was organized and directed by Dr. Robert I. Wise.

Employing bacteriophage typing for identifying the penicillin-
resistant strains responsible for our epidemic, we made a comprehensive review for the hospital staff (Wise, Cranny, and Spink, 1956). By
1951 over 50 percent of the isolated hospital strains of coagulase-
positive staphylococci were highly resistant not only to penicillin but
to streptomycin as well. Increasing resistance was established for the
tetracycline drugs and for chloramphenicol. More important, the incidence of resistant strains isolated from patients within the hospital
was considerably greater than that found in patients in the outpatient
dispensary. The crux of the problem was the carrier rate of resistant
strains in hospital personnel charged with the care of patients, including physicians, surgeons, nurses, ward attendants, and
housekeepers. That is to say, patients and hospital personnel were
heavily parasitized by highly resistant strains of pathogenic
staphylococci falling principally within the bacteriophage type
Group III. Even the nasopharynges of newborn babies in the nursery
were quickly parasitized with the resistant strains harbored by the
nurses. There was also a neglect of careful aseptic techniques in the
care of patients. Isolation practices were avoided because they interfered with patient care. Under the presumed security of available
antibiotics, strict isolation was no longer believed necessary. All of
these findings paralleled the findings in other institutions throughout
the world where penicillin and other antibiotics were heavily used.

We presented all the known facts to the hospital staff and to all
personnel, including nurses, students, housekeepers, dieticians, social workers, and administrators. A major move was the establishment of an isolation unit almost in the center of the hospital (Bullock
et al., 1964). Throughout the hospital strict isolation techniques were
employed. Improvement was apparent over the next few years. Perhaps the isolation unit, watched by many, had a cautionary effect on
the hospital as a whole. Even the janitors and elevator operators were
telling us how careful one must be because of "that staph!"

Staphylococcal sepsis was brought under control through similar
efforts in most other institutions. An important contribution was the

introduction of several new antibiotics such as methicillin, oxacillin, vancomycin, dicloxacillin, and cephalothin. And, most interesting, when other antibiotics were administered instead of penicillin, the incidence of penicillin-resistant strains decreased so that penicillin could reenter as a desirable therapeutic agent. R. I. Wise (1965; 1973) has reviewed the subsequent status of staphylococcal sepsis and its control. Staphylococcal sepsis will not be eliminated as a constant threat to human health, largely because man is the major reservoir of pathogenic strains. The expanded Listerian principles of aseptic techniques should be seriously respected because of this threat. The skin and respiratory tract will remain as the major portals of entry, and staphylococcal sepsis will continue to challenge medical practice.

Suppurative Meningitis

Suppurative meningitis was probably not recognized as a clinical entity before the nineteenth century. Knowledge of this inflammatory condition evolved rapidly with the discovery of microbes as specific etiological agents, and because of studies on the pathological changes in the tissues. Interest centered on epidemic meningitis, known as "spotted fever" because of the hemorrhagic skin lesions, and later identified as meningococcal meningitis. The disease attacked the young, causing high mortality rates and extensive damage to the brain in those who recovered. It was a disease feared as much as poliomyelitis in the twentieth century.

Meningococcal Meningitis

The story of meningococcal disease is challenging for the medical historian because of its complexity, which has continued into the present period. Apparently sporadic cases of meningococcal meningitis occasioned little interest in the past, although a characteristic feature of the disease that has persisted to the present time was the periodic appearance of epidemics every decade or so in civilian populations as well as in military groups.

A. Hirsch (1886) described the epidemic waves of the nineteenth century, which he divided into four periods. The first occurred during 1805 to 1830 in Europe and in the United States. The second, from

1837 to 1850, was the extension of epidemics appearing in the same geographical areas as the former. The third, 1854 to 1875, marked the spread and increased incidence of the disease in Europe, the United States, Asia, Africa, and South America. And in the last part of the century the disease appeared to a lesser degree in the United States, Germany, and Italy. Although fewer rhythmic eruptions appeared in the twentieth century, the disease was particularly intensified in the armed forces during World War I. A. L. Bloomfield (1958b) has documented the historical literature on the subject from the early nineteenth century up to World War II.

M. Vieusseux (1806) provided the first reliable description of epidemic meningitis when it occurred in Geneva, Switzerland. He called it "malignant noncontagious fever." A. Matthey (1806) performed autopsies on the victims. During this time an epidemic of the disease also occurred in the United States in the New England areas and was designated "a malignant epidemic of spotted fever" (North, 1811). Verification of the clinical findings was augmented in Elisha North's publication by the appended autopsy findings of L. Danielson and E. Mann carried out in 1806 on patients who had died in Medfield, Massachusetts.

In 1867 Professor Alfred Stillé (1867) of the University of Pennsylvania surveyed the subject and synthesized the existing knowledge about the disease, concluding that it was noncontagious. Shortly thereafter M. Clymer (1872), also of Philadelphia, described the extensive epidemic in New York City in which there were 790 reported cases with 607 deaths, mostly in children, between January 1 and June 30, 1872. Clymer sensed the contagious nature of the disease and wrote (1872, p. 33), "the effective cause of epidemic cerebro-spinal meningitis is to be sought far beyond physical and bodily conditions; that it is outside of the degree of heat, moisture, etc., and the constitutional state of the individual; and we are forced to take refuge in the assumption of an unknown specific morbific agent as the aetic factor." From the viewpoint of the historian, this statement of Clymer, written only a hundred years ago, indicated the departure from centuries of obscure medical thinking about the causes of infectious diseases to a consideration of the revelations of the new science of bacteriology.

In a little more than twenty-five years after the time of Stillé and

Clymer, a formidable scientific report on epidemic meningitis appeared in Boston in 1898 by three Harvard professors, Dr. W. T. Councilman, Dr. F. B. Mallory, and Dr. J. H. Wright (1898). They summarized the historical development of the disease and then analyzed the cases seen in the Massachusetts General Hospital, the Boston City Hospital, and the Children's Hospital. It was the first comprehensive medical treatise to appear after the discovery of the etiological agent of meningococcal meningitis. In the summary they stated (1898, p. 162), "Epidemic cerebro-spinal meningitis is an acute infectious disease, which is produced by a micrococcus characterized by its growth in pairs and by certain cultural and staining properties." They concluded with descriptions of "meningitis due to the pneumococcus," "meningitis due to streptococcus," "tubercular meningitis," and "anthrax meningitis."

The pathologist Professor A. Weichselbaum (1887a) described the characteristic *Neisseria meningitides* in both the tissues and exudate of six fatal cases of cerebral meningitis, a finding that was soon confirmed by others. For at least two decades thereafter, isolated strains were considered to be homogeneous, but biochemical and immunological investigations that intensified during the early stages of World War I revealed at least four different antigenic groups (Gordon, 1915; Gordon and Murray, 1915). This differentiation was important for epidemiological studies, serving as a basis for antiserum therapy and for the subsequent preparation of prophylactic vaccines.

The experience of British investigators in the military forces and in civilian populations between 1915 and 1919 during extensive epidemics of meningococcemia and meningitis has been well summarized (Gordon, 1920). Since it was known that the natural reservoir of the meningococcus was in the nasopharynx of a healthy carrier, the source of epidemics could be more closely followed. The British concluded that there was a critical level of a carrier rate — at which point an epidemic could be anticipated — and that this occurred when 20 percent or more of a population were carriers. In ensuing years this quantitative relationship was not fully confirmed, however, and it was seriously questioned during World War II. The second aspect of the British experience was the high mortality rate of the disease. In civilian life during those four years the death rate between the ages of 20 and 30 years was approximately 60 percent, whereas in the armed forces it was slightly above 40 percent. The difference was ascribed to the use of immune serum in the armed forces, a factor that will be discussed shortly.

In the United States Army during World War I "Cerebralspinal meningitis was of serious importance . . , not because of its incidence, which was comparatively low — in fact this disease ranked seventy-sixth as a cause for admission to hospital — but because of its high case mortality" (Simmons and Michie, 1928, p. 203). Of the 4,831 cases, 1,836 died, or 38 percent, but the mortality rates varied from area to area.

After World War I certain concepts relating to meningococcal infections became firmly established. It was confirmed that the portal of entry was the nasopharynx and that acute illness occurred when the bloodstream was invaded by meningococci. The meninges and other organs and tissues became secondarily involved. Sporadic cases of meningitis continued to appear, and intermittent epidemic disease still occurred about every decade in the United States, as noted in Figure 14.

Continuous investigations of the biology of meningococci resulted

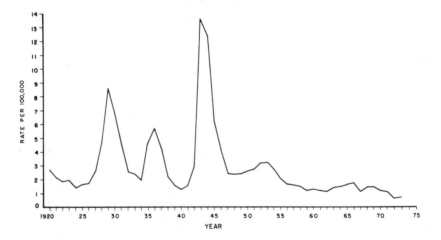

Figure 14. Meningococcal infections. Reported cases per 100,000 population by year, United States, 1920–1973. Reproduced from Weekly Report for Year Ending December 29, 1973, Reported Morbidity and Mortality in the U.S., Volume 22, No. 53, July 15, 1974. Center for Disease Control, Atlanta, Georgia (p. 44).

in a new international classification of isolated strains, based on the antigenic carbohydrate moiety of the cell and serological immune reactions. Meningococci were then assigned to Group A, B, C, or D, the first three being of major significance.

Until the twentieth century therapy for meningococcal infections was largely supportive and, at times, without benefit and even harmful. The widespread use of bleeding had abated by the late nineteenth century, but purging, emetics, and blistering were still advised, and a variety of stimulants was recommended. The successful use of diphtheria antitoxin serum aroused a similar hope for meningococcal infection.

Shortly after the 1904–1905 epidemic in Germany, G. Jochmann (1906) in Breslau and A. Wassermann (1907) in Berlin reported on the use of antiserum administered intrathecally. Doctor Simon Flexner (1907) soon followed with a long series of investigations in serotherapy at the Rockefeller Institute for Medical Research, having been consulted on an epidemic in New York City in 1904–1905 in which four thousand cases were reported with 3,429 deaths! S. Flexner and J. W. Jobling (1908) cited the results of serotherapy in 47 patients in whom the serum had been injected intrathecally. Even though the recovery rate was 80 percent, they were cautious in their conclusions. British authorities expressed enthusiasm over the use of antimeningococcus serum during World War I; between World War I and World War II extensive clinical studies suggested that it was of some benefit. Shortly after the outbreak of World War II, however, J. Dingle and M. Finland (1942) published an extensive review on the subject, and at that time the definitive treatment of meningitis still had not been achieved.

As stated above, one of the most dramatic periods in all of medical history was the introduction of the sulfonamides in 1937. We received the drug for investigational purposes in 1936 and were amazed at its success in the treatment of acute gonorrhea in the male. Within twenty-four hours of initiating oral therapy, gonococci could no longer be identified in the purulent urethral discharge. The gonococcus is closely related biologically to the meningococcus, and there was every anticipation that sulfanilamide would be similarly effective in meningococcal infection. One of the earliest reports on the use of sulfanilamide in meningitis was by F. Schwentker and his associates

(Schwentker, Gelman, and Long 1937), who stated that a mortality rate of about 9 percent had been achieved. Subsequent reports confirmed this highly successful attack on a severe disease. Other sulfonamides were introduced, such as sulfapyridine, sulfathiazole, and then sulfadiazine. The drugs could be given orally or parenterally, and it was not necessary to administer them intrathecally. During World War II my colleagues and I at the University of Minnesota participated in investigations on sulfonamide therapy during an epidemic of meningococcal meningitis that had appeared in a contingent of young army recruits. As in gonococcal urethritis, the prompt use of sulfadiazine resulted in the rapid disappearance of the meningococci from the cerebrospinal fluid and blood within twenty-four hours. All of the patients recovered, even those who had been comatose when they entered the hospital, and there were no demonstrable sequelae after recovery. Small prophylactic doses of sulfadiazine given orally to healthy contacts quickly brought the epidemic to a close, although the high carrier rate was not appreciably affected.

Unfortunately, after a few years, as with gonorrhea, sulfonamide-resistant strains of meningococci began to appear (Alexander et al., 1968). But penicillin and other antibiotics proved equally effective, and have remained so, although penicillin-resistant strains have been encountered. Rifampin appears to be an antibiotic highly useful for prophylactic purposes.

There remained an urgent need for a prophylactic vaccine, particularly in view of the disastrous recurring epidemics that involved thousands of people in Africa and — more recently — in Brazil. United States military authorities were also haunted by the fear of epidemics. In response to this need, intensive investigations were undertaken, which yielded promising results. In a series of important reports from the Walter Reed Army Institute of Research in Washington, D.C., a number of basic concepts toward this end were established (Artenstein et al., 1970; Goldschneider, Gotschlich, and Artenstein, 1969; Gotschlich, Liu, and Artenstein, 1969). The researchers found that "the occurrence of meningococcal disease is related more to the unique susceptibility of the individual host than to the innate virulence of the infecting organism" (Goldschneider, Gotschlich, and Artenstein, 1969, Part I, p. 1307).

This group also found that natural immunization occurred between two and twelve years of age and resulted principally from parasitization of the nasopharynx by meningococci. Polysaccharides from Groups A and C meningococci were successfully prepared and volunteers immunized. Immunized recruits established a carrier state in the nasopharynx to a lesser extent than controls. Recruits immunized with Group C had significantly lower attack rates than controls, but they were not protected against Group B infections. The immunizing process was Group specific.

Meningococcal disease continued to pose a serious threat in different areas in the world, including the United States. In 1962 a troublesome epidemic spot in the United States appeared at a United States Army installation for new recruits located at Fort Ord, California (Brown and Condit, 1965). This epidemic was due to Group B meningococci. Beginning in 1960 and rising to a peak in 1964, there was a total of 213 cases of meningococcal infections in the recruits and in their dependents. In the latter year the death rate rose to 13.3 percent, an increase due largely to fulminating cases of meningococcemia. The carrier rate at the beginning of training was 10 to 15 percent, and by the seventh week it was 100 percent! Furthermore the isolated strains of Type B were sulfonamide-resistant. The unusual features of this epidemic were the shift to Group B organisms in contrast to Group A commonly found previously, and the appearance of sulfonamide-resistant organisms. Assignment of new recruits to Fort Ord was discontinued late in 1964. Unfortunately there had been some distribution of these Group B organisms to other areas in California at this time. Simultaneously an outbreak of Group B meningitis occurred in the isolated Eskimo village of Barrow, Alaska, bordering on the Arctic Ocean, possibly coming indirectly from Fort Ord (Reed et al., 1966).

One of the most challenging problems in international health is the persistence of epidemic meningococcal disease in some large areas of the world. For over a quarter of a century a "meningitis belt" has existed in several African countries, known geographically as the Sahel and lying between the Sahara to the North and the equatorial forest to the South (World Health Organization, 1969b). Approximately ten thousand cases of meningitis have occurred annually within this area with a mortality rate of 12 percent. This mortality rate is to be compared with the presulfonamide rate of 85 percent in Niger in the period between 1921 and 1924. The epidemics have been associated with Group A meningococci, which unfortunately have become sulfonamide-resistant. The World Health Organization has been participating vigorously toward a resolution of the problem, as L. Lapeyssonnie has summarized (1963). It is in this area that studies with prophylactic vaccine were undertaken after 1970 (Erwa et al., 1973; Wahdan et al., 1973).

A second area of major importance for epidemic meningococcal infections is Sao Paulo in Brazil. An epidemic there, due largely to Groups C and A meningococci, attacked mostly children and young adults. In July and August of 1974, 13,141 suspected cases were admitted to Sao Paulo hospitals (Center for Disease Control, 1974b). In 1971 and 1972 there were 2,005 cases of sulfonamide-resistant Group C infections with a mortality rate of 9.2 percent. "The São Paulo outbreak, . . . is the first large citywide outbreak known to be caused by this meningococcal serogroup" (Souza de Morais et al., 1974, p. 571). Approximately seven hundred thousand doses of Group A, and some Group C vaccine, were administered to school children in Brazil late in 1974 (Center for Disease Control, 1974b).

The successful prevention and treatment of meningococcal infections has been one of the most encouraging developments in modern medicine (Feldman, 1972). Reduced mortality rates are highly desirable, but prevention of the disease is essential because many who recover are rendered blind or deaf, and long-term follow-up studies have demonstrated brain damage in some.

There remain other groups of infections in which suppurative meningitis may develop and constitute a grave disease with a high mortality rate in untreated patients. Because these cases of meningitis occur sporadically rather than in epidemics, therapeutic efforts do not carry the drama that surrounds the success with epidemic meningococcal meningitis. These include *Haemophilis influenzae* meningitis, pneumococcal meningitis, tuberculous meningitis, and staphylococcal and streptococcal meningitis.

Haemophilus[2] influenzae *Meningitis*

Haemophilus influenzae is a major cause of suppurative meningitis in infants. The microorganism was first identified during the pandemic of influenza in 1889–1892 by Richard Pfeiffer, who considered it to be the etiological agent. In 1933, however, this disease was shown to be caused by a virus. In more recent years *H. influenzae* has become an important factor in chronic respiratory disease (Turk and May, 1967). Slawyk (1899), a pupil of Pfeiffer, described the first case of suppurative meningitis in infants, and therafter sporadic case reports appeared. The year 1911 marked the first of an important series of reports on research on this disease. Martha Wollstein (1911a; 1911b) reviewed the subject and reported on a series of eight cases. She also cited the reproduction of the disease in monkeys, and the successful experimental use of an anti-influenza goat serum. Josephine Neal (1921) of the New York City Department of Health in one report summarized 32 cases with only one recovery, and in a second report only four patients survived out of 111 (Neal, Jackson, and Appelbaum, 1934). Margaret Pittman (1931) of the Rockefeller Institute for Medical Research classified strains of *H. influenzae* into six types, the encapsulated type B strain being the one implicated in suppurative meningitis in children. She also proceeded to prepare specific immune serum for human use.

By the early 1930s certain basic clinical facts had been established. The majority of the cases occurred in infants and children from three months to three years of age with a mortality rate of over 90 cent. The disease was sudden in onset with fever, restlessness, vomiting, and diarrhea, and meningitis was not always suspected. A pharyngitis with evidence of otitis media often alerted the physician to perform a lumbar puncture, which resulted in a precise diagnosis of meningitis. But why did the disease occur largely in very young children and rarely in older children and adults?

L. Fothergill and J. Wright (1933) in Boston demonstrated specific antibodies against *H. influenzae* in the bloods of newborns and infants up to two months of age, but these antibodies were absent in children between two months and three years. The disease had its highest incidence and most severe mortality rate in the latter group because of the lack of immunity. The early protection was passively transferred from the mother to the infant, whereas immunity after three years was established because the *H. influenzae* organisms had become part of the nasopharyngeal flora of healthy individuals. It is significant that up to 1930 in Boston the most common form of suppurative meningitis in this young age group was tuberculous. But between 1933 and 1936, just before the sulfonamide era, Type B *H. influenzae* meningitis became the leading cause. This form of suppurative meningitis is rare in adults.

Within a little more than a decade medical science was to provide a therapy for this infectious desease. In 1939 Dr. Hattie Alexander (1939) introduced type B anti-influenzal rabbit serum, which significantly reduced the mortality rate. When a sulfonamide and antiserum were used simultaneously, further reduction was achieved. But the residuals in those who recovered often included mental retardation, blindness, and hydrocephalus (Koch and Carson, 1955). Sulfonamides were then combined with streptomycin, and immune serum was no longer employed. Chloramphenicol with sulfonamides were then recommended by some authorities, as was ampicillin. It became increasingly clear that the important features in the management of type B influenzae meningitis were early diagnosis and prompt therapy. When these were accomplished a disastrous infection with a mortality rate approaching 100 percent was converted into a disease having a death rate of less than 5 percent (McGowan, Jr. et al., 1974). Early treatment also thwarted the appearance of serious sequelae after recovery.

Pneumococcal, Staphylococcal, and Streptococcal Meningitis

Before the introduction of the sulfonamides in 1936, recovery from pneumococcal meningitis was rare. In the years between 1930 and 1939 I had never seen a patient recover. In his extensive survey of pneumococcal pneumonia and its complications, R. Heffron (1939) pointed out that the overall mortality rate of meningitis was 95 to 100 percent. He concluded that reports of recoveries often contained insufficent laboratory data on which to base such a diagnosis.

Studies on the pathogenesis of pneumococcal pneumonia revealed that only a small minority of the cases of pneumococcal meningitis were associated with this disease. The most frequent portal of entry was an infected middle ear, with and without mastoiditis.

A significant historical report on pneumococcal meningitis appeared in 1938 from the Boston City Hospital (Finland, Brown, and Rauh, 1938). Nine-nine patients had been observed between 1929 and

1936 at that institution, and all had died. But in 1938 six patients recovered following the use of sulfanilamide and type-specific anti-pneumococcal rabbit serum. In 1939 we had attempted to treat three patients at the University of Minnesota Hospitals with sulfapyridine and specific antiserum, without success. Following investigations with pencillin we reviewed the many reports that had appeared, and reported on our own results with 17 patients, 13 of whom recovered (Hall et al., 1946). In these patients a sulfonamide drug was adminis-tered and penicillin was given parenterally and intrathecally. In addi-tion surgical drainage of otitis media and mastoiditis was carried out in some patients. But the devastating effects of this type of menin-gitis, even though recovery took place, were the residuals of loss of vision or hearing, and severe brain damage. Our experience was a confirmation of the experience of many other clinical investigators.

Fortunately pneumococcal meningitis has become an uncommon disease, principally because the premeningitis suppurative conditions have responded to antibiotic therapy. Successful management of meningitis is dependent upon early diagnosis and the use of large amounts of penicillin for up to two weeks in a hospital, with surgical drainage of localized suppuration.

Streptococcal meningitis, like that of pneumococcal origin, often begins in the nasopharynx with the suppurative complications of otitis media and mastoiditis. Group A streptococci are usually in-volved. Before the modern era of sulfonamides and antibiotics no therapy was available, and the mortality rates, especially in infants and children, approximated those of pneumococcal meningitis. Again, the early recognition of the suppurative complications and prompt treatment with antibiotics have resulted in streptococcal meningitis becoming a rare complication. When recognized early, treatment with antibiotics is highly successful.

Staphylococcal meningitis often occurs as a complication of bac-teremia arising from a suppurative focus. Traumatic fractures of the skull precede involvement of the brain and meninges, or localized paravertebral abscesses can be associated with extension to the meninges. Three important factors that have reduced the threat to life of this type of meningitis are early diagnosis, surgical drainage of abscesses, and prompt antibiotic therapy.

Tuberculous Meningitis

In 1768 Dr. Robert Whytt, professor of medicine at Edinburgh, presented the first clinical description of tuberculous meningitis, emphasizing the *"hydrocephalus*, or dropsy of the brain." He described the rapid progression of the disease and concluded (1768, p. 46), "I freely own that I have never been so lucky as to cure one patient . . . (of) this disease." Sixty years later John Cheyne (1808) wrote on the autopsy findings of dropsy of the brain. He related the disease to the "strumous" taint or "scrophula" in families, but cautioned that "hydrocephalus cannot well be considered as an effect of the scrophula . . . we are not warranted in admitting more than a great affinity between the two actions . . ." (Cheyne, 1808, p. 85). His treatment consisted of bleeding, blistering, leeching, counter-irritation, and digitalis, William Withering having introduced digitalis in 1785 for dropsy!

As early as 1813 Dr. W. Gerhard of Philadelphia delineated the tuberculous type of cerebral meningitis. He described the clinical course and autopsy findings in ten cases that he had observed in one year at the Children's Hospital in Paris. He concluded (1833–1834, Vol. 14, p. 104), "In every case analyzed, there was evidence of the existence of tubercles in one or more organs; the subjects were therefore all tuberculous."

For nearly one hundred fifty years tuberculous meningitis was looked upon as a dreary and hopeless disease. Doctor M. W. Barr of Philadelphia wrote (1892, p. 70), "The prognosis of tubercular meningitis is most grave. There can be but one termination — death." In 1901 Osler remarked on this type of meningitis in the fourth edition of his textbook (1901, p. 280), "I have never seen a case which I regarded as tuberculous recover." And Russell L. Cecil, in the first edition of his *Text-book of Medicine*, published in 1928, stated (p. 190), "In no disease is the prognosis more hopeless." As late as 1963 it was stated, "Meningitis is the most dreaded complication of tuberculosis and the most common cause of death from tuberculosis in childhood. . . . [it is] a swift killer" (Lincoln and Sewell, 1963, p. 161).

The turning point in the specific therapy of tuberculosis came in 1944 with the discovery of streptomycin (Schatz, Bugie, and Waksman, 1944). In the following year, with the aid of an excellent experimental model of tuberculosis in the guinea pig, it was demonstrated that therapy with streptomycin would prevent a lethal out-come (Feldman, Hinshaw, and Mann, 1945). Streptomycin was speedily evaluated in tuberculous meningitis, and by 1954 J. Lorber (1954) in Sheffield, England reported on 549 treated cases of which 246, or 48.4 percent, survived for more than a year. He concluded that there was no difference in the mortality rate of patients between 3 and 14 years of age and those more than 14 years of age. Nevertheless further studies with streptomycin used in combination with other drugs showed that the mortality rate in children under 2 years of age was 75 percent, while in older patients, 70 percent recovered (Lepper and Spies, 1959).

One of the most auspicious and successful cooperative investiga-tions carried out on the treatment of tuberculosis with chemotherapy was by the United States Veterans Administration-Armed Forces groups. A. Falk (1965) has given an illuminating follow-up on tuber-culous meningitis treated in this combined study, not only with re-spect to survival but also concerning the neurological residuals and work status of the patients. He was very careful to distinguish mili-ary tuberculosis with meningitis from meningitis with a localized ce-rebral focus. His most significant finding related to the comparative mortality statistics of two six-year periods. From 1946 to 1951, strep-tomycin alone, or with para-aminobenzoic acid, was used in 236 pa-tients, of whom 162 died, or 69 percent. Between 1952 and 1957, when isoniazid, which first became available in 1952, was added to the therapeutic regimes in 129 patients, only 20 percent died. In all the patients followed for more than a year after the start of chemotherapy, up to 25 percent had neurologic residuals, often se-vere enough to hamper physical activity.

Tuberculous meningitis is becoming less common, principally through the recognition of early pulmonary tuberculosis and its prompt treatment. Successful results in tuberculous meningitis, how-ever, can be anticipated only when the disease is recognized and treated early in the acute phase with combinations of drugs, including isoniazid, for several months.

Tetanus [3]

Tetanus is due to an anaerobic microbe, *Clostridium tetani*. E. Behring and S. Kitasato (1890) reported on the lethal action of tetanus exotoxin and the protective action of tetanus antiserum in their report on diphtheria toxin. Unlike diphtheria, tetanus is not an epidemic disease but usually afflicts susceptible humans following the accidental traumatization of the skin and underlying tissues with the entrance of the tetanus spores into anaerobic and ischemic tissues. An important feature of the pathogenesis of tetanus is that the tetanus spores evolve into the toxin-producing vegetative stage; this phenomenon is abetted by the suppuration and necrosis induced by contaminating Group A hemolytic streptococci and staphylococci. Tetanus spores abound in the soil, especially around farmyards. Neonatal tetanus results from tetanus spores that invade the umbilical stump and is associated with a high death rate.

Following an incubation period of several days, there is an onset of fever with spasmodic contraction of the muscles ("lockjaw"). Opisthotonus, or contraction of the large back muscles, may be severe and frequent, and respiratory action may be impeded, leading to death from aspiration pneumonia. Another feature is vascular collapse, which may result in death.

For many years at the University of Minnesota Hospitals I attended up to a dozen cases of tetanus a year, mostly in adults, none of whom had received a completed course of tetanus immunization prior to injury. Most of these patients had sustained their accidents on farms, and their wounds had become contaminated with Cl. tetani. Prognosis was extremely guarded in those individuals in whom the incubation period was less than seven days or who were 50 years or more of age. In such persons the mortality rate was around 50 percent, a rate that agreed with that for the United States (Figure 15).

Reliable statistics on the incidence of tetanus in warfare did not appear until World War I. Since tetanus toxoid for prophylactic purposes did not become available until after this war, it is informative to compare the incidence of the disease in the two World Wars of the twentieth century. Much of World War I in the western sector was fought across the farm lands of France, where exposure to Cl. tetani must have been considerable. The total number of British wounded on all fronts was 2,032,142, of whom 2,385 developed tetanus, an incidence of 1.17 per thousand wounded (Wilson and Miles, 1964b). On the western front alone there was an incidence of 0.06 per

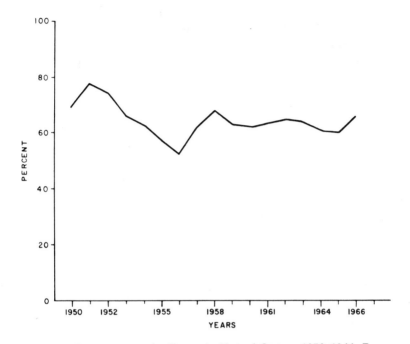

Figure 15. Tetanus case fatality ratio United States, 1950–1966. Repro-
duced from Tetanus Surveillance Report No. 1, February 1, 1968.
Bureau of Disease Prevention and Environmental Control,
National Communicable Disease Center, Atlanta,
Georgia (Figure 2, p. 3).

thousand. The relatively low incidence under the circumstances was probably due to the excellence of the surgical teams.

The very low incidence of tetanus among United States personnel during World War II can be attributed to tetanus immunization of all military personnel. During 1939–1945, including all fronts, the United States forces had half a million wounded, and only one case of tetanus (Wilson and Miles, 1964b)! The total number of cases in over twelve million persons in the United States armed forces was only twelve.

There is no question that prophylactic immunization for tetanus is one of the outstanding advances in the control of infectious diseases. Following childhood immunization it is not necessary to repeat the procedure more often than every seven to ten years. It is of no value to give the toxoid to an active case. I have always had reservations about the efficacy of prophylactic antiserum given simultaneously with tetanus toxoid in accident cases. There remains some doubt, too, about the efficacy of antitoxin administered therapeutically. Selective therapy with antibiotics is advocated both prophylactically and after the onset of tetanus. One of the interesting features of immunity is that recovery does not offer sufficient protection for the future; patients should be immunized after they have convalesced. Treatment of all tetanus patients must be supervised carefully in intensive care units because of the dangers of respiratory failure or cardiovascular collapse. L. Eckmann (1963) has written a critical summary of the prophylaxis and treatment of tetanus.

Gas Gangrene

Although the incidence of gas gangrene has been reduced considerably because of improved surgical techniques, the problem has not been eliminated. The era of modern surgery dates from the latter part of the nineteenth century with the introduction of anesthesia and the aseptic principles of Lister and Semmelweis. It is interesting to read of the difficulties encountered by the early surgeons at the Boston City Hospital (Cheever, 1906). Doctor David Cheever was one of the first surgeons on the staff. He related the constant challenge of sepsis and pyemia with mortality rates of 50 percent and higher. But by 1904 he wrote movingly (1906, p. 276), "These are happy days for the surgeon. Although misfortunes happen, they are rare. . . . It is a cause of satisfaction, if not of pride, that our Hospital is fully abreast of others in the improvements, the sanitation, the asepsis of this golden age of surgery."

Nevertheless, between 1932 and 1937 in the same hospital I witnessed the continuing toll of lives because of the septic complications of surgery. Although gas gangrene was limited, it still prevailed, and thoracic surgery was in its infancy. The "golden age of surgery" was still to come.

Gas gangrene was a serious problem during World War I. One of the finest treatises on the disease is in the medical report of the United States Army for World War I (Coupal, 1929). Of the 224,080 men in the Army wounded in France, 13,691 died of their wounds. Of the 1,329 cases of bone fractures with gas gangrene, 593 died, or 44.62

percent, a rate approaching that of Dr. Cheever's time. The opening paragraph of this monograph merits quoting (p. 407):

Gas gangrene is a spreading, moist gangrene produced by gas-forming anaerobic bacteria in extensively traumatized tissues. It is characterized by a gaseous infiltration and edema of the part affected, and by changes in the color and contractility of the muscle. The infection may remain strictly localized or it may tend to spread and involve a single muscle group or an entire limb or other part of the body; in the latter type the onset and course are generally rapid and accompanied by profound toxemia and high mortality. The condition is practically always associated with a mixed infection and the clinical picture varies according to the combined characteristic activities of the etiologic agents present. With a certain type of bacterium dominant, we may have, as one extreme, a gaseous infiltration; as another, edema without gas; and as another, rapid digestion and dissolution of tissue with neither edema nor gas. Most frequently the dominance is only partial, and edema, gaseous infiltration, and rapid tissue destruction go hand in hand with profound intoxication. The aerobic bacteria which usually are present are either ancillary, through preparing a more favorable substratum for the anerobic bacilli which constitute the determining factor in the production of gas gangrene, form a part of the process affecting the wounded tissues, or both.

The most common anaerobic Clostridia associated with gas gangrene are *Cl. welchii*, *Cl. oedematiens*, and *Cl. septicum*. Of the aerobic organisms the most important are hemolytic streptococci and staphylococci. It is essential to recognize that true gas gangrene must be differentiated from cellulitis caused by the same Clostridia, which is much less severe. Even Clostridia bacteremia without gangrene is not always a severe illness. Septic abortion due to Clostridia with necrosis of the uterus is a devastating infection because of the toxemia and shock. Modern therapy calls for hysterectomy as soon as possible.

After World War I gas gangrene occurred much less frequently, and the mortality rates decreased. This was due largely to prompt surgical intervention and the debridement of wounds. With the introduction of the sulfonamides and antibiotics, the contaminating streptococci and staphylococci were eliminated, and gas gangrene was not a serious problem in World War II or in civilian life thereafter. Intensive care units provided supportive measurements and constant nursing care. Although antisera had become available before World War II, its effectiveness was always difficult to ascertain.

CHAPTER 17

Venereal Infections

Gonorrhea[1] and syphilis[2] are strictly human infections, usually transmitted from human to human through direct contact. Although the precise nature of these two diseases was poorly understood until the nineteenth century, there is evidence that gonorrhea was recognized during the early stages of human history (Finger, 1893, translation 1894). Gonorrhea was considered to be contagious in the Biblical days of Moses. The early evidence for syphilis is not so evident, but the disease attracted attention in the fifteenth century, when epidemics occurred throughout Europe. Any serious historical delineation of these two diseases before this period is not possible. When the alarming incidence of syphilitic disease occurred, there was little concern for gonorrhea.

The origin of epidemic syphilis in Europe remains controversial. Some believe the disease was introduced into Europe by sailors of Columbus returning from the New World, who joined mercenaries roaming Europe, including those from France and Italy, rapidly disseminating the disease (Pusey, 1933a). Another popular concept is that syphilis was endemic in Africa for centuries and that the disease was introduced into Portugal and Spain as a result of the slave trade. According to this theory the disease was introduced in the same way to the Americas. Finally many support the hypothesis that the treponemes had smoldered in man for a long while as benign forms of the disease, and then suddenly mutated to a more virulent state, resulting in the eruption of severe epidemics. This explanation appeared reasonable to Zinsser, who wrote (1935, p. 74):

The infection as it occurred in Naples was to all intents and purposes a *new disease* in representing a completely altered relationship between parasite and host, with consequent profound changes of symptoms. Something must have happened at that time, apart from war and promiscuity, — both of which had been present to an equal degree many times before, — which converted a relatively benign infection into a highly virulent one. The history of the subsequent fifty years strikingly illustrates the rapidity with which adaptive changes may take place. It is probable that in all parasitisms these alterations of mutual adjustment begin with considerable velocity, the curve flattening out progressively with the increasing number of passages of the parasite through the same species of host.

Perhaps the most scholarly investigation on the origin of syphilis is that of C. J. Hackett (1963), whose hypotheses extend Zinsser's. According to Hackett there are four clinical forms of human treponematoses: pinta (*Treponema carateum*), yaws (*Treponema pertenue*), endemic syphilis, and venereal syphilis (*Treponema pallidum*). Man is the reservoir for the foregoing microbes. "The only treponeme in animals which is microscopically indistinguishable from the human *pallidum/pertenue* treponeme is *T. cuniculi*" (Hackett, 1963, p. 18), the cause of a venereal disease in rabbits.

Pinta, yaws, and endemic syphilis are nonvenereal contagious diseases that result from contact and primarily afflict children. Pinta, which localizes in the skin and causes chronic lesions, abounds in the tropical areas of Central and South America. Yaws is also a chronic disease of the skin, but produces destructive lesions in the deeper tissues, including bones. Bejel (endemic syphilis), which is found most frequently in the eastern Mediterranean areas and North Africa, but not in the Western Hemisphere, causes chronic skin lesions and later disseminates in the body, including the bones, but rarely results in the late cardiovascular and neurological lesions of venereal syphilis.

The cause of venereal syphilis is *Treponema pallidum*.[3] The disease is usually transmitted sexually, with a primary chancre appearing on the genitals about three weeks after contact and with the simultaneous appearance of enlarged regional lymph nodes. About six weeks after exposure, systemic manifestations due to dissemination of the organisms in the blood include fever, painful joints, skin rashes, mucocutaneous lesions, and generalized enlarged lymph nodes. Then a latent period of many years ensues, during which time the treponemes lurk in the tissues and intermittently in the blood and spinal fluid, with or without obvious evidence of the disease. The most serious and common late manifestations are inflammatory reactions of the heart and vessels or of the central nervous system, which can lead to death.

Because syphilis has such a long latent period between the time of the primary lesion and the appearance of the tertiary complications, it has been difficult to ascertain the incidence of the complications, especially in untreated patients. In a revealing follow-up study in Oslo, Norway, Dr. Trygve Gjestland (1955) determined that only 15 percent of untreated patients with primary and secondary syphilis had serious late complications. These patients had been followed for 15 to 40 years. It is an outstanding investigation of the natural history of syphilis.

Congenital syphilis arises *in utero* through transmission of the treponema from the mother's blood to the infant via the placenta. Disseminated syphilis in the infant often causes death *in utero*. Those who survive are weak, develop poorly, and usually succumb at an early age. An untreated mother can continue to have other "stillborn" infants due to a persistent infection. The important feature of untreated syphilis is that it can be a chronic, lifelong, active infection.

Although the origins of the treponematoses are uncertain, C. J. Hackett (1963) indicated that pinta was the first of the diseases. Pinta was perhaps disseminated as a result of human contact about 15,000 B.C. Appearing in the warm, humid climate of Afro-Asia, a mutation of the pinta treponemes occurred about 10,000 B.C., which caused the disease yaws. Referring to endemic, nonvenereal syphilis, Hackett states (1963, p. 27), "It is proposed here that mutants of the yaws treponeme were selected by arid, warm climates resulting from the retreat of the last glaciation and that by about 7000 B.C. yaws in such areas had changed into endemic syphilis, while in humid warm climates yaws has continued unchanged."

The change from endemic to venereal syphilis is probably a product of civilization, with the building of large cities and the use of more clothing. Such developments took place in the now arid countries of the eastern Mediterranean and southwestern Asia about 3000 B.C. There was a decrease in childhood contact disease and a resultant increase of nonimmune adult populations. "The social conditions, customs and habits of the congested urban populations of Europe in the fifteenth and sixteenth centuries would have assisted in spreading venereal syphilis" (Hackett, 1963, p. 30).

In summary, out of the controversy on the origins of syphilis a certain pattern has been established. There is a need for persistent investigations of the type now being carried out on anthropological excavations and findings with the aid of the discipline of paleobiology. The concept appears reasonable that the different human treponeme diseases evolved from the treponeme of pinta through mutations of the organisms brought about by climate, geography, the mobility and concentration of people, and the changing customs and conducts of society (Hackett, 1963; Hudson, 1963).

During the pandemic of syphilis in the fifteenth and sixteenth centuries concepts of the disease reflected a modern viewpoint. It was looked upon as a contagious malady of venereal origin. After a long incubation period the secondary features of the cutaneous lesions appeared, and then a tertiary stage in which the bones and soft palate were involved. Gum of guaiac and mercury were used in treatment. These concepts were expressed by Girolamo Fracastoro (1934) in a Latin poem on syphilis, "Syphilis Sive Morbus Gallicus," published in 1530. It has been called "the most famous of all medical poems" (Morton, 1970, p. 280). The poem, based on mythology, relates that Syphilus was a shepherd who decided to worship his king rather than the gods, whom he could not see. This infuriated Apollo, who visited Syphilus and bestowed painful ulcers on his body.

William Van Wyck has presented an English translation of Fracastoro's poem, "The Sinister Shepherd." The incubation period and initial stages of the disease are thus described (Fracastoro, 1934, p. 18):

> The epidemic bursting, very soon,
> Shutting her disc four times, a frightened moon
> Showed by the signs that she would manifest
> That this new evil would become a pest.
> Within the body, long its ferment rests,
> To nourish at some hidden source of breasts.

> Then suddenly, beneath a langor's weight,
> The victim creeps about in fearful state,
> The heart defective and the slightest strain
> Tiring the limbs, while energies remain
> All sapped. A gloomy eye and saddened face
> Of sickly pallor bend to this disgrace,
> And soon a vicious ulcer eats its way
> Into the privates. And a vengeful sway
> Takes cancerous possession to remain
> Extended to the groin is its fell bane.

He praises as the best of therapy an infusion of the leaf and bark of the tree that yields guaiac (p. 57):

> Vainly gold glitters there, a greater treasure
> Is this tree that pours riches without measure,
> The *lignum sanctum*, what a precious name!
> And for its gifts it has a mighty fame.

A contemporary of Fracastoro was Paracelsus, probably the greatest medical figure of the sixteenth century. He too contributed to the knowledge and confusion of syphilis and gonorrhea. He concluded that syphilis was transmitted through heredity and advocated mercury taken internally as a form of treatment. Unfortunately he called syphilis the "French gonorrhea." William Clowes (1596 and 1971), the leading Elizabethan surgeon, also advocated mercury for syphilis and wrote the first English monograph on the disease. He emphasized the prevalence of syphilis, stating that fifteen out of every twenty patients entering St. Bartholomew's Hospital were syphilitic.

The confusion over the nature of gonorrhea and syphilis was accentuated by the experiment of the greatest surgeon of the eighteenth century, John Hunter (1835). He described experiments on himself in which he attempted to differentiate between gonorrhea and syphilis. He related the symptoms and performed a courageous but foolish procedure, coming to an erroneous conclusion that was to influence medical thought for several decades. He wrote that in May 1769, "two punctures were made on the penis with a lancet dipped in venereal matter from a gonorrhoea; one puncture was on the glans, the other on the prepuce" (p. 417). These observations on himself ended in the conclusion, "It proves, first, that matter from a gonorrhoea will produce chancres" (p. 419). He was absolutely wrong. What he had done was to take purulent material from a patient having gonorrhea and syphilis and unknowingly infected himself with both diseases. Possibly he proved for his own benefit that mercurial inunctions were beneficial (for syphilis), but it took him three years to achieve a cure.

Venereal diseases appeared to command the attention of surgeons. Following Hunter an Edinburgh surgeon, Benjamin Bell (1795), published a two-volume work on "Gonorrhoea Virulenta" and "Lues Venerea." Considering the state of knowledge on the subject at the time it was a masterful clinical delineation of the two diseases. He emphasized the complications of gonorrhea, such as urethral stricture in the male. Unfortunately he confused the nomenclature by referring to "gonorrhoea virulente" as *the* specific contagious disease resulting from sexual contact, but he also described "gonorrhoea simplex" as a benign disease resulting from many causes. He also introduced the term "gleet" as a form of thin mucous discharge from the urethra that persists for a long period after the acute stage of "gonorrhoea virulente." Bell's recognition of syphilis and its complications as a distinct clinical entity resulted from his wide experience with the disease. He clearly recognized congenital syphilis and emphasized the value of mercury in the treatment of syphilis.

The confusion between gonorrhoea and syphilis continued into the nineteenth century, although the Parisian surgeon Phillippe Ricord (1838, translation 1848) did clarify the clinical features of syphilis after extensive observations. He designated the three stages of syphilis primary, secondary, and tertiary. He described the primary chancre ("Ricord's chancre") and showed that the viable, contagious material that resided in the ulcerating chancre could induce a similar one when injected into the skin of the thigh. Ricord carried out over six hundred inoculations in humans in corroborating the findings of Hunter, whom he highly respected. But he did not consider gonorrhea a contagious disease, because he could not reproduce an ulceration in the skin after inoculating the area with purulent material. This method of inoculation constituted a means of differentiating the two diseases, according to Ricord. Knowledge of syphilis was considerably enhanced by the pathological studies of Rudolph Virchow (1858) when he demonstrated that the disease was widely disseminated throughout the body to many different tissues and organs.

Like syphilis, gonorrhea is acquired through human contact but with a much shorter incubation period, usually three to seven days. In the male there is little systemic reaction, the infection remaining localized to the anterior urethra and associated with purulent discharge. Manifestations in the female are less pronounced, and any local discomfort or discharge of the genitalia is often attributed to other factors or irritants.[4]

The complications of untreated gonorrhea can be serious and debilitating (Spink, 1939b). Gonococcal arthritis is a suppurative and destructive joint disease, with ankylosis occurring in the larger joints. In the male there is also the late complication of urethral stricture, and in the female, of pelvic inflammatory disease, which often leads to sterility. Asymptomatic chronic carriers of the gonococcus in the genitalia of females and at times in males makes complete control of the disease difficult.

Congenital gonorrhea does not afflict the infant, but a very serious complication is gonorrheal ophthalmic neonatorum. Unrecognized and untreated infections often result in blindness. Infection of the conjunctivae with *Neisseria gonorrhoeae* is acquired during birth through contact with gonococcal exudate in the mother's pelvic outlet, a condition that usually occurs in infants when prophylactic drops of silver nitrate have not been instilled into the conjunctival sacs at birth. Fortunately the problem is not common in contemporary medicine, but it has not been completely prevented (Thatcher and Pettit, 1971).

The distinction between gonorrhea and syphilis was made etiologically when Albert Neisser (1879) discovered the gonococcus (*Neisseria gonococcus*) in the purulent urethral discharge. The etiological spirochete of syphilis was identified by Fritz Schaudinn and Erich Hoffmann (1905). Syphilis was transmitted experimentally from human material to apes (Klebs, 1879; Metchnikoff and Roux, 1903–1904), to the rabbit's eye (Haensell, 1881), and to rabbits' testicles (Parodi, 1907). Gonorrhea had been transmitted experimentally from human to human in isolated instances (Hill, 1943); more definitive evidence of human transmission was offered by J. F. Mahoney et al. (1946). Gonococcal urethritis was established in the chimpanzee from the exudate of a human male patient (Lucas et al., 1971). The diagnosis of human syphilis was further clarified by serological tests (Wassermann, Neisser, and Bruck, 1906), particularly in the later stages of the disease, when the spirochete could not be demonstrated.

Venereal infections illustrate the slow process of acquiring knowledge about the basic nature and precise causes of diseases, a story repeated time and time again. The growth of knowledge depended on new ideas, a scientific approach, and refined technological skills and procedures. After the two principal venereal diseases could be delineated etiologically, more accurate epidemiological investigations were possible, a more intelligent approach to prophylactic measures could be made, and more scientific means were available for evaluating therapy. In the first part of the twentieth century millions of persons throughout the world were to suffer from these diseases before adequate therapeutic regimes were discovered.

The control of many epidemic diseases is dependent on precise epidemiological data, which include geographical location of the foci of active disease, information on the mode of spread, temporary segregation and treatment of individual cases, and prophylactic procedures, including intensive public health education. The highly successful campaign against tuberculosis operated along these lines. In the case of venereal diseases, many factors militated against the accumulation of such information, even though scientific medical knowledge had advanced considerably so that through intense effort the diseases could be controlled. A person with venereal disease was considered to be highly immoral, since the infection was most commonly acquired through sexual intercourse and often involved promiscuity and prostitution. Attending physicians in a civilian population were, and still are, reluctant to report acute cases. In the armed forces of the United States until World War II officers and noncommissioned personnel were discredited if they reported to sick call with a venereal infection. In addition precise diagnostic criteria were not always available, nor were efforts always made to seek out laboratory aids. Serological tests for syphilis remained in a chaotic state of standardization for several years.

Effective treatment became available for gonorrhea in 1937 and for syphilis in 1943. Nevertheless the incidence of these diseases contitued to rise to epidemic proportions. One important factor was a succession of major wars during this period. Herding healthy young males into the armed services and then sending them to foreign shores where the only relaxation with the opposite sex was with prostitutes resulted in an alarming dissemination of venereal diseases. In the civilian population the fear of pregnancy had been a major deterrent against sexual promiscuity, but with the advent of highly publicized birth control measures and available abortions this fear was greatly reduced. Restraint was further diminished by the availability of effective and relatively inexpensive therapeutic agents.

Society has been universally dislocated by a succession of wars during the twentieth century: World War I, 1914–1918; World War II, 1939–1945; the Korean War, 1950–1953; and the war in Vietnam, 1965–1973. Fairly reliable statistical data are available on the incidence of venereal infections among military personnel. This information parallels the occurrence of disease in the civilian population. During World War I the United States Armed Forces had a mean strength of 4 million. The total number of admissions for sickness was 3.5 million, of which 357,969, or 10.2 percent, were for venereal disease (Michie 1928c). It has been estimated that the ratio of gonorrhea to syphilis usually is around ten to one (Anderson, Arnstein, and Lester, 1962). Since no specific therapy was available except arsenicals and bismuth for syphilis, a large amount of disability resulted.

In World War II military personnel and support were dispersed around the globe with a mean strength of 16 million, and the incidence of venereal disease varied in different areas. The rate of venereal infections in the Army, which include only gonorrhea and syphilis, was 49.20 per thousand in the continental United States, and the overall army rate was 51.96 (Gordon, 1958). The highest rate of 104.51 occurred in the Mediterranean Theater, including North Africa.

Perhaps the most alarming and revealing statistics pertained to the Korean War (McNinch, 1955). Figure 16 shows the Army incidence in 1951–1953. The rather steep rise over a brief period was due to the fact that prostitutes learned quickly where the newly arrived troops were based. This is certainly applicable to the rates in two groups of personnel as seen in Figure 17. After the hostilities ended a large occupational force was stationed in South Korea and the incidence of gonorrhea occasioned great concern. In 1961, as a consultant for the United States Air Force, I visited bases in the Far East, including those in Japan, Korea, Okinawa, and the Philippines. Authorities

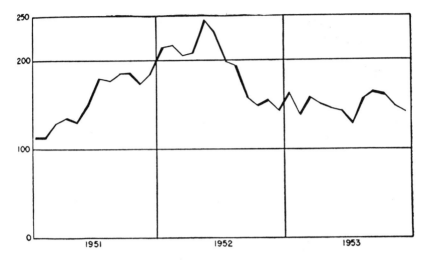

Figure 16. Venereal disease, United States Army forces, Far East 1951–1953. Reproduced with permission of the author from Colonel Joseph H. McNinch, "Venereal Disease Problems, U.S. Army Forces, Far East 1950–1953," in *Recent Advances in Medicine and Surgery Based on Professional Medical Experiences in Japan and Korea 1950–53*, Medical Science Publication No. 4, published by the United States Army Service Graduate School, Walter Reed Army Medical Center, Washington, D.C., 1955, Vol. II, pp. 144–158 (Figure 1, p. 147).

were alarmed by the vast number of cases of gonorrhea and by the threat of penicillin-resistant strains of gonococci, which would not only incapacitate the men, but could be carried back home and become disseminated in the United States. Although a slight increase in the resistance of the gonococcus to the killing effect of penicillin could be demonstrated *in vitro*, these findings did not preclude the effective use of the antibiotic when the doses of the drug were increased.

The epidemiological status of venereal diseases in the United States between 1919 and 1973 is shown in Figure 18. Around 1940 there was a sharp rise in the incidence of syphilis. This was due to an intensive campaign instituted by the United States Public Health Service to bring syphilis out into the open and to wage a cooperative attack against the disease. Following this rise there has been a steady decline. On the other hand there has been a constant rise in the incidence of gonorrhea, approaching epidemic proportions, mostly in

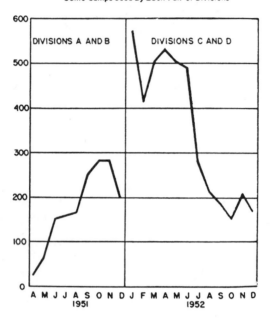

Divisions A and B Arrived From The United States
Divisions C and D Returned From Korea
Same Camps Used By Each Pair of Divisions

Figure 17. Incidence of venereal disease in four
United States Army divisions after arrival in
Japan. Reproduced with permission of the
author from Colonel Joseph H. McNinch,
"Venereal Disease Problems, U.S. Army
Forces, Far East 1950–1953," in *Recent Advances
in Medicine and Surgery Based on Professional
Medical Experiences in Japan and Korea 1950–53*,
Medical Science Publication No. 4 published
by the United States Army Service Gradu-
ate School, Walter Reed Army Medi-
cal Center, Washington, D.C.,
Vol. II, pp. 144–158 (Fig-
ure 2, p. 148).

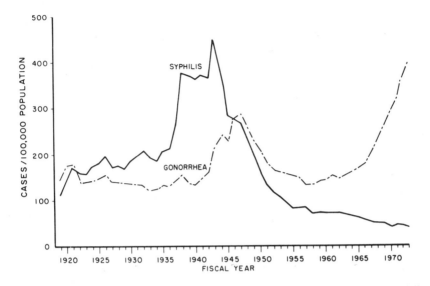

Figure 18. Venereal disease. Reported cases of gonorrhea and syphilis (all stages) per 100,000 population by year, United States, fiscal years 1919–1973. Reproduced from Weekly Report for Year Ending December 29, 1973, Reported Morbidity and Mortality in the U.S., Volume 22, No. 53, July 15, 1974. Center for Disease Control, Atlanta, Georgia (p. 59). Beginning in 1939 all states are included in the reporting area (military cases are included for 1919–1940 and are excluded thereafter).

young people. In the past the number of reported new cases of gonorrhea and syphilis had a ratio of ten to one respectively. In 1964 this ratio was considerably distorted when there were 300,667 cases of gonorrhea and 114,314 of syphilis. But the 10:1 ratio was restored in 1973 when there were 842,621 cases of gonorrhea and 87,469 of syphilis. However alarming the reported incidence of gonorrhea may be, one can be reasonably certain that the actual number of cases was much higher.

Treatment of syphilis has remained a challenge for medical science ever since the days of Paracelsus, when mercury was used. Bismuth and then the arsenicals were added in the twentieth century. The arsenicals were effective in the early stages of syphilis, but there is little evidence that the spirochoetes were totally eliminated from the tissues following such treatment. The use of the arsenicals in the later tertiary stages was also difficult to evaluate. The iodides were successful in the treatment of the syphilitic gumma, which is a localized, expanding lesion in certain organs, such as the liver.

The history of therapy for chronic syphilis has been one of hopes and frustrations. The resulting slow but progressive deterioration of human health has challenged physicians. One of the most fascinating discoveries was that of the influence of induced fever on the course of the manifestations in the central nervous system. Julius Wagner-Jauregg (1921), a Viennese psychiatrist in the latter part of the nineteenth century, had a patient with severe dementia, who recovered from her illness following an attack of typhoid fever. This observation led him to propose fever therapy for syphilis. He suggested the induction of malaria in patients with syphilitic tabes and paresis. Encouraged by the results, others joined in similar investigations. Further clinical studies included the evaluation of fever induced radiothermically (Hinsie and Carpenter, 1931). This precluded the necessity of provoking fever with another infection or by material that produced a febrile response, such as that following the injection of vaccines. Investigations in rabbits with experimental testicular syphilis and the satisfactory response to fever therapy supported this approach, as did work on the thermal death point of spirochoetes (Boak, Carpenter, and Warren, 1932; Carpenter, Boak, and Warren, 1932). Subsequently, induced fever was combined with arsenical therapy, but these procedures were very difficult to evaluate.

Additional investigations were made with fever therapy in gonococcal infections utilizing the improved and unique Kettering hypertherm cabinet (Carpenter, Boak, and Warren, 1938). The thermal death point of the gonococcus was found to be at 106° F., a temperature that could be attained and sustained in a patient for several hours without harm, despite obvious discomfort (Warren, Scott, and Carpenter, 1937).

As a member of a research committee at the University of Minnesota Hospitals on the evaluation of fever therapy induced by malaria, and of the hyperthermic cabinet for gonorrhea and syphilis, I was not impressed with the results. Further long-range studies were interrupted because of the successful therapeutic results with the sulfonamides and penicillin (Dees and Colston, 1937; Mahoney, Arnold, and Harris, 1943).

One of the most dramatic therapeutic triumphs was the advent of the sulfonamides, and then of penicillin, for the treatment of gonorrhea and syphilis. Although gonorrhea continued in epidemic proportions, the severe, disabling, and even lethal complications were largely prevented. Early in 1936 we received a supply of sulfanilamide for research purposes at the Boston City Hospital and elected to evaluate treatment of patients with gonococcal suppurative arthritis, a painful, disabling, and chronic illness for which there was no specific therapy. The first case, a male with a purulent penile discharge and suppuration of a knee joint, received sulfanilamide orally. The results were almost beyond belief. Within twenty-four hours of initiating treatment the urethral discharge was free of gonococci, microscopically and culturally, and by the third day gonococci were absent from the knee effusion. The patient left the hospital in the second week without any disability of the joint. The details were presented at the annual meeting of the American Medical Association in June 1937 (Keefer and Spink, 1937). In previous experience such patients had remained for weeks in the hospital and then had permanent disability due to ankylosis of the joint. Our observations were to be repeated on many occasions.

Neonatal gonococcal conjunctivitis has been controlled but not eliminated. In the female the incidence of pelvic inflammatory disease has been reduced, but not eradicated by any means.

Although sulfonamide therapy for gonorrhea proved highly successful, within a few years strains of gonococci had become resistant to the killing action of all the sulfonamide preparations and the resistant organisms were widely disseminated in the population. Fortunately penicillin became available and proved to be highly effective.[5]

Penicillin became equally effective in the treatment of syphilis. Within a few days of the beginning of therapy, spirochoetes can no longer be seen in the exudate of the primary chancre. More important, the late and serious manifestations of syphilis that occur after several years are being encountered with less and less frequency. Penicillin and the requirement of premarital serological tests for syphilis have made congenital syphilis a rare affliction. There still remains the question of how effective penicillin is in the treatment of the well-established late cardiovascular and central nervous system complications. In these instances penicillin must be administered for a much longer period and in larger doses than in the primary stage of the disease.

An informative follow-up study on penicillin therapy for syphilis has described the results in 225 patients with endemic syphilis in Bosnia, Yugoslavia (Nadaždin and Karlovac, 1977). This endemic form was introduced into the country as an epidemic, nonvenereal family disease that became intensified during World War II. Under the auspices of WHO and UNICEF, Yugoslavia health teams systematically treated patients between 1948 and 1953 with 4 to 8.6 megaunits of penicillin, and the disease was eradicated. No clinical evidence of syphilis was present in 225 studied serologically 20 years after treatment. Up to 195 individuals or 86.7 percent had seropositive reactions, however. It was not clear to the investigators whether the persistence of specific antibodies was due to the presence of living organisms or "residual treponemal material which has not been entirely metabolised." Because of these residual titers in patients treated with penicillin they suggested the possibility that venereal syphilis differs from endemic syphilis.

At the present time the control of gonorrhea and syphilis is within the power of medical science. The causes of both diseases have been established, and tests are readily available for early diagnosis. The reservoir of the disease resides strictly in human beings, and the modes of transmission are clearly known. Why, then, does syphilis remain so prevalent, and why do we have gonorrhea as a leading epidemic disease?

Several years ago a wise clinician told me that whenever a highly effective therapeutic agent becomes generally available for a serious major disease, a period of carelessness ensues in the control of that disease. He illustrated his point with diabetes and insulin. Research on diabetes abated for a decade after this discovery. Patients and physicians depended on the single therapeutic expediency of insulin. We now know that diabetes remains a common and complex metabolic problem, and major research in the field is again being conducted. In the case of gonorrhea and syphilis, a philosophy of living without restraint has helped to maintain the high attack rate. Since pregnancy can be avoided with rather simple procedures and drugs, and since there is highly successful treatment for venereal infections available to all, is there any reason why one of man's basic instincts should not be obeyed? Prevention of venereal diseases is more than a medical or public health problem; it involves society at large, and intensive educational efforts with children and adolescents are essential.

Other less common venereal infections in which inflammatory lesions are quite localized to the genito-anal regions include *chancroid*, *granuloma inguinale*, and *lymphogranuloma venereum*. These diseases are more common in some of the developing countries. In the United States in 1973 the combined reported cases of these three diseases was a total of 1,635. Effective therapy includes sulfonamides and antibiotics.

There is growing recognition that venereal diseases can be caused by other recognized infections such as cytomegalic virus (CMV), herpes simplex virus, Chlamydia, and Mycoplasma. Chlamydia is one of a group of intracellular agents that causes not only lymphogranuloma venereum but also psittacosis, trachoma, and inclusion conjunctivitis.

CHAPTER 18

Rickettsioses

The human rickettsial diseases are characterized by fever, rash, and disturbances of the central nervous system. The causative microbes occupy a place between bacteria and viruses and can be visualized by a light microscope. They can be described as small, intracellular, gram-negative, bacterium-like organisms. The reservoirs are principally small rodents, but man and other vertebrates are involved as well. These diseases are also transmitted by arthropods, an important factor in successful prevention.

The generic term Rickettsia was introduced in 1916 by H. da Rocha-Lima in honor of Dr. Howard Taylor Ricketts of the University of Chicago, who in 1906 first transmitted the rickettsial disease Rocky Mountain spotted fever to guinea pigs and monkeys. During World War II and thereafter major advances were made in the control and treatment of these diseases. In that period I observed classic, louseborne epidemic typhus in Central America, tsutsugamushi or scrub typhus in the Pacific area, fièvre boutonneuse in Africa, and Rocky Mountain spotted fever in the United States. The contemporary clinical details of these diseases are reviewed in modern textbooks of medicine (Woodward, 1974). To aid in understanding the rickettsioses, Table 5 has been constructed after Burrows (1968).

Table 5. Rickettsial Diseases of Man

Group	Disease	Etiology	Reservoir	Vector
Typhus	Epidemic typhus	*Rickettsia prowazeki*	Man	Human lice
	Brill's disease			
	Murine typhus	*Rickettsia mooseri*	Wild rats	Fleas
			Field mice	Rat lice
Spotted fever	Rocky Mountain spotted fever	*Rickettsia rickettsii*	Probably rabbits, small rodents, dogs	Ticks (wood, dog, etc.)
	Boutonneuse fever	*Rickettsia conorii*	Dogs	Ticks (several species)
	Indian tick typhus		Rodents?	
	Kenya typhus			
	South African tick bite fever			
	North Asian tick-borne rickettsiosis	*Rickettsia sibirica*	Wild rodents	Ticks (several species)
	North Queensland tick typhus	*Rickettsia australis*	Rats?	Tick?
			Marsupials?	
Tsutsugamushi	Rickettsialpox	*Rickettsia akari*	House mice	Mites
	Tsutsugamushi	*Rickettsia tsutsugamushi*	Rodents	Mites
	Japanese river fever		Birds?	
	Kedani disease			
	Scrub typhus			
	Rural typhus			
	Q fever	*Coxiella burnetii*	Bandicoots	Ticks (several species)
			Birds?	
			Sheep, cattle, goats	
	Trench fever	*Rickettsia quintana*	?	Human lice

Source: Adapted with permission of publisher and author from table of "Rickettsial Diseases of Man," Burrows, 1968, pp. 832–833.

Epidemic Typhus

Epidemic typhus is a major pandemic disease, subject to maritime quarantine, as were plague, leprosy, smallpox, yellow fever, and cholera. Epidemic or classic typhus is transmitted from human to human by the human louse *Pediculus humanis*. Zinsser, in his incomparable *Rats, Lice and History* wrote (1935, p. 237), "Typhus fever was born when the first infected rat flea fed upon man. This accident probably took place — most likely somewhere in the East — centuries before the disease reached the crowded centres and armies of mediaeval Europe." He also stated that the human louse had learned to live with man in a state of parasitic existence long before typhus. "The human louse was possibly the last of the series of hosts to acquire the virus. . . . The infected louse always dies" (p. 238). He believed that the murine virus was the original typhus.

Epidemic typhus was first recognized as a malady of serious proportions in the fifteenth century. Very likely sporadic cases appeared before that period, but not enough to attract the attention of physicians or historians. Perhaps the disease was not differentiated from other febrile conditions. With the expansion of trade and the movement of large numbers of soldiers, typhus became a major epidemic disease.

Typhus was probably transmitted by soldiers from Cyprus to Spain; epidemics raged amongst the troops at Granada in 1489–1490. From there the disease was carried across Europe in the following century by wandering soldiers causing epidemics in Italy. Spaniards possibly carried the disease to Mexico at the same time, where it became known as *tabardillo*.[1]

Fracastoro, in his travels about Europe, probably recognized the disease in Italy in the sixteenth century (Fracastoro, 1930). He succinctly described typhus in 1546 under the title "De Febre Quam Lenticulas vel Puncticulas, Vocant" (the fever called lenticulae or puncticulae). Concerning the characteristic rash he stated (p. 103), "About the fourth or seventh day, red, or often purplish-red spots broke out on the arms, back and chest, looking like flea-bites (punctiform), though they were often larger and in the shape of lentils, whence arose the name of the fever." Fracastoro believed that the disease had existed since antiquity in Cyprus and the neighboring islands.

Tobias Cober first recognized the role of fleas in the genesis of epidemics in 1606 while he was with the Hungarian troops in the wars with Turkey (Garrison, 1922b; see p. 130). The disastrous inroads in the armies of World War I by typhus dramatized the persistent foci of the disease in Southeastern Europe since the time of Cober.

In the sixteenth and seventeenth centuries typhus became known as "gaol-fever" because it was commonly associated with those confined within jails, where filth and lousiness abounded. Creighton records the contents of an old manuscript as follows (1891a, p. 375):

In the 13th year of Henry VIII [1552] at the Assize[2] held in the Castle of Cambridge in Lent, "the justices and all the gentlemen, bailiffs and other, resorting thither, took such an infection, whether it were of the savour of the prisoners, or of the filth of the house, that many gentlemen, as Sir John Cut, Sir Giles Arlington, Knights, and many other honest yeomen, thereof died, and almost all which were present were sore sick, and narrowly escaped with their lives."

Similar "Black Assizes" occurred at Oxford in 1577 at Exeter in 1586. It is apparent that the infected fleas of the prisoners found susceptible typhus victims amongst those who had come to judge them in court. Not until the eighteenth century did improved jail conditions result in a reduction of typhus victims. This change was largely due to the Quaker humanitarian John Howard (1792), whose recommendations on cleanliness in prisons and hospitals are also discussed in relation to the origins of the British public health movement (see Section I, · Chapter 3).

The contributions of Sir John Pringle, surgeon-general of the British Army during the eighteenth century, have been cited elsewhere (see Section I, Chapter 1). He recognized typhus as a disease associated with filth and poor hygiene, and his principles of cleanliness in living quarters on land and sea did much to control typhus in the armed forces. In the same period James Lind of the Royal British Navy campaigned for hygienic conditions on ships and in hospitals.

During the nineteenth century in the migration of large numbers of people across Europe, and during a succession of wars and famine, typhus took a large toll of lives. Poor crops and famine in Ireland from 1816 to 1819 resulted in seven hundred thousand cases among six million inhabitants (Zinsser, 1935). In 1847 the young doctor Rudolph Virchow, then twenty-six, was sent by the German government into

Upper Silesia in Prussia to survey the conditions during a severe epidemic of typhus. He was appalled by the suffering, misery, and poverty of the people. In 1868 he delivered a lecture on behalf of the victims in which he described the history of typhus and "the neglect of public cleanliness in towns and villages, as also in private dwelling-houses" (Virchow, 1868, p. 42). He also became involved in the problem of cholera epidemics. As a result he acquired considerable influence as a statesman and worked for social and prison reform through education and legislation. Public health problems engaged much of his attention.

Epidemics of typhus also occurred in the United States during the nineteenth century. It was during such an epidemic in the summer of 1836 in Philadelphia that W. W. Gerhard (1836–1837) correctly distinguished typhus from typhoid fever. Further epidemics along the eastern seaboard appeared in 1846 and 1847, the disease probably being introduced by Irish immigrants.

During the early years of the twentieth century isolated foci of epidemic typhus continued in Eastern Europe. Little had been contributed to the scientific understanding of the disease before World War I except for the fundamental discoveries of Charles Nicolle (Nicolle, Comte, and Conseil, 1909). Working in Algiers, Nicolle succeeded in transmitting typhus to chimpanzees by means of infected human blood and proved the transmission of human typhus by the body louse *Pediculus corporis*, a discovery for which he received the Nobel Prize.

Since typhus had been endemic in the Balkan countries of southeastern Europe, epidemics occurred among the civilian population and troops during World War I. An American Red Cross Commission composed of personnel from Harvard University under the direction of Dr. Richard Strong (Strong et al., 1920) provided a vivid description of the horrors of the epidemic in Serbia in 1915. Up to twenty-five hundred new cases entered the military hospitals within one day; it is estimated that there were three times that number among civilians. The mortality rate was 30 to 60 percent, with more than a hundred fifty thousand deaths.

A second Harvard group comprised the Typhus Research Commission of the League of Red Cross Societies to Poland. Their main concern was the investigation of the etiology and pathology of typhus in a Warsaw hospital in 1920. Studying selected severe cases, they issued a superb report (Wolbach, Todd, and Palfrey, 1922), extending the earlier observations of Ricketts and Wilder (1910), of Prowazek (1915), and of Rocha-Lima (1916), and showing that *Rickettsia prowazeki* was the cause of typhus. They dissected lice and in histological studies displayed the role of the body louse as a vector of the disease. Finally they delineated the vascular lesions of human typhus.

Russia suffered considerably from typhus and other diseases between 1917 and 1921. There were probably more than 25 million cases in the territories controlled by the Soviet Republic with from two and one-half to three million deaths (Zinsser, 1935)! Typhus raged on the eastern front of Europe during World War I. On the other hand, there was an almost unbelievable rarity of the disease on the western front, a fact to which military authorities have devoted only a few lines. The official report of the United States Army medical department on typhus stated (Tasker, 1928, p. 483), "Its incidence in the Army during the World War was as follows: United States, 15; Europe, 7; other countries, 19; officers, 1; total 42." This is in contrast to the threat that appeared in World War II, as will be discussed shortly.

In concluding his book on typhus Zinsser wrote (1935, p. 301): "Typhus is not dead. It will live on for centuries, and it will continue to break into the open whenever human stupidity and brutality give it a chance, as most likely they occasionally will. But its freedom of action is being restricted, and more and more it will be confined, like other savage creatures, in the zoölogical gardens of controlled diseases." Zinsser had an unusual insight into biological phenomena, and it is unfortunate that he did not live to see typhus controlled during World War II. The medical department of the United States Army was alerted for the worst and the preparations achieved a brilliant success in the restriction of typhus, particularly in the Mediterranean Theater of Operations (Bayne-Jones, 1948).

The United States Typhus Commission, a joint undertaking of the Army, Navy, and United States Public Health Service, was formed in 1942. Information collected by this group revealed an alarming increase of typhus in North Africa and in Iran, which were the locations of many American and British military personnel. In 1942 twenty-eight thousand Polish refugees had arrived in Iran from Russia, and in 1943–1944 there were twenty-five thousand cases of typhus with mortality rates of 12 to 37 percent. The Persian Gulf Command of American forces in Iran was a sizeable undertaking, and the situation was potentially serious. In Egypt from 1940 to 1944 there were ninety-six thousand cases with a mortality rate of 15 percent. In Morocco in the first ten months of 1942 there were twenty thousand cases among civilians, and thirty thousand in Algiers. Among hundreds of thousands of American troops in North Africa and Iran, however, there were only nine cases of typhus and no deaths, because of the use of the highly effective Cox-Craigie typhus vaccine (Cox and Bell, 1940; Craigie, 1945) and the availability of DDT as an insecticide.

The acme in the successful control of typhus occurred in Naples in 1943–1944 among a population of five hundred thousand living along with lice in the bombed-out ruins. The first case of typhus in Italy was recognized in Bari in March 1943, and the first case in Naples in July 1943. By January 1944 there were 723 cases in Naples. After this the numbers declined rapidly, and by April 1944 the epidemic had terminated. For the first time in history an epidemic of typhus had been abruptly terminated with control methods, especially with DDT and vaccination (Bayne-Jones, 1948). Similarly epidemic typhus became a serious menace amidst the ruins in Germany (Gordon, 1948), and also in Japan and in Korea (Scoville, Jr., 1948); but again control measures avoided catastrophes. An important symposium on the status of the rickettsial diseases in man was published after World War II (Moulton, 1948).

Recurrent Epidemic Typhus — Brill-Zinsser Disease

Doctor Nathan Brill, an attending physician at Mount Sinai Hospital in New York City in 1896, worked on an active service with typhoid fever patients. He began to see individuals who had an illness closely resembling typhoid, but the diagnosis could not be supported by definitive laboratory data. The disease also simulated typhus, but it was milder. Brill reported his clinical findings on 221 cases under the heading of "An Acute Infectious Disease of Unknown Origin." His discussion concluded (1910, p. 501):

Clinically this disease resembles typhus fever more than it does any other disease, and I should have felt that I had offered nothing to our nosology if it had been proved that typhus fever had lost its virulence, that it was constantly present in a community, that it was not communicable, that when it was present epidemics of it did not occur, and that it was no longer a grave and fatal disease. But with typhus fever, as the great masters of medicine have taught, and as I have seen it, such a conception would be unjustifiable; therefore, I believe this disease not to be typhus fever.

Similar groups of cases were reported from Boston and New York. In 1912 it was demonstrated through experimental studies in monkeys that Brill's disease was related to the Mexican type of typhus (Anderson and Goldberger, 1912). Doctor Kenneth Maxcy (1926) of the United States Public Health Service had reported on 114 cases of mild endemic typhus in the southeastern part of the United States, which he reluctantly called "Brill's disease." In reality he had described murine typhus. Zinsser (1934) had isolated from patients with Brill's disease the strain of rickettsia that caused classic epidemic typhus, and it was different from the murine strain of Mexico. He concluded that Brill's disease was a recrudescence of classic typhus in persons who had originally contracted the disease in endemic areas in southeastern Europe and Russia. This thesis was fully confirmed, with the additional notation that Brill's disease could be transmitted from human to human under circumstances where the human louse was prevalent (Murray et al., 1950; Murray and Snyder, 1951).

Typhus is a disease of intracellular parasitism. Under such conditions latent disease can continue in a host for a long period without apparent ill effects for either the parasite or the host. This is also seen in other intracellular parasitic diseases such as tuberculosis and varicella-herpes zoster infections. In typhus there is not a solid immunity against the invading parasite following an acute infection, but sufficient protection is present so that relapses are mild.

Murine Typhus

Mexican typhus, or *tabardillo*, simulates epidemic typhus, and also Rocky Mountain spotted fever except for the distribution of the rash. During the first decade of the twentieth century there were several unanswered problems that related to the rickettsioses. Was tabardillo in reality the disease of classic European epidemic typhus, and was the mode of transmission the same? And was Rocky Mountain spotted fever either epidemic typhus or tabardillo? Answers to these questions came quickly. H. T. Ricketts and R. M. Wilder (1910) proved that tabardillo and spotted fever were two different diseases, and members of the United States Public Health Service established that tabardillo was transmitted by fleas from infected rats, distinctly unlike the transmission of epidemic typhus from human to human through the human body louse (Dyer, Rumreich, and Badger, 1931). S. B. Wolbach and his associates (Wolbach, Todd and Palfrey, 1922) had demonstrated that *Rickettsia prowazeki* caused only a mild inflammatory reaction of the tunica vaginalis of the testicles of the guinea pig, whereas H. Mooser (1928) showed that an intense inflammatory reaction was caused by the murine strain, now known as *Rickettsia mooseri*. These pathological reactions are specific and consistent differential factors.

Murine typhus has continued to prevail in the Southeastern and Gulf areas of the United States. It is a relatively mild disease associated with rats and their fleas, and the incidence is not remarkable, fewer than a hundred cases having been reported since 1964.

Rocky Mountain Spotted Fever

During the latter part of the nineteenth century sporadic cases of a febrile disease with a rash were noted in parts of Montana, Idaho, and Utah. It varied from a mild infection to one with a highly fatal outcome, such as the one that occurred in the Bitter Root Valley of Montana, which had mortality rates of 80 to 90 percent. In an address before the Oregon State Medical Society in June 1899, Dr. Edward Maxey, a general practitioner from Boise, Idaho, first described the disease as follows (1899, p. 433): "an acute endemic, non-contagious, but probably infectious, febrile disease, characterized clinically by a continuous moderately high fever, severe arthritic and muscular pains, and a profuse petechial or puerperal eruption in the skin, appearing first on the ankles, wrists, and forehead, but rapidly spreading to all parts of the body." Mild cases simulate typhoid fever, whereas the more severely ill patients have a rash that mimics typhus. There is one important distinction between the rash of spotted fever and that of typhus. In the former the rash appears first on the hands, arms, feet, and legs, whereas in typhus the eruption begins on the body and spreads peripherally.

When Dr. Howard Ricketts went to Montana in April 1906 to restore his health, he made two basic observations on spotted fever (1911). First, he demonstrated that the disease was transmitted to man by the wood tick *Dermacentor andersoni*. Unlike the louse, which transmits typhus and is itself killed by the disease, the wood tick harbors the parasite of spotted fever for many months, and the female transmits the microbes to her progeny. Rodents probably play a part in maintaining the parasite in nature. Second, in transmitting the infection to male guinea pigs with the blood of patients, Ricketts noted the marked inflammatory reaction of the testicle, a distinguishing diagnostic test for spotted fever. He died from typhus at forty years of age while working in Mexico City.

S. B. Wolbach (1919) presented the early history and defined the vector and histopathology of Rocky Mountain spotted fever. Members of the United States Public Health Service carried out extensive studies on ticks and the transmission of the disease to man, demonstrating the organisms in tick smears, and also prepared the first effective prophylactic vaccine for man (Parker, 1938; Parker and Spencer, 1926).

Subsequently it was shown that Rocky Mountain spotted fever was widely disseminated, but occurred rarely in Minnesota (Spink, 1941a). The disease was identified in the Eastern part of the United States (Badger, Dyer, and Rumreich, 1931). In the latter area the dog tick, *Dermacentor variabilis*, was implicated in the transmission of the disease.

From an epidemiological point of view it is of considerable importance that in the decade 1963–1973 there was an increased incidence of Rocky Mountain spotted fever. The vast majority of the cases occurred in the South Central states and along the eastern border, especially in the South Atlantic states. Few cases were encountered in the western states. Most of the cases in the East occurred in children.

Control of Rocky Mountain spotted fever has been accomplished through preventive measures, such as the wearing of appropriate clothing in tick-infested areas, the use of repellants, and a careful daily search for ticks that may have become attached to the body.

Specific vaccine is available for those whose occupations are particularly hazardous, such as stockmen, shepherds, and foresters. Antibiotic therapy is effective with tetracycline or chloramphenicol.

Other members of the spotted fever group as shown in Table 5 are boutonneuse fever, Indian tick fever, Kenya typhus, South African tick bite fever, and North Asian tick-borne rickettsiosis. All have similar clinical manifestations, are transmitted by ticks, and have biologically related etiological parasites. The measures for controlling and treating the diseases are similar to those for Rocky Mountain spotted fever.

Rickettsialpox

The causative rickettsia is *Rickettsia akari*.[3] The natural reservoir is in mites carried by house mice (Huebner, Jellison, and Pomerantz, 1946). It is a mild, self-limiting, febrile illness of about one week's duration, characterized by a lesion from the mite bite and a rash. The disease is prevented by the extermination of house mice and elimination of mites.

Rickettsialpox was discovered in 1946. A review of rickettsialpox has been presented by M. Greenberg (1948). An excellent description of the discovery of the role of mites and mice in the spread of the disease has been written by the science writer Berton Roueché (1954). Entitled "The Alerting of Mr. Pomerantz," it reads like a detective story. Doctor Benjamin Shankman (1946), a general practitioner, saw the first human case of rickettsialpox in the Kew Gardens section of New York City on February 23, 1946. Mites and mice were present in the dwellings where further cases were seen. Mr. Pomerantz was a clothing manufacturer whose hobby was exterminating insects. He zealously gathered up the mites and supplied them to investigators of the United States Public Health Service, who then isolated the causative agent, *R. akari*. Ironically, "the cause of rickettsialpox and its means of transmission were established just seven months and seven days [after the first case was seen]" (Roueché, 1954, p. 49).

Tsutsugamushi[4] Disease, or Scrub Typhus

If epidemic typhus was of serious concern in the armed forces and civilian population during and after World War I, little attention had been devoted to tsutsugamushi disease. In fact a leading American textbook of medicine devoted only a brief paragraph in 1928 to this disease with the opening statement (Baldwin, 1928, p. 338), "Tsutsugamushi fever is an acute, endemic, febrile disease limited to the island of Nippon, Japan." The reference to the geography of the disease was optimistic. The first substantial work to appear in English was from the Kitasato Institute of Infectious Diseases in 1917 (Miyajima and Okumura, 1917). During World War II the United States Army was made aware of the widespread distribution of the disease in the Far East. The affected area extended as a triangle in Asia and the Pacific and included the area of Japan, India, and Australia (Zarafonetis and Baker, 1963). One of the most comprehensive reviews related to the war was that of F. G. Blake and his associates (Blake et al., 1945) in the Office of the Surgeon General of the United States.

The disease was recognized by missionaries in Japan and in China early in the nineteenth century. The characteristic feature was a febrile illness with a mild erythematous body rash, but the most singular manifestation was a necrotic area or eschar surrounding a bite by an infected mite. N. Ogata (1931) had discovered *Rickettsia tsutsugamushi* in 1927 as the cause of the disease. Extensive epidemiological studies revealed rodents in the fields as the host, the disease being transmitted by mites.

During World War II, between January 1943 and August 1945, in the Southwest Pacific area there were 5,663 cases of scrub typhus in the United States Army with 234 deaths. At that time there was no satisfactory vaccine for prophylactic purposes, and no specific therapy was available (Zarafonetis and Baker, 1963).

In the postwar period effective therapy was achieved with chloramphenicol and the tetracyclines. In a Pacific area I saw United States military personnel during the acute phase of the disease. The response to antibiotic treatment was remarkable, with a decline in fever and improvement within 24 to 48 hours. No satisfactory prophylactic vaccine has been achieved. But effective preventive measures include the use of proper protective clothing and miticides.

Q Fever

This disease was designated Q fever because it was first recognized in abattoir workers in Queensland, Australia (Derrick, 1937). The causative agent was a rickettsia (Burnet and Freeman, 1937), and at first it was termed *Rickettsia burneti*. A similar strain in ticks was later isolated in Montana, with the etiological agent then called *Coxiella burnetii* (Cox, 1940; Cox, Tesar, and Irans, 1947).

During laboratory studies on Q fever at the United States National Institutes of Health, sixteen cases appeared among the workers (Hornibrook and Nelson, 1940). I saw patients who had acquired the disease in the laboratory at Fort Bragg, North Carolina during World War II (Commission on Acute Respiratory Diseases, Fort Bragg, North Carolina, 1946). The clinical features, the epidemiology, and the occurrence of the disease in troops during World War II in the Mediterranean area, especially in Italy and Greece, were reviewed by F. C. Robbins (1948).

The disease is marked by fever, chilly sensations, severe headache, and prostration. Many cases demonstrate pulmonary infiltrates with a paucity of clinical findings. This is a rickettsial disease without an accompanying rash, and it is rarely fatal. Q fever is probably not transmitted from human to human, but through inhalation of the organisms (in laboratories) and from contaminated dust in the neighborhood of infected cattle, sheep, and goats (Cox, Tesar, and Irans, 1947). Contaminated cow's milk may be another source. It is enzootic in bandicoots in Australia, and principally in cattle in the United States, and is transmitted from animal to animal by ticks, including *Dermacentor andersoni* and *Amblyomma americanum*.

The disease occurs sporadically in civilian life and epidemically only in certain areas in the United States, such as Texas and California. A serological survey carried out in Minnesota on cows from the surrounding states showed no sign of the disease. Probably this is the reason that an indigenous human case of Q fever in Minnesota has never been recognized.

Control measures include a vaccine for workers in endemic areas as well as protection of infected domestic animals from atmospheric dusts in contaminated areas. Chloramphenicol and tetracycline drugs are effective in therapy.

Trench Fever

During World War I an acute febrile disease appeared along the western front in Europe that temporarily incapacitated up to a million men

(Swift, 1921). It was associated with trench warfare, and its transmission was due to the human body louse, *Pediculus humanis corporis*. There was an acute onset of chills, fever, headache, an erythematous macular rash, and severe pain in the legs. The illness lasted for several days; convalescence was prolonged, but there were no deaths. The affliction appeared to originate in Russia. A rickettsia organism was isolated from lice found on patients and termed *Rickettsia quintana* [5] (Mooser, Marti, and Leemann, 1949). The disease has also been reported from Mexico. During World War II cases were encountered on the Eastern front in Europe, but not on the scale as in World War I.

CHAPTER 19

Infections of the Central Nervous System Due to Viruses

Encephalitis and Hemorrhagic Fever Caused by Arboviruses and Arenoviruses

Encephalitis, like pneumonia, is caused by a wide variety of microbes, parasites, chemicals, and metabolic derangements. With the development of refined techniques and expanding knowledge, a spectrum of viruses has been shown to cause inflammation of the brain, including the viruses of rubeola, rubella, varicella, and pertussis, all of which have been considered elsewhere (see Section III, Chapter 13). The present discussion is concerned with encephalitis and the systemic complications due to arboviruses and slow viruses.

Arboviruses, as defined by a WHO scientific group, "are viruses which are maintained in nature principally, or to an important extent, through biological transmission between susceptible vertebrate hosts by haematophagous arthropods; they multiply and produce viraemia in the vertebrates by the bite of arthropods after a period of extrinsic incubation" (World Health Organization, 1967a, p. 9). Vectors include mosquitoes, flies, and ticks. In 1942 the term "arthropod-borne" virus was introduced, and then changed to "arborvirus." But *arbor* is Latin for tree, so this term implied that the group consisted of plant or tree viruses. Finally in 1963 the designation "arbovirus" was accepted internationally.

Knowledge of the complexity of the amazing number of arboviruses, the geographical distribution, mode of transmission, resulting diseases, and methods of identification is a product of intense investigations beginning in 1930. There are at least 250 arboviruses, divided into at least 28 groups, with the two largest containing 20 to 36 different viruses. To complicate matters still more, the natural reservoirs of many of the viruses are in animals, birds, and perhaps reptiles, some causing epizootics in domestic animals, such as the equine encephalomyelitides. Since some of the human diseases have animals as reservoirs, they may be properly called zoonoses. The zoonoses occupy a separate chapter in this volume; the major arbovirus diseases are discussed here (Section III, Chapter 22). Although yellow fever is an arbovirus infection, it has been presented as one of the epidemic diseases subject to international quarantine (see Section III, Chapter 12).

It is not my purpose to detail the classification of the arboviruses, nor to describe the clinical features of the diseases they cause and the methods of diagnosis, but rather to discuss the development of knowledge about them, particularly with reference to the control and treatment of the diseases. Additional information can be readily obtained from standard textbooks of microbiology and clinical medicine. A brief but authoritative summary of the basic features of arboviruses and their classification is available (Casals, 1971).

It is probable that down through the centuries encephalitis and hemorrhagic complications were observed among the contagious virus diseases of childhood such as measles, mumps, chickenpox, and pertussis. It is also possible that chronic encephalitis, as exhibited by Parkinsonism in young adults, was observed.

Isolated and sporadic cases of encephalitis are difficult to evaluate clinically. When cases occur in epidemic form, however, the basic features of the disease become apparent. In the individual infection there are three possible stages varying from mild to severe. First there is a systemic febrile condition followed by rapid recovery; in these cases a precise diagnosis is often lacking. Second, a rash and hemorrhage may be associated with fever, lethal vascular collapse, and renal failure. And third, an acute febrile period is associated with the manifestations of encephalomeningitis followed by complete recovery, chronic encephalitis, or death.

In the latter part of the nineteenth century there was only sporadic interest in outbreaks of acute encephalitis in Europe, especially in relation to influenza. During World War I epidemic encephalitis appeared in Central Europe and France. Understanding at that time culminated in the historic reports of Baron von Economo, an Austrian aviator and neurologist in the psychiatric clinic of Dr. J. Wagner-Jauregg in Vienna. Von Economo carefully described thirteen cases of "encephalitis lethargica"[1] (Economo, 1917). Other cases occurred in the winter of 1917–1918, in many areas — including the United States — in association with the 1918 pandemic of influenza (Smith, 1921). Encephalitis lethargica was not recognized in the statistical tables of the Office of the Surgeon-General of the United States Army until 1920, so only meager information became available (Michie, 1928a). By 1942 the scientific consensus was that no direct relationship existed between influenza and epidemic encephalitis, but the etiology of von Economo's "encephalitis lethargica" has continued to remain obscure (Neal et al., 1942).

The first successful attempt to understand the etiology and mode of transmission of arbovirus encephalitis began with the St. Louis epidemic in 1933. During August, September, and October there were 1,097 cases with a mortality rate of 20.1 percent, occurring mostly in children under 15 years and in adults over 40. Investigators sought for the source in food and water and probed the possibility of human-to-human transmission. L. Lumsden (1958), an epidemiologist with the United States Public Health Service, recorded his experiences during the epidemic and postulated insects as a mode of transmission. The first demonstration of arbovirus as a cause of human encephalitis was made simultaneously by two groups (Muckenfuss, Armstrong, and McCordock, 1933; Webster and Fite, 1933) during the St. Louis epidemic. Subsequent epidemics of St. Louis virus encephalitis were recorded from other parts of the United States (Barrett, Yow, and Phillips, 1965; Luby, Sulkin, and Sanford, 1969).

Almost coincidentally with the St. Louis epidemic, interest was directed to epidemic encephalitis in Japan. Encephalitis — including von Economo's encephalitis lethargica, now known as Japanese A encephalitis — had been recognized in that area during the nineteenth century. Another type of encephalitis had recurred periodically during the hot seasons ever since 1871 (Kaneko and Aoki, 1928). During the summer of 1924 there were six thousand cases of this type, with a mortality rate of 62 percent; in 1935 there were five thousand, with 42 percent dying. It was during the latter epidemic that the causative arbovirus for Japanese B was isolated and proved to be distinct from the St. Louis virus (Taniguchi, Hosokawa, and Kuga, 1936).

Japanese B encephalitis was of concern among United States military personnel in Okinawa during World War II because of the simultaneous appearance of epidemic disease among the civilian population. The attack rate among the Americans was small. Albert Sabin (1947) administered mouse-brain preparations of prophylactic vaccine to thousands of troops and civilians, but under the circumstances it was difficult to draw any conclusions as to its efficacy.

Another chain of events involving the arboviruses was under way simultaneously in California. In the summer of 1930 investigators at the Hooper Foundation of the University of California encountered a large epidemic of equine encephalomyelitis and reported a virus as the causal agent (Meyer, Haring, and Howitt, 1931). Subsequently substantial evidence was presented that a human and often fatal disease arose from this source.

Epidemic equine encephalomyelitis had been recognized in Minnesota since 1934 (Eklund and Blumstein, 1938). During the summer of 1937, among 737,000 horses, 41,159 became infected and 9,200 died. At the same time human encephalitis occurred in the state, and it was proved that the human disease was due to the western strain of equine encephalomyelitis. In the summer of 1941 a severe human epidemic of equine western encephalomyelitis appeared in the Red River Valley area of North Dakota and Minnesota with 1,700 cases and 150 deaths (Eklund, 1946). In the meantime the mosquito was clearly implicated as the vector. Many of the patients were treated at the University of Minnesota Hospitals during this period. Although the mortality rates did not exceed 10 percent, the sequelae of brain damage were severe (Baker and Noran, 1942; Noran and Baker, 1945).

Advances in scientific knowledge often occur rapidly, almost as if nature had set the stage for them to be made at a particular time. Within a decade the first three arbovirus epidemic diseases had been identified etiologically — St. Louis, Japanese B, and western equine encephalitis. A second type of equine encephalomyelitis in the United States was discovered during the summer of 1938 among horses in Massachusetts. L. D. Fothergill and his associates (Fothergill et al., 1938) defined a virus antigenically different from the western strain, and the disease became known as eastern equine encephalomyelitis. The mosquito was the most likely vector, with the tick *Dermacentor andersoni* also implicated. Natural reservoirs included horses, pigeons, and ring-tailed pheasants. Several clinical reports described a series of human cases with autopsy findings (Farber et al., 1940; Feemster, 1938; Howitt, 1938; Wesselhoeft, Smith, and Branch, 1938).

Besides western and eastern equine encephalomyelitis, a third form of equine encephalomyelitis was described in 1939, known as the Venezuelan type (Kubes and Ríos, 1939). But this occasioned little interest as far as human disease was concerned until 1943, when two series of human cases were reported as a result of accidental laboratory infections (Casals, Curnen, and Thomas, 1943; Lennette and Koprowski, 1943). Epidemic human disease was reported in Venezuela in 1962. Under natural circumstances the mosquito was the vector. The first human case infected under natural conditions in the United States was seen in 1968 near Miami (Ehrenkranz et al., 1970). Interest in the potential of Venezuelan equine encephalomyelitis as a source of human disease was intensified in 1971 when a large equine epidemic erupted in Mexico. The disease spread to Texas with potentially serious consequences, and human cases were detected along the lower Rio Grande Valley. Intensive control programs were immediately organized by the United States Department of Agriculture. The vaccination of a million horses in Texas, adjacent states, and Mexico was carried out, together with aerial spraying with ultra-low volume malathion to reduce the mosquito population. The successful results of these programs illustrate that prompt international control could be put into force, based on modern epidemiological knowledge and the availability of effective prophylactic agents and competent personnel. Fortunately Venezuelan human encephalomyelitis is a relatively mild disease with a low mortality rate, and severe neurological disturbances are not common.

Neurotropic viruses in man can have clinical manifestations such as encephalitis, encephalomeningitis, and "aseptic meningitis." Following the initial surge of information about new agents and vectors as the cause of encephalitis in the 1930s, a continued search was made for other viruses in relation to human disease. Although serological and virological diagnostic techniques became available for known diseases, it soon became apparent that the etiology of many human infections had not been identified. Public health authorities, epidemiologists, entymologists, virologists, and clinicians combined in continued investigations before, during, and after World War II. Since various mosquitoes were implicated in the transmission of arboviruses to humans, careful programs for screening these potential vectors were carried out.

During World War II and thereafter W. McD. Hammon and W. C. Reeves (1952) in California were able to identify a new group of antigenically related arboviruses causing encephalitis, particularly in children, with known species of mosquitoes as vectors. The mortality rate has been low, but the neurological sequelae have not been thoroughly evaluated. Subsequent epidemiological studies by other investigators revealed the widespread distribution of "California" virus throughout the United States, including New York, Florida, and — especially — Wisconsin, Minnesota, and Ohio (Cramblett, Stegmiller, and Spencer, 1966; Monath et al., 1970; Thompson and Inhorn, 1967).

Studies of California virus encephalitis led to valuable new information concerning the distribution of the disease, as well as to basic epidemiological information. Of particular epidemiological interest were the clusters of cases along the Mississippi River in the environs of the two adjacent communities just south of Minneapolis — La Crosse, Wisconsin and Winona, Minnesota [2] — and also in the wildlife workers in Wisconsin (Thompson et al., 1963). A source of diagnostic antigen for epidemiological purposes was the brain of a child who contracted the disease in Minnesota, but who died in La Crosse (Thompson, Kalfayan, and Anslow, 1965).

Hammon and Reeves (1952) originally isolated the California virus from the mosquito species *Aedes dorsalis* and *Culex tarsalis*. In the midwest, however, the major vector proved to be *Aedes triseriatus*, a species living in forests of hardwood trees. Small wild mammals, including rabbits, acquired the disease through this channel. The female *triseriatus* transmits the virus to her eggs, an important reser-

voir. J. Sanford (1974) emphasized the importance of California encephalitis in the United States, stating that it was the most common
form identified in the laboratory but was second to the meningoen-
cephalitides of the enterovirus group in Minnesota (Balfour, Jr., 1974).

The St. Louis epidemic led to the first implication and isolation of
an arbovirus as the cause of epidemic encephalitis. Probably the first
recognition of such a virus as the cause of human disease occurred
when an Austrian military commission defined sandfly (Phlebotomus
or pappataci) fever in 1908 (Doerr, Franz, and Taussig, 1909). The
commission demonstrated that the agent was filtrable and that the
disease could be readily produced by injecting the filtrate into healthy
human beings. They correctly designated flies (*Phlebotomus papatasii*)
as the vectors. Since then little further knowledge has been acquired
concerning the disease, which is characterized by fever, myalgia, and
headaches of brief duration. There is no known reservoir other than
man. The infection is quite prevalent throughout tropical areas in the
world, but does not occur in the United States. During World War II
this febrile disease afflicted thousands of troops, especially in the
Mediterranean area (Fleming, Bignall, and Blades, 1947; Sabin,
Philip, and Paul, 1944).

All of the foregoing arbovirus infections are transmitted to man
through mosquito bites, with the exception of sandfly fever. In various parts of the world a major group of human infections is transmitted through ticks, including Murray Valley (Australia) and West Nile
diseases, which involve viruses related to Japanese B virus. Russian
spring-summer encephalitis is a severe tickborne disease. A group of
tickborne human encephalitides with rodents as reservoirs involve
louping ill (sheep) in the British Isles, European tickborne disease,
Omsk hemorrhagic fever, and Kyasamur forest disease in India.

Apparently the only known tick-transmitted virus disease in the
western hemisphere is Colorado tick fever (Eklund, Kohls, and Brennan, 1955). Following a tick bite there is a sudden onset of malaise
and myalgia, a few days of fever, a second bout of fever, and finally
recovery. The disease simulates dengue and influenza, and convalescence may be prolonged. For over a hundred years pioneers in the
western United States had recognized this illness; they called it
"mountain fever." Undoubtedly there was diagnostic confusion in
the designation, but most medical historians agree that Colorado tick

fever was included. F. E. Becker (1930) clearly distinguished the entity of Colorado tick fever, and in 1946 the viral etiology was defined (Florio, Stewart, and Mugrage, 1946). This common infection is distributed widely in the western states, with tourists who enter these states becoming infected. Fortunately the prognosis is excellent. There is no known vaccine, nor is it essential. The most efficient prophylaxis is dressing appropriately in the tick-infested areas and removing ticks from the body promptly.

The complex nature of arbovirus infections presents further problems in the interpretation of the pathogenesis of diseases because of the syndrome of hemorrhagic fever, which occurs especially with dengue. In a comprehensive review of three hundred cases, Colonel G. M. Powell of the United States Army stated (1954, p. 99), "In 1951, hemorrhagic fever — a disease never before encountered by physicians of the Western World — broke out among the United Nations Forces in Korea. At the time, except for a few short paragraphs in official documents, the English literature was completely devoid of any reference to such an entity."

The syndrome has a general pattern of three defined stages: first, the signs of a nonspecific febrile illness; second, a toxic stage with hemorrhage, vascular collapse, and renal failure; third, a prolonged convalescent stage, usually with complete recovery. When death occurs it is commonly during shock in the second stage. One cannot restrict hemorrhagic fever to arboviruses alone, because many species of microbes other than viruses can initiate the syndrome. Our own investigations over a decade on "septic shock" at the University of Minnesota have revealed many of the obscure features of vascular collapse that occur in conjunction with bacterial infections. There is no question, however, that arboviruses were associated with epidemics of the syndrome in the Far East shortly before, during, and after World War II. A well-documented survey was made by Russian investigators (Smorodintsev, Kazbintsev, and Chudakov, 1964). Professor Susumu Hotta (1969) of Japan discussed the relationship of dengue to hemorrhagic diseases.

In 1958 a severe epidemic of hemorrhagic fever with high morbidity and mortality rates was observed for the first time in Thailand (Nelson, 1960). Perhaps the most authoritative and comprehensive review of the subject was incorporated in a symposium on "Mosquito-borne

Haemorrhagic fevers of South-east Asia and the Western Pacific," sponsored by WHO in 1964 (Halstead, 1966). This problem is of recent origin and has grown to serious proportions in many areas since 1950. D. C. Gajdusek (1962) has reviewed the arboviruses related to hemorrhagic fever and has proposed a classification based on the vector and agent. He has also pointed out that extensive epidemics of hemorrhagic fever were recognized by the Russians in various parts of their country two decades previously. Because dengue and dengue-like viruses are implicated more than any other known viruses in the genesis of the syndrome, a brief review of the development of knowledge about dengue is pertinent.

Dengue,[3] or "break-bone fever," is a common infection around the world in tropical and subtropical areas. The illness is manifested in a spectrum of symptoms varying from an undefined mild febrile disease of short duration, to that of severe joint pains and myalgia, a maculo-papular rash with hemorrhage, nausea and vomiting, and a saddle-type of febrile response. A minority of cases progress to severe hemorrhage, vascular collapse, and death. The disease has been of serious consequence among military personnel because of the epidemic proportions and the duration of debility before complete recovery. For this reason many of the advances in knowledge of dengue have been made through investigations by army officers in the medical service.

In 1922 the surgeon-general of the United States Army recommended the formation of a medical department research board in the Philippines. A group headed by Colonel J. F. Siler provided much of the past and present knowledge of dengue and of the role of *Aedes aegypti* as a vector (Siler, Hall, and Hitchens, 1926). They cited early epidemics of the disease in 1779 in Cairo, Egypt and in Batavia (Jakarta), Java. The eighteenth-century botanist-physician Carl Linnaeus had first described the mosquito *Aedes aegypti* in Cairo in 1762 that subsequently was found to be the vector for dengue and yellow fever. The Siler board also pointed out that Benjamin Rush described an epidemic of dengue in Philadelphia in 1780. Ironically both yellow fever and dengue had appeared in Philadelphia simultaneously. But these two diseases, both transmitted by the *aegypti*, occurred together only in the western hemisphere. Yellow fever has never been recognized in Asia or in the East Pacific areas, but epidemic dengue has continued there in severe form.

Shortly after the work of the Siler Commission, another Army commission carried out intensive research on dengue in the Philippines under the direction of Major James S. Simmons, who as General Simmons was to play a leading part in directing preventive medicine in World War II in the United States Army (Simmons, St. John, and Reynolds, 1926). P. M. Ashburn and C. F. Craig (1907), also in the United States Army Medical Corps, proved that dengue could be experimentally transmitted to healthy men with a filtrate of blood from acutely ill patients.

Because of the importance of dengue in military campaigns during World War II, extensive research was undertaken, principally under the direction of Colonel Albert Sabin (1952). The most significant results of these efforts were the propagation of the virus in mice and the discovery of subtypes of dengue virus, thus explaining recurrent infections. The search for a prophylactic vaccine, which had been successful in the case of yellow fever, was fruitless. There are now four known types of dengue virus. To date, no dengue vaccine has been placed in general use.

During the post-World War II period extensive civilian epidemics of dengue, accompanied by the hemorrhagic fever syndrome, occurred in the East Pacific and South Pacific areas, especially in children. Even though dengue was a mild disease with complete recovery in most cases, the pathogenesis of the severe complication, hemorrhagic fever, was not understood. Doctor Scott Halstead (1970) vigorously pursued this problem under United States Army auspices. He suggested that the syndrome was caused by previous exposure to the disease, resulting in cell-mediated hypersensitivity or circulating antibody to the virus. The cellular or humoral antibody-antigen reaction initiated the vascular phenomena essential for the appearance of collapse, which often was not reversible.

It must be emphasized that dengue virus is not the only causative agent for the hemorrhagic fever syndrome. Other arboviruses, known and unknown, can initiate the reaction. Among the others is the dengue-like arbovirus Chikungunya, first isolated in Tanganyika, causing a dengue-like illness and hemorrhagic fever elsewhere in Africa, southeast Asia, and India.

The development of the knowledge and techniques of virology has continued to bring forth new information about virus diseases in man, as illustrated by the discovery in South America of Argentinian and Bolivian hemorrhagic fevers in 1953 and 1959, and about their causative agents, known as the Junin and Machupo viruses respectively (Mackenzie et al., 1964). They have been designated arenoviruses;[4] since the reservoir is in rodents, the resulting diseases have been called zoonotic hemorrhagic fevers.

The progress of virology is dramatized by the recent discovery of two new viruses causing the hemorrhagic fever syndrome and carrying high mortality rates (Monath, 1974). In 1969 a missionary nurse in Lassa, Nigeria became acutely ill and died. Two other nurses developed the same illness, and one of them died (Buckley and Casals, 1970; Frame et al., 1970; Troup et al., 1970).[5, 6] Two laboratory workers studying the disease also became ill, and one died. The virus belongs to the arenoviruses. The disease is possibly a zoonosis, since rodents are suspected as a reservoir; it is very likely airborne. Epidemics involving over a hundred people in West Africa occurred between 1969 and 1973, with mortality rates from 36 to 67 percent. The disease frequently occurs among medical attendants. Further discussion on Lassa fever has been presented by Casals and Buckley (1974).

In 1967 about twenty-five laboratory workers in Marburg and Frankfurt-am-Main, Germany and in Belgrade, Yugoslavia became severely ill after handling tissues of a species of monkey, *Cercopithecus aethiops* (green monkeys), from Uganda (Monath, 1974). The illness simulated yellow fever, with a mortality rate of 29 percent. A virus has been isolated and grown in guinea pigs, but has not been definitely classified (Smith et al., 1967). Electron micrographic studies of the virus have revealed a doughnut type of configuration, also called the torus form, and this may suggest that the Marburg agent belongs to a new group called Toroviruses (Almeida, Waterson, and Simpson, 1971). Serological studies indicate infections in the monkey population of Uganda and in other primates in Kenya as well. Possible vectors have not been identified. Human-to-human transmission is probable. Epidemiological studies indicate that the mortality rate in monkeys is not high, a fact interesting to me in relation to the experimental studies on endotoxin shock carried out by my associates on the same species of imported monkeys. We found the green monkey more resistant to endotoxin shock than related species.

The control of arbovirus and arenovirus diseases, including encephalitis and hemorrhagic fever, poses a major problem in public health. One could postulate that elimination of these diseases could be managed by the development of prophylactic vaccines for human and animal use and by eradication of the animal reservoirs and arthropod vectors. Such procedures have been successful in the case of yellow fever, in which a successful prophylactic human vaccine and effective mosquito control have been used. In the case of the equine encephalitides (eastern, western, and Venezuelan), successful programs have included the use of equine vaccines and the slaughter of infected animals.[7] Because of the formidable number of arboviruses, however, and because of the reservoirs and vectors involved, progress has been limited, particularly in the developing countries. Continuing efforts, requiring adequate financing and trained personnel, are necessary as with malaria, smallpox, typhus, and other epidemic diseases. Unfortunately no specific therapy is available for viral diseases. Treatment for hemorrhagic fever is largely supportive. Greater effort must be made in investigating the pathogenesis of the syndrome of shock and renal failure. Finally it is probable that continued research will identify other arboviruses that affect public health.

Slow Virus Disease

The concept of slow virus diseases in the pathogenesis of animal and human diseases is one of the most exciting and challenging in the rapidly advancing discipline of virology (Kimberlin, 1976). In the evolution of knowledge on the subject attention has continued to center on a disease in sheep known as scrapie. Doctor Bjorn Sigurdsson, a veterinarian in Iceland, first defined slow virus disease in describing such diseases in sheep; a type of proliferative pneumonia called maedi; and visna, a chronic and slow demyelating disease of the central nervous system (Sigurdsson, 1954a; Sigurdsson and Pálsson, 1958). A third disease, rida, was probably a variant of scrapie (Sigurdsson, 1954b).

The following criteria for slow virus disease were suggested

(Sigurdsson, 1954b, p. 351): "A very long initial period of latency lasting from several months to several years. . . . A rather regular protracted course after clinical signs have appeared usually ending in serious disease or death. . . . Limitation of the infection to a single host species and anatomical lesions in only a single organ or tissue system. These last statements may have to be modified as knowledge increases."

Sigurdsson's concept of slow virus diseases was extended as a result of subsequent investigations (Eklund and Hadlow, 1973). Fever was not associated with the localized or systemic manifestations. The pathological changes were not inflammatory, but rather degenerative and proliferative. The genetic makeup of the host was a major factor in the disease. There was no detectable immune response to the causative virus, but an increased humoral production of globulins could occur, as well as an exaggerated cellular response. Sigurdsson's studies on visna and maedi were extended by his associates and the viruses of each were isolated and grown in tissue culture (Thormar and Pálsson, 1967). There is considerable similarity in the two viruses, and possibly visna is a variant of the maedi virus.

Scrapie was first recognized as a disease in certain breeds of sheep over two hundred years ago. The disease derived its name because itching was a prominent symptom, the animals relieving their distress by rubbing up against any fixed object. The incubation period can extend from eighteen months to five years, but the acute manifestations usually appear at two years of age. The onset is insidious, with tremors and generalized pruritis. Cerebral lesions are reflected by abnormal gait, epileptic convulsions, and paralysis of the limbs. The disease terminates fatally in six weeks to six months. There is a prominent vacuolization of the brain tissue *without* inflammation. The disease is transmitted orally; some breeds of goats can be afflicted. Scrapie has been extensively studied experimentally in mice and in other animal species (Hotchin, 1971) and has been transmitted to the cynomolgus monkey (*Macaca fascicularis*) with an incubation period of five years (Gibbs and Gajdusek, 1972)! Scrapie is now present in most of the sheep-breeding areas in the world.

Isolation of the scrapie virus from brain tissue has been extremely difficult. It is a very stable virus against heat, cold, and chemicals. Perhaps the difficulty in isolation and replication in pure culture is due to the fact that the virus is tightly incorporated within the host's membranes (Gajdusek and Gibbs, 1973). Does this mean, one may ask, that only a fragmented portion of a virus with genetic material is bound within the host's tissues (virion)?

In 1947 a lethal encephalopathy was observed on mink farms in Wisconsin, particularly in the Aleutian strain of mink. Increased numbers of mink became afflicted, which prompted reports on the disease from that state (Burger and Hartsough, 1965; Hartsough and Burger, 1965). The cerebral lesions as well as the virus were found to be similar to that of scrapie. In fact the disease first appeared in Wisconsin about the same time that scrapie in sheep was recognized there. Infection of mink possibly was caused by feeding them sheep carcasses. The incubation period is about a year, and death occurs within three to eight weeks. Transmission is oral.

In addition to the neurological lesions of mink encephalopathy ("Aleutian mink disease"), there are certain generalized pathological lesions that have occasioned many investigations because of the similarity of the humoral response and of the pathology to certain human diseases. There is a generalized lymphocytic proliferation with the production of plasma cells and hypergammaglobulinemia, mainly 19S globulin. Necrotizing arteritis and glomerulitis occur. The glomerular lesions probably result from the deposition of antigen-antibody complexes similar to that found in glomerulonephritis caused by lymphocytic choriomeningitis virus. Bence Jones proteins have been recovered in the urine. Mink disease may be an auto-immune disease (Hanson and Marsh, 1974; Marsh, Burger, and Hanson, 1969).

Doctor W. J. Hadlow (1959), a prominent investigator of scrapie, first called attention to the similarity of scrapie and kuru. Kuru is an endemic chronic and progressive neurological disease that existed in a primitive cannibalistic tribe among the Fore people in New Guinea. The elegant studies of Dr. D. C. Gajdusek and C. J. Gibbs, Jr. (1973) of the United States National Institutes of Health, Bethesda, demonstrated the relationship of scrapie and kuru. During their investigations almost twenty-five hundred people died of the disease, mostly young women and young children. In the ritual exercises of cannibalism it was the females and children who ate the highly infectious brain tissue of their close kinsmen. The close intermarriage system possibly contributed to a genetic susceptibility to the virus, but this genetic factor remains controversial.

The incubation of kuru varies between a few months to several years, and the disease usually appears in young adults. After the onset of symptoms, death occurs in three to six months. The clinical manifestations are tremors, ataxia, extraocular movements, and dementia. Kuru has been successfully transmitted to chimpanzees, which developed a kuru-like syndrome (Gajdusek, Gibbs, and Alpers, 1966).

In a review of unconventional viruses that cause chronic disease (Gajdusek and Gibbs, 1973), attention was called to those diseases in which there is a subacute spongiform encephalopathy. This unusual cytopathic reaction involved animals with scrapie and mink with encephalopathy. The counterparts of these diseases in humans are kuru and Creutzfeldt-Jakob disease, or C-J disease. Doctor H. G. Creutzfeldt was a neuropathologist at the University of Breslau, where he worked under Professor Alzheimer. He described for the first time the histology of C-J disease (Creutzfeldt, 1920). This report was soon followed by that of Dr. A. Jakob (1921), a pathologist in a state mental institution in Hamburg. Jakob described what he called spastic pseudosclerosis or encephalomyelopathy with disseminated degeneration. The clinical features of these and succeeding investigations consisted of dementia, spasticity, and weakness, with muscular atrophy. The disease rarely appears before middle age and probably has often been mistaken for presenile dementia with a rapid and lethal course after the onset.

It was generally known that C-J disease simulates the spongiform encephalopathy characteristic of kuru. Following their success in the study of kuru, D. C. Gajdusek and C. J. Gibbs, Jr. turned their attention to C-J disease and successfully transmitted the disease with brain tissue from a 59-year-old white male to a chimpanzee after an incubation period of thirteen months (Gibbs et al., 1968). In subsequent studies the similarities of kuru and C-J disease extended to the biological nature of the viruses. Indeed, the spongiform virus encephalopathies were to include the two diseases of animals, scrapie and mink encephalopathy, and the human diseases, kuru and C-J disease.

Clinical and pathological studies on C-J disease were extended by

Gajdusek and Gibbs (1973). They investigated eighty patients, including their tissues, obtained from different areas of the world. They continued to transmit the disease with tissues to chimpanzees and several species of monkeys. In remarkable studies on one family, the authors also discovered a hereditary trait for the disease. They concluded that they now had information on eight families with the disease and "what appears to be an autosomal dominant form of inheritance" (Gajdusek and Gibbs, 1973, p. 296).

In discussing the biology of kuru and C-J disease, Gibbs and Gajdusek (1974) pointed out the similarities of the familial Alzheimer's disease and kuru. They suggested that further consideration as a slow virus should be given not only to Alzheimer's disease but also to Huntington's chorea and Pick's disease.[8]

The foregoing slow virus diseases caused by "unconventional agents" should be distinguished from those diseases of *persistent* infection caused by the classic viruses (Johnson, 1974). The virus of measles has been implicated in neurological disorders such as multiple sclerosis (Adams and Imagawa, 1962); this virus has been isolated from the brain of patients with subacute sclerosis panencephalitis (Horta-Barbosa et al., 1969; Payne, Baublis, and Itabashi, 1969). ASV40 type of virus has been recovered from patients with progressive multifocal encephalopathy (Weiner et al., 1972). And a papova-like virus was found in the brain of a patient with progressive multifocal leukoencephalopathy (Padjett et al., 1971). To complicate the problem further it is well established that bacteria and parasites may remain dormant in the nervous tissue for years before activating an acute and lethal disease. It is entirely possible that with further intensive research on viruses, other viruses will be associated with obscure neurological disorders.

CHAPTER 20

Parasitic Diseases

While bacteriology was achieving scientific status in the nineteenth century, so was the related discipline of parasitology, concerned chiefly with protozoan and helminthic infections and with the vectors that transmit the diseases. It had been known for centuries that man and animals harbored worms. Their appearance in the intestinal tract and other tissues was assumed to have originated through spontaneous generation. Almost two hundred years elapsed before definitive scientific advances were achieved in parasitology.

Doctor Theobald Smith was one of America's most productive medical scientists. He had a broad interest in parasitism, viewing it as a universal biological phenomenon, an expression of "the interdependence of all living organisms" (Smith, 1934, p. 2). Subsequently Dr. Thomas Cameron expanded the meaning of parasitism and also presented a useful annotated bibliography on the subject. He defined a parasite as "an organism which at some stage of its life requires some vital factor which it can obtain only from another living organism" (Cameron, 1956, Introduction, p. xv). This broad biological definition can rightfully include man as a parasite.

During the nineteenth century cattlemen in the midwestern United States observed a devastating disease in their stock popularly known as "Texas Tick Fever." The animals developed an acute fever, severe anemia, and cachexia, after which they died. In the warmer months each year thousands of cattle were driven north from Texas to Illinois and Missouri on their way to feeding and slaughter. The disease created an economic hazard for the livestock industry and the loss of a valuable source of human food.

The Commissioners of the Illinois State Agricultural Society (1868), as a result of an inquiry, issued a report that pointed to the possible role of ticks in the transmission of the disease. The Texas cattle were often covered with the insects. When the cattle arrived in the northern states, these ticks would fall to the grazing ground of the northern cattle. Shortly thereafter the latter appeared weak and malnourished and eventually succumbed to a febrile disease.

In 1883 the veterinary division of the United States Department of Agriculture was organized under the direction of Dr. Daniel E. Salmon. It was designated in 1884 as the Bureau of Animal Industry and was headed by Dr. Salmon, who appointed Dr. Theobald Smith, a physician, head of the pathological laboratory. Soon thereafter Smith and the veterinarian Dr. F. L. Kilborne carried out their classical studies on Texas tick fever, also known as piroplasmosis (Smith and Kilborne, 1893). They identified the protozoa *Babesia bigemina* in the blood of cattle, which destroys red blood cells causing a severe anemia and eventual death. The protozoa were carried in the tick *Boophilus annulatus*, which invaded the skin of healthy cattle and fed on the blood. The ticks transmitted the disease from animal to animal. This soon led to a process of dipping the cattle in a solution that killed the ticks and virtually eliminated Texas tick fever. This research is one of several projects carried out subsequently by the bureau; others include investigations on bovine tuberculosis and brucellosis.[1]

My own interest in parasitology extended over a long period in research, teaching, and patient care. I did my initial research as a medical student at Harvard University under the direction of Professor Donald Augustine in the department of comparative pathology. Working in the same laboratory where Dr. Theobald Smith had formerly worked, I investigated the parasitic disease trichinosis. Using the guinea pig as an experimental model I studied the pathogenesis of the disease with especial reference to the blood and tissue eosinophilia, a characteristic hematological response in the disease (Spink, 1934). Immunological tests for diagnostic purposes in humans suspected of the disease were successfully used, and a surprising number of patients were discovered to have contracted the illness through the ingestion of improperly prepared pork products (Spink and Augustine, 1935a; 1935b).

Certain examples of the major parasitic diseases are selected here to illustrate the development of knowledge that has contributed to the control of many of these infectious diseases. These preventive measures have been and continue to be of major importance in many developing countries. Table 6 is a summary of information on some of the protozoal and helminthic infections, many of which still threaten the health of millions of people throughout the world.

Protozoal Diseases

Amoebiasis

Amoebic dysentery, due to a protozoan, *Entamoeba histolytica*, was first described by F. Lösch (1875) in St. Petersburg, Russia. A good source for a documented historical background of the disease and an authoritative description of the biological features is that of C. F. Craig and E. C. Faust (1945a).

The disease occurs primarily in tropical and subtropical areas, with man as the principal host. Amoebae in the form of cysts are eliminated in human feces and contaminate food or water, the disease being acquired through the ingestion of the cysts. A serious common source has been traced to food handlers who may continue to pass cysts in the feces for a long time, with or without a history of an acute attack. The classic pathological picture in the gut was described by W. T. Councilman and H. A. Lafleur (1891) of Johns Hopkins University. The most serious complication, hepatic amoeba abscess, was reviewed by A. Ochsner and M. DeBakey (1943) of Tulane University. The disease has occurred in epidemic proportion in military personnel and civilians stationed in the tropics.

The most severe civilian epidemic of amoebic dysentery in modern society occurred in Chicago during the World Fair in 1933 (United States Public Health Service, 1936). The outbreak, which resulted in 1,409 cases with 98 deaths, was traced to contaminated drinking water. Since the majority of patients came from all parts of the United States there was often a delay before medical advice was sought, and incorrect diagnoses were frequently made, including appendicitis or malignancy of the cecum. Investigations by the United States Public

Table 6. Classification of Parasitic Diseases

Disease and Parasite	Primary Reservoir	Vector or Intermediary Host	Mode of Transmission to Man
Protozoal Diseases			
Amoebiasis (*Entamoeba histolytica*)	Man		Man to man through fecal contamination of water and food
Leishmaniasis			
Kala-azar (*Leishmania donovani*)	Man, dog, fox	*Phlebotomus* species (sandfly)	Man to man or other reservoir to man through vector
Oriental sore Old world (*L. tropica*) New world (*L. braziliensis*)	Dog, man, rodents	*Phlebotomus* species	Man to man or other reservoirs through vectors
Trypanosomiasis African sleeping sickness	Principally man	Several species of Glossina (tsetse flies)	Man to man through vector
American-Chagas' disease	Man	Reduvid "bugs"	Man to man
Malaria (*Plasmodium* species)	Man	Many species of Anopheles mosquitoes	Man to man through vector
Helminthic Diseases			
Schistosomiasis (*Schistosoma* species)	Man	Snail families — intermediary hosts	Man to man through contaminated water containing appropriate snail intermediary host
Filariasis (*Wuchereria bancrofti* and *Wuchereria malayi*)	Man	Several species of mosquitoes — Culex, Aedes and Anopheles	Man to man through mosquitoes
Onchocerciasis "blinding filariasis" (*Onchocerca volvulus*)	Man	Simulium species of black flies	Man to man through flies
Trichinosis (*Trichinella spiralis*)	Swine and bear		Animal to man through ingestion of meat containing viable larvae
Ancylostomiasis (hookworm disease) (*Necator americanus* and *Ancylostoma duodenale*)	Man		Fecal contamination of soil and water
Diphyllobothriasis	Man	Cyclops Diaptomus	Ingestion of infected fish
Taeniasis (*Taenia saginata* and *Taenia solium*)	Man		Ingestion of improperly cooked beef or pork
Ascariasis	Man		Contamination of hands, food, and water by ascaris eggs

Health Service traced the source of infection to two hotels employing twenty-three hundred persons, and in this large group 37.8 percent in one hotel and 47.4 percent in the other were found to be carriers of E. histolytica.

In most of the cases arising in the United States since 1933, the infection has been acquired outside the country. Statistics have revealed the occurrence of from two to three thousand cases between 1964 and 1973. Fortunately effective chemotherapy is now available, including emetine hydrochloride, tetracycline, chloroquin, and metronidazole. The last is probably the least toxic and can be given orally. Surgical intervention and chloroquin are recommended for hepatic abscesses.

Contemporary physicians in the developed nations of the temperate zones look upon the Trypanosomidae as the cause of exotic diseases, which they rarely encounter. But protozoan flagellates that localize in the blood and tissues of human hosts are the major causes of diseases in the tropical and subtropical areas of the world. The present discussion centers on the significant diseases under leishmaniasis and trypanosomiasis as outlined in Table 6.

For the medical historian tracing the growth of knowledge about these diseases, the task is intriguing and exciting, but somewhat difficult. Their history simulates the course of discoveries that occurred in the studies of malaria, particularly in the struggles for priority. Just as tuberculosis was a major infectious disease in the nineteenth century because of the industrial revolution and the resulting crowding and poor hygiene in the large urban areas, there was in this period an acceleration of epidemics of trypanosomal diseases. An increase in the incidence and severity of African sleeping sickness occurred because under an expanding colonialism ruthless mercenaries and adventurers exploited the countries and promoted the slave trade. Knowledge of these old diseases accumulated rapidly in the nineteenth century as a result of observations made by a few intrepid missionaries and the dedicated efforts and skills of military and civilian scientists working under the most primitive conditions and encountering constant hardships.

Scientific progress in medicine during the latter part of the nineteenth and early twentieth century owed much to those military doctors trained in pathology and surgery at The Royal Army Medical

College at Netley, England. This institution was founded in 1863, largely through the efforts of Florence Nightingale. Netley physicians included David Bruce, Ronald Ross, William Leishman, Timothy Lewis, Almroth Wright, David Semple, and Charles Donovan.

Leishmaniasis

Kala-azar, also called "black disease," was known to have existed for centuries in India, North China, the Mediterranean littoral, Africa, Sumatra, and China (Scott, 1939c). In 1934 endemic kala-azar was recognized in South America. This chronic and debilitating condition has a mortality rate of over 90 percent. For a long period kala-azar was confused with malaria. It was known to spread slowly over large, well-traveled areas, about ten miles per year. Children were particularly susceptible to the disease.

The major aspects of the disease are a long incubation period of several weeks, followed by fever with swelling of the lymph nodes, marked enlargement of the spleen and liver, anemia, weakness, and emaciation; and then collapse and death after periods of intermittent fever.

Pertinent to knowledge of kala-azar was the basic discovery by Surgeon-Major Timothy Lewis of Britain. As an assistant to the sanitary commissioner of India, he reported on the presence of flagellated trypanosomes in the blood of healthy rats, later called *Trypanosoma lewisi* (Lewis, 1878). This initial finding of trypanosomes in a mammal provided a link to the discovery of related parasites in kala-azar and other human diseases. On May 30, 1903, Major W. B. Leishman, then at Netley, published a paper describing trypanosomes in the splenic pulp of a fatal case of Dumdum fever. The patient had been invalided home to England from India suffering from the disease. Leishman stated (1903, p. 1252), "The recent discovery of trypanosomiasis in man by Dr. Dutton and Dr. Forde, and the report of further cases by Dr. Manson, naturally lead one to question the possibility of the occurrence of this disease in other parts of the world than those originally reported — viz. the Congo and the Gambia." In this report he referred to his brief experience at Dumdum near Calcutta, from which many cachectic soldiers had to be sent home to England and Netley Hospital, only to die. He concluded his paper by suggesting that both kala-azar and sleeping sickness may be "due to trypanosomiasis" (Leishman, 1903, p. 1254).

Within six weeks, on July 11, 1903, Captain C. Donovan (1903) recorded that while stationed in Madras, India he had punctured the spleen of a 12-year-old boy and had observed the parasites in smears of the pulp, as described by Leishman. The independent observations of Leishman and Donovan on the parasite that causes kala-azar resulted in the major diagnostic procedure for identifying the disease by aspirating splenic pulp and observing the "Leishman-Donovan bodies." This procedure, together with the hypergammaglobulinemia in the chronic cases, constitute pertinent diagnostic findings in kala-azar.

Further progress on the nature of kala-azar was made by two Indian commissions, that of the Calcutta School of Tropical Medicine and the Indian Kala-azar Commission. The cause of kala-azar being known, it was gradually learned that the disease occurred in widely separated geographical areas. The mode of transmission as worked out by the Indian commission showed that the fly *Phlebotomus argentipes* was responsible (Shortt et al., 1931). Elsewhere other members of the Phlebotomus were found to be the vectors.

One of the modern scientific achievements in tropical medicine is the reduction of the mortality rate of kala-azar from around 90 percent to 2 to 5 percent with the use of antimony compounds, especially sodium antimony gluconate, and to a lesser extent with pentamidine isethionate (Imperato, 1974a). Prevention of the disease has resulted largely from eliminating the phlebotomus flies. This has been accomplished by the use of insecticide sprays such as those used in malaria control. In areas where malaria and kala-azar are both endemic, control measures used against the mosquito for malaria have simultaneously reduced the incidence of kala-azar.

Oriental Sore

This ailment, characterized by discrete and superficial ulcerations of the face, ears, and extremities, was observed for many centuries. Probably the earliest description of the specific clinical entity of this leishmaniasis disease was that given in a travel volume on Aleppo, Syria by A. Russell (1756). In the concluding pages he cited the "Mal d'Aleppo," which was an indigenous skin disease observed in that city, hence the synonym "Aleppo sore." He thought it was caused by water. It was not usually a serious affliction, but the more severe cases were undoubtedly complicated by secondary infection. The sores were also recognized in dogs. The disease still occurs in many parts of the world, and in India is known as "Delhi sore." In Central and South America it can be quite severe, in one form called "espundia," involving the muco-cutaneous areas of the nose and mouth. When the disease is associated with secondary microbial invasion, large areas of tissue necrosis occur.

Some controversy has surrounded the discovery of the causative agent, now known as *Leishmania tropica*. Cecil A. Hoare has brought to light a report of 1898 by the Russian military surgeon Peter F. Borovsky, who clearly described the parasite obtained from the lesions. Hoare concludes (1938, p. 71), "To Borovsky thus belongs the credit of being the first to give a recognizable description of *Leismania tropica* — and indeed of leishmanias in general — and of assigning it to the Protozoa."

Although United States military personnel during World War II were deployed to many areas in the world where leishmaniasis was indigenous, there was relatively little disability caused by these diseases. There were not more than 50 to 75 cases of kala-azar and only one death (Most, 1968). During the war I learned about a United States military installation in Iran along the Persian Gulf, known as the Persian Gulf Command. This group was concerned with the transportation of military supplies from the United States to Russia. It was estimated that there were a thousand to fifteen hundred cases of cutaneous leishmaniasis, or oriental sore, in American troops during the war, and the vast majority occurred in the Persian Gulf Command. The circumscribed lesions appeared on the extremities, face, neck, and ears. Most of the patients were treated in dispensaries; all recovered completely.

But cutaneous, and especially muco-cutaneous, leishmaniasis in Central and South America is more serious. Neglected lesions with ulceration are often invaded with bacterial pathogens, such as streptococci and staphylococci. Treatment demands antibiotic therapy as well as parenteral neostibosan.

Because of the magnitude of the problem of leishmaniasis the World

Health Organization has taken steps to review knowledge on the subject and to offer authoritative recommendations for treatment and prevention. As a result of an international conference in Russia, a significant report was issued (World Health Organization, 1971b). The variety of Leishmania species in animals and man, and their clinical manifestations, were emphasized. Significant was the fact that the reservoir of disease is in animals, making leishmaniasis one of the zoonoses. Recommended control measures simulate those for malaria.

Trypanosomiasis

African trypanosomiasis or "sleeping sickness" provides for the student of comparative medicine an example of the contributions of veterinary science and human medicine to the understanding of the nature of a disease or group of diseases. Probably the earliest known description of African trypanosomiasis was that given by John Atkins, an English naval surgeon who was on the Guinea Coast in 1721. He wrote of the common manifestation of somnolence in the African population there, and of the associated high mortality rate (Atkins, 1742; Scott, 1939b).

Another important observer was the physician Thomas Winterbottom (1803), who described the lethargy in Africans in Sierra Leone in western Africa. He called attention to one of the most important physical signs occurring early in the disease, the swelling of the posterior cervical lymph nodes, now known as "Winterbottom's sign." Practically every textbook of tropical medicine carries an illustration of this sign. The Portuguese and Arab slave-traders recognized this ominous sign in young and otherwise healthy Africans and even went to the extreme of excising the nodes before selling the youths for shipment to the western hemisphere. The traders knew that these swellings portended a lazy and sleepy individual.

As stated above, the spread of sleeping sickness in Africa was due to the slave trade and to the opening up of commerce. Severe epidemic disease prevailed around Lake Victoria. Neither the cause nor the mode of spread of the disease was known at the time. It is now realized that the disease was spread by infected humans travelling into isolated areas where the Glossina (tsetse fly) was prevalent.

The disease became such an economic threat to spreading colonialism in the nineteenth century that interested nations, including Germany, France, Portugal, Spain, and Belgium, organized scientific commissions to study the problem. There were two British commissions, one from the Liverpool School of Tropical Medicine and one from the Royal Society of London.

But economic disaster of another type beset the slave traders, explorers, and entrepreneurs in Africa. The horses and oxen that were used for transporting supplies were often afflicted by a strange and fatal disease known as *nagana*,[2] a name given by the Zulu tribes. Similarly *surra* decimated both horses and cattle. These were trypanosomal infections; *dourine* in the horse was another. Losses of domestic animals due to these diseases deprived the natives of food and of sources of power and transportation. The exploiting groups then turned to human beings as a means of transporting supplies, which in turn led to the spread of human trypanosomiasis. By the end of the nineteenth century trypanosomiasis was ravaging both animal and human populations, comprising a complex biological and medical challenge that would be resolved only by veterinary and medical scientists in the twentieth century.

By the mid-nineteenth century observers saw a vague relationship between nagana and the tsetse fly.[3] In 1857 the description of the missionary travels of Dr. David Livingstone appeared, in which his shrewd and important observations on nagana and the tsetse fly were recorded. He wrote (1857, p. 80), "A few remarks on the Tsetse, or *Glossina moristans*, may here be appropriate. . . . Its peculiar buzz when once heard can never be forgotten by the traveller whose means of locomotion are domestic animals; for it is well known that the bite of this poisonous insect is certain death to the ox, horse, and dog." He continued (p. 81), "A most remarkable feature in the bite of the tsetse is its perfect harmlessness in man and wild animals." The importance of the tsetse fly to Livingstone was demonstrated by the fact that his volume on travels in Africa had an enlarged engraving of the fly on the title page, and also several views of the insect within the volume. Livingstone's observations were scientifically correct and were to influence the work of the famous Sleeping Sickness Commission of the Royal Society fifty years later (Great Britain. Royal Society of London, 1903 and 1905).

With the developing interest in the relationship of nagana to the tsetse fly, the next step was to define the etiology of the disease. This was accomplished in 1895 by Sir David Bruce, who, together with his competent wife, Lady Bruce, devoted a lifetime to an army career. Their careers are summarized in the discussion on brucellosis (see Section III, Chapter 22). Their first Army assignment took them from Netley to Malta, where between 1883 and 1885 Sir David discovered the etiology of Malta fever, or brucellosis. Upon returning to England he met with his friend Sir Walter Hely-Hutchinson, who had been lieutenant governor of Malta and who had then become governor of Zululand and Natal. Sir Walter persuaded the Bruce team to accept an appointment in Natal where epidemics of nagana were severe. Tulloch, in writing of their distinguished service of two years in Zululand on investigating the etiology of nagana, stated (1955, p. 84), "This devoted couple during these years lived and worked under truly primitive conditions; their housing differed in no way from that of the native population, for food they had to rely on their capabilities as hunters." In a series of brilliant but simple experiments Bruce isolated a trypanosome (*Trypanosoma brucei*) from diseased cattle and proved that the tsetse fly (*Glossina morsitans*) was the vector. Wild game, though not suffering from the disease, were the reservoirs of *T. brucei*.

Bruce's initial report (1895) on nagana was published in Durban in what is now South Africa. It is a beautiful model of scientific discovery, with Lady Bruce's drawings in color as well as her detailed sketches of the trypanosomes in the blood of horses, cows, and dogs. Bruce began (1895, p. 1):

Definition — The Fly Disease or Nagana is a specific disease which occurs in the horse, donkey, ox and dog, and varies in duration from a few weeks to many months. It is invariably fatal in the horse, donkey and dog, but a small percentage of cattle recover. It is characterized by fever, infiltration of co-agulable lymph into the subcutaneous tissue of the neck, abdomen or extremities, giving rise to swelling in these regions, by more or less rapid destruction of the Red Blood Corpuscles, extreme emaciation, and the constant occurrence in the blood of an infusorial parasite, either identical with or closely resembling the Trypanosoma Evansi found in Surra, a disease of India and Burmah.

At the end the report asks (p. 28), "from what source does the fly obtain the living virus?" This was the missing link in the epidemiology of nagana.

Near the Thames River in London, and adjacent to the Tate Art Gallery, stands the Royal Army Medical College. On a fall afternoon in 1955, the Centenary year of the birth of Bruce, I entered the library to study Bruce's original data on nagana. There, laid out for me on a long table in the quiet of a beautiful room, were his notes; photographs of their rude hut and primitive laboratory, and of the surrounding countryside; and photographs of a variety of animals, living and dead. Included were the exquisite drawings and sketches by Lady Bruce. It was as though medical history had come alive, an eloquent expression of the courage and perseverance of this dedicated and competent husband and wife, alone with a few natives in the wilds of Africa.

The serious problem of African sleeping sickness gained increasing attention. Was it related to nagana, even though the trypanosome of *T. brucei* was not implicated? Since the disease did occur in the "fly country," was another trypanosome involved and transmitted by Glossina? The connecting link between a trypanosome and Glossina was forged by the famous report on the patient Mr. K by Dr. J. Everett Dutton (1902) of the Liverpool School of Tropical Medicine. Mr. K was an English boatman on the River Gambia and was suffering from sleeping sickness, unknown to himself or others. Dutton had seen him in Africa and again when, as a patient, Mr. K had been invalided home to die in Liverpool. Dutton isolated a trypanosome from the patient's blood just before death, and meticulously described the morphology. He concluded (1902, p. 884):

The discovery of a parasite — evidently of the genus trypanosoma — in the blood of a patient presenting symptoms markedly similar in very many points to those of the two or more diseases of lower animals which have been definitely proved to be caused by the presence of different species of the genus trypanosoma forces one to the conclusion that the parasite found in this patient is a new species, and is also the cause of the disease from which the patient is suffering. I would therefore suggest that the name of *Trypanosoma gambiense* be given to this trypanosoma.

The etiology of sleeping sickness had been discovered.[4]

The most significant advances in the study of African sleeping sickness were made between 1903 and 1905 through the Sleeping Sickness Commission of the Royal Society of London, of which Bruce was a leading member. Seven reports were published within that period. The Commission arrived in Uganda in March 1903. Doctor Aldo Castellani had been sent ahead a year before, during which time he had made a significant finding. His first sentence in the first report of the Commission reads, "On the 12th of November, 1902, when examining a specimen of cerebro-spinal fluid taken by lumbar puncture during life from a well-marked case of *sleeping sickness*, I was surprised to observe a living Trypanosoma" (Great Britain-Royal Society of London 1903 and 1905, Report No. I, p. 3). But he did not consider this parasite the cause of sleeping sickness.

It is extraordinary that within a few months of the arrival of Bruce and his associates, the Report No. IV of November 1903 (Great Britain-Royal Society of London 1903 and 1905) established Dutton's *Trypanosoma gambiense* as the cause of sleeping sickness, and the tsetse fly *Glossina palpalis* as the vector of disease. Doctor L. Everard Napier, the director of the Calcutta School of Tropical Medicine and an authority on the disease, was moved to write (1946b, p. 199), "Not unnaturally Bruce, remembering his experience with nagana and the findings of Forde and Dutton in the blood and of Castellani in the cerebrospinal fluid, pieced together the whole story, but probably no other medical investigation has been carried through so methodically and with such painstaking restraint as the work of this commission." Bruce (1915) summarized the subject of trypanosomiasis in Central Africa in his Croonian Lectures.

Napier continued (ibid.), "In 1910, Stephens and Fantham found trypanosomes in the blood of a man who had come from Rhodesia; they considered that it differed from *T. gambiense* and named it *Trypanosoma rhodesiense*. In the following year, Kinghorn and Yorke showed this trypanosome was transmitted by another tsetse, *Glossina morsitans*." Thus there were two forms of African sleeping sickness, each due to a different trypanosome and each transmitted by different species of tsetse fly.

In the succeeding years efforts have been devoted to extensive epidemiological studies, to effective treatment, and to the prevention of the disease. Emphasis in therapy is based on early diagnosis. Pentamidine isethionate is indicated for the Gambian, and suramin (Bayer 205) for the Rhodesian, form of the disease. The trivalent arsenical melarsoprol can be employed for both.

The World Health Organization has maintained an active interest in trypanosomiasis, especially on a regional basis. A report of an expert group reviewed progress in controlling the disease in Kenya, where *Glossina pallidipes* is the sole vector for cattle, sheep, and goats, and *T. congolense* is the most frequently encountered trypanosome (World Health Organization, 1972b). Control measures have centered on destroying the tsetse flies by spraying insecticides, such as dieldron, from helicopters.

But control measures in Africa are far from successful. J. Ford (1971) reviewed the problem and cast much doubt on the preventive measures to date. He did make some pertinent suggestions for the future, pointing out that the colonial period in Africa began in 1878 with the Congress of Berlin and ended about 1960. Therefore Africans themselves have not had much opportunity to resolve the problem of trypanosomiasis. A sound control policy, according to Ford, should include "(1) An assessment of the nature and rate of development expected in each ecological area, regardless of the presence of tsetse and trypanosomiasis. (2) A much more profound understanding than exists at present, of the causes of epidemics and epizootics of tsetse-borne disease" (Ford, 1971, p. 491). He continued (p. 492), "What ought to be avoided are all forms of mass treatment, whether by mass injection of curative or prophylactic drugs, or by blanket spraying with insecticides, or by large-scale felling of vegetation, or destruction of wild life. All sorts of biological as well as mechanical bulldozing may, on occasion, control the spread of disease but at a cost to future generations that cannot be fully assessed." But he equally decried the conservationists in their attempt to preserve wildlife in areas where human pathogenic populations of trypanosomes reside. W. E. Ormerod (1961) has detailed the spread of Rhodesian sleeping sickness between 1908 and 1960.

Finally, in a comprehensive review edited by H. W. Mulligan (1970), Professor W. E. Kershaw emphasized the magnitude of the contemporary problem of African trypanosomiasis (Foreword, p. viii):

With the sometimes stormy advent of independence of the African territories in the 1950s and 60s, these control organizations became gradually less reliable for many reasons and the control of human trypanosomiases deteriorated until, in 1969, it was believed that there were up to a million cases of sleeping sickness in the Congo and that epidemics of vast proportions might well break out in other territories. Research, as well as control, in the field suffered from unstable political conditions.

Similar apprehension has been expressed by WHO authorities (World Health Organization, 1969a).

Trypanosomiases are found in Central and South America, and the problems there appear to approach the severity of those in Africa. In 1907 a railroad was under construction in a province of Brazil. Dr. Carlos Chagas was sent to evaluate and to make recommendations for the control of malaria in the area (Scott, 1939a). While there he heard of the barbeiro, or biting Reduviid[5] bug, that hides in the crevices of the human dwellings during the day and comes out at night and bites the faces of humans. It is also called the "kissing bug" and the "assassin." It was this biting bug that Darwin so vividly described in The Voyage of the Beagle. Chagas found flagellates in the bugs and sent specimens on to Oswald Cruz, who observed that the insects transmitted the flagellates to monkeys and to many other hosts, such as the armadillo. He demonstrated the flagellate in the blood of humans, especially children, who had been bitten. Thus the existence of Chagas' disease was established in South America with Trypanosome cruzi as the cause. The disease extends from Chile and Argentina to Mexico, and by 1969 up to seven million people were estimated to harbor the infection (World Health Organization, 1969c).

When T. cruzi is introduced into the human host the flagellates appear in the bloodstream, where, unlike African trypanosomes, they do not multiply, but localize in several tissues and organs. During the acute phase they can cause meningoencephalitis, which in the very young is fatal. A more chronic disease, myocarditis, occurs and may endure for years. A comprehensive report from Brazil on this complication cites over a thousand acute and chronic cases of myocarditis (Laranja et al., 1956). In chronic myocarditis, which occurs mostly in males over 50 years of age, parasites have been found in the myocardium. There is no treatment for Chagas' disease, but it can be readily prevented by employing a residual insecticide in the dwellings, especially benzene hexachloride.

In the rural areas of Guatemala in 1943 I encountered school children who had been bitten by the barbeiro. A few doubtful cases of the myocardial complication were observed. At my request some of the children quickly supplied me with a quantity of bugs, which were used later for teaching purposes at the University of Minnesota.

Malaria

When I was a medical student in 1930 an international authority on malaria remarked to our class, "There is no disease more important than malaria." Laughter ran through the group because most of us, nearing completion of medical school training, had never seen a case of malaria. Within a few years many of us were to learn the truth of that statement during World War II. By then I was teaching clinical parasitology and fortifying my lectures by quoting Dr. F. Macfarlane Burnet (1940, p. 282), "If we take as our standard of importance the greatest harm to the greatest number, then there is no question that malaria is the most important of all infectious diseases." I also quoted Professor Ernest Faust (1939) of Tulane University, who estimated that the annual cost of malaria to the South in the United States was a total of 1.5 million cases, costing a hundred million dollars!

As the war progressed more and more military personnel were sent into areas where malaria and other parasitic diseases confronted them. There was an urgent need for military people adequately trained in medicine to meet these problems. There was also a dearth of teachers in the medical schools who had suffcient clinical experience in this field of infectious diseases. To meet this emergency, teachers from each of the medical schools in the United States were given intensive laboratory and clinical training in tropical medicine. Selected from the University of Minnesota in 1943, I journeyed to a United Fruit Hospital at Quiruga, Guatemala, where I gained an unusual experience working with Dr. Neal MacPhail, the director and the acknowledged "Dean of Tropical Medicine" in Central America.[6] Malaria was rampant in that area and was the major cause of physical disability. We studied hundreds of cases, including those with the dreaded complication, black water fever. In surveys carried out among the civilian population, blood films were reviewed microscopically for malaria parasites on up to five hundred persons daily. Stool examinations revealed the common intestinal worms of ascariasis, enterobiasis, and hookworm. Hundreds of cases of onchocerciasis were observed in other surveys. There was much malnutrition, principally due to protein deprivation. In the highlands the devastation of classic epidemic typhus was seen among an Indian population.

For several centuries febrile syndromes consistent with malaria had been known to physicians. The disease was often designated as the "agues," and at least two febrile forms were noted, intermittent and continuous. Living in the Mediterranean basin where the disease was common, Hippocrates presented clinical descriptions consistent with the different forms in his "Epidemics." Malaria was long an affliction of the environs of Rome. Sydenham recognized the disease in England and wrote favorably on the use of quinine for treatment. As the world opened up further to travel in the seventeenth and eighteenth centuries, it was recognized that malaria occurred in many temperate, as well as tropical, zones (Boyd, 1949). One of the important features of the early descriptions of malaria was its relation to certain geographical and meteorological conditions such as the marshes adjacent to Rome and London. Daniel Drake (1850), in his topography of the interior of North America, described this association. J. K. Mitchell (1849) stated, without proof, that malaria was a parasitic fungal disease that was worse near marshes, and stressed the fact that the disease was usually acquired at night. E. H. Ackerknecht (1945) traced the course of malaria during the periods of migration in the upper Mississippi Valley from 1760–1900. Malaria was the primary disease of the lower Ohio and Mississippi valleys. The disease gradually abated in these areas with the clearing and drainage of the land for producing cattle, the use of quinine, and the replacement of the older and parasitized settlers with new uninfected healthy groups.

Advances in scientific understanding are often followed by a scramble of investigators to mount the ladder of priority, so that each can announce, "I was the first ———." This occurred with the basic discoveries on malaria. "It happens that some of the characters involved in the solving of the malaria problem were of a jealous and acrimonious disposition and scarcely any topic of medical research has excited so much controversy over matters of priority and credit" (Foster, 1965, p. 158). In order to understand the historical features of the priority entanglements, the nature of the disease and of its parasites should be briefly reviewed.

Malaria is caused by protozoa of the genus *Plasmodium*. Four species produce disease in man: *P. vivax* (benign tertian or *vivax* malaria); *P. falciparum* (malignant or *estivo-autumnal* malaria); *P. malariae* (quartan or *malariae* malaria); and *P. ovale* (or *ovale* malaria). Of the four, *P. vivax* and *P. falciparum* occur most frequently in man. In the older clinical literature it is probable that intermittent febrile attacks were associated with *P. vivax* and a continuous fever with *P. falciparum*. The latter form is confined to the tropics; one of its synonyms, *estivo-autumnal*, suggests that it occurred during the summer and autumn. Malaria due to *P. malariae* and *P. ovale* is relatively rare. Malaria due to *P. vivax* is encountered in the tropics and also in the subtropical and temperate zones. I have seen endemic cases of *vivax* malaria in Minnesota without a known exposure outside the state, and with no history of the patients having received blood transfusions.

The life cycle of the malaria parasite is complex, consisting of an exogenous sexual phase (sporogony) with multiplication in the mosquito, and an endogenous asexual phase (schizogony) occurring in man. Thus three factors are essential for the perpetuation of human malaria. First, an infected population with parasitemia — such individuals often manifest no illness, and a state of host-parasite balance may endure for long periods; second, a susceptible uninfected population; and third, appropriate species of mosquitoes that will complete the life cycle of the parasite and act as vectors in the transmission. Malaria is transmitted by mosquitoes but can often be transmitted from human to human through blood transfusions without the participation of the insect.

The classical clinical features of malaria are an acute or chronic febrile illness with anemia and weakness, an enlarged spleen, and sometimes fatal complications. The outstanding finding is anemia due to parasitization and the destruction of red blood cells as a part of the parasite's life cycle. Before these aspects of the disease were known, physicians ascribed malaria to certain geographical areas where mosquitoes were abundant, but the precise relationship was not proved until the nineteenth century. Following the report of Patrick Manson (1877) on the role of the mosquito in filariasis and the hypothetical relationship advanced by C. J. Finlay (1937) for yellow fever in 1881, Professor A. F. A. King suggested in an address in Washington, D.C. in 1882 that mosquitoes were possibly the vectors for malaria, and if this were true "the means of prophylaxis from malarial disease will not be difficult" (King, 1883, p. 657). He then went on to advise mosquito netting for personal use and for housing. He also recommended that municipalities drain swamps and pools, a suggestion made before the discovery of the parasite and proof that the mosquito was the vector.

The discovery of the malarial parasite in human blood was made in Algiers by the French army surgeon Charles Louis Alphonse Laveran (1880). He named the parasite *Oscillaria malariae*, because the parasite was a protozoon and because he was impressed by its amoeboid movements in specimens of fresh blood. Shortly thereafter he published a monograph in which he described the parasites in detail with excellent drawings (Laveran, 1893). Laveran outlined the epidemiology and alluded to the endemicity of the disease in marshy areas. He referred to the role of mosquitoes in the propagation of disease. He also suggested quinine as a prophylactic and therapeutic agent.

Laveran also called attention to malaria in the marshy areas of Rome and noted that the disease appeared each year at the same time. The Roman school of malariologists was of excellent caliber and was led by Professor E. Marchiafava, who with his assistant A. Bignami confirmed Laveran's findings (Marchiafava and Bignami, 1894). About the same time Major G. M. Sternberg of the United States Army had Marchiafava demonstrate the parasites to him. Returning to Johns Hopkins University, Sternberg showed his preparations to Dr. W. Welch in 1886; in 1887 Professor W. Councilman, also at Johns Hopkins, confirmed Marchiafava's work, as did Dr. William Osler in 1887. G. M. Sternberg (1884) wrote a comprehensive volume on malaria. He cited Laveran's discovery but did not record with conviction that the definitive cause of malaria was known. Camillo Golgi (1886), also in the same Italian group, discovered another species, *P. malariae*.

Ronald Ross worked out the life cycle of the malaria parasite and the role of the mosquito in transmitting the disease from human to human. Ross was an unusual person. Born in the Himalayan Mountains while his Scottish father was in the British military forces, he was a "poet, novelist, musician, scientist and reluctant physician" (Talbott, 1970, p. 770). Educated as a physician, with training in bacteriology and public health, he joined the Indian Medical Service in

1881. Malaria became of intense interest to him. During his time it was estimated that up to a million deaths occurred annually because of malaria. His life as a medical practitioner was boring, and he plodded on alone in his studies. Ross returned to England in 1894, where he met Manson, who encouraged him to study the role of mosquitoes in malaria. For several months Ross allowed mosquitoes to feed on febrile patients and learned to dissect mosquitoes skillfully. He related his final successes in the *Indian Medical Gazette* as follows (1898, p. 401): "In a report to the Director-General, Indian Medical Service, dated 19th September 1897, I described some peculiar pigmented cells found by me in August 1897 in two dappled-winged mosquitos fed on blood containing crescents, and anticipated that they were a stage of the parasite of malaria in those insects." This report appeared in the *British Medical Journal* for December 18, 1897 under the heading "On Some Peculiar Pigmented Cells Found in Two Mosquitos Fed on Malarial Blood" (Ross, 1897).

Appended to the article were favorable comments by Patrick Manson, who included some drawings of the parasites. Encouragement also came from Sir John Bland-Sutton, who was a distinguished London surgeon and a naturalist interested in malaria. He recognized the value of Ross's observations and wrote to the *British Medical Journal* supporting him (Bett, 1956). After years of laborious work Ross received a Nobel Prize for his findings. But continuing his report in the *Indian Medical Gazette*, he turned to avian malaria and wrote of his continued success "in producing these pigmented cells at will in grey mosquitoes by feeding them on birds infected by proteosoma, Labbé — a parasite very similar and close related to the haemamoebae of malaria in man. . . . There is no doubt then that these parasites are a development in the mosquito of proteosoma in birds" (Ross, 1898, p. 401). He continued with detailed descriptions of his experiments in birds. But quite independently and almost simultaneously, G. Grassi (1899) in Rome described the sexual phase of the malaria parasite in the mosquito in his beautifully illustrated monograph on malaria, which he dedicated to Patrick Manson. As a medical student at Johns Hopkins University, W. G. MacCallum (1897), a future professor of pathology in that institution, described the conjugation of male and female gametocytes in pigeon malaria.

Many investigators contributed to knowledge of the life cycle of the malarial parasite. Some were considered more deserving of the Nobel Prize than Laveran and Ross were. The sensitive Ross was scarred by the criticisms he incurred for not sharing the award with his friend and mentor, Manson. Others believed that Italian scholars should have been recognized. The controversy has been tempered by time but not resolved. Ross (1923) wrote almost bitterly of his feelings about the dispute, but he later paid tribute to Manson (Ross, 1930).

Knowledge of the role of the mosquito in the transmission of filariasis and malaria helped in the control of these diseases. Nevertheless Dr. J. D. Gillett (1973), writing with authority almost a hundred years after Manson's discovery, headed his paper with the title, "The Mosquito: Still Man's Worst Enemy." He stated that over a million and a half people in the world still died annually from malaria.

Reliable epidemiological statistics on the incidence and distribution of malaria in the world did not become available until the twentieth century. The disease has always had a severe impact on the efficiency of troops operating in endemic areas. F. H. Mowrey (1963) dates the military experience of the United States with malaria from the year 1776, when the Continental Congress ordered the medical committee to forward three hundred pounds of Peruvian bark to the southern department. During the Civil War one-half of the white troops and four-fifths of the black troops in the northern armies had malaria annually; in the Spanish-American War there were 90,461 hospital admissions for malaria, with 349 deaths.

In World War I and World War II the incidence of malaria in the United States Army was a study in marked contrast. During the first war, from April 1, 1917 to December 31, 1919 there were 15,555 cases of malaria with 36 deaths occurring in troops stationed in the United States, while only 950 cases were reported in Europe. This is a relatively low incidence among approximately four million participants.

During World War II, however, the attack rate of malaria in the United States Army was considerable. American troops were dispersed in many areas where malaria existed as a major endemic disease.[7] Such areas included the South Pacific Islands, the China-Burma-India area, North Africa, Sicily, and Italy. During the early battles in Guadalcanal in 1943 between the Japanese and Americans, there were 10,206 primary cases of malaria among American troops. The 1st Marine Division was ineffective for months because 80 percent of the command was hospitalized with malaria, an experience repeated in many other units. Malaria was particularly severe in the China-Burma-India Theater. In the North African Theater there were sixty-nine thousand cases during 1943–1944. "During the Sicilian campaign, the Seventh U.S. and British Eighth Armies lost, from malaria alone, the equivalent of . . . two infantry divisions" (Mowrey, 1963, p. 453). In summary, from 1942–1945 in the United States Army there was a total of 492,299 cases of malaria, mostly of the *vivax* variety. Fortunately the death rate was relatively low.

One of the distressing features of malaria control became apparent in the Korean war, 1950–1953. During World War II a tropical form of *vivax* malaria was encountered in the Southwest Pacific, whereas in the temperate zone of Korea a different form of *vivax* occurred (Alving, 1955). A characteristic of the clinical course in those infected with the latter type was an initial febrile attack followed by a long latent period of ten to eighteen months of good health and then a relapse. The attack rate of malaria in Korea was severe. In August 1951 there were as many as 629 cases a week, and this was reflected in the incidence of malaria in the continental United States. Until 1951 there were relatively few cases in the United States, but by that summer there were ten thousand cases, mostly among Korean veterans who had completed their tour of duty. Several of these veterans were encountered at the United States Veterans Administration Hospital in Minneapolis and at the University of Minnesota Hospitals. A consistent pattern was seen on the campus of the University in Korean War veterans who were back in school. During a summer of good health many of these men had a sudden onset of chills and fever, which was a relapse of *vivax* malaria. Some had no history of an initial attack because they had become infected in Korea while on suppressive antimalaria therapy. This sudden turn of events was recognized by the medical department of the United States Army. To combat the possibility of a relapse, every individual returning home after discharge from the army was given fourteen daily doses of primaquine. The program was successful (Alving, 1955).

It could have been predicted that malaria would be a military problem in the Vietnam War, 1964–1973. The incidence in United States troops was quite high, especially amongst those located in Vietnam central highlands, where 90 percent of the cases were due to *P. fal-*

ciparum. But *P. vivax* was responsible for 80 percent of the relapses that occurred in individuals after returning to the United States (Khan, Zinneman, and Hall, 1970). Figure 19 shows the distribution of military and civilian cases in the United States between 1959–1973 (Center for Disease Control, 1974c). Note that the number of civilian cases remained constant during that time. In 1973 there were 175 civilian cases, of whom only two had contracted their disease in the United States! One was the result of disease transmitted by a blood transfusion. The second case was a newborn infant treated at the University of Minnesota Hospitals, who contracted the illness con-

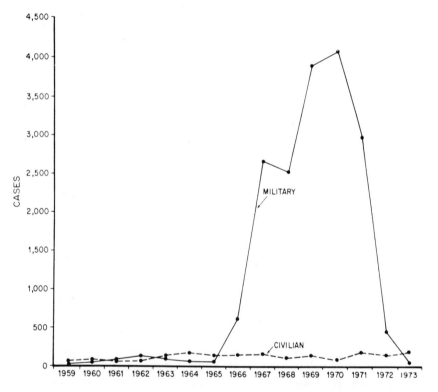

Figure 19. Military and civilian cases of malaria, United States, 1959–1973. Reproduced from Center for Disease Control Malaria Surveillance, Annual Summary 1973, issued August 1974. Center for Disease Control-Public Health Service, United States Department of Health, Education and Welfare, Atlanta, Georgia (Figure 1, p. 3).

genitally from its parasitized mother, the wife of a returned mission-ary.

The problem in the United States posed by relapsing malaria in Vietnam veterans is reflected in the experience at the United States Veterans Administration Hospital in Minneapolis (Khan, Zinneman, and Hall, 1970). Fifty patients were seen over a period of three years. The dominant feature in the relapses was that the prophylactic regime of chloraquine-primaquine for eight weeks had not been properly followed in these individuals. The majority of cases were of *vivax* origin and all responded to chloroquine-primaquine therapy, whereas the *falciparum*-resistant cases responded to a combination of quinine and other agents.

At the beginning of the twentieth century most of the fundamental knowledge on the transmission of malaria was known, but efforts to eradicate, or even to control, the disease were often ineffective. Again, the three major factors in the dissemination of malaria are individuals with parasitemia, the mosquito vector, and a susceptible population. Among the first major control programs were those in Cuba shortly after the Spanish-American War and in Panama during the building of the Canal. The only therapeutic and prophylactic agent at the time was quinine, which was and remains a valuable drug. With the passage of time intensive therapeutic regimes with newer drugs have aided considerably in eliminating the human sources of the disease in those with parasitemia.

Probably the most significant achievement in malaria control was the suppression of mosquitoes through massive drainage programs and the use of larvicides such as the lighter petroleum oils. This attack was accompanied by an intensive educational program to eliminate mosquitoes from living quarters through proper screening. The sus-ceptible population was partially protected with proper clothing and netting. The programs were stepped up in the southern United States during the economic depression in the 1930s through the Work Progress Administration (WPA) and through federal and state efforts connected with the electric power developments under the Tennessee Valley Administration (TVA). In the late 1930s state and county an-timalarial programs were accelerated in the south, resulting in large areas of environmental control of malaria.

The need for persistent vigilance in the control of malaria was dramatically emphasized in Brazil in 1930 when the dreaded mosquito vector *Anopheles gambiae* was introduced from Africa. This species is to malaria what *Aedes aegypti* is to yellow fever; knowledgeable people predicted that if *A. gambiae* were to be disseminated widely in Brazil and adjacent areas, serious epidemic disease and high mortality rates would ensue because *A. gambiae* fed largely, if not completely, on human beings and lived and reproduced near human dwellings.

These predictions were borne out. Large numbers of people were infected, and many died. Fortunately the International Health Division of the Rockefeller Foundation had successfully attacked the vector of yellow fever, *A. aegypti*, under the direction of such leaders as Dr. Fred Soper. The Rockefeller Foundation, in cooperation with Brazilian health personnel, waged a successful campaign against the vector and its breeding areas so that within a decade the morbidity and mortality rates of malaria rapidly declined (Soper and Wilson, 1943).

With the advent of World War II increased efforts were made to control malaria in the environment of Army training camps and bases and in adjacent communities. The Office of Malaria Control in War Areas was established in 1942 under the United States Public Health Service with headquarters in Atlanta. This program involved extensive drainage; the use of larvicides such as oil, Paris green, and DDT (chlorophenothane) in kerosene or as an emulsion; spraying of homes with DDT; and mosquito-proofing of buildings and homes. It is estimated that a hundred million dollars was disbursed over a decade for the control program, a small price to pay for a highly successful eradication effort compared with the sickness and disability that had afflicted millions of people.

All through the twentieth century attempts to control malaria involved administrative, educational, and technological factors requiring considerable financial aid. For this reason, at the time of the outbreak of World War II, success had been mostly limited to the subtropical and temperate regions. The war would be waged in many tropical areas, where malaria raged and control measures had never even been attempted. Doctor Mark Boyd (1939), the malariologist of the Rockefeller Foundation, remarked that knowledge of the control of malaria was at hand but that this information could not be applied in heavily infested areas because of primitive conditions. The inroads of malaria on the health of military personnel during World War II stimulated research and resulted in prophylactic and therapeutic advances, as well as in refined technological methods and new insecticides for breaking the transmission of the disease from human to human. This information was to aid the attack on malaria after the war, principally through the coordinated efforts of the World Health Organization, which will be summarized shortly.

For centuries quinine was used in both the prevention and treatment of malaria. The basis for its administration was empirical. Because quinine played such a major therapeutic role before the contemporary advances with other synthetic chemicals, the history of quinine is reviewed briefly here.[8]

In 1639 an Augustinian monk in Lima, Peru published a religious book containing this paragraph (Duran-Reynals, 1946, p. 24): "A tree grows which they call the 'fever tree' [árbol de calenturas] in the country of Loxa whose bark, of the color of cinnamon, made into powder amounting to the weight of two small silver coins and given as a beverage, cures the fevers and tertianas; it has produced miraculous results in Lima." In 1650 Peruvian bark was imported at Rome through a Jesuit priest, Cardinal De Lugo, and distributed among the people. It was also known as "Jesuit's powder" or "Jesuit bark."

Ague was rampant in England in 1650. But the possibility of importing quinine as a remedy was negated by Oliver Cromwell, the most influential person in Parliament, who was both anti-papist and anti-Spanish. He stated, "no one would undertake to bring into England a medicine coming from the Spanish colonies, sponsored by the Vatican, and known by the abhorrent name of the Jesuits' powder" (Duran-Reynals, 1946, p. 55). Ironically Cromwell died in 1658 of the ague. The story of quinine continues with Sir Robert Talbor, not a physician, but an out-and-out quack, who defied Galen and the British medical profession and successfully treated Charles II and the son of Louis XIV for ague with quinine. Thus quinine was introduced into Europe by two nonmedical men. A. W. Haggis (1941) has recently exploded the myth that the Countess of Cinchona, Spain, whose husband was Viceroy to Peru, was cured of malaria with quinine and was responsible for its introduction into Europe. The first wife of the Count of Cinchona died before he was appointed Viceroy, and it was his second wife who went to Peru with him. There is no mention of any illness or remedy in connection with the Countess in the official Diary of the Court. The Count's second wife never returned to Spain and died in Colombia in 1641. Thus she could not have brought the remedy to Europe and distributed it to the poor in her native country.

At the time of the outbreak of hostilities in World War II quinine was the most widely used antimalarial drug. After the Japanese Armed Forces had driven into the Southwest Pacific, however, the supplies of quinine were cut off and another drug or drugs became necessary. Out of a screening program in the 1920s for antimalarials in the famed research laboratories of the I. G. Farbenindustrie in Germany, quinacrine or atabrine, an acridine derivative had been developed. (This was the same laboratory that, a decade later, brought forth prontosil, the precursor of sulfanilamide.) Synthesis of atabrine on a large scale allowed its general use in military personnel in lieu of quinine in 1943. But it neither cured nor acted as a satisfactory prophylactic, and furthermore it was toxic. Chloraquine, one of the several of the series 4-aminoquinolines screened during the war, proved superior to atabrine and was especially effective in the treatment of the *P. falciparum* infections. Prophylactically chloroquine acted more as a suppressive than as a completely preventive agent. Unfortunately a significant number of *P. falciparum* strains became resistant to chloroquine.

Primaquine, another aminoquinoline derivative that was a result of wartime screening for antimalarials, is particularly effective for relapsing *P. vivax* infections. A more recent addition has been pyrimethamine, which is useful for the chloroquine-resistant *P. falciparum* infections. Chloroquine and primaquine have both been recommended as suppressive agents, but not to be administered simultaneously. The chemotherapy of malaria has been reviewed by G. Covell et al. (1955) for the World Health Organization. Under certain conditions combinations of drugs are recommended in the therapy of malaria. Sometimes quinine is used with another drug in patients with severe disease. Combinations are useful in infections due to chloraquine-resistant *P. falciparum* and in recurrent *P. vivax* infections (World Health Organization, 1967b; 1973). The several hundred cases of malaria that I observed in Guatemala in 1943 were due to *P. falciparum* and *P. vivax*, many of them of the chronic, recurring type, and were treated with combinations of quinine, atabrine, and plasmochin. I saw patients with black water fever, which is a dramatic complication of malaria, usually occurring in those with chronic *P. falciparum* infections being treated with quinine. There is a sudden massive hemolysis of erythrocytes with collapse and the passing of hemolyzed blood (black) in the urine.

Control programs for malaria call not only for the treatment of patients but also, in highly endemic areas, for the administration of selected drugs to every member of a given population, including children. In this manner the source of the disease, the individual with parasitemia, is brought under control (World Health Organization, 1973).

A significant factor in the control of malaria was the research on insecticides and pesticides that was conducted before and during World War II. The major insecticides were derived from two chemical groups: the chlorinated hydrocarbons, which included DDT, and the organic phosphorus series, including malathion and parathion. DDT had been synthesized in Germany in the nineteenth century, but in 1939 Paul Müller of Switzerland discovered the extraordinary features of DDT as an insecticide, for which contribution he received the Nobel Prize. During World War II DDT was highly effective as a powder in destroying lice; hence it was invaluable in the control of typhus. In this form it is nontoxic, since the powder form does not penetrate the skin. But when DDT is dissolved in oil it is toxic upon being swallowed or inhaled. It is fat-soluble and localizes in the fatty tissues of the body. DDT does not deteriorate, but remains active and toxic for long periods of time.

Mosquitoes and other insects are highly susceptible to the lethal action of DDT, which penetrates the cuticle and localizes in the central nervous system, resulting in paralysis of the extremities. When used as sprays in dwellings, the effective residue remains for a long time. Since DDT was so effective in small quantities, extensive aerial spraying was eventually carried out in malaria-control programs. DDT was distributed in waters and streams in the effort to destroy mosquitoes. Eventually the ecology was seriously disturbed and DDT was making its way into humans through water and food. Finally a sensitive and scholarly biologist, Rachel Carson (1962), published her volume, *Silent Spring*, which alarmed not only ecologists, environmentalists, and public health officials, but the general public as well. She inveighed against the pollution of the environment by DDT and other toxic pesticides with documented details. Not surprisingly she was severely criticized by the chemical industry and others, but she had made her point.

DDT was — and still is — an excellent agent for the eradication of the highly susceptible mosquito. But the indiscriminate use of DDT had to be stopped. The final outcome was that DDT was banned in many areas, especially in the United States. WHO experts were disturbed by the threat presented by the banning of DDT in highly endemic areas of malaria because of its effectiveness in the battle against the disease. It is an age-old story that the use of any prophylactic or therapeutic agent will lead to disaster if not properly controlled.

Other hydrocarbons, such as the chlorinated naphthalenes, found their way into chemical warfare against insects. These included dieldrin, aldrin, and the highly toxic endrin. Dieldrin was successfully used by WHO personnel in areas where DDT-resistant mosquitoes occurred. The toxicity of these agents is similar to that of DDT, acting on the central nervous system. Again these chemicals were extensively used, especially in crop control in agriculture. People began to be alarmed about the toxicity of such agents, and after it was found that cancer developed in experimental animals when they were exposed to the drugs, the sale and use of aldrin and dieldrin were prohibited by the Environmental Protection Administration of the United States on October 1, 1974.

The organic phosphates, including parathion and malathion are also highly toxic for insects, and they decompose rapidly after spraying. However, they do offer potential hazards.

It became apparent after World War II that malaria was destroying the health and lives of millions of people. If the disease were to be controlled, a centralized international organization would be necessary that would bring together the world's authorities for advice on dealing with the disease on an area basis. The World Health Organization was quick to respond to this challenge. The enthusiasm was so marked that a program defined by the Eighth WHO Assembly in 1955 had as its goal "the world-wide eradication of malaria" (World Health Organization, 1955, p. 31). For the following fifteen years the program was as follows (World Health Organization, Director General, 1972, p. 485): "A malaria eradication programme is divided into four phases: the preparatory phase, characterized principally by geographical reconnaissance and training of staff; the attack phase, during which total-coverage house-spraying or other attack methods are applied; the consolidation phase, during which total-coverage spraying has ceased and surveillance is carried out; and lastly, from the time malaria is eradicated in the country, the maintenance phase." The intensity of the program is reflected in twenty-two reports on malaria published before 1971 in the WHO Technical Report Series since 1950 (World Health Organization, 1972a). These include the reports of expert committees and major regional conferences.

The results were encouraging (World Health Organization-Director General 1972). By December 31, 1971, of the estimated 1,827 million people living in previously malarial areas, 1,346 million (74 percent) were in areas where malaria had been eradicated or eradication programs were in progress. Although progress had been considerable, there still remained large areas where malaria had not been restrained, especially in Africa. Nor was there any room for complacency once malaria had been subdued, as the example of Ceylon (Sri Lanka) illustrated. In that country, as a result of a vigorous campaign, there were only a hundred cases in 1963, but with relaxed programming more than a million cases occurred in 1968. Presently WHO officials and experts are taking a more realistic attitude toward malaria eradication. The hope for a world without malaria is a long way off.

Helminthic Diseases

The helminthic diseases, or illness caused by worms, constitute a major group of human parasitic diseases. From an etiological viewpoint these diseases can be divided into three main groups. The *trematodes* include the flukes that cause fascioliasis and schistosomiasis. Fascioliasis, due to the liver fluke *Fasciola hepatica* was recognized for centuries as "liver rot" in sheep, and its etiology challenged many zoologists and parasitologists. Since the affliction is not a common human disease, it is not reviewed here; but for those interested, such a presentation is available (Foster, 1965).

The second group of helminthic diseases are those due to the *ces-*

todes, or tapeworms, and include diphyllobothriasis (fish tapeworm), taeniasis (beef and pork tapeworms), and echinococciasis. The third group, due to *nematodes*, consists of diseases caused by roundworms such as ancylostomiasis (hookworm), filariasis, trichinosis, and ascariasis.

Schistosomiasis

Schistosomiasis [9] is a disease that has existed along the Nile Valley from very ancient times, as revealed by evidence found in mummies (Craig and Faust, 1945a). In 1851 Dr. Theodor Maximilian Bilharz (1852), professor of zoology at Cairo University, discovered in the mesenteric veins of an Egyptian the worms that cause the disease. Hence the synonym often used for the disease, bilharziasis.

Before World War I Lord Kitchener, the high commissioner of Egypt, recognized the serious nature of schistosomiasis in that country and recommended that measures should be undertaken to control the disease. Just before the outbreak of World War I investigators in Japan had defined the life cycle of *Schistosoma japonicum*. With the outbreak of the war, Lieutenant Colonel R. T. Leiper, a helminthologist at the University of London, headed a British Army medical unit to study schistosomiasis in Egypt. In an informative series of reports his group described the life cycles of *S. haematobium* and *S. mansoni*; identified the mollusca as the intermediary host; and recommended methods of prevention (Leiper, 1915–1918). Other extensive reports on bilharziasis have been documented (Khalil, 1931; World Health Organization, 1960).

The human schistosomes, which belong to the phylum of flatworms (Platyhelminthes) known as trematodes or blood flukes, consist of three species: *Schistosoma japonicum*, *S. mansoni*, and *S. haematobium*. They are distributed around the world in tropical and subtropical areas. *Schistosoma japonicum* is found in the Far East, *S. mansoni* occurs in Central and South America, and both *S. haematobium* and *S. mansoni* are widely distributed in Africa.

The life cycle of the schistosomes is complex. Man is the definitive host for the male and female worms, which localize and copulate in the vascular tissues of the intestinal tract and bladder. The ova or eggs are passed in the urine and feces. Largely through unhygienic practices and poor sewage disposal the freshly passed ova are transported to bodies of water used for bathing and drinking purposes. The eggs soon hatch out as *miracidia* or free-swimming organisms, which must find their way into a proper species of snails for further development. After four to eight weeks *cercariae*, or fork-tailed, free-swimming larvae emerge from the snails. Man contracts the disease while bathing in or drinking the polluted water, the *cercariae* penetrating the skin or mucous membrane and entering the bloodstream. After they enter the body, the larvae begin an odyssey through the bloodstream on the venous side, entering the right side of the heart and from there passing through to the pulmonary venules and going on to the left side of the heart. The larvae are then pumped into the arterial system, largely into the abdominal artery. Upon reaching the mesenteric artery, they travel to the portal circulation of the liver, where sexual differentiation takes place.

Traveling back against the liver bloodstream, the larvae find access to the mesentery veins and thence to the veins of the lower intestine and bladder, where they mature, copulate, and deposit their eggs. It is in these sites that inflammation occurs, which continues for long periods, inducing intestinal disorders with blood in the stools and inflammation of the bladder wall with the passage of bloody urine. The constant inflammation and proliferation of tissue are often associated with the development of carcinoma of the colon and bladder. Obviously, in traveling through such a circuitous route in the body, occasional larvae may localize in other parts, such as in the brain, causing neurological manifestations that simulate brain tumor. Chronic hepatic cirrhosis is a common complication. In recent years the pathogenesis of the disease has been approached through immunological studies. The clinical features are weakness, anemia, debilitation, and secondary complications from other diseases, all of which are described in any modern textbook of medicine. Pathological disturbances and the functional disability resulting from chronic disease have been described elsewhere (Mostofi, 1967). Diagnosis of the individual case is made by searching for the characteristic ova in the feces and urine. A simple procedure for detecting the ova in the tissues is carried out through a biopsy of the rectal mucosa.

Ever since World War II schistosomiasis has been of major concern to health authorities, especially the World Health Organization. The estimated number of cases in the world is between 150 and 200 million. The United States Army medical department had had little experience with the disease until the invasion of Leyte in the Philippines in October 1944. Many soldiers had contact with the parasite in the water and by 1946, thirteen hundred cases of *S. japonicum* infections had been diagnosed as a result of this campaign (Bang and Billings, 1968). Withdrawal from the areas of infection and prompt treatment resulted in recovery.

A little-known story of World War II involved the plans of Mao Tsetung's Chinese Communists to invade Taiwan. For this purpose thousands of carefully selected men were trained in the canals of China preparing for this invasion. The plan failed because the canals were infested with *S. japonicum* and between thirty and fifty thousand men became incapacitated (Kierman, Jr., 1959).

The incidence of schistosomiasis in developing nations has been influenced — unexpectedly — by large-scale engineering projects that disturb ecological relationships. Such a project in Africa is the Aswan High Dam on the Nile and the Lake Nasser Development Center. Before the dam was built, 14 million of 30 million people in the area had schistosomiasis; since its completion the infection rate along the new canals has ranged up to 80 percent (Sterling, 1972). The explanation is that the construction has introduced the intermediary snail hosts into new areas. Such construction is causing a serious threat in many areas from other diseases as well.

The control of schistosomiasis has posed a serious public health program because of the incredible financial burden, and because prophylactic measures for a mass population are inadequate (Ansari, 1973). Most advances in control have involved the use of molluscides for eradicating the snails in contaminated waters. These are effective and include niclosamide (an ethonolamine salt of 5, 2'-dichloro-4'-nitrosalicylicanilide), NaPCP (sodium pentachlorophenate), copper sulphate, and N-tritylmorpholine. The primary difficulty with these agents has been the expense in undertaking the necessary large-scale trials.

The treatment of the individual patient is based on another method for breaking the cycle of transmission. There is no question that proper therapy does restore a patient to health, as seen in the Leyte veterans. Trivalent organic antimonial compounds such as tartar emetic have been successfully used, but these drugs are toxic and must be administered intramuscularly and intravenously. I have treated sporadic cases, including returned missionaries and their families, and can attest to the difficulties attached to a long-range therapeutic program. What is really needed is effective oral therapy. Several nonantimony compounds are under investigation such as the thioxanthones, lucanthone hydrochloride, hycanthone, and niridazole. But toxicity continues to be a difficult problem. Because of the severity of schistosomiasis, WHO is encouraging further research on control and therapeutic programs.

Filariasis

Filariasis is a helminthic infection found principally in tropical and subtropical areas in Africa, and in the South Pacific regions. The disease is transmitted from man to man through several genera and species of mosquitoes. The acute disease is manifested by recurrent chills and fever and by visible swelling or nodules of the lymphatics and redness of the overlying skin due to parasitic involvement. The illness usually subsides gradually with or without therapy. But in those who have been repeatedly infected and are chronically ill, the inflammatory reaction and scarring of the tissues surrounding the vessels may impede the flow of lymph and blood, and mammoth enlargement ("elephantiasis") of the arms, legs, scrotum and breasts can occur. During World War II approximately fifteen thousand American military personnel became infected, but prompt withdrawal of these patients from the endemic zones prevented chronic disease and elephantiasis.

Filariasis was the first human disease described in which transmission through the skin was caused by the bites of arthropods. Doctor O. Wucherer (1868) found the embryonic filaria worms in the urine of a patient in Bahia, Brazil. T. R. Lewis (1872), working in India, observed the embryos in the urine and also in the blood, and Joseph Bancroft (1878) in Brisbane, Australia first described the adult worm. The parasite has been designated *Wuchereria bancrofti*.

The momentous discovery of the role of the mosquito in transmitting the disease was made by the Scotsman Patrick Manson (1877) while he was practicing medicine in the Far East with the Chinese

Imperial Maritime Customs. He became interested in the diseases that confronted him, including filariasis. In that disease he recognized the parasites in peripheral blood films and also in postmortem material. He noted the nocturnal appearance of the parasites in the peripheral blood and postulated that a blood-sucking insect might be responsible for transmitting the infection. Manson proved the presence of the microfilaria in the mosquito *Culex fatigans*, thus supplying the missing link in the life cycle of the disease. In his communication to the Linnean Society he chose the title, "On the Development of *Filaria sanguinis hominis*, and on the Mosquito Considered as a Nurse" (Manson, 1879). While at Amoy, China, he brought together his observations on filariasis in a well-illustrated volume (Manson, 1877). He carried out many other parasitological studies. After he returned to London he became a distinguished leader of tropical medicine and befriended young Ronald Ross in his studies on malaria.

Filariasis constitutes a severe health problem in the warmer climates. In 1974 it was estimated by WHO authorities that there were 250 million cases of the disease (World Health Organization Expert Committee on Filariasis, 1974). Control of the disease is dependent on the treatment of patients; hetrazan (diethylcarbazine) is highly effective. Also, as in malaria, mosquito control is essential.

Onchocerciasis

Onchocerciasis is due to the filaria parasite *Onchocerca volvulus* and is transmitted from man to man through the bites of the black flies of the family *Simuliidae*. Embedded in the subcutaneous tissue of the scalp and upper part of the body, the adult worms produce elevated nodules. Invasion of the bloodstream is not prominent, however, if it does occur. Blindness in chronic disease is the most serious complication, one that can usually be prevented by surgical removal of the nodules. A group from Harvard University made important studies on the disease in South America (Strong, 1938; Strong et al., 1934). The magnitude of the contemporary problem is emphasized by a report of the World Health Organization (1974b) to the effect that among the ten million inhabitants of the Volta River basin in East Africa, more than one million are infected with onchocerciasis, of whom many thousands have serious visual deficiency.

Trichinosis

Trichinosis is an interesting infectious disease, clinically and historically. It is due to the helminth *Trichinella spiralis*, which causes an acute febrile disease with gastrointestinal manifestations and painful muscles. It is usually transmitted to man through the ingestion of pork as well as the meat of black and polar bears and of the walrus, particularly when the meat has been improperly cooked. The encapsulated larvae are contained in the striated muscles of the infected animals. Refrigeration at 5° F. or −15° C. for 20 days destroys the parasite. The hog and black bear become infected through eating pork scraps in garbage and offal, but the route is not clearly known for polar bears or for the walrus. S. E. Gould (1970) has edited a monograph on the subject.

Trichinosis has been called a "medical student's disease" because several of the fundamental discoveries about it were made by students. James Paget, a medical student in London, first recognized the encysted larvae in the muscles of man during anatomical dissections when he was 21 years old. This discovery was first recorded by Richard Owen (1835), but Paget (1866) later related that he had first made the discovery and called this to Owen's attention. James Leidy (1846), an anatomist at the University of Pennsylvania, as an undergraduate student discovered the parasite in the muscles of the hog. The life cycle and the nature of the parasite were described by R. Leuckart (1860), R. Virchow (1864) and by F. A. Zenker (1866), who reported a fatal case in man. Thomas Brown (1897), as a student at Johns Hopkins University, first described the diagnostic importance of peripheral blood eosinophils in man, and Channing Frothingham, Jr. (1906), while a student at Harvard Medical School, recognized the disseminated nature of the infection in a fatal case. As cited previously (Section III, Chapter 20, page 351) I participated in epidemiological, clinical, and immunological research on the disease while a student at Harvard Medical School.

It was observed by German investigators that several epidemics of trichinosis had occurred in that country in the latter part of the nineteenth century. Largely through the efforts of Virchow, the government instituted methods for inspecting pork for the disease in 1866. In 1879 and 1880, the governments of Italy, Austria, Hungary, and Germany prohibited the importation of pork and pork products from the United States because of the danger of trichinosis. At that time such exports from the United States amounted to over 84 million dollars. The United States Congress was upset by this embargo, and the surgeon-general of the then United States Marine Hospital Service was directed by the secretary of the treasury in 1879 to investigate the presence of trichinae in American pork. This prompt report, prepared by Dr. W. C. W. Glazier (1881) of the Service, exonerated the meat producers. Later, when the Untied States Public Health Service was organized, this constituted the first scientific report of the Service and was given the title of "Public Health Bulletin No. 1 on Trichinae and Trichinosis." Fortunately the crisis quickly abated, to the economic advantage of the United States.

Trichinosis remains a threat to human health, largely because of negligence. The disease in the Arctic has been graphically detailed in the historically accurate novel *The Flight of the Eagle* (Sundman, 1970), which tells the story of a party of Scandinavian scientists who traveled to the Arctic in a balloon in 1897. All of them died after eating trichinous polar bear meat, their only source of food. Their frozen remains, preserved along with the frozen bear meat, still contained trichinella larvae when they were discovered thirty-three years later!

Hookworm Disease

This infection parasitizes up to one-fourth of the world's population, principally in the tropical and subtropical countries around the world. The disease has had a devastating effect on the social and economic welfare in the afflicted areas. Its control, the result in part of the cooperation of the Rockefeller Foundation with many public health agencies, has constituted one of the brilliant achievements in modern medicine.

Two species of the worm are *Ancylostoma duodenale* (European) and *Necator americanus*. Man is the natural host, harboring the adult parasites in the intestinal tract, where fertilization occurs; eggs are passed in the feces. The larvae develop in the soil and invade man, principally through the skin of the feet. Millions of people during the nineteenth and early twentieth centuries were afflicted by the disease in the southern United States, Central America, the Caribbean Islands, South America, Africa, the Pacific, and the Far East. The symptoms are weakness and lassitude from a severe iron-deficiency anemia due to the fact that the worms obtain their daily intake of blood from the gut. Hookworm disease is often compounded by severe malnutrition, particularly in children. A proper diagnosis is readily made by examining feces for the presence of the eggs.

Historically the disease was not recognized as an important clinical entity until 1880, when the Saint Gotthard Tunnel through the Alps was under construction. Thousands of sick Italian laborers were found to be harboring the worms. Diagnosis was simplified by identifying hookworm eggs in the feces, a procedure put forth by the Italian scientist known for his work on malaria, Giovanni Grassi (1878). The disease was also found in miners throughout Europe.

Definitive work on the life cycle of the parasites and on the disease was carried out by Dr. Arthur Looss (1901), a parasitologist in Cairo, Egypt. While working with a culture of hookworm larvae in the laboratory in 1898, he accidentally spilled the contents on his hands, where a dermatitis ensued. Subsequently he found hookworm ova in his stools. One of the cardinal signs of hookworm infection is a dermatitis between the toes due to contact with larvae in the soil that has been contaminated with human feces. Thus by a fortunate accident the life cycle of the parasites, as well as the pathogenesis of the disease, were determined.

Doctor Charles W. Stiles (1903), a zoologist in the United States Bureau of Animal Industry, discovered the American species of hookworm. Lieutenant Bailey Ashford (1900) of the United States Army had supplied Stiles with the specimens and had reported on the widespread presence of the disease in Puerto Rico. Doctor Maurice C. Hall (1921), another zoologist in the Bureau of Animal Industry, discovered that carbon tetrachloride, when administered orally to dogs, quickly exterminated canine hookworms. Even though the canine parasite does not cause disease in man, carbon tetrachloride was thus shown to be a potential therapeutic agent. Dr. S. M. Lambert (1941) of the Rockefeller International Health Board in the Pacific demonstrated that carbon tetrachloride was also effective in human hookworm disease.

During the first quarter of the twentieth century, then, the etiology, epidemiology, pathogenesis, clinical and laboratory findings, and treatment for hookworm diseases were established. These discoveries were associated with a worldwide campaign against the disease. In 1913 the Rockefeller International Health Board provided expert personnel and finances toward its control. Cooperating with the United States Public Health Service and the state health boards, the Rockefeller Board made extensive surveys of the population, an effort that was extended to other countries. Success was achieved largely through education about the spread of the disease. The threat posed by polluted soil was emphasized; one of the main results was the building of latrines and privies. Treatment was undertaken for the infected. The magnitude of the interest across the world in the disease is shown by the bibliography on hookworm disease accumulated by the Rockefeller Foundation International Health Board (1922) up to 1922, amounting to 5,680 references. Another 4,213 references were made available in a publication of the World Health Organization (1965). The story of hookworm control in the Pacific, under the auspices of the Rockefeller Foundation, has been engagingly written by Dr. S. M. Lambert (1941) in *A Yankee Doctor in Paradise*. In the technologically advanced countries hookworm disease has been largely eliminated, but it is still a major menace in developing areas.

Diphyllobothriasis

Because of their size and unique morphology, segmented tapeworms were recognized in the intestinal tract and feces of ancient man. Diphyllobothriasis is due to the fish tapeworm, *Diphyllobothrium latum*; the broad segments of this worm were a distinctive characteristic for early parasitologists. The fairly complex life cycle was not recognized until the nineteenth century, however. The eggs of the adult worm, residing in the human intestinal tract, are deposited with the feces in fresh water lakes, where the larvae are liberated. After the larvae pass through two intermediate hosts, *Cyclops* or *Diaptomus*, they are taken up by fish. Humans contract the disease by ingesting the larvae in insufficiently cooked fish. A widely known source of the disease is said to be the dish known as gefüllte fish. An outstanding clinical feature of the human disease is the appearance of megaloblastic anemia. Modern therapy depends mostly on the administration of niclosamide; the disease is prevented by the thorough cooking of fish.

It is often stated in textbooks that diphyllobothriasis is endemic in the Great Lakes region of Minnesota, Wisconsin, and Michigan. Experience at the University of Minnesota Hospitals, however, indicates that this is a rather uncommon form of tapeworm disease in this area. There is some evidence that the reservoir of the disease is in wild animal life, suggesting that diphyllobothriasis is one of the zoonoses.

Taeniasis

There are two forms of taeniasis. *Taenia saginata* is the cause of beef tapeworm disease, and *T. solium* of pork tapeworm disease. Humans are the definitive reservoir of these infections, with animals acting as intermediary hosts. Two stages of each of the diseases occur in the animal hosts. After the ingestion of larvae by the animals, the adult worms develop in the intestinal tract. In addition to the intestinal stage there is a larval stage, in which the parasite finds its way into the general circulation and localizes in various tissues and organs, especially the muscles, where encystment of the larvae occurs. People contract the disease through eating improperly cooked meat. The ancient Greeks, Arabs, and Jews recognized these parasitic diseases in animals, including the intestinal phase and the cystic stage; but it was not until the nineteenth century that the two were traced to a common source.

Beef tapeworm in humans exists only in the alimentary tract; a cystic stage rarely occurs. The symptoms are mild and indistinct, and the diagnosis is established by finding the segmented worms in the feces. The disease is relatively rare in the United States because of good animal husbandry. Less than 1 percent of cattle have been found infected by federal meat inspectors.

Taeniasis in man due to the pork tapeworm, *T. solium*, is a more serious infection because the encystment of larvae in the tissues (cysticercosis) occurs more frequently. Localization in the brain can cause epilepsy and the manifestations of brain tumor. During my student days I saw Dr. Harvey Cushing remove an encysted larvae of *T. solium* from the brain of a patient presumed to have had a malignant brain tumor. Calcified encysted areas due to *T. solium* have been demonstrated in X-ray films of patients residing in mental institutions. X-ray findings have also revealed such areas in the large skeletal muscles, especially those of the legs and buttocks.

Since man is the definitive host, both beef and pork tapeworm disease in animals are propagated by the dissemination of contaminated human feces in the feeding areas of cattle and swine. The incidence of the human diseases is thus related to the sanitary habits of people. Prevention of the disease involves careful disposal of human feces, proper examination of animals in abattoirs, and thorough cooking of meat.

Ascariasis [10]

Any primary textbook of parasitology includes a discussion of the common worm infections of enterobiasis or pinworm disease (*Enterobius vermicularis*), trichuriasis or whipworm infection (*Trichuris trichiura*), and ascariasis (*Ascaris lumbricoides*). The worms, especially *ascaris*, were known to the ancients, and the diseases abound in many areas of the world today where the climate is mild and where there is careless disposal of human feces. Man is the definitive host of these parasites.

Ascariasis is the more severe of these diseases. Large roundworms of *Ascaris lumbricoides* reside in the human intestinal tract, and ova passed in the feces contaminate soil, and thence water and food for human use. The ingested ova have a life cycle similar to that found in hookworm disease. After passage through the circulation via the portal system and the lungs, the larvae are coughed up, swallowed, and come to rest in the intestine, where they develop into adults. The cycle of further environmental contamination and infection is then repeated.

The disease is manifested by pulmonary symptoms during the early stages. In the later stages the large worms may cause intestinal obstruction and actually may perforate the gut, causing peritonitis. Exceedingly high incidences of the disease are found in children in some areas of the world due to contamination of the hands and ingestion of the ova. Several effective drugs for therapeutic and preventative purposes are available, including the widely used piperazine citrate.

CHAPTER 21

Infections Due to Fungi
and Actinomyces

The word "fungus" is derived from Latin and means "mushroom," while "mycology" is Greek and means "the study of fungi." Fungi include molds and yeasts, but the actinomyces are now classified as bacteria, which tend to form branching filaments. A typical fungus has a thallus with branching hyphae, called mycelia, although some nonmycelial forms do occur. There are at least a hundred thousand species of fungi. They are plantlike but possess no chlorophyll; for nutrition they utilize the organic material of decaying plants and animals, and the latter in turn is converted into humus. Fungi do not form roots, stems, or leaves. They reproduce by means of spores.

Fungi are the cause of many infectious diseases. Agostino Bassi (1835–36, translation 1958) described muscardine, a fungal disease of silkworms. This was not only the first discovery of a fungal disease, but, more generally, the first definitive evidence that a microbe caused disease. In the same period Professor Johann Schoenlein (1839, translation 1933) in a two-hundred-word report described favus, or ringworm of the scalp, also caused by a fungus. The history of mycology represents another one of those tantalizing mysteries of medical history in which a considerable lapse of time took place between the initial discovery of a scientific fact or technique and its application to further research. Leeuwenhoek had discovered the microscope in the seventeenth century, and in his letter No. 39 to the Royal Society of London had accurately observed and illustrated the microorganisms found in the scrapings of his teeth. And yet almost two hundred years elapsed before Schoenlein made the simple observation of examining the scrapings from the lesions of the scalp and identifying a fungus. Schoenlein's findings were confirmed by Dr. David Gruby (1842; 1844; Pusey 1933b) of Paris, whose work laid the foundation for future mycotic medical research. He identified the variety of fungi responsible for ringworm of the scalp and the beard, and described the trichophytons. Gruby's peregrinations from Hungary to Vienna and thence to Paris, and his professional life as a physician and scientist, have been described by T. Rosenthal (1932).

Mycology, something of a stepchild of medical science, was adopted by dermatology because of the concern within that discipline for superficial mycoses of the skin. Dermatology emerged as a medical specialty when Dr. Robert Willan (1809) issued the first volume of his work *On Cutaneous Diseases*, which attempted to classify diseases of the skin and included localized lesions as well as the exanthemata of the systemic diseases, such as scarlatina, erysipelas, and leprosy. Willan's volume was extended by T. Bateman (1813), but the contents were mostly descriptive and devoid of any knowledge of the underlying pathology. Almost a hundred years later Dr. J. F. Schamberg, a distinguished dermatologist of Philadelphia, published a widely-used textbook of dermatology and practically restated the basic thesis of Willan and Bateman as follows (1908, Preface, p. 9): "The study of dermatology in its broadest sense embraces the consideration of all morbid processes that are characterized by cutaneous manifestations. . . . The specialist in diseases of the skin should be skilled in the diagnosis not only of the ordinary dermatoses, but of the rashes of the various eruptive fevers."

Mycological investigations in dermatology were enhanced by the work of Ferdinand Hebra (1856–76; 1874–76) in Vienna, considered the founder of modern mycology, who incorporated a new nomenclature and classification of skin diseases in his textbook. Further advances included histopathological descriptions, especially by Paul Unna (1896) at Hamburg.

Fifty years were to intervene between Gruby's findings and the major work of Professor Raimond J. A. Sabouraud (1894a), who practically rediscovered Gruby. Sabouraud's great contribution was his precise delineation of the dermatophytes such as the Microsporum and Trichophyton species (Sabouraud, 1894b). He published a comprehensive volume on the fungus diseases of the skin with a historical review of the subject (Sabouraud, 1910). Every modern mycology laboratory utilizes the simple Sabouraud culture medium, which consists of glucose, peptone, agar, and water for growing fungi and identifying the morphological characteristics. Yet one finds only sparse reference to Sabouraud in histories of dermatology (Pusey, 1933b; Shelley and Crissey, 1953).

Mycologists, on the other hand, universally remember and respect Sabouraud. On the occasion of the Eighth International Botanical Congress in Paris in 1954, the International Society for Human and Animal Mycology was founded, and the society's annual journal was named "Sabouraudia." The preface of Volume I states (Gentles, 1961, p. 1):

The outstanding names in the history of any branch of science are not always those of the men who made the primary observations. The prevailing climate of opinion and the available techniques greatly affect the contemporary significance attributed to any novel discovery and the historical landmarks are frequently the reputations of subsequent workers who were men of their time, who showed singleness of purpose, and who crystallized ideas which were nearing supersaturation. Raimond Sabouraud, the French dermatologist, was such a man. In the early eighteen-nineties by re-making observations which had been on record for fifty years but not universally accepted he was able to silence finally the view that the association of fungi with ringworm was incidental. Using the recently developed pure-culture techniques he was able to establish convincingly the "plurality" of the ringworm fungi, and his medical training enabled him to integrate the mycological and the clinical aspects of ringworm.

Another distinguished scientist was Professor Emile Brumpt at the University of Paris. He was notable not only as a parasitologist, but also for his definitive work, *Précis de Parasitologie*, which was published in 1910 and incorporated over two hundred pages on mycology.

Mycology developed as a scientific discipline not so much in a medical context as it did through the disciplines of botany and agriculture. Because of the frequent failure of crops due to the destructive action of fungi, human health was indirectly affected. One need only recall Ireland's suffering in 1845–1847 when a fungus, *Phytophthora infestans*, destroyed much of the potato crop and led to half a million deaths and the migration of two million people. The devastating effect of fungi on fruit, vegetables, and cereal grains in the nineteenth and twentieth centuries provided a stimulus for further investigations.

Medical mycology continued to evolve slowly. Doctor Herbert Fox (1923), a physician and pathologist of the Zoological Society of Philadelphia, described fungal diseases in animals and in birds. A valuable contribution in medical mycology was a review of the literature since 1900, which appeared in the *Botanical Review* and was written by C. W. Emmons (1940), senior mycologist of the United States National Institutes of Health.

During my years in medical school, 1928–1932, mycology was brushed over lightly in the curriculum. J. G. Hopkins (1927), writing in Zinsser's *A Textbook of Bacteriology*, had 31 pages on the subject, and F. T. Lord (1928) devoted 7 pages to it in Cecil's *A Textbook of Medicine* for students and practitioners. But upon joining the faculty of the University of Minnesota in 1937 I found mycology a lively science in the college of agriculture and in the medical school. Professor Elvin Stakman, a distinguished plant pathologist, and his students were concerned with the problems of wheat rust caused by fungi, and Professor C. M. Christensen continued the tradition. In the medical school Professor Arthur T. Henrici (1930) stimulated the interest of many medical students in basic and medical mycology. His handbook on the subject, published in 1930, is a classic and has been revised subsequently by his students. The introductory chapter of the first edition is still valuable — and current — reading today. Later Professor Henrici, with Professor Selman Waksman (1943), defined the nomenclature and classification of the actinomyces.

Mycoses

There are about fifty potential fungal pathogens that can afflict man. The present discussion will concentrate on the more common superficial and systemic diseases as shown in Table 7. For additional information monographs and textbooks are available (Conant et al., 1971; Emmons, Binford, and Utz, 1970). Introductory works on mycology include the monograph for the general reader by C. M. Christensen (1961). There are sophisticated and detailed works for the advanced student (Ainsworth and Sussman, 1965 to 1973; Burnett, 1968). D. B. Louria (1967) has offered a helpful review of the literature for 1957–1967 on the pathogenesis, clinical manifestations, and immunology of the deep-seated mycoses.

The tabulated causative organisms have their reservoir in decaying organic matter in the soil *outside* man, except for *Candida albicans*, which is harbored by man. The dermatophytes, which cause the cutaneous infections, parasitize and reproduce in man, utilizing keratin for nutrition. These diseases can be transmitted from man to man or from animals to man.

Two species of actinomyces of medical interest are *Actinomyces bovis*, which is a facultative anaerobe and infects only cattle, causing "lumpy jaw"; and *Actinomyces israeli*, which is aerobic and is endogenous in the oropharynx of man, and which occasionally can infect cattle. The related *Nocardia asteroides* is aerobic, is found widely in nature, and causes systemic disease in animals and man, especially

Table 7. Mycoses

Type of Infection	Disease	Etiology
Cutaneous	Ringworm of scalp, glabrous skin, nails	Dermatophytes (*Microsporum* sp., *Trichophyton* sp., *Epidermophyton* sp.)
	Candidosis of skin, mucous membranes [of throat and vagina], and nails	*Candida albicans* and related species
Subcutaneous	Mycotic mycetoma (also actino-mycotic in origin)	*Madurella mycetomii, Allescheria boydii*, etc.
	Sporotrichosis	*Sporothrix schenckii*
Systemic	Histoplasmosis	*Histoplasma capsulatum*
	Blastomycosis	*Blastomyces dermatitidis*
	Coccidioidomycosis	*Coccidioides immitis*
	Cryptococcosis	*Cryptococcus neoformans*
	Aspergillosis	*Aspergillus fumigatus*
	Mucormycosis	*Mucor* sp., *Absidia* sp., *Rhizopus* sp.
	Systemic candidosis	*Candida albicans*

Source: Excerpted with permission of publisher and author from J. W. Rippon, *Medical Mycology. The Pathogenic Fungi and the Pathogenic Actinomycetes*, W. B. Saunders Co., Philadelphia, 1974, Table 1, p. 4.

chronic pulmonary infections simulating tuberculosis. A separate species, probably more invasive, is *Nocardia brasiliensis*.

Cutaneous Mycoses

The dermatophytes commonly cause uncomfortable and chronic skin inflammation, sometimes occurring in epidemic form (dermatophytosis), and the lesions are potentially dangerous, serving as a portal of entry for more pathogenic organisms such as streptococci and staphylococci. These mycoses have always offered a therapeutic challenge to the physician. E. L. Hazen and R. Brown (1950) isolated an antifungal agent, Nystatin, from *Streptomyces noursei*, which was used locally with some degree of success in ointments or solutions. It was too toxic for systemic administration. But the search for antifungicides continued. J. C. Gentles (1958), working in Glasgow, produced skin lesions in guinea pigs with *Trichophyton* species, and successfully treated the disease with an oral preparation of griseofulvin, which was derived from a *Penicillium* species. Subsequently this drug was effective in human disease (Anderson, 1965). In chronic nail infections (onychomycosis), griseofulvin does result in improvement but relapses do occur.

Candidiasis, due principally to *Candida albicans*, can be a severe and lethal disease. The organisms, harbored in the normal mouth, vagina, and intestinal tract, can give rise to localized inflammatory disease. Thrush in malnourished infants involves the mouth and nasal mucous membrane, often resulting in severe destruction of the tissues. Systemic candidiasis with invasion of the bloodstream has become a major problem, especially in hospitals. It is a severe handicap in post-transplantation patients and in open-heart surgery. Patients with immune deficiencies, either acquired or induced by immunosuppressive drugs, have become victims of the fungus. Localization of the monilia in the kidneys provides a severe prognosis, even with modern drug therapy. Implantation of the fungi on artificial heart valves or previously damaged valves causes a severe type of endocarditis, which has been cured only by removing the infected valves and replacing them with clean artificial valves. Pulmonary moniliasis is severe because of the invasion of the vascular walls of the bronchioles. Infusions of amphotericin B have been successful in some instances.

Amphotericin B was first isolated from *Streptomyces nodosus* and initially used as an antifungal agent for coccidioidomycosis (Littman, Horowitz, and Swadey, 1958; Vandeputte, Wachtel, and Stiller, 1956). Unfortunately the drug is toxic, causing damage to the renal tubules and nitrogen retention. Another handicap is that the agent must be administered for many days. Favorable results have followed the use of 5-fluorocytosine (Tassel and Madoff, 1968).

Subcutaneous Mycoses

(1) Mycetoma. Doctor H. Vandyke Carter (1861) at Bombay Medical College wrote a report on a new disease of India. His very interesting paper is significant in the history of medical mycology not only because his two cases represent the first description of mycetoma, but also because included is a letter from the Rev. M. J. Berkeley. Berkeley was England's most distinguished mycologist in the nineteenth century, and it was he who determined the fungal cause for the destruction of the Irish potato crop in 1845. Carter sent specimens of the fresh tissues to Berkeley at a time of long sea travel and poor refrigeration. Berkeley's response (Carter 1861), in which he described the results of his examination, should be read carefully because it expresses his striving for precision in scientific inquiry as well as his wide-ranging interest in new information.

Mycetoma is a localized swollen lesion, usually on a foot or hand, less often on shoulders, buttocks, head, or any site that has been subjected to trauma. It involves skin, subcutaneous tissue, fascia, and bone. The lesion contains granulomas and abscesses that suppurate and drain through sinus tracts (Rippon, 1974). The disease is not due to any specific species of fungus, since many different organisms can invoke the lesion. Mycetoma in man and animals is caused by *Actinomyces*, such as *A. israeli*, *N. asteroides*, *N. brasiliensis*, and *Actinomadura madurae*. About half are actinomycotic in origin; the other half are caused by *Eumycotic* organisms. Occurring primarily in the tropical and subtropical zones, it is also observed in the temperate zones. Secondary bacterial invasion often complicates the clinical picture. Treatment calls for antifungal therapy, including amphotericin B, and antibacterial agents, often to no avail. Amputation frequently becomes necessary in the more chronic cases.

(2) Sporotrichosis. B. R. Schenck published a report on subcutane-

ous abscesses and wrote as follows (1898, p. 286): "On November 30, 1896, A. W. presented himself at the surgical clinic of the Johns Hopkins Hospital with an infection of the right hand and arm of an unusual nature. The primary point of infection was on the index finger, whence it extended up the radial side of the arm, following the lymph channels, and giving rise to several circumscribed indurations, which were in part broken down and ulcerated." The patient had advanced pulmonary tuberculosis "refractory to treatment." We do not know what happened to the patient. Schenck was working in the pathological laboratory at Johns Hopkins, and he meticulously studied a fungus isolated from the lesions of the arm. The fungus proved to be the cause of sporotrichosis. His report contains excellent illustrations of *Sporothrix schenkii*.

There is little question that sporotrichosis was often overlooked in the past because of its confusion with tuberculous ulcers and lymphangitis. On May 26, 1904 Dr. E. P. Quain (1904) presented a paper at the North Dakota Medical Association on "Report of Six Cases of Tubercular Ulcers and Tubercular Lymphangitis of the Upper Extremity." He unknowingly described six cases of classical sporotrichosis, a diagnosis that was later correctly made. This confusion is further emphasized by the case report made sixty years after Quain's, in which a California rose gardener was thought to have had tuberculous synovitis for months until the correct diagnosis was made and proper treatment resulted in cure (Kedes, Siemienski, and Braude, 1964).

G. F. Ruediger, working in the North Dakota Public Health Laboratory, reviewed the status of sporotrichosis in the United States in 1912. "Ten years ago we were of the opinion that infection of the human subject with the sporothrix fungus was so rare as to be a pathological curiosity. At that time only three cases had been mentioned in the literature of America and no cases had been recognized in any other country . . . a total of 57 cases [has been] . . . observed [within the past decade] in the United States" (Ruediger, 1912, p. 193). He cited the relatively high frequency of the infection in the region of the upper Missouri Valley. D. J. Davis (1919), studying the beneficial effect of the iodides for treating sporotrichosis, carried out experiments in the rat and proved that the administration of potassium iodide was followed by prompt recovery. He suggested that the drug should be used in more chronic disease.

Sporotrichosis has now been recognized in many parts of the world. The most extensive number of cases in a single geographic area involved over twenty-eight hundred workers who had been preparing timbers for the gold mines of South Africa (Transvaal Mine Medical Officers' Association Proceedings, 1947). Although localized skin lesions are most common, attention has also been directed to involvement of the lungs (Baum et al., 1969). This possibility should be considered an occupational hazard to gardeners and agricultural workers.

Systemic Mycoses

(1) Histoplasmosis. While working in the Ancon Hospital in the Canal Zone of the Isthmus of Panama, Dr. S. T. Darling (1906) recorded the first case of histoplasmosis. He described a 27-year-old male patient in whom he initially considered the diagnosis of miliary tuberculosis. But in his report he cited the pulmonary lesions as pseudo-tubercles and called attention to the necrotic lesions in the liver, spleen, and lymph nodes with intracellular inclusion bodies. He called it a protozoan disease and named the etiological agent *Histoplasma capsulatum*. In a subsequent report he described the morphology of the parasite, called it a disease of the tropics, presented the clinical course, and pointed out that the lesions suggested those of kala-azar (Darling, 1909). Cecil J. Watson and W. A. Riley (1926) at the University of Minnesota described the first case of histoplasmosis in the United States, at first mistaken for kala-azar. The patient had lived for forty-five years in Minnesota and had not been exposed to kala-azar in an endemic area.

In the following years histoplasmosis was found to be widely distributed in the United States, and the calcified pulmonary nodules suggested healed miliary tuberculosis (Furcolow and Grayston, 1953). Furthermore the reservoir was in soil, and epidemics of respiratory disease with pulmonary lesions were traced to exposure to contaminated dust, especially that emanating from the sites of chicken coops and bird nestings.

W. A. DeMonbreun (1934) at Vanderbilt University first cultured and studied *Histoplasma capsulatum*. His pediatric colleague A. Christie called attention to the frequency of benign histoplasmosis and pulmonary calcification in children (Christie and Peterson, 1946). Amphotericin B has proved to be effective in the more severe cases with complications, such as meningitis. As will be noted later, the differential diagnosis between tuberculosis and a fungal disease often is quite difficult.

(2) Blastomycosis. In 1894 at a meeting of the American Dermatological Association in Washington, D.C., Dr. T. C. Gilchrist reported on a 33-year-old male patient seen at Johns Hopkins Hospital with an unusual proliferative facial eruption. He had been examined by Dr. Louis Duhring, a dermatologist in Philadelphia, who called it "a typical example of scrofuloderma," and he was sent to the surgeon Dr. William Halsted at Johns Hopkins. Histopathological sections of biopsied lesions did not appear to be tuberculous in origin. After consulting with Dr. William Welch, Gilchrist (1896) published the first report of blastomycetic dermatitis with excellent illustrations.

Two years later Gilchrist and W. R. Stokes (1898) published a second report on the same case. They had advanced their studies considerably in the interim by carrying out meticulous cultural and animal studies. They named the organism *Blastomyces dermatitis* and made a pertinent concluding statement (1898, p. 76): "It would be advisable to examine more carefully all tuberculous lesions of the skin, and especially those of tuberculosis verrucosa cutis, for the presence of blastomycetes. This can be readily and rapidly done by soaking the unstained sections in ordinary liquor potassae, when the organisms if present will stand out as doubly contoured refractive bodies." As in cryptococcosis, yeast-like forms of blastomycosis are present in the tissues of patients.

Blastomycosis appeared to be limited to the western hemisphere. Patients whom I saw with the disease and who were treated at the University of Minnesota originated from a focus in the northern part of the state. Although the disease is relatively uncommon, D. S. Martin and D. T. Smith (1939) at Duke University were able to collect a total of 347 cases from the literature, and included 13 of their own patients. They pointed out that sodium iodide caused marked improvement and recovery in the chronic facial cases. In the systemic disease, however, with involvement of lungs, bone, and the central nervous system, the mortality reached almost 100 percent. They considered that combined therapy with vaccine and iodide improved the prognosis.

Some recoveries from systemic disease occurred after the use of 2-hydroxystilbamidine, but the treatment of choice is now amphotericin B. The antibiotic saramycetin is being evaluated for the dermal lesions.

Adolpho Lutz (1908) and A. Splendore (1909) of Brazil have described a form of blastomycosis known as South American blastomycosis caused by *B. braziliensis*.

(3) Coccidioidomycosis. Dr. E. C. Dickson wrote on a new disease in California as follows (1937, p. 151): "A febrile disease which has been recognized in the San Joaquin Valley for many years has occurred so frequently that it is known locally as 'valley fever.' It is characterized by a cold or bronchopneumonia, often with a relatively high fever . . . the appearance of very painful erythema nodosum . . . and usually rather prompt recovery." He reported five cases with laboratory investigations and suggested the disease be named "coccidioidomycosis." Subsequently he described the granulomatous tissue reaction that occurred in the disease (Dickson, 1938).

Epidemiological studies revealed a high attack rate of the disease in the southwestern part of the United States, with most of the patients recovering (Smith, 1943). Occasionally patients developed a progressive pulmonary disease simulating tuberculosis, however. During World War II the morbidity rate was considerable in military personnel training in the southwestern desert area, although the disease was not severe. The etiological agent *Coccidioides immitis* is a dustborne microbe that enters the body through the respiratory tract. It is remarkable how brief an exposure in an endemic area will result in infection. M. J. Fiese (1958) has prepared an authoritative monograph on the subject.

An informative report on the disease was made in 1964 by Dr. Wendell Hall and his associates at the United States Veterans Administration Hospital in Minneapolis (Strom, Hall, and Casey, 1964). The disease is not endemic in Minnesota, and yet they had observed twenty cases since 1948. Four of the twenty patients died, one of disseminated disease and three of meningitis. The authors emphasized that the infection was frequently acquired elsewhere in the country by tourists visiting the endemic areas in the southwestern

United States, and recovery usually occurred without ill effects. For those with serious disease amphotericin B is the drug of choice. The prognosis is extremely poor in patients with disseminated disease and in those with meningitis.

(4) Cryptococcosis. Like blastomycosis, cryptococcosis is caused by an encapsulated yeast, in this case *Cryptococcus neoformans*. It has a predilection for the central nervous system and produces a chronic, and usually fatal, disease. The characteristic feature of the cerebral lesion is a lytic effect on the tissues with little inflammatory reaction. Therefore the cerebrospinal fluid reveals a high concentration of protein, but few cells. The principal reservoir is in pigeons, which contaminate the soil, where viable organisms may reside for long periods of time.

The first recorded case of cryptococcosis has an unusual history, which is not generally known. A 31-year-old female had multiple abscesses of the lungs, spleen, kidney, and bones, and died after a prolonged illness. Encapsulated yeastlike organisms were recovered from the lesions before and after death (Buschke, 1895; Busse, 1894). Before she died the isolated organisms, after being injected into her own skin, produced an inflammatory reaction. For many years the precise nature of this organism remained unknown, but a surviving culture was finally restudied by Rhoda Benham (1935) at Columbia University and identified as *Cryptococcus hominis*, and later defined as *Cryptococcus neoformans*.

The nomenclature of the disease and the causative organism remained in a confused state for a number of years. In Europe *Cryptococcus* was known as "European blastomycosis." J. L. Stoddard and E. C. Cutler (1916) reported on two cases of suspected brain tumor from the clinic of Dr. Harvey Cushing in Boston, for which the autopsy material suggested a fungus infection; but none were recovered for culture. The photographs of the cerebral sections provide beautiful demonstrations of the fungus within the brain. L. Frothingham (1902), also in Boston, had reported on a tumor removed from a horse in 1902 and had isolated a Blastomyces (Torula) from the lesion. J. L. Stoddard and E. C. Cutler injected Frothingham's equine culture into animals and reproduced the same type of lesion they had studied in the human. They named the organism *Torula histolytica*, and the disease became known as torulosis. The fungus produces a curious gelatinous mass within the tissues. An excellent monograph on *Human Torulosis* was written by Australian investigators (Cox and Tolhurst, 1946), and a definitive and well-illustrated volume on cryptococcosis was published by M. L. Littman and L. E. Zimmerman (1956). Neither the term torulosis nor the name *Torula histolytica* is in use today. Stoddard and Cutler had mistakenly interpreted the mucoid capsular material of the fungus as histolysis.

Cryptococcosis has also been called a signal disease, "malade signal," because the fungus invades the central nervous system with clinical manifestations in patients who have underlying debilitating diseases, such as Hodgkin's disease and chronic leukemia. An examination of cerebrospinal fluid in such patients may reveal the characteristic encapsulated *C. neoformans* when the fluid is stained with India ink and examined microscopically. Amphotericin B has been used successfully for meningitis and pulmonary lesions; 5-fluorocytosine has been administered with some degree of success.

(5) Aspergillosis. Many species of the *Aspergillus* group are widely distributed in nature and were the cause of the first human fungus diseases to be described. Virchow (1856) wrote a lengthy paper on human pulmonary disease due to aspergillosis. His illustrations show spores, mycelia, and hyphae. Animals as well as man were invaded by this "plant parasite." Shortly thereafter others described infection of the external ear by *Aspergillus* ("maladies de l'oreille"). Pseudotuberculosis in young pigeons was described as a "vegetation d'un champignon" with typical tuberculous granulomas, but the cultures revealed *Aspergillus fumigatus* (Dieulafoy, Chantemesse, and Widal, 1890). Pigeons were infected experimentally with this fungus. *Aspergillus* infection is one of the major causes of disease in birds.

Louis Renon, in a remarkable student thesis (1893) for the Faculty of Medicine of Paris on *Pseudo-tuberculose Aspergillaire*, described a large series of experiments in animals and defined the tissue reactions. Since this original work was written, about three hundred species of *Aspergillus* have been identified, and the fungus has been found in abundance in all parts of the world. Modern investigations have revealed that *A. fumigatus* is a common cause of pulmonary allergies, such as asthma, caused by the inhalation of spores. Disseminated disease is relatively uncommon and rarely the primary cause of death. Opportunistic infections caused by *Aspergillus* can be serious in debilitated patients, those undergoing organ transplantation, and those receiving immunosuppressive drugs and antibiotics. An informative modern review of aspergillosis has been made by Sydney M. Finegold and his associates (Finegold, Will, and Murray, 1959). A major development has been the elucidation of the role of the mycotoxins of *Aspergillus* in human and animal economy, as will be pointed out shortly. The treatment of aspergillosis is a surgical approach whenever feasible, and the use of amphotericin B. Nystatin has also been used locally with success.

(6) Mucormycosis. This mycotic disease is due to various species in the *Mucorales* group, found widely distributed in the soil, the spores being disseminated in the air. Its importance derives from the destructive inflammatory disease that involves the rhino-facial-cranial area, the skin, and the lungs. Two species are commonly involved, *Rhizopus arrhizus* and *R. oryzae*. The infection was probably known for many years before the nature of the disease was recognized. Recognition did not really take place until J. E. Gregory, A. Golden, and W. Haymaker (1943) reviewed the subject and called attention to three cases of brain and meninges involvement that had originated through orbital infections. All three patients had diabetes.

It is now generally understood that mucormycosis is a disease of debilitated individuals, especially those with diabetes, and those with leukemia and lymphoma. Malnourished children and adults also are susceptible. Surgery combined with amphotericin B has been effective.

The treatment of the systemic mycoses continues to be a challenge. Chronic suppurative lesions require surgical drainage. Doctor Robert Abernathy (1973) has written a contemporary review of treatment citing the drugs that can be used.

Diseases Due to Actinomyces

Actinomycosis

When A. T. Henrici introduced the subject of *Actinomycetes* in his manual he stated (1930, p. 234), "No group of microorganisms presents so much difficulty in classification as that now generally designated Actinomycetes." Henrici and Waksman were considered the leading taxonomists of mycology in the United States, and both labored hard for clarification. Responsible for *Actinomyces* in the sixth edition of *Bergey's Manual of Determinative Bacteriology*, they formulated a classification that clarified the subject (Waksman and Henrici, 1943). As an example of the difficulties encountered by experts, A. T. Henrici and E. L. Gardner (1921) cultured an organism from the sputum of a patient with chronic lung disease and described what they considered a new species of *Actinomyces*, calling it *A. gypsoides* because it appeared chalky white on culture. This acid-fast organism later proved to belong to *Nocardia*, however. C. H. Drake and A. T. Henrici (1943) in a definitive paper pointed out that although *Nocardia* and *Mycobacterium* are closely related culturally and morphologically, *M. tuberculosis* pulmonary disease could not be distinguished clinically from diseases of *Nocardia* origin, and there was no basic immunological activity that related these two acid-fast species. Clarification of the bacterial groups of *Actinomyces* and *Nocardia* has arrived only slowly.

Otto Bollinger (1877) first isolated *A. bovis* from a bovine lesion. The following year James Israel (1878, translation 1886), working in the Jewish Hospital in Berlin, described thirty-eight cases of human suppurative disease of fungal origin. The lesions were localized in the mouth and pharynx, respiratory tract, and intestinal tract. Shortly thereafter Israel isolated the organism *A. israeli* in pure culture. Confusion increased when Professor Edmond Nocard (1888), the distinguished French veterinarian, described a lesion in cattle in Guadeloupe called "farcin du boeuf"; the causative aerobic actinomycete was called *Nocardia farcinica*.

A few years later Hans Eppinger (1891) described pseudo-tubercles in abscesses of the human central nervous system due to what later became known as *Nocardia asteroides*. The designation *asteroides* was chosen because of the beautiful starlike growth of the culture on agar plates. Thus by the end of the nineteenth century the three principal species of actinomycetes of concern to clinicians had been isolated, grown, and identified. *Nocardia brasiliensis* was added later, largely because it appeared to be more pathogenic. With the passage of time more human and animal cases were encountered. The difficulty of identifying the isolated cultures led to taxonomic confusion, but this has gradually been clarified.

Actinomycosis is not a common disease in animals or man. In a comprehensive review on human infections the British surgeon Zachary Cope (1938) collected 1,330 cases from the literature. His review included a discussion of the cervico-facial, thoracic, and abdominal cases. Treatment consisted of multiple drugs, radiation, vaccine, and surgical intervention. It is difficult to ascertain the mortality rates from his review, but the outlook was most favorable in the cervico-facial cases, the most common form of the disease. Another review by an American surgeon at approximately the same time was by my colleague Dr. Owen H. Wangensteen (1936) at the University of Minnesota. He recorded the details of 30 cases. In the cervico-facial cases, there were 14 with 11 recoveries, while the thoracic and abdominal cases did poorly. Wangensteen emphasized the primary need for extensive surgical drainage and excision of necrotic tissues. These two informative reports appeared just before the antibiotic era and provided a basis for therapeutic evaluation of subsequent cases.

Except for the control of secondary infections, therapy with the sulfonamides was not very successful. Penicillin, however, and later chlortetracycline, proved to be beneficial. D. R. Nichols and W. E. Herrell (1948) at the Mayo Clinic reviewed the results with penicillin, in which 38 out of 46 cases recovered.

Nocardiosis

Nocardiosis has been extensively studied by L. A. Weed et al. (1955) at the Mayo Clinic and by R. Raich, F. Casey, and W. H. Hall (1961) at the University of Minnesota. The most common manifestation is pulmonary involvement, which may be associated with dissemination of the disease to other organs and tissues, including the brain. Pulmonary inflammation is readily confused with tuberculosis unless meticulous sputum studies are carried out. We have seen excellent results follow a course of intensive sulfonamide therapy, especially sulfadiazine. Ampicillin is also effective and may be combined with the sulfonamide.

The Mycotoxins

Fungi not only invade the tissues of animals and man, but they also produce toxins, the significance of which is just being realized. It has long been known that mushrooms belonging to the genus Amanita, especially *A. phalloides* and *A. muscaria*, are poisonous for man. In reviewing this subject William W. Ford concluded (1911, p. 317), "Poisonous fungi may be divided into three groups. A. Those containing poisons acting on the nerve centers. Example, *Amanita muscaria*. B. Those producing degenerative changes in the internal organs. Examples, *Amanita phalloides, verna*, etc. C. Those causing gastro-intestinal disturbances of a more or less violent character. Example, *Lactarius torminosus.*" Despite general health and food warnings on this subject mushroom poisoning of humans continues to occur.

The mycotoxins are being intensively investigated because of the startling revelations of their dangers to livestock and poultry, and possibly to humans. It has been known for almost a hundred years that moldy feed can have deleterious effect on animals, but no serious attention was aroused by these sporadic events. As C. M. Christensen and H. H. Kaufmann (1969) have pointed out, however, five thousand horses died in 1933–34 in Illinois from moldy corn disease; and in 1952–1953 fifteen hundred swine were poisoned in the southwestern United States with a mortality rate of 22 percent, with moldy corn again the cause. As a result of competent investigations by J. E. Burnside et al. (1957) in Georgia, causative mycotoxins were associated with *Aspergillus flavus* and *Penicillium rubrum*, especially the former. When toxins were prepared from the isolates and injected into healthy swine, horses, and mice, the animals developed hepatic necrosis and jaundice with a lethal outcome. These investigators cited a report by Gajdusek stating that the Russians had observed similar epidemic disease.

Still these revelations did not arouse general interest until the English disaster in turkeys (Christensen and Kaufmann, 1969). One hundred thousand turkey poults died suddenly in England in 1960. The cause was first suspected to be a virus or bacteria, but was finally proved to be due to a feed prepared from peanuts imported from Brazil, with contamination of the nuts by *Aspergillus flavus*. Because the *aspergillus* group appeared to be the chief offender the mycotoxins became known as "aflatoxins." Not only were Brazilian peanuts involved, but also some peanuts in the United States and elsewhere in the world; grain food was also implicated.

The occurrence of a biological catastrophe, especially when the possibilities of human disasters are entertained, usually arouses the attention of scientists. Between 1962 and 1969 almost a thousand papers were published on the aflatoxins. By 1964 an important International Symposium on Mycotoxins in Foodstuffs was held at the Massachusetts Institute of Technology (Wogan, 1965). By that time the mycotoxins had been extracted and identified chemically. But the most disturbing feature was that chronic ingestion of the aflatoxins in experimental animals resulted in carcinoma of the liver. The aflatoxins had proved to be carcinogenic. The story of aflatoxins was also soon recorded in a scientific monograph (Goldblatt 1969), and J. M. Barnes (1970) of the British Medical Research Council Toxicology Unit reviewed "Aflatoxin as a Health Hazard." Finally the American Veterinary Medical Association devoted an entire issue of its publication to twelve papers on "Mycotoxicoses of Domestic Animals" (Mycotoxicoses, 1973).

At this stage it is obvious that prevention of contamination of animal feeds by fungi is the key to the problem. But the health hazard resides not in the technically advanced countries but in the developing nations, where grains for human as well as animal consumption are known to be parasitized. "Like malaria, aflatoxin and other mycotoxins are the greatest hazard to those who live in countries least able to afford to take those measures needed to control it" (Barnes, 1970, p. 286). As in many other health hazards of microbial origin, the mycotoxins are of international importance. Fortunately scientists can and do reach across boundaries to exchange information on mutual human health problems.

Ergotism [1] (*Ignis sacer*; St. Anthony's Fire)

The fungus *Claviceps purpurea* parasitizes grains, especially rye, and reproduces as a red-purple spur at the tip of the stem. The fungus forms a number of alkaloids used medicinally, including those with the oxytocic property of inducing uterine contractions in pregnancy. It is the cause of a severe epidemic disease known as ergotism, which has occurred for centuries among people who eat rye bread. Rye is particularly parasitized because the flowers are open-pollinated and remain exposed to infection for several days (Christensen, 1961). Rye bread was a staple food of the poor in Europe. In France, Germany, and Russia the moist and prolonged foggy weather in spring lengthened the growth period of rye and offered more of an opportunity for contamination by the fungus. The plant infection usually resulted in a poor crop. Wheat was the preferred source for bread in England and among the upper classes. Since wheat is not parasitized so readily, ergotism was less prevalent among such people.

The historian Charles Creighton presented a lucid picture of ergotism (1891b, p. 54):

It is almost exclusively among the peasantry that symptoms of ergotism have been seen, and among children particularly. The attack usually began with intense pains in the legs or feet, causing the victims to writhe and scream. A fire seemed to burn between the flesh and the bones; and, at a later stage, even in the bowels, the surface of the body being all the while cold as ice. Sometimes the skin of affected limbs became livid or black; now and then large blebs or blisters arose upon it, as in bad kinds of erysipelas. Gangrene or sloughing of the extremities followed; a foot or a hand fell off, or the flesh of a whole limb was destroyed down to the bones, by a process which began in the deeper textures. The spontaneous separation of a gangrenous hand or foot was on the whole a good sign for the recovery of the patient. Such was the *ignis sacer*, or *ignis S. Antonii* which figures prominently, I am told, in the French legends of the Saints, and of which epidemics are recorded in the French medieval chronicles.

Ergotism was known as St. Anthony's fire during the Middle Ages, although erysipelas probably was occasionally included in the term. St. Anthony of Padua was the Saint of the Poor, and it was the poor peasants suffering from the disease who flocked to the shrine of St. Anthony for relief. Hans von Gersdorff (1517) in his *Field-Book of Wound Surgery* (Feldtbuch der Wundartzney) has a magnificent illustration of a victim appealing to St. Anthony (Figure 20). The person has lost a foot, and flames are shooting from his left hand.

The malady attracted notice and pity and is discussed in the old French legends of the Saints (Creighton, 1891b). These date back to 857 with epidemics cited from the tenth to sixteenth centuries. During the sixteenth and seventeenth centuries, however, extensive epidemics also occurred in Germany, Sweden, and Russia. Even modern epidemics have been reported from Russia in 1926, Ireland in 1929, and France in 1953.

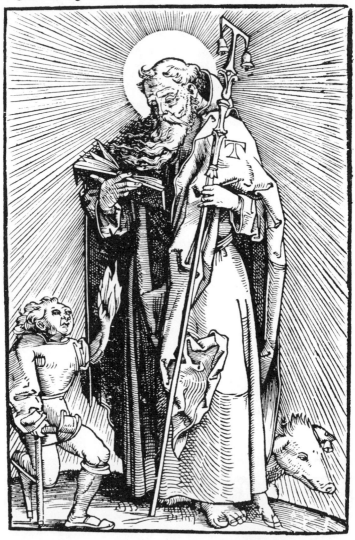

O heylger herr Antony groß /
Erwürb vns gnad on vnderloß /

Abloß der sünd / gots huld vñ gunst /
Behüt vns vor deim schweré brüst.

Figure 20. St. Anthony's fire or ergotism. Reproduced with permission of publisher from Hans von Gersdorff, *Feldtbuch der Wundartzney*, 1st edition, Strassburg: J. Schott, 1517, reprinted by Wissenschaftliche Buchgesellschaft, Darmstadt, Germany, 1967 (opposite p. 66).

Because of the feared toxic effects of ergot, recognition of its medical value was delayed in Europe. Since America used much less rye in the diet, ergotism was not an epidemic disease. For this reason the medicinal properties of ergot were accepted earlier. At a meeting of the Massachusetts Medical Society on June 2, 1813, Dr. Oliver Prescott presented a paper on the medical history of ergot, which was published and widely disseminated (Barger, 1931). Inspection of grain for human use by regulatory authorities has reduced the incidence of ergotism except for small, spasmodic outbreaks.

CHAPTER 22

Zoonoses

On December 11–16, 1950 a joint WHO/FAO Expert Committee on Zoonoses met for the first time to formulate guidelines on the interrelationships between human health and animal diseases. Zoonoses were defined as "those diseases which are naturally transmitted between vertebrate animals and man." This field was considered one of the major branches of veterinary public health, and the professional aim involved "all the community efforts influencing and influenced by the veterinary medical arts and sciences applied to the prevention of disease, protection of life, and promotion of the well-being and efficiency of man" (World Health Organization Expert Committee on Zoonoses, 1951, p. 3). A list of eighty animal diseases was formulated.

Nine years later the committee extended the list of zoonoses to more than a hundred (World Health Organization Expert Committee on Zoonoses, 1959). A third meeting in 1967 concluded, "More than 150 zoonoses are now recognized" (World Health Organization Expert Committee on Zoonoses, 1967, p. 7). Very likely the list will extend still further in later years.

The term *zoonoses* was first introduced by Virchow (1855) in a long discussion of the literature on the pathology of animal diseases transmitted to man. He emphasized anthrax and glanders, and the suppuration of wounds due to animal bites. Virchow was writing just before the discoveries made by Pasteur and Koch of the specific microbial causes of diseases. He brought together some of the empirical observations that had been made over the centuries, particularly those of wounds of animals and man caused by animal bites, which were often followed by local suppuration and even death.

Precise information about zoonoses was dependent largely on the evolution of veterinary medical science. Formal veterinary medical education remained undeveloped from the Roman period until the eighteenth century, when, because of severe epidemic diseases in animals in Europe, two veterinary schools — Lyons and Alfort — were founded in France. Other such schools soon were established in Berlin, Copenhagen, London, and Edinburgh. The first veterinary school in North America was the Ontario Veterinary College in Canada, founded in 1862. The first college of veterinary medicine in the United States was opened in 1879 at Iowa State College. Veterinary medicine was organized principally around the institutions serving agriculture and the mechanical arts that benefited from the Federal Land-Grant Act of 1862.

In the United States the forerunner of the veterinarian was the farrier, charged principally with the care and shoeing of horses. In 1792, by congressional authority, specially trained farriers were assigned to the United States Army as animal nurses (Miller, 1961). The slow evolution of veterinary medical care is underscored by the fact that in 1861, at the beginning of the Civil War, a total of $168.50 was allotted for civilian veterinarians in the quartermaster department of the Army. In World War II, however, there were 2,116 veterinary officers in the United States army with a supporting group of six to eight thousand enlisted personnel.

An early and vigorous advocate for a more scientific veterinary profession in the United States was Dr. Frank Billings, who had graduated from the Royal Veterinary Institute of Berlin. His volume on *The Relation of Animal Diseases to the Public Health, and Their Prevention* (Billings, 1884) reflected the German scientific and scholarly attitude at the time. His works suggest that he must have been an abrasive personality in American veterinary medicine. In rambling prose he castigated the veterinary profession for their scientific ignorance and for following the principles and teachings of human medicine, rather than developing their own discipline. Billings scolded his peers for naming diseases on the sole basis of clinical manifestations. Classification of disease, he maintained, should always relate to the causes. He interspersed scientific information on diseases with philosophical discussions of scholarly teaching, the proper selection of students for a school of veterinary medicine, and the contents of a curriculum for such a school. Billings provided detailed information on such diseases as trichinosis, bovine tuberculosis, anthrax, rabies, and glanders. His section on the history of veterinary medicine is informative.

The same year that Billings was attempting to arouse the veterinary profession to a more scientific approach, one of the most significant developments in veterinary public health took place in the establishment of the Bureau of Animal Industry in the United States Department of Agriculture. The first director was the veterinarian Dr. D. E. Salmon. Associated with him was the physician Dr. Theobald Smith. They were the first to use a heat-killed culture of bacteria (*Salmonella choleraesuis*) successfully for prophylactic immunization (Salmon and Smith, 1886). In later years the public health movement in the United States was greatly influenced by the brilliant scientists who followed Salmon and Smith. The annual reports of this bureau detail the research that led to the discoveries and recommendations for the control of the zoonoses.

Veterinary public health gradually became a specific discipline for the protection of human and animal public health (Steele, 1973). After World War II there was a growing interest in the zoonoses. Not only was this subject of concern to public health, but the economic costs of diseases in domestic animals were also recognized (Hambidge, 1942; Stefferud, 1956). A major symposium on the zoonoses in the United States pointed out that the estimated costs of these diseases to the livestock industry in 1942 amounted to almost a half billion dollars (Miner, 1947).

In more recent years investigations on the zoonoses were accelerated at state and national levels through the Center for Disease Control of the United States Public Health Service, coordinated with each of the state health departments. Periodic CDC epidemiological reports and recommended control measures on the zoonoses were issued, usually monthly. Internationally the World Health Organization and the Food and Agricultural Organization of the United Nations convened expert groups for the purpose of reviewing information and making recommendations on the zoonoses. International centers were established, such as the Pan American Zoonoses Center in Azul, Argentina, to serve the Americas, and the International Salmonella and Escherichia Centre in Copenhagen.

The subject of man and his pets is currently of growing concern in public health (Bisseru, 1967). In contemporary urban settings the range of pets varies from snakes and hedgehogs to lions. The magnitude of the pet problem from the viewpoint of health and economics is revealed in the fact that in the United States humans own 66 to 80 million pets. Whereas "approximately 415 human beings are born each hour in the United States, 2000 to 3500 dogs and cats are born" (Djerassi, Israel, and Jochle, 1973, p. 10). The threats to human health from pets include leptospirosis, toxoplasmosis, *Toxocara canis* disease, cat scratch fever, and rabies. "Costs incurred with rabies control, dog bite care, sanitation, and public health care related to dog- and cat-borne diseases amount to at least $50 million. . . . the annual total voluntary financial output for these pets now exceeds $4.5 billion." (Djerassi, Israel and Jochle, 1973, pp. 11–12). The authors recommend birth control for dogs and cats, but there is no other obvious solution to the problem.

By the 1950s interest in the zoonoses and in veterinary public health had expanded considerably. Authoritative monographs on the zoonoses demonstrate the increase in knowledge (Hull, 1955). There is also greater emphasis on infectious diseases in wild mammals (Davis, Karstad, and Trainer, 1970), and on the relation of the zoonoses to rural health (Meyer, 1956b). Calvin W. Schwabe (1969) has written a scholarly textbook on veterinary medicine as it relates to human health. Veterinarians, like physicians in human medicine, have entered a wide-ranging effort in basic research, as well as applied investigations in public health, the preservation of the health of domestic and wild animals, and problems relating veterinary medicine to agriculture. There has also been a recent resurgence of the discipline of comparative medicine, in which the basic knowledge and techniques of human and veterinary medical science are joined for a more comprehensive understanding of human and animal health and the nature of diseases common to both.

The diversity of the zoonoses is illustrated in Table 8. Calvin

Table 8. Zoonoses*

Viruses

Arbovirus infection
Influenza
Rabies
Lymphocytic choriomeningitis

Rickettsial Diseases

Murine (endemic typhus)
Rickettsialpox
Tsutsugamushi (scrub typhus)
Rocky Mountain spotted fever
Q fever

Bedsonia Infection

Psittacosis

Bacterial Diseases

Anthrax
Brucellosis
Salmonellosis
Leptospirosis
Tularemia

Protozoal Diseases

Leishmaniasis
   Kala-azar
   Oriental sore
   American
Trypanosomiasis
Toxoplasmosis

Helminthic Diseases

Echinococcosis
Trichinosis

---

*Because of the diversity of the etiology and epidemiology of the zoonoses, several listed in the table have been discussed elsewhere in the present study, as indicated in the index.

Schwabe (1969) has suggested a further classification of the diseases into the following four categories:

(1) Direct zoonoses that are transmitted from the reservoir to susceptibles by direct contact, fomite contact, or mechanical vector. These include rabies, trichinosis, and brucellosis.

(2) Cyclo-zoonoses, such as human taeniases and echinococcosis, which require in their cycle more than one vertebrate host species.

(3) Meta-zoonoses, which require both vertebrates and invertebrates; these include arbovirus infections, plague, and schistosomiasis.

(4) Sapro-zoonoses, such as larva migrans and some mycoses,

which have a vertebrate host and nonanimal reservoir (food, soil, and plants).

Rabies

No infectious disease has been feared more than rabies. Since the early Christian era it was recognized that a person bitten by a mad dog would develop foaming at the mouth and would inevitably die. People also believed that such victims of animal bites would develop hydrophobia, or fear of water; we now know that this happens only infrequently. It was also learned that there were other species of rabid domestic and wild animals and that the "poison" transmitted to man was contained in the saliva. It is difficult to ascertain the incidence of human rabies before the nineteenth century, but compared to the frequency of animal bites the number of cases was not large. The alarming feature was that the onset of human rabies, with its neurological manifestations, meant certain death. In any community the death of one individual from rabies excited the population at large.

One of the early prophylactic measures employed in human rabies after a person had been bitten by a rabid animal was the local excision and cauterization of the injured tissue. Doctor James Thacher (1812) of Plymouth, Massachusetts published a remarkable series of seventeen letters on rabies written to a friend. The concepts he articulated are twentieth-century in vision. As treatment he recommended the excision and cauterization of the wounded area. It is now known that not all humans bitten by rabid animals will develop rabies. And not all dogs roaming wildly about and biting people have rabies. Thacher suggested that a dog who had bitten a person should be incarcerated and observed rather than killed. He also recommended that a series of normal dogs should be inoculated with the saliva of a rabid animal, and that the injected areas should be excised periodically to determine how long the inoculated material would have to remain in place before a lethal illness ensued. Thacher implied that death might be prevented by early excision of the tissue around the wound, but that during the time the poison was allowed to remain in the tissues immunity against the disease would be acquired. He stated that he had patterned his thinking after Jenner as "an attempt to mitigate the horrors attending one of the greatest of all human calamities"

(Thacher, 1812, p. 301). Shortly thereafter the Swedish surgeon Baron Ekström (1830) described an "epidemic" of human rabies in Stockholm and commented on the value of excision and cauterization.[1]

Little progress was made on understanding the nature of rabies until the germ theory of disease had been established. Rabies had always been of great interest to Pasteur. "Amidst the various researches undertaken in his laboratory, one study was placed by Pasteur above every other, one mystery constantly haunted his mind — that of hydrophobia [rabies]" (Vallery-Radot, 1923, p. 390). Madame Pasteur, in writing to her children on May 20, 1884 about her husband's concern for rabies, stated (Vallery-Radot, 1923, p. 396), "The Commission on rabies met to-day and elected M. Bouley as chairman. Nothing is settled as to commencing experiments. Your father is absorbed in his thoughts, talks little, sleeps little, rises at dawn, and, in one word, continues the life I began with this day thirty-five years ago."

The most significant development in the twentieth century with respect to the control of animal rabies was a series of epidemiological studies on a worldwide basis, which were encouraged and aided largely by the World Health Organization. The studies involved seeking out the animal reservoirs of the disease and the means of transmission of the disease to other animals and humans. In describing the histopathology of the central nervous system lesions, A. Negri (1903) had provided a diagnostic criterion for establishing the disease in animals suspected of having rabies; this work was helpful in epidemiological surveys of the disease in domestic and wild animals.

Epidemiological information on the contemporary status of rabies in various parts of the world are contained in the reports of the World Health Organization — for example, in the fifth report of the WHO Expert Committee on Rabies (World Health Organization Expert Committee on Rabies, 1966). Extensive data for the United States are available in the surveillance studies of the Center for Disease Control of the United States Department of Health, Education and Welfare, such as annual summaries (Center for Disease Control, 1974d). An extensive and comprehensive description of the natural history of rabies is available (Baer, 1975).

There are two epidemiological forms of rabies: the urban type,

Table 9. Incidence of Rabies in the United States by Type of Animal, 1953–1973*

Year	Dogs	Cats	Farm Animals	Foxes	Skunks	Bats	Other Animals	Man	Total
1953	5,688	538	1,118	1,033	319	8	119	14	8,837
1954	4,083	462	1,032	1,028	547	4	118	8	7,282
1955	2,657	343	924	1,223	580	14	98	5	5,844
1956	2,592	371	794	1,281	631	41	126	10	5,846
1957	1,758	382	714	1,021	775	31	115	6	4,802
1958	1,643	353	737	845	1,005	68	157	6	4,814
1959	1,119	292	751	920	789	80	126	6	4,083
1960	697	277	645	915	725	88	108	2	3,457
1961	594	217	482	614	1,254	186	120	3	3,470
1962	565	232	614	594	1,449	157	114	2	3,727
1963	573	217	531	622	1,462	303	224	1	3,933
1964	409	220	594	1,061	1,909	352	238	1	4,784
1965	412	289	625	1,038	1,582	484	153	1	4,584
1966	412	252	587	864	1,522	377	183	1	4,198
1967	412	293	691	979	1,568	414	250	2	4,609
1968	296	157	457	801	1,400	291	210	1	3,613
1969	256	165	428	888	1,156	321	307	1	3,522
1970	185	135	399	771	1,235	296	252	3**	3,276
1971	235	222	484	677	2,018	465	289	2	4,392
1972	232	184	547	645	2,095	504	218	2	4,427
1973	180	139	488	477	1,851	432	170	1	3,698

Source: Reproduced from Center for Disease Control Annual Summary-Rabies 1973, Zoonosis Surveillance, issued July 1974, Center for Disease Control, United States Department of Health, Education and Welfare, Atlanta, Georgia (Table 1).

*Data prior to 1960 from USDA [United States Department of Agriculture], ARS [Agricultural Research Service]. Subsequent data from PHS [Public Health Service], CDC [Center for Disease Control].

**1 patient recovered.

existing principally in dogs; and wildlife rabies, especially in foxes, jackals, wolves, coyotes, skunks, mongooses, weasels, and bats. When the wildlife animal reservoirs become overpopulated, as in the mid-nineteenth century, epizootics of the disease occur in enzootic foci. This biological cycle was repeated in the mid-twentieth century in Europe, Asia, Africa, and North and South America. Because of the recent epizootics, surveillance studies have been intensified. The data for the United States for the period 1953–1973 are particularly revealing in depicting a decline in all animal reservoirs, except for bats and skunks, as noted in Table 9. The distribution of laboratory confirmed cases of rabies reported in the United States in 1973 is seen in Figure 21. Seventy-nine percent of the cases occurred in wild animals, and the remainder in domestic animals, with the exception of one human case. The incidence of human rabies in the United States between 1950 and 1973 is found in Figure 22. Fortunately, when an epizootic occurs in wildlife, the one or more infected overpopulated species are diminished through death from the disease. However, the overpopulated canines and felines in urban areas must be controlled through legislation and immunization.

In the 1973 annual summary of rabies in the United States (Center for Disease Control, 1974d), it was pointed out that although bat rabies accounted for only 15 percent of wildlife rabies, bat bites have been the most frequent source of human rabies since 1970. In 1929 an epidemic of ascending myelitis on the island of Trinidad involved seventeen humans, all of whom died (Hurst and Pawan, 1931). They were suspected of having Landry's paralysis, but histological studies revealed the cause to be rabies. Coincidentally in the same area since 1925 there had been a fatal epidemic disease in cattle, presumed to be

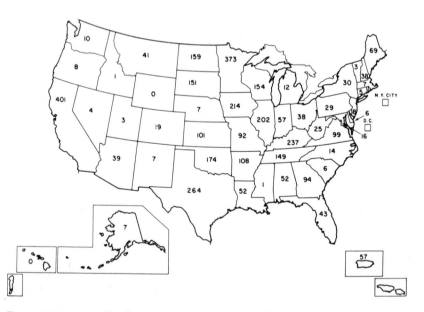

Figure 21. *Legend*: Confirmed rabies cases in the United States by state, 1973. Reproduced from Center for Disease Control Annual Summary-Rabies 1973, Zoonosis Surveillance, issued July 1974. Center for Disease Control, United States Department of Health, Education and Welfare, Atlanta, Georgia (Figure 2).

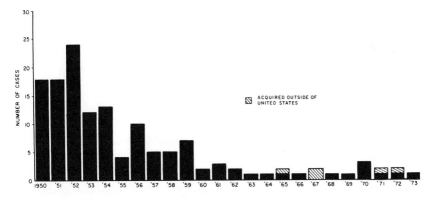

Figure 22. Reported cases of human rabies, 1950–1973. Reproduced from Center for Disease Control Annual Summary-Rabies 1973, Zoonosis Surveillance, issued July 1974. Center for Disease Control, United States Department of Health, Education and Welfare, Atlanta, Georgia (Figure 4).

botulism, but bovine rabies was also present. The vector for both the human and animal cases was unknown, but E. W. Haupt and J. L. Rehaag (1921), investigating a severe enzootic disease in cattle and horses that had occurred in Brazil since 1908, proved it to be rabies and suggested that the vampire bat was the vector. This bat was suspected through further studies in Trinidad (Hurst and Pawan, 1932), and finally this was proved (Pawan, 1936a; 1936b). By 1966 there were 160 human rabies deaths caused by the bites of vampire bats in six countries following the Trinidad outbreak (World Health Organization Expert Committee on Rabies, 1966).

The first report on the presence of rabid vampire bats in the United States appeared when a boy was bitten by such a bat and recovered following antirabies vaccine treatment (Venters et al., 1954). Under most unusual circumstances bat rabies was found in Minnesota.[2] On August 30, 1956 Dr. E. A. Rogers of the Nebraska Department of Health and Dr. James H. Steele of the United States Public Health Service were walking through the University of Minnesota campus while in attendance at a meeting of the State and Territorial Health Officers Association. They saw a living, but paralyzed, bat on the sidewalk and took it to the state health laboratories, where rabies was identified in the bat. The species was a hoary bat (*Lasiurus Cenereus*) found infrequently during the summer months in Minnesota while migrating from Canada to warmer climates.

A human case of bat rabies that attracted universal attention in the news media involved a six-year-old boy in Ohio, bitten by a bat on October 10, 1970. The bat was proved to have rabies, and although the patient was promptly given prophylactic vaccine he developed signs of rabies within three weeks. He was treated in an intensive care unit of a hospital and recovered. His recovery was remarkable because he was the first patient known to survive rabies after an illness of over a month.

The only case of human rabies acquired from a domestic animal in the United States between 1963 and 1974 occurred in Minnesota. A farmer was bitten by a stray cat on November 8, 1974; he began receiving prophylactic rabies vaccine on November 29, 1974. He died on January 15, 1975, and the presence of rabies virus in the brain was proved. The cat had escaped and could not be located.

The prevention of human rabies is dependent on the control of the disease in wild and domestic animals, including bats. Rabies can be controlled on a national basis; eradication of the disease has been accomplished in the British Isles, the Scandinavian countries, Australia, New Zealand, and the Hawaiian Islands. Animal rabies is common in Africa, Asia, and the United States, however. During the summer of 1963, 4,371 people in Rome were bitten by dogs known or suspected to be rabid (Bisseru, 1967). Control and eradication of the disease in wildlife and in bats are very difficult ecological problems and should be associated with intensive educational programs.

Prompt prophylactic vaccine should be administered to an individual bitten by a suspected rabid animal or by a bat. For those bitten about the face or neck, antirabies horse serum should also be used. Wherever possible, the suspected animal or bat should be observed, and after death a search for rabies virus and tissue lesions should be made.

Immunization of dogs and cats should be mandatory, and neither cats nor dogs should be permitted to roam urban areas. Stray dogs should be incarcerated. For economic reasons cattle should be immunized in certain areas of the world. In persons whose activities involve a high risk of acquiring the disease, preexposure immunization should be carried out; such persons include veterinarians, laboratory personnel working with rabies virus, dog handlers, and naturalists.

Lymphocytic Choriomeningitis

In 1925 the Swedish pediatrician Dr. Arvid Wallgren (1925) reported on a disease that he termed acute aseptic meningitis. The outstanding features were an abrupt onset of fever with meningeal signs and quick recovery. The cerebrospinal fluid showed polymorphonuclear leukocytes during the initial phase, followed by replacement with lymphocytes. Later this was also termed benign lymphocytic meningitis, a condition associated with several viruses, including poliomyelitis, mumps, Coxsackie, lymphocytic choriomeningitis, and the ECHO group of viruses. The virus of lymphocytic choriomeningitis (LCM) was first isolated from a monkey during studies of an epidemic of St. Louis encephalitis (Armstrong and Lillie, 1934), and subsequently from mice (Traub, 1935) and from human patients (Rivers and Scott, 1935).

The reservoir of the LCM virus is in mice, although epidemic human disease has also been traced to pet hamsters (Biggar et al., 1975). The number of reported human cases is not large, but the unusual pathogenesis of the disease in mice has excited the interest of many investigators (Volkert, 1965). The mouse disease has two distinct clinical courses, depending on the age of the animals. A vertical transmission of the disease to the fetus can take place either *in utero* or shortly after birth from a mother who has symptomless viremia. The offspring grow to maturity without any subsequent ill effects, but an abundance of LCM virus persists in the blood and tissues. No antibodies can be demonstrated, but mice are resistant to large challenge doses of virus. The state of host-parasite balance has been designated as acquired immunological tolerance to the virus. The second type of clinical course involves the primary infection of adult mice. Under these conditions the mice either die or recover. Persistent antibodies are found in the recovered animals as well as small numbers of virus in the blood and tissues. LCM virus is excreted in the urine of mice and is the source of human disease through direct or indirect channels of contamination.

Brucellosis

As people learned more about zoonoses in the twentieth century, it became apparent that brucellosis caused more human disability than any other animal disease. Brucellosis also caused severe economic losses in livestock, involving cattle, sheep, goats, and swine. Our investigations on this disease at the University of Minnesota have been summarized elsewhere (Spink, 1956).

Brucellosis must have existed for many centuries in the Mediterranean area, but the disease remained undifferentiated because human patients exhibited few distinguishing clinical characteristics. It certainly simulated two other common conditions, typhoid and malaria. For this reason many synonyms appeared that suggested a disease with the chief characteristics of weakness and fatigue, and an undulating type of fever. Some of the designations included intermittent typhoid, typho-malarial fever, Mediterranean fever, Rock or Gibraltar fever, Malta fever, Neapolitan fever, Cyprus fever, and undulant fever.

The identity of the common Mediterranean fever was established in 1887 by the young British Army surgeon David Bruce (1888).[3] Bruce was born in Australia but received his education in Scotland, graduating in medicine at Edinburgh. Shortly thereafter he married Mary Steele, the daughter of a successful Scottish physician. She was an artist, and she provided the illustrations for many of his scientific discoveries (MacArthur, 1955). Bruce decided on an army career and trained further at the military hospital at Netley. His first official assignment was in Valetta, Malta, where he first encountered cases of Malta fever. Possessed of a restless and inquiring mind, he discovered the bacterial cause of Malta fever when 32 years of age and called the organism *Micrococcus melitensis*. The species was later designated *Brucella* in his honor. Another young medical officer, M. Louis Hughes (1897), published a classical monograph on the subject when he was 30 years old.

Because brucellosis was a serious affliction of British military personnel, every effort was made by scientists and military administrators to gain knowledge of its epidemiology and the mode of transmission so that the disease could be controlled. For this purpose the Mediterranean Fever Commission was organized through the Royal

Society of London, including personnel from the British Army and Navy and the civilian Public Health personnel of Malta. Under Bruce's leadership this group prepared one of the most brilliant series of reports on the epidemiology of a disease in medical history (Great Britain Royal Society of London. Mediterranean Fever Commission Reports, 1905–1907). The reservoir of the disease was in the Maltese goat; human illness was contracted through drinking goats' milk. Goats' milk was promptly prohibited for use by British military personnel, and the incidence of the disease decreased dramatically. Bruce (1908) was so elated by the course of events that he delivered a paper on "The Extinction of Malta Fever." But other observers in the following fifty years did not share his optimism.

Shortly after the Commission on Mediterranean Fever carried out their investigations, a little-known practitioner, Dr. Paul Cantaloube (1911) in southern France, published a classic monograph on *La Fièvre de Malte en France* (Malta Fever in France). He reported on the clinical findings in two hundred cases occurring in epidemic form in 1909.

Brucellosis also occurs in domestic animals and can cause abortions in them. Such abortions had been known for centuries and were the cause of severe economic losses. Not long after Bruce made his discovery in Malta, Dr. O. Bang, a veterinarian in Denmark, announced the bacterial cause of contagious bovine abortion (Bang, 1897). The etiological agent was appropriately named *Bacillus abortus*, later *Brucella abortus*, and the disease in cattle was called Bang's disease. It was not until 1921 that human disease was traced to this source in Africa, and not until 1926 in the United States (Carpenter and Merriam, 1926). These findings of animal and human brucellosis rising from diseased cattle were to have widespread repercussions in the following quarter century. A. W. Stableforth (1959) has reviewed the brucella group and the veterinary aspects of the disease in several animal species.

A final major epidemiological work was on the isolation of *Brucella suis* from swine, by Jacob Traum in the United States Bureau of Animal Industry (Melvin, 1914). Chester Keefer (1924) reported the first case of human disease due to this porcine strain.

Before World War II public health officials, livestock producers, and veterinarians were increasingly alarmed about the serious nature of brucellosis in animals and in man. The League of Nations fostered a brucellosis research center at Montpellier, France supported by the Rockefeller Foundation under the direction of Dr. R. M. Taylor (Taylor et al., 1938). Serious efforts were made in the United States and elsewhere to control and eradicate the disease in the animal reservoirs. But the demands of the war for increased supplies of meat and animal products seriously intervened with practically all attempts to control the disease. During and after the war it had spread into new areas and had intensified in others.

Recognizing the threat of brucellosis to food supplies and animal health, the World Health Organization and the Food and Agriculture Organization of the newly organized United Nations set up expert committees to coordinate information on the disease and to make recommendations for eliminating it in animals. The activities of WHO and FAO through these expert committees can be found in the periodic reports that were issued (World Health Organization Expert Panel on Brucellosis, 1951, 1953, 1958, 1964, 1971). The United States took an active part in brucellosis control, largely through the United States Bureau of Animal Industry (1913), the United States National Institutes of Health (Hardy et al., 1931), and the recommendations of the National Research Council's Agriculture Board and Committee on Brucellosis. The Bureau of Animal Industry, under the leadership of Dr. B. T. Simms, was greatly responsible for the remarkable eradication programs that were organized in each state. The appeal for the support of programs had to be made along two lines, the economic gains to livestock producers and the protection of human health.

The cooperative pattern of the states and the federal government for the control of bovine brucellosis in the United States has been highly successful and has been carried out with modifications in other countries. Essentially the program has consisted of the serological testing of individual herds, the elimination of the positive reactors, and the vaccination of young animals. The vaccine, known as attenuated, live strain 19, *Br. abortus*, was introduced by the United States Bureau of Animal Industry (Graves, 1943). A successful program entails adequate public financial support, which fortunately was supplied by state legislatures and the federal government.

The control of brucellosis in sheep and goats at international levels has met with less success, largely because of inadequate financing. An effective, attenuated, live vaccine known as Rev. I has been developed, principally through the efforts of Dr. Sanford Elberg and his group at the University of California in Berkeley (Alton and Elberg, 1967).

The control of swine brucellosis still poses a major problem, though confined to smaller areas. No prophylactic vaccine is available. Human brucellosis from this source is limited to occupational groups, especially in meat-processing plants (Buchanan et al., 1974).

Wherever animal brucellosis is endemic, human disease occurs. Other reservoirs of animal species include caribou and reindeer in Siberia and Alaska, involving a *suis* species. Because brucellosis can cause a chronic and debilitating disease in humans, continuing for months and years, investigations have been directed at treating the acutely ill patient. At first a combination of streptomycin and sulfadiazine was used, with good results. This was later replaced by the tetracycline drugs, with or without added streptomycin (Spink, Braude, Castaneda, and Goytia, 1948; Spink, Hall, Shaffer, and Braude, 1948). Prophylactic vaccines for human use have been evaluated, but the side effects have thwarted continued application (Spink et al., 1962). It should be pointed out that only a very limited number of human infections have resulted from the prophylactic use of strain 19, *Br. abortus* in cattle. These infections have occurred in veterinarians or their aids who have been accidentally injected with the organisms while vaccinating animals (Spink and Thompson, 1953). The disease is short-lived and can be treated successfully with tetracyclines.

Two other brucella species have been recognized as causing animal brucellosis. *Brucella ovis* causes infection in sheep, especially rams (Buddle and Boyes, 1953). *Brucella canis* has caused widespread abortions in the beagle species in the United States, but rarely human disease (Carmichael and Kenney, 1968; Morisset and Spink, 1969).

Leptospirosis

Human leptospirosis is a spirochaetal disease caused by a variety of serotypes of the genus *Leptospira*. The characteristic clinical features are a sudden onset with a biphasic type of fever, the first phase enduring from three to ten days, followed by a remission for a day or two; and then another febrile period of two to four days, ending with convalescence. The course may be mild or severe, and even fatal. The manifestations include headache with meningitis, muscle aches, ocular lesions, skin eruptions, and jaundice. Because the organisms localize in the kidneys, albuminuria is common.

The natural reservoirs of the disease include domestic animals, such as cattle, swine, sheep, horses, and dogs; and wild rodents, including field mice, rats, and voles. Healthy animals excrete the leptospira in urine, contaminating the environment and water. The disease is occupational, affecting farmers, livestock personnel, rice field workers, those in abattoirs, and individuals working in and about sewers. Excellent reviews on leptospirosis are available and include those of J. M. Alston and J. C. Broom (1958), O. Gsell (1952), G. A. Edwards and B. M. Domm (1960), and the United States Army Medical Service Graduate School (1953).

The classification of the leptospira has been a taxonomic nightmare. A WHO expert group described 18 serogroups containing 130 serotypes (World Health Organization Report of a WHO Expert Group, 1967). However, the authoritative *Bergey's Manual of Determinative Bacteriology*, eighth edition, 1974, concludes that "strains of *Leptospira* cannot be accommodated satisfactorily and with confidence" (Turner, 1974, p. 192). Therefore two long-recognized "complexes" are used, the pathogenic group under *L. interrogans*, and the saprophytic group, *L. biflexa*.

Although a certain amount of taxonomic confusion does exist it is still possible to consider some of the clinical entities caused by recognized serotypes and thus to approach the history of the understanding of leptospirosis. For this purpose disease due to *L. icterohaemorrhagiae*, *L. canicola*, and *L. autumnalis* will be considered.

Professor Adolf Weil (1886) of Heidelberg discussed the clinical manifestations in four male patients with fever, jaundice, nervous symptoms, enlargement of the liver and spleen, and evidence of renal involvement. They all recovered. Weil did not determine the etiology, but he did express confidence in the conclusion that he had observed a new clinical entity; he distinguished it from that group of cases known as "epidemic jaundice," now recognized as the virus disease hepatitis-A. Japanese workers supported Weil's conclusion and were convinced from their own experience that "Weil's disease" was a distinct clinical entity (Ido et al., 1917; Inada et al., 1916). They succeeded in isolating a spirochaete from the blood of patients after it had been injected into guinea pigs. They reported that the rat was the reservoir for the disease. This disease is known as "autumnal fever" in Japan because of the annual appearance of the disease at that time.

In the twentieth century Weil's disease was recognized as existing throughout the world. During World War I it was reported among British troops fighting in the trenches of France, which were infested with rats. In the Fall of 1952 I observed an epidemic of Weil's disease in Barcelona, Spain. Most of the individuals affected had contracted the disease while working in the rice fields where the water had been contaminated with the urine of rats and mice. There were also some children with the disease who had become infected while playing and bathing around the sewer outlets of the city. No fatalities were seen. Penicillin was effective when administered early during the disease, at a time when leptospira were in the blood.

Recognition of the disease depends on modern bacteriological techniques of blood cultures during the first phase, and urine cultures during the second phase of fever. Serodiagnosis is also an aid. Preventive measures are largely educational and also involve rat control in abattoirs and around municipal sewers and garbage disposal sites. The disease is not common in the United States.

The sequence of events that led to the discovery of leptospirosis due to *L. autumnalis* in the United States constitutes an interesting tale in the modern history of infectious diseases. In 1942 an obscure form of fever with a rash over the pretibial area afflicted army troops at Fort Bragg, North Carolina. Forty persons became ill; all recovered. Attempts to obtain the etiological agent from the blood of the patients were fruitless. The disease could not be transmitted experimentally to human volunteers. W. B. Daniels and H. A. Grennan (1943) reported the clinical and experimental observations as "Pretibial Fever: An Obscure Disease." H. Tatlock (1947) thought a virus was the cause and found that the blood from one of the patients produced death in hamsters and a mild disease in guinea pigs and rabbits, and that the agent reproduced in embryonated eggs. He also successfully transmitted the disease to human volunteers. The agent was carried along intermittently in many laboratories after the initial epidemic. Finally investigators at the Walter Reed Army Medical Research installation reported on the isolation of *L. autumnalis* after several hundred previous passages in hamsters, guinea pigs, and eggs (Gochenour, Jr. et al., 1952). They also obtained the preserved blood specimens of chimpanzees injected with blood from patients (which had been studied by J. L. Melnick and J. R. Paul, 1948) as well as the blood of human volunteers who had been injected by Tatlock. Serological evidence of *L. autumnalis* was found in both the human and the chimpanzees' blood.

Leptospirosis in dogs was first recognized in Holland when a specific strain was implicated (Schüffner, 1934). It had become known in Europe as "Stuttgart disease" and also as canine typhus. Human disease due to this strain was first identified in Europe in 1937 and in the United States in 1941 (Ashe, Pratt-Thomas, and Kumpe, 1941). Karl Meyer and his group in California (Meyer, Stewart-Anderson, and Eddie, 1939) estimated that up to 25 percent of dogs were infected with *Leptospira canicola*, a finding suggested by investigators in Minnesota (Stavitsky and Green, 1945).

Although a relatively high incidence of canine leptospirosis does appear to exist, the number of recognized human cases is small. This is borne out in the report of the first human case in Minnesota by R. T. Pearson and W. H. Hall (1952). In their review they emphasized the difficulties in diagnosing the sporadic case. Jaundice and meningitis were not prominent features. It is possible that an acute febrile disease due to *L. canicola* is readily overlooked, terminating rather quickly in recovery either spontaneously or with the aid of antibiotic therapy.

In 1951, as a consultant for the World Health Organization, I witnessed in Rijeka, Yugoslavia an epidemic disease known in Europe as "Swineherd's disease" or "maladies des porchers." The outstanding features were an acute onset of fever with severe headache, weakness, conjunctivitis, and meningitis. Jaundice was unusual, and recovery occurred within two weeks. Most of the patients were male farmers. The apparent reservoir of the disease was in swine, although cattle and horses have also been implicated.

The disease was first recognized in a dairy farmer in 1937 in the town of Pomona in Australia (Clayton and Derrick, 1937). In the next few years it was found in Europe. After my experience in Yugoslavia I visited Professor O. Gsell (1952) of Basel University in Switzerland, who had studied 217 cases of *L. pomona* human disease. He pointed out that the tetracycline drugs were quite effective therapeutically during the first stages of the disease.

Upon returning to the University of Minnesota with this newly acquired information I saw an employee of an abattoir who was thought to have brucellosis, but who in fact had aseptic meningitis. I was mindful of L. *pomona* disease, and investigations proved this to be the first recognized case of that illness in Minnesota (Spink, 1952a). P. Beeson and his associates (Beeson, Hankey, and Cooper, Jr., 1951) had reported the first human infection in the United States from Atlanta; a waterborne epidemic in Mississippi with swine as the source had also been described (Schaeffer, 1951).

Although leptospirosis appears to be widespread in domestic and wild animals, the true incidence in the human population is difficult to ascertain. Probably many cases remain unrecognized, terminating uneventfully, with or without antibiotic therapy. Over a period of several years fewer than a hundred cases a year have been reported for the United States.

Tularemia [4]

In spite of the similarity between tularemia and plague, which will be described shortly, the present discussion of tularemia has been placed with the zoonoses. The etiological agent of tularemia has been a taxonomic puzzle. It was first called *Bacterium tularense*, then *Pasteurella tularensis*, and is now known as *Francisella tularensis*. The basic knowledge of the nature of tularemia is due principally to the personnel of the United States Public Health Service, and especially to the dedicated efforts of the bacteriologist Dr. Edward Francis.

The discovery of tularemia grew out of apprehension over plague following the San Francisco earthquake in 1906. A significant number of human cases of plague appeared in and around that area. Doctor George McCoy (1911) of the United States Public Health Service was assigned to direct a plague laboratory in San Francisco, and, as a result of investigating rodents, reported on a plaguelike illness in ground squirrels. He later described the disease as being due to *Bacterium tularense* (McCoy and Chapin, 1912). The first proven human case of tularemia was described by W. B. Wherry and B. H. Lamb (1914) at the University of Cincinnati. This occurred in a meat cutter, working in a restaurant, who had an ocular lesion. He probably contracted the disease dressing rabbits, which are highly susceptible to the disease (an epidemic appeared among rabbits in Ohio). Since then it has been well established that ocular tissue can be infected directly by contaminated fingers.

But the natural reservoirs of the disease and the modes of transmission remained to be worked out, and it was Dr. Edward Francis of the United States Public Health Service who directed the studies. A debilitating disease was known to afflict the ranchers and farmers in the Pahvant Valley adjacent to Delta, Utah. For years the disease in this area was called "deer fly fever" because it was presumed that the blood-sucking fly commonly seen on horses conveyed the illness to man. Doctor R. A. Pearse (1911), a local medical practitioner, had described six human cases, which constituted the first description of the disease in the literature. In 1919 Dr. T. B. Beatty, state health commissioner of Utah, requested aid from the United States Public Health Service in studying the disease. Dr. Francis was assigned from the Hygienic Laboratory, the precursor of the National Institutes of Health. A field laboratory with appropriate experimental animals was established.

Two comprehensive reviews of the important contributions made by Francis and his associates are available. The first is a monograph, *Tularaemia Francis 1921. A New Disease of Man*, consisting of eight papers and published as a bulletin by the Hygienic Laboratory (Francis, 1922). The second is a comprehensive review in a single paper (Francis, 1925). DeKruif (1928) has presented a description of the man, his methods of work, and his accomplishments.

Francis pointed out that the major reservoir is in several species of wild rabbits, and also ground squirrels in California. The disease is transmitted from rabbit to rabbit by a rabbit tick and a rabbit louse, neither of which bites man. Man is infected by direct contact with infected rabbit tissues, through the skin and gastro-intestinal tract, and — rarely — through the conjunctivae. Man is also infected by the wood tick *Dermacentor andersoni*, which can transmit the bacteria transovarially to the progeny, and by the deer fly. Francis also described the highly infectious nature of *tularens*. He himself, along with several other laboratory workers, contracted the disease and suffered from prolonged physical disability. Diagnostic bacteriological and serological procedures were also perfected. Francis and his colleagues concluded by saying that the disease was widespread in the United States but had not been reported from other countries.

The clinical features of the disease are fundamentally two types of illness. The first, the ulcero-glandular form, consists of a localized ulcerating lesion, usually of the finger, as a result of handling infected tissues, and enlargement of the regional lymph nodes, particularly axillary. The natural course is usually uncomplicated, and recovery ensues. The second type resembles typhoid, usually tickborne, and often without a localized lesion. Toxemia is prominent with generalized weakness. Pneumonia and pericarditis are severe and lethal complications. Convalescence is prolonged, often requiring several months.

During the 1930s and 1940s I attended several outpatient cases of the ulcero-glandular type of tularemia at the University of Minnesota Hospitals. Most of them occurred in housewives and hunters who had handled infected rabbit carcasses. The second and more severe form, seen usually in the spring and summer, was tickborne and had lethal complications of pneumonia and pericarditis. No specific therapy was available. *Francisella tularensis* is highly infectious in the laboratory, but I never saw a human-to-human infection, even though attendants dressed suppurating wounds and nurses cared for patients with pneumonia. I was unable to obtain any information about such transmission at the time from authorities on the disease.

Further studies revealed a widespread distribution of the disease in the United States, and a wide range of possible reservoirs, including rodents, carnivores, ungulates, birds, and arthropods. The cottontail rabbit is the most important reservoir in the United States. Infected carcasses contaminate waters, so that the disease has been described in beavers (Jellison et al., 1942) and in muskrats (Young et al., 1969). An epidemic in Vermont in 1968 involved forty-seven cases among people who had trapped or handled muskrats.

The incidence of the disease in the United States from 1950 to 1973 is shown in Figure 23. The majority of 171 cases in 1973 occurred in Arkansas and Oklahoma. In Minnesota between 1930 and 1945 there were 430 cases with 28 deaths, mostly traced to cottontail and snow-shoe rabbits. Between 1960 and 1973 there were only nine reported cases and no deaths. As is generally the case, a high incidence of

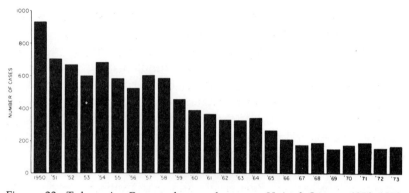

Figure 23. Tularemia. Reported cases by year, United States, 1950–1973.
Reproduced from Weekly Report for Year Ending December 29, 1973,
Reported Morbidity and Mortality in the U.S., Volume 22, No.
53, July 15, 1974. Center for Disease Control, Atlanta,
Georgia (p. 57).

human disease can be associated with epizootics in nature; but as the
wildlife population is decimated by the disease, the incidence of
human disease diminishes.

Since tularemia was first described, it has been recognized in many
other countries. First described in Japan by Ohara (1930), the disease
is known there as "Ohara's disease." The disease has been controlled
in many large areas by natural ecological factors, as discussed above,
and through public health educational programs that warn hunters,
campers, and housewives about the reservoirs of the disease and the
mode of transmission. Fortunately streptomycin is a specific and effective therapeutic agent.

Toxoplasmosis

Toxoplasmosis is one of the most challenging of all the zoonoses
because of its widespread distribution. It constitutes a notorious
example of lifelong intracellular parasitization of the healthy human
host. Although 30 to 35 percent of adult populations in the United
States are infected, the incidence of recognized active disease is small
(Feldman, 1968).

Two forms of the disease are encountered, the congenital infection
and the acquired type (Krugman and Ward, 1973d). Infection of the

infant occurs *in utero* as a result of parasitemia in the mother. The classical clinical picture in early life is that of a generalized infection with involvement of the central nervous system, revealing chorioretinitis, cerebral calcification, and hydrocephalus or microcephalus. One hundred and fifty cases of this type have been reported in the United States (Eichenwald, 1957). The acquired type, which occurs in later life, manifests itself with fever, a generalized rash, lymphadenitis simulating infectious mononucleosis, gastrointestinal manifestations, myocarditis, and pneumonitis. Extensive reviews and symposia on the subject have been presented by H. A. Feldman (1968), D. Hentsch (1971), and J. Siim (1961).

The etiological agent of toxoplasmosis is *Toxoplasma gondii*, an obligate intracellular protozoa. The parasite can successfully invade and remain viable in every cell in the human body with the exception of the erythrocyte. C. Nicolle and L. Manceaux (1908) discovered the parasite in the *gondi*, a small African rodent. In the same year A. Splendore (1908) in Brazil isolated the organisms from a rabbit. A. B. Sabin and P. K. Olitsky (1937) obtained *T. gondii* for the first time in the United States from a guinea pig at the Rockefeller Institute for Medical Research, and A. Wolf and D. Cowen (1937) reported the first human infant with the disease.

Toxoplasma gondii is found in a wide range of wild mammals, birds, and reptiles throughout the world, and in domestic species, including cats, dogs, sheep, goats, swine, cattle, rabbits, rats, guinea pigs, and chickens. The oocysts of *T. gondii* can remain viable in the soil for several weeks, and mice have been successfully infected. An exciting aspect of recent epidemiological studies involves the cat as a major reservoir. The ova of the feline nematode *Toxocara cati* becomes parasitized through the ingestion of *T. gondii* cysts in contaminated food, and the ova passed in the feces of the cat can remain viable for months under proper conditions (Hutchison, 1967).

Many cases of toxoplasmosis in infants have been reported, but the disease is relatively rare in adults. This discrepancy between widespread infection and active disease is difficult to comprehend. It is likely that many cases of toxoplasmosis are not recognized. Diagnosis depends on the Sabin-Feldman dye test, which denotes past infection, and on the complement-fixation test with a rising titer that occurs during an acute attack (Sabin and Feldman, 1948). Reports of adult cases have been so uncommon that up to 1953 only five cases were known; then R. C. Sexton, Jr., D. E. Eyles, and R. E. Dillman (1953) reported the sixth case.

When Dr. Anne Kimball worked in the laboratories of the Minnesota State Department of Health, she supervised the diagnostic screening of thousands of persons for toxoplasmosis, and we at the University of Minnesota Hospitals sought her aid in suspected cases. In this manner congenital infantile cases were recognized, and adults with chronic inflammatory ocular lesions, pneumonitis, and lymphadenitis were correctly diagnosed. It is little wonder, then, that when she went to New York Hospital in 1963, toxoplasmosis was recognized there. In fact, carrying on with her interest, she examined the blood of three thousand pregnant women with the Sabin-Feldman dye test and found antibodies in 32.8 percent! In 1965 six adult cases were reported from that source, and in 1969 a unique epidemic of the acute disease was described (Jones, Kean, and Kimball, 1965; Kean, Kimball, and Christenson, 1969). Five medical students became ill within the same week and complained of fever, headache, myalgia, lymphadenopathy, splenomegaly, and laboratory evidence of acute toxoplasmosis. This report, which reads like a medical saga, cited raw hamburger as the probable cause: "On March 5, a prominent surgeon gave an address at Cornell University Medical College to an overflow crowd. All five students [the patients] ate hamburgers at the dormitory snack bar on that night, prior to attending the lecture. Many students have reported that no matter how the hamburgers are ordered at this snack bar they are almost always served rare; on this particular night, because of the crush, the meat was very rare indeed" (Kean, Kimball, and Christenson, 1969, p. 1002). This was the apparent source of the epidemic. Toxoplasmosis has been traced to raw pork containing the *T. gondii* oocysts, but hamburger is usually prepared from beef, which has been an unlikely source of toxoplasmosis. There is always the possibility that beef hamburger has been contaminated in the grinder that is also used for pork, however. In fact, while investigating the source of human trichinosis several years ago, my colleagues and I suspected hamburger that had been prepared from beef as the source. But a health officer told us, "When beef is high (in price), and pork is low, the latter is 'boot-legged' into the beef." In relation to the Cornell-New

York epidemic of toxoplasmosis it is of interest that in 1965, G. Desmonts et al. (1965) found a rising incidence of toxoplasma antibody titers among children in a tuberculosis institution where raw or undercooked meat was served to the patients. The incidence was five times that which was anticipated.

There is an increasing incidence of active adult disease arising from other sources. This increase of active disease is caused by endogenous latent parasitization of the tissues activated by immunosuppressive chemotherapy for transplantation and malignancies (Reynolds, Walls, and Pfeiffer, 1966; Theologides, Osterberg, and Kennedy, 1966).[5]

There is an urgent need for more intensive epidemiological studies for a disease having such a high incidence in humans, so that preventive measures can be undertaken. Prolonged administration of pyrimethamine (Daraprim) and sulfadiazine has led to improvement in acute cases.

Echinococcosis[6] (Hydatid Disease; Hydatidosis)

Echinococcosis is due to the larvae of the tapeworms *Echinococcus granulosus* or *E. multilocularis*. The former causes cystic, expanding lesions of the lung, liver, and abdominal cavity, whereas the latter has invasive and destructive capacities for tissues.

Echinococcal cysts were known to the ancient Greeks and Romans. The identity of *E. granulosus* was established in 1786 by August Johann Georg Carl Batsch, and *E. multilocularis* in 1863 by R. Leuckart (Craig and Faust, 1945b). The life cycle of the *E. granulosus* tapeworm is usually a sheep-dog cycle, with man contracting the disease from sheepdogs. Cystic disease in sheep is the source of infection for dogs — the canine ingests the discarded viscera of slaughtered parasitized sheep. Mature adult tapeworms develop in the intestine of the dog, and infective ova are passed in the feces.

Man acquires the disease through the ingestion of food or drink contaminated with the ova. The eggs hatch in the human duodenum, and larvae enter the bloodstream and localize in the liver and lung to form encapsulated cysts, which enlarge. The inner membranes of the cysts produce budding daughter cysts and fill with fluid. Symptoms are due to the pressure of an expanding lesion, usually in the liver; or the cyst may become secondarily infected with pyogenic bacteria, producing the signs and symptoms of a hepatic abscess. On occasion a cyst may rupture into the abdominal cavity, thus producing additional cysts, or the escaping cystic fluid may provoke fatal anaphylactic shock due to the acquired hypersensitivity to the hydatid antigen. Sometimes the cysts become fibrotic and calcified, evidence of which can be detected by X-ray. The diagnosis of echinococcosis is established by skin tests and by serological reactions with purified hydatid antigen (Casoni, 1911–12; Kagan et al., 1966).

Although sheep and dogs are the source of most human and animal infections, other reservoirs include cattle, pigs, and jackals. *Echinococcus granulosus* has been described in moose in Minnesota (Riley, 1933), and has been identified in deer and coyotes in California (Romano et al., 1974; Schwabe et al., 1972).

The life cycle of *E. multilocularis* involves the red fox (*Vulpes vulpes*) and the arctic fox (*Alopex lagopus*), with the cystic stage occurring in wild rodents (World Health Organization, 1959). The cycle in man is similar to that of *E. granulosus* except that no encapsulating cyst membrane is formed, and therefore growth does not take place inside the inner membrane but extends like a destructive malignancy into the liver, lung, and even into the bone.

While the incidence of human echinococcosis in general is not large, endemic foci with high rates have been associated with sheep-raising areas such as New Zealand, Australia, the Mediterranean countries, Iceland, Argentina, and Uruguay. In a period of almost forty years I did not recognize a case at the University of Minnesota Hospitals. Previously I had seen three patients with fatal cystic disease of the liver at the Boston City Hospital. I reviewed the cases treated there between 1916 and 1936 and found a total of eleven patients, all of them adults, nine of whom had hepatic involvement with death occurring in four of the eleven. All had apparently ac-
 ᵈ their disease in other countries, especially in Italy and in
 At that time I was informed that human echinococcosis was
 ᵉd in the United States. T. B. Magath (1937) at the Mayo
 ʰed an important paper on cases originating in Canada
 ᵈ States, however. There had been documented cases
 ᵉs as early as 1822 (Low, 1822). K. D. Fairley (1922)

reported that three hundred patients with "hydatid disease" had been seen at the Melbourne Hospital in thirteen years.

I have been in two areas where the disease was quite prevalent — Uruguay and Alaska. In Uruguay there was a sheep-dog cycle, while in Alaska the arctic fox-dog cycle prevailed. Disease due to *E. granulosus* in Alaska is milder than in other parts of the world (Wilson, Diddams, and Rausch, 1968). Illness caused by *E. multilocularis* also occurs in Alaska.

Specific therapy for echinococcosis is lacking. Surgical drainage and meticulous extirpation of cysts offer the best approach in severe cases. But control measures in animals have been quite successful in preventing human disease, especially in Iceland, New Zealand, and Tasmania. The disease has been eradicated in Iceland, where until 1880, 15 to 20 percent of human autopsies in Reykjavik had revealed the presence of cysts (World Health Organization, 1967c). Since 1900 only one known case has been identified. "An intensive 27-year educational campaign in Iceland prior to institution of specific control measures was responsible for a dramatic drop in human infections" (p. 77), and "a detailed health education booklet on echinococcosis prepared in 1864 and distributed to all families in Iceland was repeatedly read aloud in practically all rural households" (p. 125). A major factor in controlling the disease in various parts of the world has been an intensive educational program on the manner by which the disease is transmitted from animal to man and from animal to animal. Vigorous legislative steps begun in 1959 have contributed to a marked reduction in New Zealand (World Health Organization, 1967c). Before the campaign the canine infection rate was 18.5 to 37.3 percent, and by 1965 this had stabilized at about 1.3 percent. Dogs with the intestinal worms were treated with arecoline hydrobromide. An informative symposium on echinococcossis was sponsored by the World Health Organization (1968a).

CHAPTER 23

What of the Future?

In the history of the control of infectious diseases, the establishment of specific microbial causes of infections was essential for advances in therapy and prevention. This achievement has had its greatest impact in the period since World War II. A second factor in this history originated in the earliest of civilized societies. The compassion of man, ruthless as he was at times, moved him to aid the poor and the sick, an impulse that became part of many religions. This human factor flowered in the nineteenth century in the form of private and public philanthropy toward the alleviation and prevention of disease. The acquired wealth in a highly profitable industrial society, along with discerning political leadership, was channeled into the public health movement at local and national levels, culminating finally in the World Health Organization in the twentieth century.

The future of infectious diseases should be considered from two viewpoints. First, what is the outlook in those countries where the control has been most successful? And second, what can be accomplished in the less fortunate areas? Modern science has emphasized the unity of all life at the molecular level. There is also a social unity in the sense that all persons must join in a cooperative endeavor to maintain good health. An outbreak of influenza, cholera, or smallpox in any area is a potential threat to the rest of the world's population.

Maintaining the present status of disease control has become a paramount responsibility of the state. All health science resources

440

must be part of that effort. Freedom from contagious diseases in any community is contingent on preventive medicine, which is in turn dependent on a competent system of public health and on an enlightened public. This concept must be emphasized at all levels of health science education, and people should be informed as to why good public health programs are necessary, and why they cost so much. High priorities should be given to proper sewage disposal, clean water for human use, uncontaminated food, and adequate living and working environments. Intensive immunization campaigns with prophylactic vaccines must be continued.

In the foregoing pages the magnitude of the success that can be obtained, especially in the control of some major pandemic diseases and of the contagious diseases of childhood, is revealed in the reduction of morbidity and mortality rates. At the beginning of the twentieth century infectious diseases headed the list of the major causes of death in the United States, afflicting especially the young and the old. No statistic is more revealing than the fact that the life expectancy of the average male in 1900 was around 45 years, and in 1975 it was over 70 years. On the other hand, an increasing population of persons of advanced years has caused serious socioeconomic problems. Doctor R. N. Butler, director of the United States National Institute on Aging, stated in 1975 that there are "well over twenty million people over 65 years of age in the United States, comprising 10 per cent of the population. . . . In 1900 only three million, or 4 per cent of the population, were 65 and older" (Butler, 1975, page 16). Undoubtedly the numbers will increase in the future. Not only has this population shift severely challenged the health resources of the United States and other countries, but the proper care of older citizens has seriously strained the economy and constitutes one of the top priorities in government circles at all levels.

Turning to more specific immediate and future matters, prophylactic vaccines and therapeutic chemicals and antibiotics will offer continued help in the control of infectious diseases. The pandemic diseases subject to quarantine control include smallpox, typhus, yellow fever, cholera, and leprosy. It is now reasonably certain that smallpox will be completely eradicated in the near future, following the intensive campaign of universal vaccination under the direction of WHO. Typhus and yellow fever are sequestered in small pockets in the world, and experience has revealed that epidemics can be controlled and prevented through immunization and the use of pesticides and insecticides. Cholera will continue to smolder, principally in healthy carriers. It is doubtful that the widespread use of vaccines will eradicate the disease. Cholera originates chiefly in water contaminated by human feces, and only continued surveillance of water supplies and the prompt recognition of the disease will prevent epidemics. Leprosy is not highly contagious; immunization does not appear to be a method for controlling the disease. The most promising hope for success in eliminating leprosy lies in the availability of an animal model for studying the disease, for isolating and growing the microbes in large quantities, and for testing drugs.

Other pandemic diseases include plague and influenza. It is unlikely that the reservoirs of plague in rodents will be eradicated in the near future. The surveillance for human disease internationally under WHO auspices should contain any major epidemic, however. Immunization procedures do not appear to be promising. The prompt recognition of acute human cases and the availability of effective therapy should allow time to control plague at its sources.

Influenza will continue to be a major threat because of the antigenic shift that is manifested in new strains of the virus, thus negating the value of existing supplies of vaccines. It is difficult to predict the appearance of a new strain well enough in advance so that an effective vaccine can be prepared. The difficulties were observed in 1976 and 1977 with the appearance of what was termed a "swine type" of influenza virus in the United States. Millions of dollars were expended in the preparation of a vaccine, on the assumption that the 1918 pandemic might be repeated. Such an epidemic did not occur, and the volunteer immunization program had to be discontinued because of unforeseen complications with the vaccine. Future research should be directed toward the development of vaccines with an anti-virus spectrum capable of coping with new variants of the influenza virus.

The most dramatic advance in the management of infectious diseases occurred during the brief period between 1935 and 1950, when the sulfonamides and antibiotics became available. The remarkable antimicrobial activity of these agents has been marred by the fact that organisms have become resistant to the action of the drugs. Unfortunately, as newer antibiotics have become available, the problem of resistance has increased. The metabolic adjustment of the organisms, dependent on genetic factors and biochemical activity, raises serious doubts upon the continuing effectiveness of antibiotics in the future. The time and expense involved in searching for other antibiotics may yield to the expediency of synthesizing chemical compounds, such as has been done in the search for agents used in tuberculosis and parasitic diseases.

Closely related to the problem of microbial resistance is resistance that has occurred with the use of insecticides and pesticides in controlling those infectious diseases transmitted through insect vectors, especially mosquitoes. Vector control has been very important for malaria, filariasis, plague, viral encephalitis, dengue, and leishmaniasis. According to WHO, two thousand chemicals have been considered in recent years, and 30 have been selected as useful. Up to 1975, 108 species of arthropods had manifested resistance to insecticides, and it is postulated that the resistance will increase. An expert WHO Committee stated in 1976 (World Health Organization, 1976, p. 7), "resistance is probably the biggest single obstacle in the struggle against vector-borne disease and is mainly responsible for preventing successful malaria eradication in many countries."

In the search for further chemicals for human therapy and for vector control, not only must the cost be considered, but the toxicity for humans must also be critically evaluated. In view of these handicaps in the case of vector control, other alternatives are being investigated and tried. These include better environmental control through drainage and filling, and improved management for the disposal of sewage. Genetic control has been tried through the sterilization of male insects and through the production of strains of vectors with translocation, leading to sterility in the progeny. Biological control has included the use of larvivorous fish and of microbial isolates, such as bacteria, fungi, and nematodes. A primary difficulty in putting any one of several alternatives into practice is the lack of finances for preliminary research and the training of personnel.

The knowledge resulting from microbiological research in the twentieth century has extended beyond anticipation. The greatest remaining challenge is the control of virus diseases. Intensive investigations have probed viruses to the molecular levels to study their form and function; the pathogenesis of many acute and chronic virus diseases has been elucidated. One of the most significant problems yet to be solved is that of therapy. Since viruses must invade cells in order to replicate, therapy must be aimed at destroying extracellular virus particles without injuring the host's cells. For this purpose chemical agents rather than biological preparations would appear to be most appropriate, even though prophylactic vaccines have been highly successful for various virus diseases. When the spectrum of viruses is considered in the etiology of upper respiratory diseases or in enteric disorders, it is difficult to envision the development of specific vaccines for each of the viruses causing the diseases. Future research should be directed toward chemical prophylaxis.

The foregoing projection of the future status of infectious diseases is based on present knowledge and on the assumption that this information is being utilized in the control and management of infectious diseases. But there are many large areas in the developing countries where such knowledge is not being used and where the level of control approximates that of the more developed nations at the start of the twentieth century. Furthermore there has been a lack of research in major diseases afflicting populations in tropical countries. As an example, WHO authorities calculate that malaria, filariasis, and schistosomiasis affect at least 200 million people, or numbers comparable to the entire population of the United States or of the USSR, or one in twenty of the world's inhabitants. Millions more are infected by cholera, typhoid, trypanosomiasis and leishmaniasis. At least five million or more children are killed by communicable diseases because of the lack of immunization programs.

Obviously infectious diseases are far from controlled in the world at large. One of the major difficulties is the delivery of health care services to those areas where they are needed most. In some developing nations governments are so unstable and finances so limited that only the most primitive health services are available. One of the chief concerns of WHO is the establishment and strengthening of a system of primary health care centers, especially in rural areas, where the immediate delivery of health resources would be possible. Top priority is being given to the immunization of children, and intensive research is being conducted on some of the major tropical diseases.

Much has been accomplished in the control of infectious diseases;

much more remains to be done. One of the unusual and brighter developments in the twentieth century is a concept of health that is shared universally. Undoubtedly the social benefits that have accrued as a result of the control of infectious diseases have contributed to this general awareness of the importance of good health. To recapitulate, the constitution of WHO, adopted in 1948, contained the following statement (see Appendix II): "Health is a state of complete physical, mental and social well-being and not merely the absence of disease or infirmity. . . . Governments have a responsibility for the health of their peoples which can be fulfilled only by the provision of adequate health and social measures." This concept should help immeasurably in the future control of infectious diseases.

Appendixes

Appendix I. Shattuck Report
of Massachusetts, 1850

I. *State and Municipal Measures Recommended.*

Under this class of recommendations are to be included such measures as require, for their sanction, regulation and control, the legislative authority of the State, or the municipal authority of cities and towns. They may be called the legal measures — the *Sanitary Police* of the State,

> I. We recommend that the laws of the State relating to Public Health be thoroughly revised, and that a new and improved act be passed in their stead. . . .

> II. We recommend that a GENERAL BOARD OF HEALTH be established, which shall be charged with the general execution of the laws of the State, relating to the enumeration, the vital statistics, and the public health of the inhabitants. . . .

> III. We recommend that the Board, as far as practicable, be composed of two physicians, one counsellor at law, one chemist or natural philosopher, one civil engineer, and two persons of other professions or occupations; all properly qualified for the office by their talents, their education, their experience, and their wisdom. . . .

> IV. We recommend that the Board be authorized to appoint some suitable and competent person to be the Secretary of

the Board, who should be required to devote his whole time and energies to the discharge of the duties of his office, and be paid a proper salary for his services. . . .

V. We recommend that a LOCAL BOARD OF HEALTH be appointed in every city and town, who shall be charged with the particular execution of the laws of the State, and the municipal ordinances and regulations, relating to public health, within their respective jurisdictions. . . .

VI. We recommend that each local Board of Health appoint a Secretary; and also, if occasion require, a Surveyor and Health Officer. . . .

VII. We recommend that local Boards of Health endeavor to ascertain, with as much exactness as possible, the circumstances of the cities and towns, and of the inhabitants under their jurisdictions; and that they issue such local sanitary orders and make such regulations as are best adapted to these circumstances. . . .

VIII. We recommend that local Boards of Health endeavor to carry into effect all their orders and regulations in a conciliatory manner; and that they resort to compulsory process only when the public good requires it. . . .

IX. We recommend that an appropriation be made annually by the State, for the purchase of books for the use of the general Board of Health; and by each city and town for the purchase of books for the use of each local Board of Health. . . .

X. We recommend that each local Board of Health be required to make a written report annually to the town, concerning its sanitary condition during the next preceding year; and to transmit a written or printed copy of the same to the General Board of Health. . . .

XI. We recommend that the sanitary and other reports and statements of the affairs of cities and towns which may be printed should be in octavo form, on paper and page of uniform size (similar to the public documents of the State,) and designed to be bound together, as THE ANNUAL REPORTS OF THE TOWN: and that five copies be preserved by the Board of Health, one copy be furnished to the General Board of Health, one to the State Library, and that others be given to Boards of Health elsewhere in exchange for their publications. . . .

XII. We recommend that the successive enumerations of the inhabitants of the State be so made, abstracted, and published, that the most useful and desirable information concerning the population may be ascertained. . . .

XIII. We recommend that the Constitution of the State be so altered, that the State Census shall be taken in 1855, and at the end of every subsequent period of ten years. . . .

XIV. We recommend that the laws relating to the public registration of births, marriages, and deaths, be perfected and carried into effect in every city and town of the State.

XV. We recommend that provision be made for obtaining observations of the atmospheric phenomena, on a systematic and uniform plan, at different stations in the Commonwealth.

XVI. We recommend that, as far as practicable, there be used in all sanitary investigations and regulations, a uniform nomenclature for the causes of death, and for the causes of disease. . . .

XVII. We recommend that, in laying out new towns and villages, and in extending those already laid out, ample provision be made for a supply, in purity and abundance, of light, air, and water; for drainage and sewerage, for paving, and for cleanliness. . . .

XVIII. We recommend that, in erecting schoolhouses, churches, and other public buildings, health should be regarded in their site, structure, heating apparatus, and ventilation. . . .

XIX. We recommend that, before erecting any new dwelling-house, manufactory, or other building, for personal accommodation, either as a lodging-house or place of business, the owner or builder be required to give notice to the local Board of Health, of his intention and of the sanitary arrangements he proposes to adopt. . . .

XX. We recommend that local Boards of Health endeavor to prevent or mitigate the sanitary evils arising from overcrowded lodging-houses and cellar-dwellings. . . .

XXI. We recommend that open spaces be preserved, in cities and villages, for public walks; that wide streets be laid out; and that both be ornamented with trees. . . .

XXII. We recommend that special sanitary surveys of particular cities, towns, and localities, be made, from time to time, under the direction of the General Board of Health. . . .

XXIII. We recommend that local Boards of Health, and other persons interested, endeavor to ascertain, by exact observation, the effect of mill-ponds, and other collections or streams of water, and of their rise and fall, upon the health of the neighboring inhabitants. . . .

XXIV. We recommend that the local Boards of Health provide for periodical house-to-house visitation, for the prevention of epidemic diseases, and for other sanitary purposes. . . .

XXV. We recommend that measures be taken to ascertain the amount of sickness suffered in different localities; and among persons of different classes, professions, and occupations. . . .

XXVI. We recommend that measures be taken to ascertain the amount of sickness suffered, among the scholars who attend the public schools and other seminaries of learning in the Commonwealth. . . .

XXVII. We recommend that every city and town in the State be REQUIRED to provide means for the periodical vaccination of the inhabitants. . . .

XXVIII. We recommend that the causes of consumption, and the circumstances under which it occurs, be made the subject of particular observation and investigation. . . .

XXIX. We recommend that nuisances endangering human life or health, be prevented, destroyed, or mitigated. . . .

XXX. We recommend that measures be taken to prevent or mitigate the sanitary evils arising from the use of intoxicating drinks, and from haunts of dissipation. . . .

XXXI. We recommend that the laws for taking inquests upon the view of dead bodies, now imposed upon coroners, be revised. . . .

XXXII. We recommend that the authority now vested in justices of the peace, relating to insane and idiotic persons, not arrested or indicted for crime, be transferred to the local Boards of Health. . . .

XXXIII. We recommend that the general management of cemeteries and other places of burial, and of the interment of the dead, be regulated by the local Boards of Health. . . .

XXXIV. We recommend that measures be taken to preserve the lives and the health of passengers at sea, and of seamen engaged in the merchant service. . . .

XXXV. We recommend that the authority to make regulations for the quarantine of vessels be intrusted to the local Boards of Health. . . .

XXXVI. We recommend that measures be adopted for preventing or mitigating the sanitary evils arising from foreign emigration. . . .

II. Social and Personal Measures Recommended.

XXXVII. We recommend that a sanitary association be formed in every city and town in the State, for the purpose of collecting and diffusing information relating to public and personal health. . . .

XXXVIII. We recommend that tenements for the better accommodation of the poor, be erected in cities and villages. . . .

XXXIX. We recommend that public bathing-houses and wash-houses be established in all cities and villages. . . .

XL. We recommend that, whenever practicable, the refuse and sewage of cities and towns be collected, and applied to the purposes of agriculture. . . .

XLI. We recommend that measures be taken to prevent, as far as practicable, the smoke nuisance. . . .

XLII. We recommend that the sanitary effects of patent medicines and other nostrums, and secret remedies, be observed; that physicians in their prescriptions and names of medicines, and apothecaries in their compounds, use great caution and care; and that medical compounds advertised for sale be avoided, unless the material of which they are composed be known, or unless manufactured and sold by a person of known honesty and integrity. . . .

XLIII. We recommend that local Boards of Health, and others interested, endeavor to prevent the sale and use of unwholesome, spurious, and adulterated articles, dangerous to the public health, designed for food, drink, or medicine. . . .

XLIV. We recommend that institutions be formed to educate and qualify females to be nurses of the sick. . . .

XLV. We recommend that persons be specially educated in sanitary science, as preventive advisers as well as curative advisers. . . .

XLVI. We recommend that physicians keep records of cases professionally attended. . . .

XLVII. We recommend that clergymen of all religious denominations make public health the subject of one or more discourses annually, before their congregations. . . .

XLVIII. We recommend that each family keep such records as will show the physical and sanitary condition of its members. . . .

XLIX. We recommend that parents, and others to whom the care of those in infancy and childhood are intrusted, endeavor to understand and discharge their duties so that a good foundation may be laid for vigorous manhood and old age. . . .

L. We recommend that individuals make frequent sanitary examinations of themselves, and endeavor to promote personal health, and prevent personal disease. . . .

Report of the Sanitary Commission of Massachusetts, 1850, Dutton and Wentworth State Printers, Boston, 1850. Reprinted by Harvard University Press, Cambridge (Mass.), 1948. Part I, pp. 109–206; Part II, pp. 206–241.)

Appendix II

Constitution of The World Health Organization

THE STATES Parties to this Constitution declare, in conformity with the Charter of the United Nations, that the following principles are basic to the happiness, harmonious relations and security of all peoples:

Health is a state of complete physical, mental and social well-being and not merely the absence of disease or infirmity.

The enjoyment of the highest attainable standard of health is one of the fundamental rights of every human being without distinction of race, religion, political belief, economic or social condition.

The health of all peoples is fundamental to the attainment of peace and security and is dependent upon the fullest co-operation of individuals and States.

The achievement of any State in the promotion and protection of health is of value to all. Unequal development in different countries in the promotion of health and control of disease, especially communicable disease, is a common danger.

Healthy development of the child is of basic importance; the ability to live harmoniously in a changing total environment is essential to such development.

The extension to all peoples of the benefits of medical, psychological and related knowledge is essential to the fullest attainment of health.

455

Informed opinion and active co-operation on the part of the public are of the utmost importance in the improvement of the health of the people.

Governments have a responsibility for the health of their peoples which can be fulfilled only by the provision of adequate health and social measures.

ACCEPTING THESE PRINCIPLES, and for the purpose of co-operation among themselves and with others to promote and protect the health of all peoples, the Contracting Parties agree to the present Constitution and hereby establish the World Health Organization as a specialized agency within the terms of Article 57 of the Charter of the United Nations.

(World Health Organization: Constitution, Off. Rec. World Hlth Org., 2:100, 1948 (meeting of June 19–July 22, 1946))

Notes

Notes

Chapter 1

1. Cotton Mather was the son of the Puritan clergyman, Increase Mather, who had been a president of Harvard College. Cotton Mather was one of the leading intellects of the American colonies. Although he participated in the Salem witchcraft trials, he was a member of the Royal Society of London and read the Society's *Transactions* regularly. He completed writing the "Angel of Bethesda" in 1724, which was "the first general treatise on medicine to be prepared in the English Colonies" (*Cotton Mather: First Significant Figure in American Medicine* by O. T. Beall, Jr. and R. H. Shryock, Johns Hopkins Press, Baltimore, 1954). "The Angel" was finally published in 1972 (*The Angel of Bethesda*, edited by G. W. Jones, Barre, Mass.: American Antiquarian Society and Barre Publishers, 1972). Mather, who was familiar with the works of Leeuwenhoek and Benjamin Marten, believed diseases were propagated by "animalculae" in the atmosphere.

2. For an informative, first-hand description of inoculation in the Massachusetts colony see *The Book of Abigail and John: Selected Letters of the Adams Family, 1762–1784*, Cambridge: Harvard University Press, 1975, pp. 136–153.

3. Grease is a chronic, inflammatory, noncontagious lesion of the horse, usually involving the hoof. It is associated with poor hygiene in stables and is due to more than one species of microbe.

4. Cowpox virus is antigenetically different from smallpox, and cows cannot be infected experimentally with smallpox.

5. The name of this journal was short-lived. It later became the *Boston Medical and Surgical Journal* and then the *New England Journal of Medicine*.

Chapter 2

1. Dr. René Dubos wrote a fascinating historical account of another mosaic disease of plants, the parasitization of tulips by the virus that leads to the exotic mixture of colors in the flower. (*Perspectives in Virology*, edited by M. Pollard, New York: John Wiley & Sons, Inc., 1959, Vol. 1, p. 291.)

Chapter 3

1. I am grateful to Helen O. Neff of CDC, Atlanta, Georgia, for much of the historical information.

2. I am indebted to Dr. Philip S. Brachman, Director, Bureau of Epidemiology, CDC, Atlanta, Georgia, for his help in obtaining information on these episodes.

3. The first comprehensive scientific reports on Legionnaires' disease are: (1) David W. Fraser et al., "Legionnaires Disease: Description of an Epidemic of Pneumonia," *New England Journal of Medicine* 297:1189, December 1, 1977; (2) Joseph E. McDade et al., "Legionnaires' Disease: Isolation of a Bacterium and Demonstration of its Role in Other Respiratory Disease," Ibid, p. 1197; (3) F. W. Chandler, Martin D. Hicklin, and J. A. Blackmon, "Demonstration of the Agent of Legionnaires' Disease in Tissue," ibid, p. 1218.

Chapter 4

1. A term coined by Wright from the Greek *opsonein*, meaning "I convert into palatable pabulum" (Wright, 1908).

2. The enthusiasm generated for vaccine therapy at the time is demonstrated by the appearance of *The Journal of Vaccine Therapy*, which endured for two years (Vols. 1 and 2, 1912 and 1913, London: H. K. Lewis).

Chapter 5

1. DDT is derived from the generic name chlorophenothane.

2. The Wellcome group introduced the famous C203 strain of Group A hemolytic streptococcus, which was used extensively in experimental streptococcal infections in many laboratories in the United States.

3. A true elixir utilizes alcohol as the solvent.

Chapter 6

1. From the Greek *lysis*, dissolution, and *deixein*, to show.

Chapter 7

1. In a patent agreement with Merck & Company Dr. Waksman did what Florey failed to do. The patent on streptomycin was taken out with Schatz, and later a substantial amount of the proceeds were assigned by Merck & Company to the Rutgers Research and Endowment Foundation, with Dr. Waksman also receiving a sum. Schatz sued Waksman in 1950 for a portion, but the case was settled out of court and Schatz received $125,000 for the assignment of all foreign patent rights and 3 percent of the royalties (see Waksman, 1954, p. 279).

2. We used this model at the University of Minnesota for studying the chemotherapy of experimental brucellosis in guinea pigs and mice (Braude, 1951).

Chapter 8

1. The trade names and the companies for tetracycline were: *achromycin*, Lederle Laboratories, Division of American Cyanamid Company; *tetracyn*, Chas. Pfizer & Company; *panmycin*, Upjohn Company; *polycycline*, Bristol Laboratories; *steclin*, E. R. Squibb & Sons, Divsion of Olin Mathieson Chemical Corporation.

Chapter 11

1. Dr. Mitchell was professor of medicine at the University of Pennsylvania.

Chapter 12

1. From the Latin *plaga*, a blow, strike.
2. One of the major by-products of plague surveillance by United States federal authorities was the discovery of the disease tularemia. This is a plague-like disease of rodents. The disease is rarely, if ever, transmitted from human to human, but arises as a result of handling infected animals. This disease is considered one of the zoonoses and is discussed in Section III, Chapter 22.
3. An informative narrative on plague by Berton Roueché, including the Denver case, appeared in *The New Yorker* magazine for November 10, 1971.
4. From the Latin *variola*, pustule, pock; from the Latin *varius*, variegated, various.
5. Doctor Donald A. Henderson, the chief medical officer for WHO in the smallpox eradication program, has written of the successful program that possibly has ended the scourge of smallpox ("The Eradication of Smallpox," *Scientific American* 235:25, October 1976).
6. From the Greek *lepra*, "elephantiasis," or thickening and corrugation of the skin.
7. The designation "cholera" derives from the Hippocratic Greek word meaning a flow of bile.

Chapter 13

1. He named the disease *diphtheritis*, from the Greek for leather, i.e., skin or membrane.
2. Healthy persons may carry diphtheria bacilli in the nasopharynx that do not produce toxin, but toxins are produced by the organisms when they are parasitized (lysogenized) by diphtheria phage B.
3. For an excellent probing of the history and pathogenesis of diphtheria see the small volume by Dr. W. Barry Wood, Jr., *From Miasmas to Molecules*, Columbia University Press, New York, 1961. Also knowledge of toxin activity at a molecular level has been summarized by A. M. Pappenheimer, Jr., "Diphtheria Toxin," *Annual Review of Biochemistry*, 46:69, 1977.
4. The etymology of *measles* is a bit obscure. It is akin to Old English *mazer*, "a spot on a maple;" Dutch *mazelen* and Old English *masel*, "little spots."
5. From the Latin *rubeus*, red.
6. *Rötheln* is idiomatic in German for "German measles," from *röt*, redness, ruddy; *rötel*, red ochre, or chalk.
7. Variola designates smallpox, from the Latin for various. Varicella is the diminutive of variola, and designates chickenpox.
8. Chicken suggests little, young; thus "little-pox," as distinct from "great-pox," or syphilis.
9. *Zoster* is from the Greek for girdle. Shingles is from the Latin *cingulum*, girdle. The eruption of zoster follows the course of infected peripheral nerves of the trunk, hence the term "shingles."
10. From the Latin *per*, very; *tussis*, cough — a term introduced by Sydenham in the seventeenth century.
11. From the Dutch *mompelen*, to mumble.
12. Poliomyelitis is derived from two Greek words, *polios* — gray, and *myelos* — marrow. The virus localizes in the gray substance of the anterior horn in the spinal cord and also in the brain.
13. The difficult problem of identifying the specific cause of enterovirus infections is ascertained from the following editorial note: "Most of the 60 'common' enterovirus serotypes that are prevalent during the summer months appear to cause localized or occasional national epidemics at irregular intervals. The clinical spectrum of disease caused by the different agents is remarkably similar" (Center for Disease Control, 1976a, p. 377).

Chapter 14

1. From the Greek *kattarhoos*, a running down.
2. Marketed as Co-pavin by Eli Lilly Co.
3. From the Greek *pneumones*, the lungs.
4. A well-documented survey of the 1918 pandemic and the sequence of investigations that followed has been written by A. W. Crosby, Jr., *Epidemic and Peace, 1918*, Greenwood Press, Westport, Conn., 1976.
5. Dr. W. I. B. Beveridge (1977) has written a concise and informative book on the present status of influenza and the future trends of research toward control of this last of the pandemic infections. A more comprehensive volume has been prepared by Sir Charles H. Stuart-Harris and Geoffrey C. Schild on *Influenza: The Viruses and the Disease*, London: Edward Arnold, 1976.
6. From the Greek *phthisis*, I waste away; hence consumption.
7. The Minneapolis venture was an outstanding success in the management of children with primary tuberculosis. Doctor F. E. Harrington, commissioner of health for the city of Minneapolis and director of hygiene of the school system, obtained a building and land from the Lyman family. He planned a school for children having positive tuberculin tests and X-ray evidence of primary pulmonary tuberculosis where they could be brought daily and educated. They were given extra nourishment and a rest period. An outpatient service was also established. Doctor J. A. Myers was placed in charge and for years observed these children from early infancy through high school, and later through the University of Minnesota, where he was a member of the staff of the University Student Health Service. This continuing surveillance over a period of twenty years was a remarkable achievement in the control and treatment of early tuberculosis.
8. For a classification and characteristics of the atypical mycobacteria, see *Bergey's Manual of Determinative Bacteriology*, 8th Ed., Baltimore: Williams and Wilkins, 1974, p. 682.
9. From the Greek *psittakos*, parrot.
10. From the Greek *trachys*, rough; *oma*, morbid affection.

Chapter 15

1. From the Greek *typhos*, stupor from fever.
2. From the Greek meaning to flow through.
3. From the Greek meaning ill or bad intestines.
4. I am indebted for this information to Dr. Barry S. Levy of the Minnesota Department of Health.
5. For a comprehensive review see Center for Disease Control: Foodborne and Waterborne Disease Outbreaks, Annual Summary 1976, issued October 1977.
6. From the Latin *botulus*, sausage.
7. Abundant staphylococci were cultured from the centers of each layer of the two cakes, but insignificant numbers were obtained from the icing and filling. Eggs used in the preparation were unrefrigerated and were possibly the source of the contamination.
8. Sir Arnold was the father of Dr. Max Theiler, the discoverer of yellow fever vaccine for human use, for which he received the Nobel Prize.
9. For a detailed discussion on the evolution of knowledge on hepatitis B, see Nobel Prize Lecture for 1976 of B. S. Blumberg, "Australia Antigen and the Biology of Hepatitis B," *Science* 197:17, July 1, 1977.
10. I am indebted to Dr. B. S. Levy, Minnesota State Department of Health, for this information.

Chapter 16

1. The penicillin was provided by the Office of Scientific Research and Development from supplies assigned by the committee on medical research for investigations recommended by the committee on chemotherapeutic and other agents of the National Research Council.

2. From the Greek *haema*, blood, and *philos*, loving; hence blood lover.

3. From the Greek *tetanos*, rigid, stretched.

Chapter 17

1. From a combination of two Greek words: *gono*, to beget, and *rhoea*, to flow. Other names are blennorrhea, also two Greek words — *blenno*, mucus, and *rhoea*, to flow; also gleet from medieval English *glet*, *glette* — slince or ooze, referring to urethral discharge.

2. See the discussion below of the poem by Fracastoro for the origin of this term.

3. Treponema is from the Greek *trepein*, to turn; *nema*, thread. Pallidum is from the Latin *pallidus*, pale. Hence "the pale spirochoete."

4. For a vivid autobiographical account of the physical and mental agony associated with repeated attacks of gonorrhea in the male, see *Boswell's London Journal, 1762–1763,* edited by F. A. Pottle, New York: McGraw-Hill, 1950.

5. But penicillin-resistant strains (penicillinase-producers) have been identified in eleven countries, including the United States. There is a spread of these strains within the civilian populations (*Morbidity and Mortality Weekly Report* 26:29, February 4, 1977).

Chapter 18

1. "The much dreaded red cloak"; the rash.

2. According to English law, judges and an entourage of lawyers and assistants travelled from parish to parish during the year holding court trials known as Assizes.

3. Akari is from the Greek for mite.

4. Tsutsugamushi is from the Japanese for dangerous mite; Akamushi — red mite of Japan.

5. Five day fever, another synonym for the disease.

Chapter 19

1. Encephalitis lethargica was also called *Nona*, for reasons not clear. Nona is from the Latin for ninth. According to Bassoe (1919) of Chicago, who wrote one of the first American reports, *nona* originated in Italy in the epidemic that followed the pandemic of influenza in 1890. He termed it a "meaningless word."

2. I am indebted to Dr. Henry Bauer, director of the Medical Laboratories of the Minnesota Department of Health, for information on California arbovirus infection in Minnesota.

3. The etymological origin of *dengue* is obscure (see the historical discussion by Siler, Hall, and Hitchens, 1926, p. 7).

4. *Arenosus* is Latin for sandy. The term derives from the sandy appearance of the virus under the electron microscope. The choriomeningitis virus with its reservoir in mice also belongs to the arenoviruses, but it does not cause hemorrhagic fever.

5. An informative and well-written popular book on Lassa fever is that of J. G. Fuller, *Fever! The Hunt for a New Killer Virus,* New York: E. P. Dutton, 1974.

6. A very comprehensive and authoritative review on Arenaviral Infections can be found in "International Symposium on Arenaviral Infections of Public Health Importance (July 14–16, 1975)," *Bulletin of the World Health Organization* 52, Nos. 4, 5, 6, 1975.

7. In 1975 epidemic western equine encephalitis in horses again appeared in North Dakota and Minnesota, with humans also involved.

8. For a detailed discussion of slow virus disease, see the Nobel Prize Lecture for 1976 of D. C. Gajdusek, "Unconventional Viruses and the Origin and Disappearance of Kuru," *Science* 197:943, September 2, 1977.

Chapter 20

1. Dr. Maurice Hall, a highly recognized parasitologist, has written a critical analysis of the basic discoveries on tick fever that preceded the work of Smith and Kilborne (M. C. Hall, "Theobald Smith as a Parasitologist," *Journal of Parasitology* 21:231, 1935).

2. *Nagana* is from the Zulu for low or depressed in spirits.

3. Tsetse received its name from the Tswana African people bordering on the Kalahari Desert, probably because of the loud buzz made by the flies in flight. J. J. McKelvey, Jr. has written an excellent volume on *Man Against Tsetse: Struggle for Africa*, Ithaca (N.Y.): Cornell University Press, 1973.

4. A colonial surgeon, R. M. Forde, had also attended Mr. K in Gambia, Africa. He had examined the patient's blood and had observed highly active wormlike bodies, but he did not realize the significance of this finding until later (R. M. Forde, "Some Clinical Notes on a European Patient in Whose Blood a Trypanosome was Observed," *Journal of Tropical Medicine and Hygiene* 5:261, 1902).

5. Reduviid is from the Latin *reduvid*, hangnail.

6. This program was initiated by the committee on teaching of tropical medicine of the Association of American Medical Colleges and financed by the John and Mary R. Markle Foundation. Intensive laboratory courses on parasitic diseases were conducted by the army medical school in Washington, D.C. and at Tulane University. The clinical training and field trips were carried out in Central America under the auspices of the health and sanitation division of the Office of Coordinator of Inter-American Affairs, and the public health departments of each country.

7. *Weekly Epidemiological Record*, No. 3, 1973, World Health Organization.

8. In my discussion of quinine I have relied principally on the history by M. L. Duran-Reynals (1946).

9. From the Greek *schistos*, to divide; *soma*, body; *iasis*, diseased condition.

10. From the Greek *ascaris*, an intestinal worm.

Chapter 21

1. From the French *ergot*, spur (cock's comb).

Chapter 22

1. It is doubtful that many of his patients were bitten by dogs that actually had rabies.

2. I am indebted to Dr. Henry Bauer of the laboratories of the Minnesota State Department of Health for the details.

3. The centenary of Bruce's birth occurred in 1855; to commemorate the occasion, his life and work were reviewed in the *Journal of the Royal Army Medical Corps* 101:79–122, April 1955.

4. Named after Tulare County, California, where the disease was first recognized in an epizootic among ground squirrels.

5. Dr. B. J. Kennedy at the University of Minnesota has informed me that his group in cancer chemotherapy have encountered four active cases in adults following treatment.

6. From the Greek *exinos*, spine, and *kokkos*, berry.

Suggested Readings

Suggested Readings

The following list of publications is recommended for those who desire further information on the history of medicine, with special reference to infectious diseases.

Bayne-Jones, S., 1968. *The Evolution of Preventive Medicine in the United States Army, 1607–1939*. Washington, D.C.: Office of the Surgeon General, Department of the Army. [A scholarly summary of progress in the control of infectious diseases during war and peace.]

Bloomfield, A. L., 1958. *A Bibliography of Internal Medicine: Communicable Diseases*. Chicago: University of Chicago Press. [Written by a physician who was a professor of medicine at Stanford University Medical School. He provides useful abstracts of pertinent literature.]

Bulloch, W., 1938. *The History of Bacteriology*. London: Oxford University Press. [A classic on the development of bacteriology and immunology written by a bacteriologist, beginning with the early concepts of contagion and ending before World War II.]

Cairns, J., Stent, G. S., and Watson, J. D., Editors, 1966. *Phage and the Origins of Molecular Biology*. Cold Spring Harbor (N.Y.): Cold Spring Harbor Laboratory of Quantitative Biology. [A delightful group of essays by scientists who contributed outstanding discoveries on molecular biology.]

Creighton, C., 1965. *A History of Epidemics in Great Britain*, Vol. 1. From A.D. 664–1666 (1891). Vol. 2. From A.D. 1666–1894 (1894). Second edition unrevised with introductions by D. E. C. Eversley, E. Ashworth Underwood, and Lynda Ovenall. London: Frank Cass. [One of the most outstanding medical histories of all time, although Creighton could not accept the established germ theory of disease and inveighed against Jenner and vaccination for smallpox. The second edition is enhanced by two introductory essays, the first by D. E. C. Eversley on Creighton's contribution to epidemiology and social history, and the second by E. A. Underwood on the life and work of Creighton. There is also a selected bibliography by L. Ovenall on epidemiological literature since 1894.]

Dobell, C., 1932. *Antony van Leeuwenhoek and His "Little Animals."* New York: Harcourt, Brace & Co. [The story of the microscope, probably the most important invention in the history of bacteriology.]

Garrison, F. H., 1922. *An Introduction to the History of Medicine with Medical Chronology,*

Suggestions for Study and Bibliographic Data. Third edition revised. Philadelphia: W. B. Saunders. [The foremost American contribution to medical history, comprehensive and detailed in biographical and bibliographical information.]

Hirsch, A., 1881–1886. *Handbuch der historisch-geographischen Pathologie*. Second edition, 3 vols. Stuttgart: F. Enke. *Handbook of Geographical and Historical Pathology*. Translated from the second German edition by Charles Creighton, The New Sydenham Society, 106:1–710, 1883 (Vol. 1); 112:1–681, 1885 (Vol. 2); 117:1–780, 1886 (Vol. 3). [A classic in epidemiology. Translated by C. Creighton before he wrote his own volumes on epidemics in Great Britain. It reflects Creighton's deep scholarship and linguistic abilities.]

Major, R. H., 1945. *Classic Descriptions of Disease*. Third Edition. Springfield (Ill.): Chas. C Thomas. [This valuable source contains some original contributions on infectious diseases, all in English.]

Major, R. H., 1954. *A History of Medicine*. 2 vols. Springfield (Ill.): Chas. C Thomas. [A chronological survey from antiquity to World War II, written by a physician, emphasizing the contributions of the medical profession to medical education and research, and to the care of the sick.]

Medical Classics compiled by Emerson Crosby Kelly, M.D. 5 vols. September 1936 thru June 1941. Baltimore: Williams & Wilkins. [A partial collection of some of the foremost writings in medical history, all in English, including Hippocrates, Rhazes, Sydenham, Koch, Lister, Panum, and Semmelweis.]

Morton, L. T., 1970. *A Medical Bibliography (Garrison and Morton)*. Third edition. Philadelphia: J. P. Lippincott. [One of the best reference sources for medical history covering the basic medical sciences and clinical discoveries.]

Scott, H. H., 1939. *A History of Tropical Medicine*. 2 vols. Based on the Fitzpatrick lectures delivered before the Royal College of Physicians of London, 1937–1938. London: Edward Arnold. [A valuable source for historical materials in a major field of medicine.]

Smith, T., 1934. *Parasitism and Disease*. Princeton (N.J.): Princeton University Press. [A medical classic by one of America's greatest bacteriologists.]

Winslow, C-E. A., 1943. *The Conquest of Epidemic Diseases; A Chapter in the History of Ideas*. Princeton (N.J.): Princeton University Press. [A thoughtful historical survey for the student of infectious diseases.]

World Health Organization, 1958. *The First Ten Years of the World Health Organization*. Geneva: World Health Organization.

World Health Organization, 1968. *The Second Ten Years of the World Health Organization 1958–1967*. Geneva: World Health Organization. [Excellent for a comprehensive understanding of the operations and achievements of international public health through WHO; one of the most significant accomplishments of the twentieth century toward better health throughout the world.]

Zinsser, H., 1935. *Rats, Lice and History*. Boston: Little, Brown and Co. [A brilliant example of exploring the history of a single disease (typhus).]

Bibliography

List of Journals and
Their Abbreviations

ACTA Dermato-Venereologica (Stockholm)	*Acta Derm Venereol.* (Stockh)
ACTA Medica Scandinavica (Stockholm)	*Acta med. Scand.*
ACTA Paediatrica (Uppsala) Later:	*Acta Paediatr.*
ACTA Paediatrica Scandinavica (Stockholm)	*Acta Paediatr. Scand.*
ACTA Pathologica et Microbiologica Scandinavica (Kobenhavn)	*Acta Pathol. Microbiol. Scand.*
Advances in Internal Medicine	*Adv. Intern. Med.*
Albrecht von Graefes Archiv für Ophthalmologie Later: *Albrecht von Graefes Archiv für Klinische und Experimentelle Ophthalmologie* (Berlin)	*Albrecht von Graefes Arch. Klin. Ophthalmol.*
American Journal of Clinical Pathology	*Am. J. Clin. Pathol.*
American Journal of Diseases of Children	*Am. J. Dis. Child.*
American Journal of Hygiene Later: *American Journal of Epidemiology*	*Am. J. Hyg.* *Am. J. Epidemiol.*
American Journal of Medicine	*Am. J. Med.*
American Journal of Pathology	*Am. J. Pathol.*
American Journal of Public Health	*Am. J. Public Health*
American Journal of Syphilis, Gonorrhea, and Venereal Diseases	*Am. J. Syph. Gonorrhea vener. Dis.*

471

American Journal of the Medical Sciences	Am. J. Med. Sci.
American Journal of Tropical Medicine Later:	Am. J. Trop. Med.
American Journal of Tropical Medicine and Hygiene	Am. J. Trop. Med. Hyg.
American Journal of Veterinary Medicine	Am. J. vet. Med.
American Journal of Veterinary Research	Am. J. Vet. Res.
American Review of Respiratory Disease	Am. Rev. Respir. Dis.
American Review of Tuberculosis Later:	Am. Rev. Tuberc.
American Review of Respiratory Disease	Am. Rev. Respir. Dis.
American Scientist	Am. Sci.
Annalen der Physik und Chemie (Leipzig)	Annln. Phys. Chem.
Annales de Chimie et de Physique (Paris)	Annls. Chim. Phys.
Annales de l'Institut Pasteur (Paris)	Annls. Inst. Pasteur
Annales. Société r. des sciences médicales et naturelles de Bruxelles.	Annls. Soc. r. Sci. méd. nat. Brux.
Annals and Magazine of Natural History (London)	Ann. Mag. nat. Hist.
Annals of Allergy	Ann. Allergy
Annals of Internal Medicine	Ann. Intern. Med.
Annals of Medical History	Ann. Med. History
Annals of Surgery	Ann. Surg.
Annals of the New York Academy of Sciences	Ann. NY Acad. Sci.
Annals of the Pickett-Thomson Research Laboratory (London)	Ann. Pickett-Thomson Res. Lab.
Annals of Tropical Medicine and Parasitology (Liverpool)	Ann. Trop. Med. Parasitol.
Annual Reports of the Department of Agriculture	Annu. Rep. Dept. Agric.
Annual Review of Biochemistry	Annu. Rev. Biochem.
Annual Review of Medicine	Annu. Rev. Med.
Annual Review of Microbiology	Annu. Rev. Microbiol.
Antibiotics and Chemotherapy (Basel)	Antibiot. Chemother.
Antibiotics Annual	Antibiot. Annu.
Arbeiten aus dem Kaiserlichen Gesundheitsamte (Berlin)	Arb. K. GesundhAmt.
Arbeiten aus dem Reichsgesundheitsamte (Berlin)	Arb. ReichsgesundhAmt.

Arbeiten aus dem Zoologischen Instituten der Universität Wien

Arb. zool. Inst. Univ. Wien

Archiv für Anatomie, Physiologie und wissenschaftliche Medicin
Later:
Archiv. für Anatomie und Physiologie, Anatomische Abteilung und Physiologische Abteilung

Arch. Anat. Physiol. wiss. Med.

Archiv für experimentelle Pathologie und Pharmakologie (Leipzig)
Later:
Archiv. fuer Pharmakologie und Experimentelle Pathologie

Arch. exp. Path. Pharmak.

Archiv für klinische Chirurgie (Berlin)
Formerly:
Deutsche Zeitschrift für Chirurgie (Leipzig)

Arch. klin. Chir.

Dtsche. Z. Chir.

Archives de Pharmacodynamie
Later:
Archives internationales de pharmacodynamie et de thérapie (Bruxelles-Paris, Gand)

Archs. Pharmacodyn.

Archs. int. Pharmacodyn. Thér.

Archives générales de Médicine (Paris)

Archs. gén. Méd.

Archives of Internal Medicine-AMA

Arch. Intern. Med.

Archives of Neurology and Psychiatry

Arch. Neurol. Psychiatry

Archives of Pathology and Laboratory Medicine

Arch. Pathol. Lab. Med.

Archives of Pediatrics

Arch. Pediat.

Archivio per le Scienze Mediche (Torino)

Arch. Sci. Med. (Torino)

Atlantic (Boston) or *Atlantic Monthly*

Atlantic (Boston) *Atlantic Mo.*

Australian Veterinary Journal (Sydney)

Aust. Vet. J.

Bacteriological Reviews

Bacteriol. Rev.

Beiträge zur Biologie der Pflanzen (Breslau)

Beitr. Biol. Pfl.

Beiträge zur Klinik der Infektionskrankheiten und zur Immunitätsforschung (Würzburg)

Beitr. Klin. InfektKrankh.

Beiträge zur pathologischen Anatomie und zur allgemeinen Pathologie (Jena)

Beitr. pathol. Anat.

Berliner klinische Wochenschrift (Berlin)

Berl. klin. Wschr.

Biochemical Journal

Biochem. J.

Boston Medical and Surgical Journal

Boston Med. Surg. J.

Botanical Review

Bot. Rev.

Brazil médico (Rio de Janeiro)

Braz.-méd.

British and Foreign Medico-Chirurgical Review

Br. and Foreign Med-chir. Rev.

Now:
Medico-Chirurgical Journal and Review

British Journal of Experimental *Pathology* (London)	*Br. J. Exp. Pathol.*
British Journal of Surgery (Bristol)	*Br. J. Surg.*
British Journal of Venereal Diseases (London)	*Br. J. Vener. Dis.*
British Medical Journal (London)	*Br. Med. J.*
British Veterinary Journal (London)	*Br. Vet. J.*
Bulletin de l'Académie de médecine (Paris) Now: *Bulletin de l'Académie Nationale* *de Médecine*	*Bull. Acad. Méd.*
Bulletin de la Société chimique de Paris	*Bull. Soc. chim. Paris*
Bulletin et mémoires de la Société *médicale des hôpitaux de Paris* (Paris)	*Bull. Mém. Soc. med. Hôp. Paris*
Bulletin of the Atomic Scientists (of Chicago)	*Bull. atom. Scient.*
Bulletin of the Health Organisation, *League of Nations, Geneva*	*Bull. Hlth. Org.*
Bulletin of the History of Medicine (Baltimore) Formerly: *Johns Hopkins University Institute of* *the History of Medicine. Bulletin.*	*Bull. Hist. Med.*
Bulletin of the Neurological Institute *of New York*	*Bull. neurol. Inst. NY*
Bulletin of the New York Academy *of Medicine*	*Bull. NY Acad. Med.*
Bulletin of the World Health *Organization* (Geneva)	*Bull. WHO*
Cairo. Egyptian University (Faculty *of Medicine) Publication* Later: *Cairo. Jāmi'at al-Qāhirah* *Kullīyat al-Tibb. Publication.*	*Cairo. Université Egyptienne Faculty* *of Med. Publ.*
California Medicine Later: *Western Journal of Medicine*	*Calif. Med.* *West. Med.*
California and Western Medicine	*Calif. west. Med.*
Canadian Journal of Research	*Can. J. Res.*
Center for Disease Control Morbidity and *Mortality Statistics*	*CDC Morbidity Mortality Statistics*
Center for Disease Control Morbidity and *Mortality Weekly Report*	*CDC Morbidity Mortality Weekly Rep.*

Center for Disease Control Veterinary Public Health Notes — CDC Vet. Public Health Notes

Chemical and Engineering News — Chem. Engng. News

Chest — Chest

Circulation: Journal of the American Heart Association — Circulation

Colorado Medicine — Colorado Med.

Comptes rendus des séances et mémoires de la Société de biologie. Paris. — C. R. Séanc. Soc. Biol.

Comptes Rendus Hebdomadaires des Séances de l'Académie des Sciences (Paris) — C. R. Acad. Sci [D] (Paris)
Later:
Comptes Rendus Hebdomadaires des Séances de l'Académie des Sciences; D: Sciences Naturelles (Paris)

Danish Medical Bulletin (Kobenhavn) — Dan. Med. Bull.

Deutsche Medizinische Wochenschrift (Stuttgart) — Dtsch. med. Wochenschr.

Deutsche Zeitschrift fuer Chirurgie (Leipzig) — Dtsche. Z. Chir.
Later:
Archiv fuer klinische Chirurgie (Berlin) — Arch. klin. Chir.

Deutsches Archiv fur klinische Medizin (Leipzig) — Dtschs. Arch. klin. Med.

Edinburgh Medical Journal (Edinburgh) — Edinb. med. J.

Encounter — Encounter

Encyclopedia Britannica — Encycloped. Brit.

Ergebnisse der Inneren Medizin und Kinderheilkunde (Berlin) — Ergeb. Inn. Med. Kinderheilkd.

Folia Clinica, Chimica et Microscopica (Salsomaggiore) — Folia clin. chim. microsc., Salsomaggiore

Fortschritte der Medicin (München) — Fortschr. Med.

Gazeta Medica da Bahia — Gazeta med. Bahia

Gazzetta medica italiana lombarda. Milano. — Gazz. med. ital. lomb.

Guy's Hospital Reports (London) — Guy's Hosp. Rep.

Harper's Magazine — Harper's Magazine

Health Service Reports (Rockville, Md.) — Health Serv. Rep.

Hospital Practice — Hosp. Practice

Hygiea. Medicinsk och Farmaceutisk Månadsskrift (Stockholm) — Hygiea

Indian Journal of Medical Research
(New Delhi)

Indian J. Med. Res.

Indian Medical Gazette (Calcutta)

Indian med. Gaz.

International Journal of Leprosy and
Other Mycobacterial Diseases

Int. J. Lepr.

International Record of Medicine —
The New York Medical Journal

Int. Record Med. — NY Med. J.

Irish Journal of Medical Sciences —
The Dublin Journal of Medical and
Chemical Science
Later:
Irish Journal of Medical Science (Dublin)

Ir. J. Med. Sci.

Jahrbuch für Kinderheilkunde (Berlin)

Jb. Kinderheilkunde

Janus (Amsterdam, Paris, Leiden)

Janus

Japanese Journal of Experimental
Medicine (Tokyo)

Jap. J. Exp. Med.

Johns Hopkins Hospital Bulletin
(Baltimore)
Later:
Johns Hopkins Medical Journal

Johns Hopkins Hosp. Bull.

Johns Hopkins Hospital Reports

Johns Hopkins Hosp. Rep.

Johns Hopkins University Institute of
the History of Medicine. Bulletin.
Later:
Bulletin of the History of Medicine
(Baltimore)

Bull. Hist. Med.

Journal de Médecine, Chirurgie,
Pharmacie (Paris)

J. Méd. Chir. Pharmacie

Journal für praktische Chemie

J. prakt. Chem.

Journal-Lancet (Minnesota)

J.-Lancet

Journal of Applied Bacteriology

J. Appl. Bacteriol.

Journal of Bacteriology

J. Bacteriol.

Journal of Biological Chemistry

J. Biol. Chem.

Journal of Bone and Joint Surgery

J. Bone Joint Surg.

Journal of Clinical Investigation

J. Clin. Invest.

Journal of Comparative Pathology and
Therapeutics (Croydon)
Later:
Journal of Comparative Pathology
(Liverpool)

J. Comp. Pathol. Therapeutics

Journal of Experimental Medicine

J. Exp. Med.

Journal of General Physiology

J. Gen. Physiol.

Journal of Hygiene
(Cambridge, England)

J. Hyg. (Camb.)

Journal of Immunology	*J. Immunol.*
Journal of Infectious Diseases	*J. Infect. Dis.*
Journal of Laboratory and Clinical Medicine	*J. Lab. Clin. Med.*
Journal of Medical Education	*J. Med. Educ.*
Journal of Medical Research	*J. Med. Res.*
Journal of Molecular Biology (London)	*J. Mol. Biol.*
Journal of Neuropathology and Experimental Neurology	*J. Neuropathol. Exp. Neurol.*
Journal of Pathology and Bacteriology (London) Later: *Journal of Pathology* (London)	*J. Pathol. Bacteriol.*
Journal of Pediatrics	*J. Pediatr.*
Journal of Pharmacology and Experimental Therapeutics	*J. Pharmacol. Exp. Ther.*
Journal of Preventive Medicine	*J. prev. Med.*
Journal of the American Chemical Society	*J. Am. Chem. Soc.*
Journal of the American Medical Association	*JAMA*
Journal of the American Veterinary Medical Association	*J. Am. Vet. Med. Assoc.*
Journal of the National Cancer Institute (Washington)	*J. Natl. Cancer Inst.*
Journal of the Proceedings of the Linnean Society (Zoology) Later: *Journal of the Linnean Society (Zoology).* London.	*J. Linn. Soc. London (Zoology)*
Journal of the Reticuloendothelial Society	*J. Reticuloendothel. Soc.*
Journal of the Royal Army Medical Corps (London)	*J.R. Army med. Cps.*
Journal of the Royal Institute of Public Health and Hygiene (London)	*J. R. Inst. publ. Hlth. Hyg.*
Journal of Wildlife Diseases	*J. Wildl. Dis.*
Kitasato Archives of Experimental Medicine (Tokyo)	*Kitasato Arch. Exp. Med.*
Klinisches Jahrbuch (Jena)	*Klin. Jb.*
Klinische Wochenschrift (Berlin)	*Klin. Wochenschr.*
Lancet (London)	*Lancet*
Lancette française. Gazette des Hôpitaux civils et militaires. Paris.	*Lancette française. Gaz. Hôp. civ. milit.,* Paris.

Lavori dell'Istituto d'igiene dell Universita di Cagliari	*Lav. Ist. Ig. Univ. Cagliari*
London Medical Gazette	*Lond. Med. Gaz.*
Medical Classics	*Med. Class.*
Medical Clinics of North America	*Med. Clin. North Am.*
Medical History (London)	*Med. Hist.*
Medical News	*Med. News*
Medical Journal of Australia (Sydney)	*Med. J. Aust.*
Medical Reports. China Imperial Maritime Customs (Shanghai)	*Med. Rep. China imp. marit. Customs*
Medical Sentinel	*Med. Sent.*
Medical Transactions. Published by the (Royal) College of Physicians of London	*Med. Trans. R. Coll. Phys. Lond.*
Medicine (Baltimore)	*Medicine*
Memoirs of the American Philosophical Society (Philadelphia)	*Mem. Am. Philos. Soc.* (Philadelphia)
Michigan Public Health	*Mich. Public Health*
Military Surgeon (Washington)	*Milit. Surg.*
Minnesota Medicine	*Minn. Med.*
Mittheilungen aus dem Kaiserlichen Gesundheitsamte (Berlin)	*Mitt. K. GesundhAmt., Berl.*
Monatsschrift für Kinderheilkunde (Berlin)	*Monatsschr. Kinderheilkd.*
Monographs of the Rockefeller Institute for Medical Research (New York)	*Monogr. Rockefeller Inst. med. Res.*
Münchener Medizinische Wochenschrift	*Münch. Med. Wochenschr.*
Nature (London)	*Nature*
Naval Medical Bulletin (Washington)	*Nav. med. Bull.*
New England Journal of Medicine	*N. Engl. J. Med.*
New England Quarterly Journal of Medicine and Surgery (Boston)	*N. Engl. Q. J. Med. Surg.*
New International Clinics (Philadelphia)	*New int. Clins.*
New Orleans Medical and Surgical Journal	*New Orl. med. surg. J.*
New York Medical and Physical Journal	*NY med. physical J.*
New York Medical Journal-International Record of Medicine	*Int. Record Med.-NY Med. J.*
New York State Journal of Medicine	*NY State J. Med.*
Northwest Medicine	*Northwest Med.*
Official Records of the World Health Organization (Geneva)	*Off. Rec. Wld. Hlth. Org.*
Osiris (Bruges, Belgium)	*Osiris*

Parent

Parent

Pathology (Sydney, Australia)

Pathology (Aust)

Pediatrics

Pediatrics

Philadelphia Medical Journal

Philad. Med. J.

Philosophical Transactions of the
Royal Society of London; B: Biological
Sciences.

Philos. Trans. R. Soc. London
[Biol. Sci.]

Physiological Reviews

Physiol. Rev.

Phytopathological Classics, published
by the American Phytopathological
Society

Phytopathol. Classics

Popular Science Monthly

Popular Sci. Monthly

Postgraduate Medical Journal (London)

Postgraduate Med. J.

Practitioner (London)

Practitioner

Presse Médicale (Paris)

Presse méd.

Proceedings of Staff Meetings of the
Mayo Clinic (Rochester, Minn.)

Proc. Staff Meet. Mayo Clin.

Proceedings of the Academy of Natural
Sciences of Philadelphia

Proc. Acad. nat. Sci. Philad.

Proceedings of the Biological Society
of Washington

Proc. biol. Soc. Wash.

Proceedings of the National Academy
of Sciences of the United States of America

Proc. Natl. Acad. Sci. USA

Proceedings of the Royal Society of
London; B: Biological Sciences

Proc. R. Soc. Lond. [Biol]

Proceedings of the Royal Society of
Medicine (London)

Proc. R. Soc. Med.

Proceedings of the Pacific Science
Congress (Java)

Proc. Pacif. Sci. Congr.

Proceedings of the Society for Experimental
Biology and Medicine (New York)

Proc. Soc. Exp. Biol. Med.

Proceedings of the United States
Livestock Sanitary Association (Chicago)
Later:
Proceedings of the United States Animal
Health Association (Richmond)

Proc. U.S. Livestock Sanit. Assoc.

U.S. Anim. Health Assoc.

Psychiatric Quarterly

Psychiatr. Q.

Public Health Laboratory

Public Health Lab.

Public Health Monographs (Washington)

Public Health Monogr.

Public Health Papers (World Health
Organization Geneva)

Publ. Hlth. Pap. WHO

Quarterly Bulletin of Sea View Hospital
(New York)

Q. Bull. Sea View Hosp.

Quarterly Journal of Medicine

Q. J. Med.

Revista da Sociedade scientifica de   Revta. Soc. scient. S. Paulo
   São Paulo

Revue française d'études cliniques et   Revue fr. Étud. clin. biol.
   biologiques (Paris)
Under:
Revue Européene d'études cliniques
   et biologiques

Rome, Reale Accademia dei Lincei   Roma, R. Accad. Lincei Mem.
   Memorie
Later:
Accademia nazionale dei Lincei, Rome

Schweizerische Zeitschrift für Pathologie   Schweiz. Z. Path. Bakt.
   und Bakteriologie (Basel)

Science   Science

Scientific American   Sci. Am.

Scientific Monthly   Sci. Mo.

Smithsonian Contributions to Knowledge   Smithson. Contr. Knowl.
   (Washington)

South African Institute for Medical   S. Afr. Inst. med. Res. Publ.
   Research. Publications.

Southern Medical Journal   South. Med. J.

St. Paul Medical Journal   St. Paul med. J.

Studies from The Rockefeller Institute   Stud. Rockefeller Inst. med. Res.
   for Medical Research (New York)

Surgery   Surgery

Surgery, Gynecology and Obstetrics   Surg. Gynecol. Obstet.

Transactions of the American   Trans. Am. Climatol. Assoc.
   Climatological Association
Later:
Transactions of the American Clinical   Trans. Am. Clin. Climatol. Assoc.
   and Climatological Association

Transactions of the Association of   Trans. Assoc. Am. Physicians
   American Physicians

Transactions of the College of Physicians   Trans. Coll. Physicians Phila.
   of Philadelphia

Transactions of the Congress of   Trans. Congr. Am. Physns. Surg.
   American Physicians and Surgeons

Transactions of the Epidemiological   Trans. Epidemiol. Soc. London
   Society of London

Transactions of the Medical and Physical   Trans. med. Phys. Soc. Bombay
   Society of Bombay

Transactions of the New York Academy   Trans. NY Acad. Sci.
   of Sciences

Transactions of the North American   Trans. N. Am. Wildl. Nat.
   Wildlife and Natural Resources   Resources Conf.
   Conference

Transactions of the Ophthalmological
Society of Australia (Sydney)

Trans. ophthalmol. Soc. Aust.

Transactions of the Pathological
Society of London

Trans. Pathol. Soc. London

Transactions of the Royal Medico-
Chirurgical Society of London

Trans. R. med.-chir. Soc. London

Transactions of the Royal Society
of Edinburgh

Trans. R. Soc. Edinb.

Transactions of the Royal Society of
Tropical Medicine and Hygiene
(London)

Trans. R. Soc. Trop. Med. Hyg.

Transactions of the Zoological Society
of London

Trans. zool. Soc. Lond.

Transplantation Reviews (Kobenhavn)

Transplant. Rev.

Proceedings of the United States
Animal Health Association (Richmond)
Formerly:
Proceedings of the United States
Livestock Sanitary Association
(Chicago)

U.S. Anim. Health Assoc.

Proc. U.S. Livestock Sanit. Assoc.

United States Hygienic Laboratory
(USPHS) Bulletin
Formerly:
United States Marine Hospital Service
Hygienic Laboratory
Later:
United States National Institutes
of Health Bulletin

U.S. Hyg. Lab. Bull.

U.S. NIH Health Bull.

United States Public Health Reports

U.S. Public Health Rep.

United States Public Health Service
Public Health Bulletin

USPHS Public Health Bull.

Verhandlungen der Deutschen
Gesellschaft für Pathologie (Stuttgart)

Verh. Dtsch. Ges. Pathol.

Veterinary Bulletin

Vet. Bull.

Veterinary Record (London)

Vet. Rec.

Virchow's Archiv für pathologische
Anatomie und Physiologie und für
klinische Medizin (Berlin)

Virchow's Arch. path. Anat. Physiol.

War Medicine

War Med.

Western Journal of Medicine
Formerly:
California Medicine

West. Med.

Calif. Med.

Wiener Klinische Wochenschrift

Wien. Klin. Wochenschr.

Wiener Medizinische Wochenschrift
(Vienna)

Wien. Med. Wochenschr.

Wisconsin Medical Journal

Wis. Med. J.

World Health Organization. Chronicle (Geneva)	WHO Chron.
World Health Organization Monograph Series (Geneva)	WHO Monogr. Ser.
World Health Organization Statistics Report (Geneva)	WHO Stat. Rep.
World Health Organization Technical Report Series (Geneva)	WHO Tech. Rep. Ser.
Yale Journal of Biology and Medicine	Yale J. Biol. Med.
Zeitschrift für die gesamte Neurologie und Psychiatrie (Berlin)	Z. ges. Neurol. Psychiat.
Zeitschrift für Hygiene (Leipzig) Later:	Z. Hyg.
Zeitschrift für Medizinische Mikrobiologie and Immunologie	Z. med. mikrobiol. Immunol.
Zeitschrift für Hygiene und Infektionskrankheiten	Z. Hyg. InfektKrankh.
Zeitschrift für Immunitätsforschung (Stuttgart)	Z. Immunitätsforsch.
Zeitschrift für Infektionskrankheiten, parasitäre Krankheiten und Hygiene der Haustiere (Berlin)	Z. InfektKrankh. parasit. Krankh. Hyg. Haustiere
Zeitschrift für Kinderheilkunde (Berlin)	Z. Kinderheilkd.
Zeitschrift für klinische Medizin (Berlin)	Z. klin. Med.
Zeitschrift für wissenschaftliche Zoologie (Leipzig)	Z. wiss. Zool.
Zentralblatt für Bakteriologie und Parasitenkunde (Jena) Later:	Zentbl. Bakt. ParasitKde.
Zentralblatt für Bakteriologie, Parasitenkunde, Infektionskrankheiten und Hygiene (Stuttgart) *Reihe A: Medizinische Mikrobiologie und Parasitologie* (beginning Vol. 217 in 1971) *Reihe B: Hygiene, Preventive Medizin* (beginning Vol. 155 in 1971)	Zentbl. Bakt. ParasitKde. Hyg.
Zentralblatt für die medizinischen Wissenschaften (Berlin)	Zentbl. med. Wiss.
Zentralblatt fuer Haut-und Geschlechts-krankheiten (Berlin)	Zentbl. Haut-u. GeschlKrankh.

Bibliography

Aberdeen's typhoid bacillus. 1973. *Lancet* 1:645.

Abernathy, R. S. 1973. Treatment of systemic mycoses. *Medicine* 52:385.

Abraham, E. P. 1971. Howard Walter Florey. In *Biographical Memoirs of Fellows of the Royal Society*. Vol. 17, p. 255. London: The Royal Society.

Abraham, E. P., and Chain, E. 1940. An enzyme from bacteria able to destroy penicillin. *Nature* 146:837.

Abraham, E. P.; Chain, C.; Fletcher, C. M.; Florey, H. W.; Gardner, A. D.; Heatley, N. G.; and Jennings, M. A. 1941. Further observations on penicillin. *Lancet* 241:177.

Abraham, E. P., and Newton, G. G. F. 1961. The structure of cephalosporin C. *Biochem. J.* 79:377.

Ackerknecht, E. H. 1945. Malaria in the upper Mississippi Valley 1760–1900. *Bull. Hist. Med., Suppl.* No. 4.

Adams, J. M., and Imagawa, D. T. 1962. Measles antibodies in multiple sclerosis. *Proc. Soc. Exp. Biol. Med.* 111:562.

Ainsworth, G. C., and Sussman, A. S., eds. 1965 to 1973. *The Fungi. An Advanced Treatise.* Vol. 1. *The Fungal Cell* (1965); Vol. 2. *The Fungal Organism* (1966); Vol. 3. *The Fungal Population* (1968); Vol. 4A. *A Taxonomic Review with Keys: Ascomycetes and Fungi Imperfecti* (1973); Vol. 4B. *A Taxonomic Review with Keys: Basidiomycetes and Lower Fungi* (1973). Vol. 4A and 4B edited by Ainsworth, G. C.; Sparrow, F. K.; and Sussman, A. S. New York: Academic Press.

Alexander, C. E.; Sanborn, W. R.; Cherriere, G.; Crocker, Jr., W. H.; Ewald, P. E.; and Kay, C. R. 1968. Sulfadiazine-resistant Group A *Neisseria meningitidis*. *Science* 161:1019.

Alexander, H. E. 1939. Type "B" anti-influenzal rabbit serum for therapeutic purposes. *Proc. Soc. Exp. Biol. Med.* 40:313.

Alexander, H. E. 1944. Treatment of type B hemophilus influenzae meningitis. *J. Pediatr.* 25:517.

Alexander, H. E., and Leidy, G. 1947. The present status of treatment for influenzal meningitis. *Am. J. Med.* 2:457.

Allbutt, T. C. 1870. Medical thermometry. *Brit. and Foreign Med-chir. Rev.* 45:429.

Allison, A. C., and Blumberg, B. S. 1961. An isoprecipitation reaction distinguishing human serum-protein types. *Lancet* 1:634.

Almeida, J. D.; Waterson, A. P.; and Simpson, D. I. H. 1971. Morphology and morphogenesis of the Marburg agent. In *Marburg Virus Diseases*, edited by G. A. Martini and R. Siegert, p. 84. New York: Springer-Verlag.

Alston, J. M., and Broom, J. C. 1958. *Leptospirosis in Man and Animals*. London: E. & S. Livingstone.

Alton, G. G., and Elberg, S. S. 1967. Rev. 1 *Brucella melitensis* vaccine. A review of ten years of study. *Vet. Bull.* 37:793.

Alving, A. S. 1955. Clinical treatment of malaria. In *Recent Advances in Medicine and Surgery* (a course held April 19–30, 1954), Vol. 2, p. 209. Medical Science Publication No. 4. Washington, D.C.: Walter Reed Army Medical Center.

American Academy of Pediatrics 1974. *Report of the Committee on Infectious Diseases 1974*. 17th ed. Evanston (Ill.): American Academy of Pediatrics.

American Public Health Association 1875. *Public Health Reports and Papers*. Presented at the meetings of the American Public Health Association in the year 1873. Cambridge (Mass.): Riverside Press.

Anderson, D. G., and Keefer, C. S. 1948. *The Therapeutic Value of Penicillin: A Study of 10,000 Cases*. Ann Arbor (Mich.): J. W. Edwards.

Anderson, D. W. 1965. Griseofulvin: Biology and clinical usefulness. *Ann. Allergy* 23:103.

Anderson, G. W. 1947. Epidemiology of poliomyelitis. *J.-Lancet* 67:10.

Anderson, G. W.; Arnstein, M. G.; and Lester, M. R. 1962. *Communicable Disease Control. A Volume for the Public Health Worker*. 4th ed. New York: Macmillan.

Anderson, J. F. 1903. Spotted fever (tick-fever) of the Rocky Mountains. A new disease. *U.S. Hyg. Lab. Bull.* No. 14.

Anderson, J. F., and Goldberger, J. 1911. Experimental measles in the monkey: A supplemental note. *U.S. Public Health Rep.* 26:887.

Anderson, J. F., and Goldberger, J. 1912. The relation of so-called Brill's disease to typhus fever. *U.S. Public Health Rep.* 27:149.

Anderson, J. S.; Cooper, K. E.; Happold, F. C.; and McLeod, J. W. 1933. Incidence and correlation with clinical severity of *gravis, mitis*, and intermediate types of diphtheria bacillus in a series of 500 cases at Leeds. *J. Pathol. Bacteriol.* 36:169.

Andrewes, C. 1965. *The Common Cold*. New York: W. W. Norton.

Andrewes, C. H. 1930. Immunity to the salivary virus of guinea-pigs studied in the living animal, and in tissue-culture. *Br. J. Exp. Pathol.* 11:23.

Ansari, N., ed. WHO 1973. *Epidemiology and Control of Schistosomiasis (Bilharziasis)*. Baltimore: University Park Press.

Armstrong, C. 1930. Psittacosis: Epidemiological considerations with reference to the 1929–30 outbreak in the United States. *U.S. Public Health Rep.* 45:2013.

Armstrong, C. 1939a. Successful transfer of the Lansing strain of poliomyelitis virus from the cotton rat to the white mouse. *U.S. Public Health Rep.* 54:2302.

Armstrong, C. 1939b. The experimental transmission of poliomyelitis to the eastern cotton rat, *Sigmodon Hispidus Hispidus*. *U.S. Public Health Rep.* 54:1719.

Armstrong, C. and Lillie, R. D. 1934. Experimental lymphocytic choriomeningitis of monkeys and mice produced by a virus encountered in studies of the 1933 St. Louis encephalitis epidemic. *U.S. Public Health Rep.* 49:1019.

Artenstein, M. S.; Gold, R.; Zimmerly, J. G.; Wyle, F. A.; Schneider, H.; and Harkins, C. 1970. Prevention of meningococcal disease by group C polysaccharide vaccine. *N. Engl. J. Med.* 282:417.

Aschoff, L. 1904, transl. 1941. Zur Myocarditisfrage. *Verh. Dtsch. Ges. Pathol.* 8:46. Translated by F. A. Willius. Concerning the question of myocarditis. In *Cardiac Classics* by F. A. Willius and T. E. Keys, p. 733. St. Louis: C. V. Mosby.

Ashburn, P. M., and Craig, C. F. 1907. Experimental investigations regarding the etiology of dengue fever. *J. Infect. Dis.* 4:440.

Ashe, W. F.; Pratt-Thomas, H. R.; and Kumpe, C. W. 1941. Weil's disease. A complete review of American literature and an abstract of the world literature. Seven case reports. *Medicine* 20:145.

Ashford, B. K. 1900. Ankylostomiasis in Puerto Rico. *Int. Record Med.-NY Med. J.* 71:552.

Atkins, E. 1960. Pathogenesis of fever. *Physiol. Rev.* 40:580.

Atkins, J. 1742. *The Navy Surgeon; or Practical System of Surgery.* London: J. Hodges.

Austrian, R. 1960. The gram stain and the etiology of lobar pneumonia, An historical note. *Bacteriol. Rev.* 24:261.

Avery, O. T. 1915. A further study on the biologic classification of pneumococci. *J. Exp. Med.* 22:804.

Avery, O. T.; Chickering, H. T.; Cole, R.; and Dochez, A. R. 1917. Acute lobar pneumonia. Prevention and serum treatment. *Monogr. Rockefeller Inst. med. Res.* No. 7 (October 16).

Badger, L. F.; Dyer, R. E.; and Rumreich, A. 1931. An infection of the Rocky Mountain spotted fever type: Identification in the eastern part of the United States. *U.S. Public Health Rep.* 46:463.

Badger, T. L., and Spink, W. W. 1937. First infection type of tuberculosis in adults: A five-year study of student nurses at the Boston City Hospital. *N. Engl. J. Med.* 217:424.

Baer, G. M., ed. 1975. *The Natural History of Rabies.* 2 vols. New York: Academic Press.

Baer, W. S. 1931. The treatment of chronic osteomyelitis with the maggot (larva of the blow fly). *J. Bone Joint Surg.* 13:438.

Baillou, G. 1736, transl. 1945. *Epidemiorum et Ephemeridum libri duo. Opera omnia,* 1, p. 155. Venice: Jeremia. Translated by Ralph H. Major. Whooping cough. In *Classic Descriptions of Disease* by Ralph H. Major. 3rd ed., p. 210. Springfield (Ill.): Chas. C Thomas.

Baker, A. B. 1949. Bulbar poliomyelitis: Its mechanism and treatment. *Am. J. Med.* 6:614.

Baker, A. B., and Noran, H. H. 1942. Western variety of equine encephalitis in man. A clinicopathologic study. *Arch. Neurol. Psychiatry* 47:565.

Baldwin, H. S. 1928. Tsutsugamushi fever. In *A Text-Book of Medicine,* edited by R. L. Cecil, p. 338. Philadelphia: W. B. Saunders.

Balfour, Jr., H. H. 1974. California (La Crosse virus) encephalitis in Minnesota. *Minn. Med.* 57:876.

Bancroft, J. 1878. Cases of filarious disease. *Trans. Pathol. Soc. London* 29:407.

Bang, B. 1897. The etiology of epizootic abortion. *J. Comp. Pathol. Therapeutics* 10:125.

Bang, F. B., and Billings, Jr., F. T. 1968. Schistosomiasis japonica: Introduction on Leyte. In *Internal Medicine in World War II* by U.S. Army Medical Department, Vol. 3, p. 91. Washington, D.C.: Office of the Surgeon-General, Department of the Army.

Barber, M., and Dutton, A. A. C. 1958. Antibiotic-resistant staphylococcal outbreaks in a medical and a surgical ward. *Lancet* 275:64.

Bard, S. 1771. *An Enquiry into the Nature, Cause and Care, of the Angina Suffocativa, or Sore Throat Distemper, as It Is Commonly Called by the Inhabitants of this City and Colony.* New York: S. Inslee and A. Car.

Barger, G. 1931. *Ergot and Ergotism.* A monograph based on the Dohme Lectures delivered in Johns Hopkins University, Baltimore. London: Gurney and Jackson.

Barnes, J. M. 1970. Aflatoxin as a health hazard. *J. Appl. Bacteriol.* 33:285.

Barr, M. W. 1892. *Cerebral Meningitis. Its History, Diagnosis, Prognosis, and Treatment.* Detroit (Mich.): George S. Davis.

Barrett, F. F.; Yow, M. D.; and Phillips, C. A. 1965. St. Louis encephalitis in children during the 1946 epidemic. *JAMA* 193:381.

Bartlett, E. 1842. *The History, Diagnosis, and Treatment of Typhoid and of Typhus Fever; with an Essay on the Diagnosis of Bilious Remittent and of Yellow Fever.* Philadelphia: Lea & Blanchard.

Bassi, A. 1835–36, transl. 1958. *Del mal del Segno, Calcinaccio o Moscardino; malattia che affligge i bachi da seta e sul modo di liberarne le bigattaje anche le piu infestate*. 2 vols. Lodi: Dalla Tipographia Orcesi. Translated by P. J. Yarrow. *On the Mark Disease, Calcinaccio or Muscardine, A Disease that Affects Silk Worms and on the Means of Freeing Therefrom Even the Most Devastated Breeding Establishments*. *Phytopathol. Classics* No. 10.

Bassoe, P. 1919. Epidemic encephalitis (Nona). *JAMA* 72:971.

Bateman, T. 1813. *A Practical Synopsis of Cutaneous Diseases*. London: Longman, Hurst, Rees, Orme and Brown.

Bauer, H. 1973. Growing problem of salmonellosis in modern society. *Medicine* 52:323.

Baum, G. L.; Donnerberg, R. L.; Stewart, D.; Mulligan, W. J.; and Putnam, L. R. 1969. Pulmonary sporotrichosis. *N. Engl. J. Med.* 280:410.

Baumgartner, L. and Ramsey, E. M. 1933–34. Johann Peter Frank and his "System Einer Vollstandigen Medicinischen Polizey." *Ann. Med. History* 5 (N.S.):525 and 6 (N.S.):69.

Bayle, G. L. 1810, transl. 1815. *Recherches sur la Phthisie Pulmonaire*. Paris: Gabon. Translated by W. Barrow. *Researches on Pulmonary Phthisis*. Liverpool: Longman, Hurst, Rees, Orme & Brown and W. Grapel.

Baylor (Univ.) Rubella Study Group, Houston, Texas 1967. Rubella: Epidemic in retrospect. *Hosp. Practice* 2 (No. 3):27.

Bayne-Jones, S. 1948. Epidemic typhus in the Mediterranean area during World War II. In *Rickettsial Diseases of Man*, edited by R. R. Moulton, p. 1. Washington, D.C.: American Association for the Advancement of Science.

Becker, F. E. 1930. Tick-borne infections in Colorado. I. The diagnosis and management of infections transmitted by the wood tick. *Colorado Med.* 27:36.

Bedson, S. P. 1959. The psittacosis-lymphogranuloma group of infective agents. The Harben Lectures, 1958. *J. R. Inst. publ. Hlth. Hyg.* 22:67.

Beeson, P., Consulting ed. 1967. Cephaloridine. Proceedings of a conference held at Oxford, March 13–16, 1967. *Postgraduate Med. J.* (London) *Suppl.* 43:1–174.

Beeson, P. B. 1943. Jaundice occurring one to four months after transfusion of blood or plasma. Report of seven cases. *JAMA* 121:1332.

Beeson, P. B.; Hankey, D. H.; and Cooper, Jr., C. F. 1951. Leptospiral iridocyclitis: Evidence of human infection with *Leptospira pomona* in the United States. *JAMA* 145:229.

Beeson, P. B.; Wintrobe, W. M.; and Jager, B. V. 1950. Reaction to injury. In *Principles of Internal Medicine*, edited by T. R. Harrison, p. 401. Philadelphia: Blakiston.

Behring, E. 1913. Ueber ein neues Diphtherieschutzmittel. *Dtsch. Med. Wochenschr.* 39:873.

Behring, E. A., and Kitasato, S. 1890. Ueber das Zustandekommen der Diphtherie-Immunität und der Tetanus-Immunität bei Thieren. *Dtsch. Med. Wochenschr.* 16:1113.

Beijerinck, M. W. 1942. Concerning a contagium vivum fluidum as a cause of the spot-disease of tobacco leaves. Translated from German by James Johnson. *Phytopathol. Classics* No. 7.

Bell, B. 1795. *A Treatise on Gonorrhoea Virulenta and Lues Venerea*. 2 vols. Philadelphia: R. Campbell.

Bender, C. E. 1967. The value of corticosteroids in the treatment of infectious mononucleosis. *JAMA* 199:529.

Benham, R. W. 1935. Cryptococci — their identification by morphology and by serology. *J. Infect. Dis.* 57:255.

Bernard, R. P. 1965. The Zermatt typhoid outbreak in 1963. *J. Hyg.* (Camb.) 63:537.

Besredka, A. 1927. *Local Immunization. Specific Dressings*. Translated by Harry Plotz. Baltimore: Williams & Wilkins.

Bett, W. R. 1956. *Sir John Bland-Sutton*. Edinburgh and London: E. & S. Livingstone.

Beveridge, W. I. B. 1977. *Influenza: The Last Great Plague*. London: Heinemann.

Beveridge, W. I. B., and Burnet, F. M. 1946. *The Cultivation of Viruses and Rickettsiae in the Chick Embryo*. Medical Research Council Special Report Series, No. 256. London: Her Majesty's Stationery Office.

Bickel, L. 1972. *Rise Up to Life. A Biography of Howard Walter Florey Who Gave Penicillin to the World*. London: Angus and Robertson.

Bier, A. 1909. *Bier's Textbook of Hyperaemia as Applied in Medicine and Surgery*. New York: Rebman.

Bietti, G., and Werner, G. H. 1967. *Trachoma. Prevention and Treatment*. Springfield (Ill.): Chas. C Thomas.

Bigelow, H. J. 1846. Insensibility during surgical operations produced by inhalation. *Boston Med. Surg. J.* 35:309.

Biggar, R. J.; Woodall, J. P.; Walter, P. D.; and Haughie, G. E. 1975. Lymphocytic choriomeningitis outbreak associated with pet hamsters. Fifty-seven cases from New York State. *JAMA* 232:494.

Bilharz, T. 1852. Ein Beitrag zur *Helminthographia humana*, aus brieflichen Mittheilungen des Dr. Bilharz in Cairo, nebst Bemerkungen von C. Th. v Siebold in Breslau. *Z. wiss. Zool.* 4:53.

Billings, F. 1914. Focal infection: Its broader application in the etiology of general disease. *JAMA* 63:899.

Billings, F. 1921. *Focal Infection*. New York: D. Appleton.

Billings, F. S. 1884. *The Relation of Animal Diseases to the Public Health, and Their Prevention*. New York: D. Appleton.

Bisseru, B. 1967. *Diseases of Man Acquired from His Pets*. Philadelphia: J. B. Lippincott.

Blake, F. G.; Maxcy, K. F.; Sadusk, Jr., J. F.; Kohls, G. M.; and Bell, E. J. 1945. Studies on tsutsugamushi disease (scrub typhus, mite-borne typhus) in New Guinea and adjacent islands. *Am. J. Hyg.* 41:243.

Blake, J. B. 1959. *Public Health in the Town of Boston: 1630–1822*. Cambridge (Mass.): Harvard University Press.

Blanden, R. V. 1971. Mechanisms of recovery from a generalized viral infection: mousepox. II. Passive transfer of recovery mechanisms with immune lymphoid cells. *J. Exp. Med.* 133:1074.

Bloomfield, A. L. 1958a. Erysipelas. In *A Bibliography of Internal Medicine: Communicable Diseases* by A. L. Bloomfield, p. 128. Chicago: University of Chicago Press.

Bloomfield, A. L. 1958b. Meningococcal infection. Ibid, p. 165.

Bloomfield, A. L. 1958c. Mumps. Ibid, p. 516.

Bloomfield, A. L. 1958d. Rheumatic fever. Ibid, p. 135.

Bloomfield, A. L. 1958e. Scarlet fever. Ibid, p. 107.

Bloomfield, A. L. 1958f. The common cold. Ibid, p. 422.

Bloomfield, A. L., and Rantz, L. A. 1943. An outbreak of streptococcic septic sore throat in an army camp. *JAMA* 121:315.

Blumberg, B. S. 1964. Polymorphisms of the serum proteins and the development of iso-precipitins in transfused patients. *Bull. N.Y. Acad. Med.* 40:377.

Blumberg, B. S.; Dray, S.; and Robinson, J. C. 1962. Antigen polymorphism of a low-density beta-lipoprotein. Allotypy in human serum. *Nature* 194:656.

Blumberg, B. S.; Sutnick, A. I.; and London, W. T. 1968. Hepatitis and leukemia: Their relation to Australia antigen. *Bull. N.Y. Acad. Med.* 44:1566.

Blumer, G. 1923a. Infectious jaundice in the United States. *JAMA* 81:353.

Blumer, G. 1923b. Subacute bacterial endocarditis. *Medicine* 2:105.

Boak, R. A.; Carpenter, C. M.; and Warren, S. L. 1932. Studies on the physiological effects of fever temperatures. III. The thermal death time of *Treponema pallidum* in vitro with special reference to fever temperatures. *J. Exp. Med.* 56:741.

Boccaccio, G. 1930. *The Decameron*. Translated by Richard Aldington. Garden City (NY): Doubleday & Co.

Boghurst, W. 1893–94. Loimographia: An account of the great plague of London in the year 1665. Now first printed from the British Museum Sloane Ms. 349 for the Epidemiological Society of London. Edited by Joseph F. Payne. *Trans. Epidemiol. Soc. London* Vol. 13 *Suppl.*

Bókay, Jr. 1909. Ueber den ätiologischen Zusammenhang der Varizellen mit gewissen Fällen von Herpes zoster. *Wien. Klin. Wochenschr.* 22:1323.

Boldt, J. 1904. *Trachoma.* Translated by J. H. Parsons and T. Snowball. London: Hodder and Stoughton.

Bollinger, O. 1877. Ueber eine neue Pilzkrankheit beim Rinde. *Zentbl. med. Wiss.* No. 27, p. 481.

Bordet, J. 1895, transl. 1909. Contribution à l'étude du sérum chez les animaux vaccinés. *Annls. Soc. r. Sci. med. nat. Brux.* 4:455. Translated by F. P. Gay. Studies on the serum of vaccinated animals. In *Studies in Immunity* by Jules Bordet et al., p. 8. New York: John Wiley & Sons.

Bordet, J., and Gengou, O. 1901, transl. 1909. Sur l'existence de substances sensibilisatrices dans la plupart des sérums antimicrobiens. *Annls. Inst. Pasteur* 15:289. Translated by Frederick P. Gay. On the existence of sensitizing substances in the majority of antimicrobial sera. In *Studies in Immunity* by Jules Bordet et al., p. 217. New York: John Wiley & Sons.

Bordet, J., and Gengou, O. 1906. Le microbe de la coqueluche. *Annls. Inst. Pasteur* 20:731.

Boring III, J. R.; Martin, W. T.; and Elliott, L. M. 1971. Isolation of *Salmonella typhimurium* from municipal water, Riverside, California, 1965. *Am. J. Epidemiol.* 93:49.

Bouillaud, J. 1837. *New Researches on Acute Articular Rheumatism in General.* Translated by J. Kitchen. Philadelphia: Haswell, Barrington, and Haswell.

Boyd, M. F. 1939. Malaria: Retrospect and prospect. *Am. J. Trop. Med.* 19:1.

Boyd, M. R., ed. 1949. *Malariology. A Comprehensive Survey of All Aspects of this Group of Diseases from a Global Standpoint.* 2 vols. Philadelphia: W. B. Saunders.

Braude, A. I. 1951. Studies in the pathology and pathogenesis of experimental brucellosis. I. A comparison of the pathogenicity of *Brucella abortus*, *Brucella melitensis* and *Brucella suis*. *J. Infect. Dis.* 89:76.

Braude, A. I. 1976. *Antimicrobial Drug Therapy.* Volume 8 of *Major Problems in Internal Medicine,* edited by Lloyd H. Smith, Jr., M.D. Philadelphia: W. B. Saunders.

Braude, A. I.; Hall, W. H.; and Spink, W. W. 1949. Aureomycin therapy in human brucellosis due to *Brucella abortus.* *JAMA* 141:831.

Braude, A. I., and Spink, W. W. 1950. The action of aureomycin and other chemotherapeutic agents in experimental brucellosis. *J. Immunol.* 65:185.

Bray, J. 1945. Isolation of antigenically homogeneous strains of *Bact. coli Neapolitanum* from summer diarrhoea of infants. *J. Pathol. Bacteriol.* 57:239.

Bretonneau, P. 1826, transl. 1859. *Des Inflammations Spéciales du Tissu Muqueux, et an Particulier de la Diphtherite, ou Inflammation Pelliculaire, connue sous le nom de croup, d'angine maligne, d'angine gangreneuse, etc.* Paris: Chez Crevot, Libraire-Editeur. Translated by R. H. Semple. *Memoirs on Diphtheria from the Writings of Bretonneau, Guersant, Trousseau, Bouchut, Empis and Deviot.* London: New Sydenham Society, Vol. 3.

Bretonneau, P. 1829. Notice sur la contagion de la dothinentérie. *Archs. gén. Méd.* 21:57.

Bright, R. 1827. *Reports of Medical Cases, selected with a view of illustrating the symptoms and cure of diseases by a reference to morbid anatomy.* London: Longman, Rees, Orme, Brown, and Green.

Brill, N. E. 1910. An acute infectious disease of unknown origin. *Am. J. Med. Sci.* 139:484.

Brodie, M., and Park, W. H. 1935. Active immunization against poliomyelitis. *NY State J. Med.* 35:815.

Brotzu, G. 1948. Richerche su di un nuovo antibiotics. *Lav. Ist. Ig. Univ. Cagliari* 3.

Brown, J. H. 1919. The use of blood agar for the study of streptococci. *Monogr. Rockefeller Inst. med. Res.* No. 9.

Brown, J. W., and Condit, P. K. 1965. Meningococcal infections: Fort Ord and California. *Calif. Med.* 102:171.

Brown, L. 1941. *The Story of Clinical Pulmonary Tuberculosis.* Baltimore: Williams & Wilkins.

Brown, T. R. 1897. Studies on trichinosis. *Johns Hopkins Hosp. Bull.* 8:79.

Bruce, D. 1888. The micrococcus of Malta fever. *Practitioner* 40:241.

Bruce, D. 1895. *Preliminary Report on the Tsetse Fly Disease or Nagana, in Zululand.* Durban: Bennett & Davis.

Bruce, D. 1908. The extinction of Malta fever. *Nature* 78:39.

Bruce, D. 1915. The Croonian Lectures on "Trypanosomes. Causing disease in man and domestic animals in Central Africa." *Lancet* 188:323, 189:1, 55, 109.

Brunell, P. A.; Ross, A.; Miller, L. H.; and Kuo, B. 1969. Prevention of varicella by zoster immune globulin. *N. Engl. J. Med.* 280:1191.

Buchanan, R. E., and Gibbons, N. E., eds. 1974. Gram-positive cocci (by various authors). In *Bergey's Manual of Determinative Bacteriology*, p. 478. 8th ed. Baltimore: Williams & Wilkins.

Buchanan, T. M., et al. 1974. Brucellosis in the United States, 1960–1972: An abattoir-associated disease. *Medicine* 53:403.

Buckley, S. M., and Casals, J. 1970. Lassa fever, a new virus disease of man from West Africa. III. Isolation and characterization of the virus. *Am. J. Trop. Med. Hyg.* 19:680.

Budd, W. 1856a. On intestinal fever: Its mode of propagation. *Lancet* 2:694.

Budd, W. 1856b. On the fever at the clergy orphan asylum. *Lancet* 2:617.

Buddle, M. B., and Boyes, B. W. 1953. A brucella mutant causing genital disease of sheep in New Zealand. *Aust. Vet. J.* 29:145.

Bull, O. B., and Hansen, G. A. 1873. *The Leprous Diseases of the Eye.* Christiania: Albert Cammermeyer.

Bulloch, W. 1938a. Discussion on pyaemia, septicaemia and surgical sepsis. In *The History of Bacteriology* by W. Bulloch, p. 139. London: Oxford University Press.

Bulloch, W. 1938b. *The History of Bacteriology.* London: Oxford University Press.

Bullock, W. E.; Fields, J. P.; and Brandriss, M. W. 1972. An evaluation of transfer factor as immunotherapy for patients with lepromatous leprosy. *N. Engl. J. Med.* 287:1053.

Bullock, W. E.; Hall, III, J. W.; Spink, W. W.; Damsky, L. J.; Greene, V. W.; Vesley, D.; and Bauer, H. 1964. A staphylococcal isolation service. Epidemiologic and clinical studies over one year. *Ann. Intern. Med.* 60:777.

Burger, D., and Hartsough, G. R. 1965. Encephalopathy of mink. II. Experimental and natural transmission. *J. Infect. Dis.* 115:393.

Burgess, P. 1940. *Who Walk Alone.* New York: Henry Holt.

Burkitt, D. 1958. A sarcoma involving the jaws in African children. *Br. J. Surg.* 46:218.

Burkitt, D. 1967. Chemotherapy of African (Burkitt) lymphoma — Clinical evidence suggesting an immunological response. *Br. J. Surg.* 54:817.

Burnet, F. M. 1935. Propagation of the virus of epidemic influenza on the developing egg. *Med. J. Aust.* 2:687.

Burnet, F. M. 1940. *Biological Aspects of Infectious Disease.* New York: Macmillan.

Burnet, F. M. 1959. *The Clonal Selection Theory of Acquired Immunity* (Abraham Flexner Lecture, 1958). Nashville: Vanderbilt Univ. Press.

Burnet, F. M. 1962. *The Integrity of the Body; A Discussion of Modern Immunological Ideas.* Cambridge (Mass.): Harvard University Press.

Burnet, F. M., and Freeman, M. 1937. Experimental studies on the virus of "Q" fever. *Med. J. Aust.* 2:299.

Burnett, J. H. 1968. *Fundamentals of Mycology.* London: Edward Arnold.

Burnside, J. E.; Sippel, W. L.; Forgacs, J.; Carll, W. T.; Atwood, M. B.; and Doll, E. R. 1957. A disease of swine and cattle caused by eating moldy corn. II. Experimental production with pure cultures of molds. *Am. J. Vet. Res.* 18:817.

Burrows, W. 1968. *Textbook of Microbiology.* 19th ed. Philadelphia: W. B. Saunders.

Burton, E. F., and Kohl, W. H. 1942. *The Electron Microscope.* New York: Reinhold Publishing.

Buschke, A. 1895. Ueber eine durch Coccidien hervorgerufene Krankheit des Menschen. *Dtsch. med. Wochenschr.* 21:14.

490   BIBLIOGRAPHY

Bushby, S. R. M. 1959. The sulphones. In *Leprosy in Theory and Practice*, edited by R. G. Cochrane. Bristol: John Wright & Sons.

Busse, O. 1894. Ueber parasitäre Zelleinschlüsse und ihre Züchtung. *Zentbl. Bakt. Hyg.*, *I. Abt.*, *Orig. B.* 16:175.

Butler, R. N. 1975. *Why Survive? Being Old in America*. New York: Harper & Row.

Buttle, G. A. H.; Gray, W. H.; and Stephenson, D. 1936. Protection of mice against streptococcal and other infections by p-aminobenzenesulphonamide and related substances. *Lancet* 230:1286.

Cagniard-Latour, C. 1838. Mémoire sur la fermentation vineuse. *Annls. Chim. Phys.* 68:206.

Cairns, J.; Stent, G. S.; and Watson, J. D., eds. 1966. *Phage and the Origins of Molecular Biology*. Cold Spring Harbor (NY): Cold Spring Harbor Laboratory of Quantitative Biology.

Callender, G. R. 1929. Pathology of acute respiratory diseases. In *The Medical Department of the United States Army in the World War* by the U.S. Surgeon-General's Office. Vol. 12, p. 1. Washington, D.C.: U.S. Govt. Printing Office.

Calmette, A. 1923. *Tubercle Bacillus Infection and Tuberculosis in Man and Animals, Processes of Infection and Resistance*. Translated by W. B. Soper and G. M. Smith. Baltimore: Williams & Wilkins.

Calmette, A.; Guerin, C.; Nègre, L.; and Boquet, A. 1927. Sur la vaccination préventive des enfants nouveau-nés contre la tuberculose par le BCG. *Annls. Inst. Pasteur* 41:201.

Cameron, T. W. M. 1956. *Parasites and Parasitism*. New York: John Wiley & Sons.

Camus, A. 1948. *The Plague*. Translated by Stuart Gilbert. New York: Modern Library.

Cantaloube, P. 1911. *La Fièvre de Malte en France*. Paris, A. Maloine.

Carmichael, L. E., and Kenney, R. M. 1968. Canine abortion caused by *Brucella canis*. *J. Am. Vet. Med. Assoc.* 152:605.

Carpenter, C. M.; Boak, R. A.; and Warren, S. L. 1932. Studies on the physiological effects of fever temperatures. IV. The healing of experimental syphilitic lesions in rabbits by short wave fevers. *J. Exp. Med.* 56:751.

Carpenter, C. M.; Boak, R. A.; and Warren, S. L. 1938. The thermal death time of the gonococcus at fever temperatures. *Am. J. Syph Gonorrhea vener. Dis.* 22:279.

Carpenter, C. M., and Merriam, H. E. 1926. Undulant fever from *Brucella abortus*. *JAMA* 87:1269.

Carson, R. L. 1962. *Silent Spring*. Boston: Houghton Mifflin.

Carter, H. R. 1931. *Yellow Fever; an Epidemiological and Historical Study of Its Place of Origin*. Baltimore: Williams & Wilkins.

Carter, H. Vandyke 1861. On 'mycetoma,' or the fungus-disease of India: Including notes of recent cases and new observations on the structure, &c. of the entophytic growth. *Trans. med. Phys. Soc. Bombay* 7 (N.S.):206.

Casals, J. 1971. Arboviruses: Incorporation in a general system of virus classification. In *Comparative Virology*, edited by K. Maramorosch and E. Kurstak, p. 307. New York: Academic Press.

Casals, J., and Buckley, S. M. 1974. Lassa fever. In *Progress in Medical Virology*, edited by J. L. Melnick. Vol. 18, p. 111. Basel: Karger.

Casels, J.; Curnen, E. C.; and Thomas, L. 1943. Venezuelan equine encephalitis in man. *J. Exp. Med.* 77:251.

Casoni, T. 1911–12. La diagnosi biologica dell' echinococcosi umana mediante l'intradermoreazione. *Folia clin. chim. microsc.*, Salsomaggiore 4 (No. 3):5.

Cassedy, J. H. 1962. *Charles V. Chapin and the Public Health Movement*. Cambridge (Mass.): Harvard University Press.

Castiglioni, A. 1933. *History of Tuberculosis*. Translated by Emilie Recht. New York: Froben Press.

Catlin, G. 1841. *Letters and Notes on the Manners, Customs, and Condition of the North American Indians*. 2 vols. London: The Author.

Caulfield, E. 1939. A history of the terrible epidemic, vulgarly called the throat distemper, as it occurred in His Majesty's New England colonies between 1735 and 1740. *Yale J. Biol. Med.* 11:219.

Caverly, C. S. 1896. Notes of an epidemic of acute anterior poliomyelitis. *JAMA* 26:1.

Cecil, R. L., ed. 1928. *Text-Book of Medicine.* Philadelphia: W. B. Saunders.

Center for Disease Control. 1970. *Plague Surveillance. Report No. 1 from the Fort Collins, Colorado Laboratory, July 1970.* Atlanta (Ga.): U.S. Dept. of Health, Education and Welfare, Public Health Service.

Center for Disease Control. 1973a. *Measles Surveillance — 1972 Summary.* CDC Report No. 9 (August). Atlanta (Ga.): Public Health Service.

Center for Disease Control. 1973b. Typhoid fever, Florida. *CDC Morbidity Mortality Weekly Rep.* 22:77 (March 3).

Center for Disease Control. 1974a. *Botulism in the United States, 1899–1973. Handbook for Epidemiologists, Clinicians, and Laboratory Workers.* DHEW Publication No. (CDC) 74-8279 (June). Atlanta (Ga.): Public Health Service.

Center for Disease Control. 1974b. Follow-up on meningococcal meningitis — Brazil. *CDC Morbidity Mortality Weekly Rep.* 23:349 (October 12).

Center for Disease Control. 1974c. *Malaria Surveillance: Annual Summary 1973.* Atlanta (Ga.): Public Health Service.

Center for Disease Control. 1974d. *Rabies Surveillance: Annual Summary 1973.* DHEW Publication No. (CDC) 75-8255 (July). Lawrenceville (Ga.): Public Health Service.

Center for Disease Control. 1974e. Salmonellosis on a Caribbean cruise ship. *CDC Morbidity Mortality Weekly Rep.* 23:333 (September 28).

Center for Disease Control. 1976a. Coxsackievirus outbreak — New York. *CDC Morbidity Mortality Weekly Rep.* No. 47, 25:377 (December 6).

Center for Disease Control. 1976b. *Hepatitis Surveillance Report No. 38.* DHEW Publication No. (CDC) 76:8261 (September). Atlanta (Ga.): Public Health Service.

Center for Disease Control. 1976c. Respiratory infection — Pennsylvania. *CDC Morbidity Mortality Weekly Rep.* No. 30, 25:244 (August 6).

Center for Disease Control. 1977a. Follow-up on respiratory disease — Pennsylvania. *CDC Morbidity Mortality Weekly Rep.* No. 12, 26:93 (March 25).

Center for Disease Control. 1977b. Follow-up on respiratory illness — Philadelphia. *CDC Morbidity Mortality Weekly Rep.* No. 2, 26:9 (January 18).

Center for Disease Control. 1977c. Follow-up on respiratory illness — Philadelphia. *CDC Morbidity Mortality Weekly Rep.* No. 6, 26:43 (February 11).

Center for Disease Control. 1977d. Legionnaires' disease — United States. *CDC Morbidity Mortality Weekly Rep.* No. 27, 26:224 (July 8).

Chadwick, H. D., and Pope, A. S. 1942. *The Modern Attack on Tuberculosis.* New York: Commonwealth Fund.

Chain, E. 1971. Thirty years of penicillin therapy. *Proc. R. Soc. Lond. (Biol.)* 179:293.

Chain, E.; Florey, H. W.; Gardner, A. D.; Heatley, N. G.; Jennings, M. A.; Orr-Ewing, J.; and Sanders, A. G. 1940. Penicillin as a chemotherapeutic agent. *Lancet* 239:226.

Chandler, C., and Hodes, H. L. 1950. Aureomycin in the treatment of experimental and clinical infections with *H. influenzae*, type B. *Pediatrics* 5:267.

Chapin, C. 1921. History of state and municipal control of disease. In *A Half Century of Public Health*, edited by Mazÿck P. Ravenel. New York: American Public Health Assn.

Chapin, C. V. 1910. *The Sources and Modes of Infection.* New York: John Wiley & Sons.

Chapin, C. V. 1916. *A Report on State Public Health Work, Based on a Survey of State Boards of Health.* Chicago: American Medical Assn.

Chaucer, G. 1934. *Canterbury Tales.* Rendered into Modern English by J. U. Nicolson. New York: Covici-Friede.

Cheadle, W. B. 1889. *The Various Manifestations of the Rheumatic State as Exemplified in Childhood and Early Life.* Harveian Lectures 1888. London: Smith, Elder & Co.

Cheever, D. W. 1906. Professional reminiscences on sepsis and gangrene. In *A History of the Boston City Hospital: 1864–1904*, edited by D. W. Cheever, G. W. Gay, A. L. Mason, and J. B. Blake, p. 271. Boston: Municipal Printing Office.

Cheyne, J. 1808. *An Essay on Hydrocephalus Acutus, or Dropsy in the Brain*. London: Mundell, Doig, & Stevenson; and J. Murray.

Cholera (Editorial). 1832. The cases of cholera successfully treated by large aqueous injections. *Lancet* 2:284.

Christensen, C. M. 1961. *The Molds and Man: An Introduction to the Fungi*, 2nd. ed. Minneapolis: University of Minnesota Press.

Christensen, C. M., and Kaufmann, H. H. 1969. *Grain Storage: The Role of Fungi in Quality Loss*. Minneapolis: University of Minnesota Press.

Christie, A., and Peterson, J. C. 1946. Benign histoplasmosis and pulmonary calcification. *Am. J. Dis. Child.* 72:460.

Ciba Foundation Study Group No. 31. 1967. *Nutrition and Infection*. Boston: Little, Brown and Co.

Cipolla, C. M. 1973. *Cristofano and the Plague. A Study in the History of Public Health in the Age of Galileo*. Berkeley: University of California Press.

Clayton, G. E. B., and Derrick, E. H. 1937. The presence of leptospirosis of a mild type (seven-day fever) in Queensland. *Med. J. Aust.* 1:647.

Clowes, W. 1596 and 1971. *A Profitable and Necessarie Booke of Observations for All Those that Are Burned with the Flame of Gun Powder, Etc. and also for curing of wounds made with musket and caliver shot, and other weapons of war commonly used at this day both by sea and land, as hereafter shall be declared: With an addition of most approved remedies, gathered for the good and comfort of many, out of divers learned men both old and new writers. Last of all is adjoyned a short treatise, for the cure of Lues Venerea by unctions and other approved ways of curing, heretofore by me collected: and now again newly corrected and augmented in the year of our Lord 1596*. London: Thomas Dawson. Reprinted in *Booke of Observations, London 1596* by Wm. Clowes. New York: Da Capo Press.

Clymer, M. 1872. *Epidemic Cerebro-Spinal Meningitis*. Philadelphia: Lindsay & Blakiston.

Cobbold, T. S. 1864. *Entozoa: An Introduction to the Study of Helminthology*. London: Groombridge and Sons.

Coburn, A. F. 1931. *The Factor of Infection in the Rheumatic State*. Baltimore: Williams & Wilkins.

Coburn, A. F., and Young, D. C. 1949. *The Epidemiology of Hemolytic Streptococcus During World War II in the United States Navy*. Baltimore: Williams & Wilkins.

Cochrane, R. G., and Davey, T. F., eds. 1964. *Leprosy in Theory and Practice*. 2nd ed. Bristol (Engl.): John Wright & Sons.

Cockayne, E. A. 1912. Catarrhal jaundice, sporadic and epidemic, and its relation to acute yellow atrophy of the liver. *Q. J. Med.* 6:1.

Coggeshall, L. T., and Craige, B. 1949. Old and new plasmodicides. In *Malariology*, edited by M. Boyd. Vol. 2, p. 1071. Philadelphia: W. B. Saunders.

Coghill, R. D., and Koch, R. S. 1945. Penicillin. A wartime accomplishment. *Chem. Engng. News* 23:2310.

Cohn, V. 1975. *Sister Kenny: The Woman Who Challenged the Doctors*. Minneapolis: University of Minnesota Press.

Cole, R., and Kuttner, A. G. 1926. A filterable virus present in the submaxillary glands of guinea pigs. *J. Exp. Med.* 44:855.

Colebrook, L., and Kenny, M. 1936. Treatment of human puerperal infections, and of experimental infections in mice, with prontosil. *Lancet* 230:1279.

Coles, A. C. 1930. Micro-organisms in psittacosis. *Lancet* 218:1011.

Collaborative Report. 1971. A waterborne epidemic of salmonellosis in Riverside, California, 1965. Epidemiologic aspects. *Am. J. Epidemiol.* 93:33.

Commission on Acute Respiratory Diseases, Fort Bragg, N.C. 1945a. A study of a food-borne epidemic of tonsillitis and pharyngitis due to β-hemolytic streptococcus, type 5. *Johns Hopkins Hosp. Bull.* 77:143.

Commission on Acute Respiratory Diseases, Fort Bragg, N.C. 1945b. Transmission of primary atypical pneumonia to human volunteers. *JAMA* 127:146.

Commission on Acute Respiratory Diseases, Fort Bragg, N.C. 1946. A laboratory outbreak of Q fever caused by the Balkan Grippe strain of *Rickettsia burneti*. *Am. J. Hyg.* 44:123.

Commission on Pneumonia, Board for the Investigation and Control of Influenza and Other Epidemic Diseases in the United States Army. 1942. Primary atypical pneumonia, etiology unknown. Prepared for the Surgeon-General of the Army. *War Med.* 2:330.

Comstock, G. W. 1975. Frost revisited: The modern epidemiology of tuberculosis. *Am. J. Epidemiol.* 101:363.

Conant, N. F.; Smith, D. T.; Baker, R. D.; and Callaway, J. L. 1971. *Manual of Clinical Mycology*. 3rd ed. Philadelphia: W. B. Saunders.

Controulis, J.; Rebstock, M. C.; and Crooks, Jr., H. M. 1949. Chloramphenicol (chloromycetin). V. Synthesis. *J. Am. Chem. Soc.* 71:2463.

Cook, E. 1913. *The Life of Florence Nightingale*. 2 vols. London: Macmillan & Co.

Cooper, G.; Rosenstein, C.; Walter, A.; and Peizer, L. 1932. The further separation of types among the pneumococci hitherto included in Group IV and the development of therapeutic antisera for these types. *J. Exp. Med.* 55:531.

Cope, Z. 1938. *Actinomycosis*. London: Oxford University Press.

Corner, G. W. 1964. *A History of the Rockefeller Institute, 1901–1953; Origins and Growth*. New York; Rockefeller Institute Press.

Couch, R. B. 1973. Mycoplasma pneumoniae. In *Viral and Mycoplasmal Infections of the Respiratory Tract*, edited by V. Knight, p. 217. Philadelphia: Lea & Febiger.

Councilman, W. T., and Lafleur, H. A. 1891. Report in pathology. I. Amoebic dysentery. *Johns Hopkins Hosp. Rep.* 2:395.

Councilman, W. T.; Mallory, F. B.; and Wright, J. H. 1898. *Epidemic Cerebro-Spinal Meningitis and Its Relation to Other Forms of Meningitis. A Report of the State Board of Health of Massachusetts*. Boston: Wright & Potter.

Coupal, J. F. 1929. Pathology of gas gangrene following war wounds. In *The Medical Department of the U.S. Army in the World War* by the U.S. Surgeon-General's Office. Vol. 12, p. 407. Washington, D.C.: U.S. Government Printing Office.

Covell, G.; Coatney, G. R.; Field, J. W.; and Singh, J. 1955. *Chemotherapy of Malaria*. Geneva: World Health Organization.

Cox, H. R. 1940. *Rickettsia diaporica* and American Q fever. *Am. J. Trop. Med.* 20:463.

Cox, H. R., and Bell, E. J. 1940. Epidemic and endemic typhus: Protective value for guinea pigs of vaccines prepared from infected tissues of the developing chick embryo. *U.S. Public Health Rep.* 55:110.

Cox, H. R.; Tesar, W. C.; and Irans, J. V. 1947. Q fever in the United States. IV. Isolation and identification of Rickettsias in an outbreak among stock handlers and slaughterhouse workers. *JAMA* 133:820.

Cox, L. B., and Tolhurst, J. C. 1946. *Human Torulosis. A Clinical, Pathological and Microbiological Study*. Melbourne: Melbourne University Press.

Craig, C. F., and Faust, E. C. 1945a. *Clinical Parasitology*. 4th ed. Philadelphia: Lea & Febiger.

Craig, C. F., and Faust, E. C. 1945b. *Echinococcus granulosus*. In *Clinical Parasitology* by C. F. Craig and E. C. Faust. 4th ed., p. 516. Philadelphia: Lea & Febiger.

Craigie, J. 1945. Application and control of ethyl-ether-water interface effects to the separation of rickettsiae from yolk sac preparations. *Can. J. Res., Section E* 23:104.

Cramblett, H. G.; Stegmiller, H.; and Spencer, C. 1966. California encephalitis virus infections in children. Clinical and laboratory studies. *JAMA* 198:108.

Creighton, C. 1889. *Jenner and Vaccination: A Strange Chapter of Medical History*. London: Swan Sonnenschein.

Creighton, C. 1891a. *A History of Epidemics in Great Britain. From A.D. 664–1666*. Vol. 1. Cambridge: University Press.

Creighton, C. 1891b. Epidemics of St. Anthony's fire, or ergotism. In *A History of Epidemics in Great Britain. From A.D. 664–1666* by C. Creighton. Vol. 1, p. 52. Cambridge: University Press.

494   BIBLIOGRAPHY

Creighton, C. 1894a. *A History of Epidemics in Great Britain. From A.D. 1666–1894.* Vol. 2. Cambridge: University Press.
Creighton, C. 1894b. Influenzas and epidemic agues. In *A History of Epidemics in Great Britain. From A.D. 1666–1894* by C. Creighton. Vol. 2, p. 300. Cambridge: University Press. 2nd ed. unrevised. 1965. 2 vols. London: Frank Cass. Informative introductions in this edition are "Epidemiology as Social History" by D. E. C. Eversley; "Charles Creighton: The Man and his Work" by E. Ashworth Underwood; and "A Select Bibliography of Epidemiological Literature since 1894" by Lynda Ovenall.
Creutzfeldt, H. G. 1920. Über eine eigenartige herdförmige Erkrankung des Zentralnervensystems. *Z. ges Neurol. Psychiat.* 57:1.
Crookshank, E. M. 1889. *History and Pathology of Vaccination,* 2 vols. London: H. K. Lewis.
Cummins, S. L. 1949. *Tuberculosis in History. From the 17th Century to our Own Times.* Introduction by Sir Arthur Salusbury Macnalty. London: Baillière, Tindall and Cox.
Currie, J. 1798. *Medical Reports, on the Effects of Water, Cold and Warm, as a Remedy in Fever and other Diseases, Whether applied to the Surface of the Body, or used Internally; Including An Inquiry into the Circumstances that render Cold Drink, or the Cold Bath, dangerous in Health. To which are added Observations on the Nature of Fever; and on the Effects of Opium, Alcohol, and Inanition.* 2nd ed. corrected and enlarged. London: Cadell Jun. and Davies.
Custer, R. P., and Smith, E. B. 1949. The pathology of infectious mononucleosis. In *G. R. Minot Symposium,* edited by W. Damashek and F. H. L. Taylor, p. 704. New York: Grune & Stratton.
Dack, G. M. 1956. Staphylococcus food poisoning. In *Food Poisoning* by G. M. Dack, p. 109. Chicago: University of Chicago Press.
Dack, G. M.; Cary, W. E.; Woolpert, O.; and Wiggers, H. 1930. An outbreak of food poisoning proved to be due to a yellow hemolytic staphylococcus. *J. prev. Med.* 4:167.
Dakin, H. D.; Cohen, J. B.; Daufresne, M.; and Kenyon, J. 1917. The antiseptic action of substances of the chloramine group. *Proc. R. Soc. London (Biol.)* 89:232.
Dale, H. 1960. Introduction. In *The Collected Papers of Paul Ehrlich,* compiled and edited by F. Himmelweit with the assistance of Martha Marquardt under the editorial direction of Sir Henry Dale. Vol. 3, p. 1. London: Pergamon Press.
Dalldorf, G., and Sickles, G. M. 1948. An unidentified, filtrable agent isolated from the feces of children with paralysis. *Science* 108:61.
Dane, D. S.; Cameron, C. H.; and Briggs, M. 1970. Virus-like particles in serum of patients with Australia-antigen-associated hepatitis. *Lancet* 1:695.
Daniels, W. B., and Grennan, H. A. 1943. Pretibial fever: An obscure disease. *JAMA* 122:361.
Danielssen, D. C., and Boeck, W. 1848. *Traité de la Spédalskhed ou Éléphantiasis des Grecs.* Translated by L. A. Cosson (de Nogaret) with M. D. Danielssen. Paris: J. B. Baillière.
Darling, S. T. 1906. A protozoon general infection producing pseudotubercles in the lungs and focal necroses in the liver, spleen and lymphnodes. *JAMA* 46:1283.
Darling, S. T. 1909. The morphology of the parasite (*Histoplasma capsulatum*) and the lesions of histoplasmosis, a fatal disease of Tropical America. *J. Exp. Med.* 11:515.
Davaine, C. 1863. Recherches sur les infusoires du sang dans la maladie connue sous le nom de sang de rate. *C. R. Acad. Sci. (D) (Paris)* 57:220.
Davidsohn, I., and Walker, P. H. 1935. The nature of the heterophilic antibodies in infectious mononucleosis. *Am. J. Clin. Pathol.* 5:455.
Davis, D. J. 1919. The effect of potassium iodid on experimental sporotrichosis. *J. Infect. Dis.* 25:124.
Davis, H. H. 1926. The present status of mercurochrome-220 soluble. *Am. J. Med. Sci.* 172:340.
Davis, J. W.; Karstad, L. H.; and Trainer, D. O., eds. 1970. *Infectious Diseases of Wild Mammals.* Ames (Iowa): Iowa State University Press.

De Beer, E. S., ed. 1955. *The Diary of John Evelyn, 1650–1672. Now first printed in full from the manuscripts belonging to Mr. John Evelyn in six volumes*. Vol. 3. Oxford: Clarendon Press.

Dees, J. E., and Colston, J. A. C. 1937. The use of sulfanilamide in gonococcic infections: Preliminary report. *JAMA* 108:1855.

DeFoe, D. 1908. *A Journal of the Plague Year, Written by a Citizen Who Continued all the While in London*. New York: E. P. Dutton.

De Kruif, P. 1928. The automatic man: Francis. In *Hunger Fighters*, p. 131. New York: Harcourt Brace.

De Lorenzo, F.; Manzillo, G.; Soscia, M.; and Balestrieri, G. G. 1974. Epidemic of cholera El Tor in Naples, 1973. *Lancet* 1:669.

De Monbreun, W. A. 1934. The cultivation and cultural characteristics of Darling's *Histoplasma capsulatum. Am. J. Trop. Med*. 14:93.

Derrick, E. H. 1937. "Q" fever, a new fever entity: Clinical features, diagnosis and laboratory investigation. *Med. J. Aust*. 2:281.

Desmonts, G.; Couvreur, J.; Alison, F.; Baudelot, J.; Gerbeaux, J.; and Lelong, M. 1965. Étude épidémiologique sur la toxoplasmose: de l'influence de la cuisson des viandes de boucherie sur la fréquence de l'infection humaine. *Revue fr. Étud. clin. biol*. 10:952.

Dévèze, J. 1794. *An Enquiry Into, and Observations Upon the Causes and Effects of the Epidemic Disease, which Raged in Philadelphia from the Month of August Till Towards the Middle of December, 1793*. Philadelphia: Parent.

D'Herelle, F. 1918. Technique de la recherche du microbe filtrant bactériophage (*Bacteriophagum intestinale*). *C. R. Séanc. Soc. Biol*. 81:1160.

Dick, G. F., and Dick, G. H. 1924. The etiology of scarlet fever. *JAMA* 82:301.

Dickson, E. C. 1937. "Valley Fever" of the San Joaquin Valley and fungus coccidioides. *Calif. west. Med*. 47:151.

Dickson, E. C. 1938. Primary coccidioidomycosis. The initial acute infection which results in coccidioidal granuloma. *Am. Rev. Tuberc*. 38:722.

Diehl, H. S. 1933. Medicinal treatment of the common cold. *JAMA* 101:2042.

Dieulafoy, Chantemesse, and Widal. 1890. Une pseudo-tuberculose mycosique. Congres. International de Berlin August 1890. *Lancette française. Gaz. Hôp. civ. milit.*, Paris. 63:821.

Dingle, J. H.; Badger, G. F.; and Jordan, Jr., W. S. 1964. *Illness in the Home. A Study of 25,000 Illnesses in a Group of Cleveland Families*. Cleveland: Press of Western Reserve University.

Dingle, J. H., and Finland, M. 1942. Diagnosis, treatment and prevention of meningococcic meningitis. With a resume of the practical aspects of treatment of other acute bacterial meningitides. *War Med*. 2:1.

Djerassi, C.; Israel, A.; and Jochle, W. 1973. Planned parenthood for pets? *Bull. atom. Scient*. 29:10.

Dobell, C. 1932. *Antony van Leeuwenhoek and His "Little Animals."* New York: Harcourt Brace.

Dochez, A. R., and Gillespie, L. J. 1913. A biological classification of pneumococci by means of immunity reactions. *JAMA* 61:727.

Dochez, A. R., and Sherman, L. 1924. The significance of *Streptococcus hemolyticus* in scarlet fever. *JAMA* 82:542.

Dochez, A. R.; Shibley, G. S.; and Mills, K. C. 1930. Studies in the common cold. IV. Experimental transmission of the common cold to anthropoid apes and human beings by means of a filtrable agent. *J. Exp. Med*. 52:701.

Doerr, R.; Franz, K.; and Taussig, S. 1909. *Das Pappataciefieber; ein endemisches Drei-Tage-Fieber im adriatischen Küstengebiete Oesterreich-Ungarns*. Leipzig: F. Deuticke.

Dolman, C. E. 1971. Paul Ehrlich. In *Dictionary of Scientific Biography*, edited by Charles C. Gillispie. Vol. 4, p. 295. New York: Chas. Scribner's Sons.

Domagk, G. 1935. Ein Beitrag zur Chemotherapie der Bakteriellen Infektionen. *Dtsch. med. Wochenschr*. 61:250.

Donovan, C. 1903. On the possibility of the occurrence of trypanosomiasis in India. *Br. Med. J.* 2:79.

Douglas, S. R.; Fleming, A.; and Colebrook, L. 1920. *Studies in Wound Infections.* Privy Council-Medical Research Council (Great Britain) Special Report Ser. No. 57. London: His Majesty's Stationery Office.

Dover, T. 1732. *The Ancient Physician's Legacy to his Country, Being What He has Collected Himself in Forty-Nine Years of Practice: Or, An Account of Several Diseases Incident to Mankind, Described in so Plain a Manner, that any Person May Know the Nature of His Own Disease, etc.* 2nd ed. London: The Author.

Dowd, H. L. 1928. Rubella. In *A Text-Book of Medicine*, edited by R. L. Cecil, p. 285. Philadelphia: W. B. Saunders.

Dowling, H. F. 1955. *Tetracycline.* Antibiotics Monographs No. 3. New York: Medical Encyclopedia.

Dowling, H. F. 1959. The history of the broad-spectrum antibiotics. In *Antibiotics Annual 1958–1959*, edited by Henry Welch and Felix Marti-Ibanez, p. 39. New York: Medical Encyclopedia.

Downey, H., and Stasney, J. 1935. Infectious mononucleosis. Part II. Hematologic studies. *JAMA* 105:764.

Downie, A. W. 1961. Chicken-pox and zoster. In *Virus and Rickettsial Diseases of Man* by S. Bedson, A. W. Downie, F. O. MacCallum, and C. H. Stuart-Harris. 3rd ed., p. 107. London: Edward Arnold.

Drake, C. H., and Henrici, A. T. 1943. Nocardia asteroides: Its pathogenicity and allergic properties. *Am. Rev. Tuberc.* 48:184.

Drake, D. 1850. *A Systematic Treatise, Historical, Etiological, and Practical, on the Principle Diseases of the Interior Valley of North America as They Appear in the Caucasian, African, Indian, and Esquimaux Varieties of Its Population.* Cincinnati: B. Smith.

Drake, M. E.; Bradley, J. E.; Imburg, J.; McCrumb, F. R.; and Woodward, T. E. 1950. Aureomycin in the Treatment of influenzal meningitis. *JAMA* 142:463.

Drinker, P., and McKhann, C. F. 1929. The use of a new apparatus for the prolonged administration of artificial respiration. I. A fatal case of poliomyelitis. *JAMA* 92:1658.

Drolet, G. J., and Lowell, A. M. 1952. *A Half Century's Progress Against Tuberculosis in New York City, 1900 to 1950.* New York: New York Tuberculosis and Health Assn.

DuBois, E. F. 1948. *Fever and the Regulation of Body Temperature.* Springfield (Ill.): Chas. C Thomas.

Dubos, R. J. 1939. Studies on a bactericidal agent extracted from a soil bacillus. I. Preparation of the agent. Its activity in vitro. II. Protective effect of the bactericidal agent against experimental pneumococcus infections in mice. *J. Exp. Med.* 70:1 and 11.

Dubos, R. J. 1940. Utilization of selective microbial agents in the study of biological problems. In *The Harvey Lectures*, Vol. 35, p. 223. Lancaster (Pa.): Science Press Printing.

Dubos, R. J. 1950. *Louis Pasteur: Free Lance of Science.* Boston: Little, Brown & Co.

Dubos, R. J., and Dubos, J. 1952. *The White Plague: Tuberculosis, Man and Society.* Boston: Little, Brown.

Duclaux, E. 1920. *Pasteur, the History of a Mind.* History of Medicine Series No. 39. Philadelphia: Saunders.

Dudgeon, L. S. 1927. *Bacterial Vaccines and Their Position in Therapeutics.* London: Constable.

Duffy, J. 1968. *A History of Public Health in New York City 1625–1866.* New York: Russell Sage Foundation.

DuPont, H. L.; Formal, S. B.; Hornick, R. B.; Snyder, M. J.; Libonati, J. P.; Sheahan, D. G.; LaBrec, E. H.; and Kalas, J. P. 1971. Pathogenesis of *Escherichia coli* diarrhea. *N. Engl. J. Med.* 285:1.

Duran-Reynals, M. L. de Ayola. 1946. *The Fever Bark Tree: The Pageant of Quinine.* New York: Doubleday.

Dutton, J. E. 1902. Note on a trypanosoma occurring in the blood of man. *Br. Med. .J.* 2:881.

Dyer, R. E.; Rumreich, A.; and Badger, L. F. 1931. Typhus fever. A virus of the typhus type derived from fleas collected from wild rats. *U.S. Public Health Rep.* 46 (Part I):334.

Eaton, M. D.; Meiklejohn, G.; and van Herick, W. 1944. Studies on the etiology of primary atypical pneumonia. A filterable agent transmissible to cotton rats, hamsters, and chick embryos. *J. Exp. Med.* 79:649.

Eberth, C. J. 1880. Die Organismen in den Organen bei Typhus abdominalis. *Virchow's Arch. path. Anat. Physiol.* 81:58.

Eckmann, L. 1963. *Tetanus. Prophylaxis and Therapy.* New York: Grune & Stratton.

Economo, C. 1917. Encephalitis lethargica. *Wien. Klin. Wochenschr.* 30:581.

Edelman, G. M. 1970. The structure and function of antibodies. *Sci. Am.* 223:34 (August).

Edelman, G. M.; Cunningham, B. A.; Gall, W. E.; Gottlieb, P. D.; Rutishauser, U.; and Waxdal, M. J. 1969. The covalent structure of an entire γG immunoglobulin molecule. *Proc. Nat. Acad. Sci. U.S.A.* 63:78.

Edwards, G. A., and Domm, B. M. 1960. Human leptospirosis. *Medicine* 39:117.

Edwards, P. Q. 1973. Is tuberculosis still a problem? *Health Serv. Rep.* 88:483 (June–July).

Edwards, P. R. 1962. *Serological Examination of Salmonella Cultures for Epidemiological Purposes.* Atlanta (Ga.): Communicable Disease Center, U.S. Department of Health, Education and Welfare (August).

Ehrenkranz, N. J.; Sinclair, M. C.; Buff, E.; and Lyman, D. O. 1970. The natural occurrence of Venezuelan equine encephalitis in the United States. First case and epidemiologic investigations. *N. Engl. J. Med.* 282:298.

Ehrlich, J.; Bartz, Q. R.; Smith, R. M.; Joslyn, D. A.; and Burkholder, P. R. 1947. Chloromycetin, a new antibiotic from a soil actinomycete. *Science* 106:417.

Ehrlich, P. 1891. Experimentelle Untersuchungen über Immunität. I. Ueber Ricin. II. Ueber Abrin. *Dtsch. med. Wochenschr.* 17:976 and 1218.

Ehrlich, P. 1897, transl. 1956. Die Wertbemessung des Diphtherieheilserums und deren theoretische Grundlagen. *Klin. Jb.* 6:299. Translated by the editors. The assay of the activity of diphtheria-curative serum and its theoretical basis. In *The Collected Papers of Paul Ehrlich*, compiled and edited by F. Himmelweit with the assistance of Martha Marquardt under the editorial direction of Sir Henry Dale. Vol. 2, p. 107. London: Pergamon Press.

Ehrlich, P. 1900. On immunity with special reference to cell life. Croonian Lecture read March 22, 1900. *Proc. R. Soc. Lond.* 66:424.

Ehrlich, P. 1960. Über Partialfunktionen der Zelle. Nobel Lecture delivered in Stockholm December 11, 1908. Reprinted from *Les Prix Nobel*, Stockholm, 1909. Translated by the editors. On partial functions of the cell. Both in *The Collected Papers of Paul Ehrlich*, compiled and edited by F. Himmelweit with the assistance of Martha Marquardt under the editorial direction of Sir Henry Dale. Vol. 3, pp. 171 and 183. London: Pergamon Press.

Ehrlich, P., and Hata, S. 1910, transl. 1960. *Die experimentelle Chemotherapie der Spirillosen.* Berlin: Springer. Translated by the editors. Closing notes to the experimental chemotherapy of Spirilloses. In *The Collected Papers of Paul Ehrlich*, compiled and edited by F. Himmelweit with the assistance of Martha Marquardt under the editorial direction of Sir Henry Dale. Vol. 3, p. 282. London: Pergamon Press.

Eichenwald, H. F. 1957. Congenital toxoplasmosis. A study of 150 cases (Abstract). *Am. J. Dis. Child.* 94:411.

Eisenberg, P. 1913. Untersuchungen über halbspezifische Desinfektionsvorgänge. I. Mitteilung. Ueber die Wirkung von Farbstoffen auf Bakterien. Vitalfärbung-Entwickelungshemmung. *Zentbl. Bakt. ParasitKde. Hyg., I. Abt. Orig.* B 71:420.

Eklund, C. M. 1946. Human encephalitis of the western equine type in Minnesota in 1941: Clinical and epidemiological study of serologically positive cases. *Am. J. Hyg.* 43:171.

Eklund, C. M., and Blumstein, A. 1938. The relation of human encephalitis to encephalomyelitis in horses. *JAMA* 111:1734.

Eklund, C. M., and Hadlow, W. J. 1973. Implications of slow viral diseases of domestic animals for human disease. *Medicine* 52:357.

Eklund, C. M.; Kohls, G. M.; and Brennan, J. M. 1955. Distribution of Colorado tick fever and virus-carrying ticks. *JAMA* 157:335.

Ekström, B. 1830. Rabies epidemic at Stockholm, in 1824. *Lond. Med. Gaz.* 6:689.

Elek, S. D. 1959. *Staphylococcus pyogenes and Its Relation to Disease.* Edinburgh and London: E. & S. Livingstone.

Emmons, C. W. 1940. Medical mycology. *Bot. Rev.* 6:474.

Emmons, C. W.; Binford, C. H.; and Utz, J. P. 1970. *Medical Mycology.* 2d ed. Philadelphia: Lea & Febiger.

Enders, J. F.; Kane, L. W.; Cohen, S.; and Levens, J. H. 1945. Immunity in mumps. I. Experiments with monkeys (Macacus mulatta). The development of complement-fixing antibody following infection and experiments on immunization by means of inactivated virus and convalescent human serum. *J. Exp. Med.* 81:93.

Enders, J. F.; Kane, L. W.; Maris, E. P.; and Stokes, Jr., J. 1946. Immunity in mumps. V. The correlation of the presence of dermal hypersensitivity and resistance to mumps. *J. Exp. Med.* 84:341.

Enders, J. F.; Katz, S. L.; Milovanovic, M. V.; and Holloway, A. 1960. Studies on an attenuated measles-virus vaccine. I. Development and preparation of the vaccine: Technics for assay of effects of vaccination. *N. Engl. J. Med.* 263:153.

Enders, J. F., and Peebles, T. C. 1954. Propagation in tissue cultures of cytopathogenic agents from patients with measles. *Proc. Soc. Exp. Biol. Med.* 86:277.

Enders, J. F.; Peebles, T. C.; McCarthy, K.; Milovanovic, M.; Mitus, A.; and Holloway, A. 1957. Measles virus: A summary of experiments concerned with isolation properties and behavior. *Am. J. Public Health* 47:275.

Enders, J. F.; Weller, T. H.; and Robbins, F. C. 1949. Cultivation of the Lansing strain of poliomyelitis virus in cultures of various human embryonic tissues. *Science* 109:85.

Eppinger, H. 1891. Ueber eine neue, pathogene Cladothrix und eine durch sie hervorgerufene Pseudotuberculosis (cladothrichica). *Beitr. pathol. Anat.* 9:287.

Epstein, L. A., and Chain, E. 1940. Some observations on the preparation and properties of the substrate of lysozyme. *Brit. J. Exp. Pathol.* 21:339.

Epstein, M. A.; Achong, B. G.; and Barr, Y. M. 1964. Virus particles in cultured lymphoblasts from Burkitt's lymphoma. *Lancet* 1:702.

Erwa, H. H.; Haseeb, M. A.; Idris, A. A.; Lapeyssonnie, L.; Sanborn, W. R.; and Sippel, J. E. 1973. A serogroup A meningococcal polysaccharide vaccine. Studies in the Sudan to combat cerebrospinal meningitis caused by *Neisseria meningitidis* group A. *Bull. WHO* 49:301.

Evans, A. S.; Niederman, J. C.; and McCollum, R. W. 1968. Seroepidemiologic studies of infectious mononucleosis with EB virus. *N. Engl. J. Med.* 279:1121.

Evans, A. S., and Robinton, E. D. 1950. An epidemiologic study of infectious mononucleosis in a New England college. *N. Engl. J. Med.* 242:492.

Ewing, H. E.; Tatum, H. W.; and Davis, B. R. 1957. The occurrence of *Escherichia coli* serotypes associated with diarrheal disease in the United States. *Public Health Lab.* 15:118.

Fahrenheit, D. G. 1724a. Araeometri novi descriptio & usus. *Philos. Trans. R. Soc. Lond. (Biol. Sci)* 33:140.

Fahrenheit, D. G. 1724b. Barometri novi descriptio. Ibid., p. 179.

Fahrenheit, D. G. 1724c. Experimenta & observationes de congelatione aquae in vacuo factae. Ibid., p. 78.

Fahrenheit, D. G. 1724d. Experimenta circa gradum caloris liquorum nonnullorum ebullientium instituta. Ibid., p. 1.

Fahrenheit, D. G. 1724e. Materiarum quarundam gravitates Specificae, diversis temporibus ad varios Scopos exploratae. Ibid., p. 114.

Fairley, K. D. 1922. Peritoneal echinococcosis. *Med. J. Aust.* 2:209.

Falk, A. 1965. U. S. Veterans Administration-Armed Forces cooperative study on the chemotherapy of tuberculosis. XIII. Tuberculous meningitis in adults, with special reference to survival, neurologic residuals, and work status. *Am. Rev. Respir. Dis.* 91:823.

Farber, R. E.; Solomon, N.; Garber, H. J.; Ashitey, G.; and Others 1970. Salmonellosis — Baltimore, Maryland. *CDC Morbidity Mortality Rep.* No. 32, 19:314 (August 15).

Farber, S.; Hill, A.; Connerly, M. L.; and Dingle, J. H. 1940. Encephalitis in infants and children. Caused by the virus of the eastern variety of equine encephalitis. *JAMA* 114:1725.

Farber, S., and Wolbach, S. B. 1932. Intranuclear and cytoplasmic inclusions ("protozoan-like bodies") in the salivary glands and other organs of infants. *Am. J. Pathol.* 8:123.

Farr, W. 1885. *Vital Statistics: A Memorial Volume of Selections from the Reports and Writings of William Farr,* edited for the Sanitary Institute of Great Britain by Noel A. Humphreys with a biographical sketch of William Farr, M.D., D.C.L., C.B., F.R.S. London: Offices of the Sanitary Institute.

Farrar, Jr., W. E., and Eidson, M. 1971. Antibiotic resistance in *Shigella* mediated by R factors. *J. Infect. Dis.* 123:477.

Faust, E. C. 1939. What the life insurance companies think of malaria. *South. Med. J.* 32:689.

Feemster, R. F. 1938. Outbreak of encephalitis in man due to the eastern virus of equine encephalomyelitis. *Am. J. Public Health* 28:1403.

Fehleisen, F. 1882, transl. 1886. Ueber Erysipel. *Dtsche. Z. Chir.* 16:391. Translated by L. Ogilvie. On erysipelas. In *Bacteria in Relation to Diseases,* edited by W. W. Cheyne. Vol. 115, p. 261. London: New Sydenham Society.

Feldberg, W. 1975. Body temperature and fever: Changes in our views during the last decade. *Proc. R. Soc. Lond. (Biol.)* 191:199.

Feldman, H. A. 1968. Toxoplasmosis. *N. Engl. J. Med.* 279:1370 and 1431.

Feldman, H. A. 1972. Meningococcal infections. *Adv. Intern. Med.* 18:117.

Feldman, W. H. 1938. *Avian Tuberculosis Infections.* Baltimore (Md.): Williams & Wilkins.

Feldman, W. H., and Hinshaw, H. C. 1945. Chemotherapeutic testing in experimental tuberculosis. *Am. Rev. Tuberc.* 51:582.

Feldman, W. H.; Hinshaw, H. C.; and Mann, F. C. 1944. Promizole in tuberculosis. *Am. Rev. Tuberc.* 50:418.

Feldman, W. H.; Hinshaw, H. C.; and Mann, F. C. 1945. Streptomycin in experimental tuberculosis. *Am. Rev. Tuberc.* 52:269.

Feldman, W. H.; Hinshaw, H. C.; and Moses, H. E. 1942. Promin in experimental tuberculosis. *Am. Rev. Tuberc.* 45:303.

Ferrell, J. A.; Smillie, W. G.; Covington, P. W.; and Mead, P. A. 1929. Health Departments of States and Provinces of the United States and Canada. *USPHS Public Health Bull.* No. 184.

Fetterman, G. H. 1952. A new laboratory aid in the clinical diagnosis of inclusion disease of infancy. *Am. J. Clin. Pathol.* 22:424.

Fiese, M. J. 1958. *Coccidioidomycosis.* Springfield (Ill.): Chas. C Thomas.

Findlay, G. M., and MacCallum, F. O. 1938. Hepatitis and jaundice associated with immunization against certain virus diseases. *Proc. R. Soc. Med.* 31:799.

Findlay, G. M.; MacCallum, F. O.; and Murgatroyd, F. 1939. Observations bearing on the aetiology of infective hepatitis (so-called epidemic catarrhal jaundice). *Trans. R. Soc. Trop. Med. Hyg.* 32:575.

Finegold, S. M.; Will, D.; and Murray, J. F. 1959. Aspergillosis. A review and report of twelve cases. *Am. J. Med.* 27:463.

Finger, E. 1893, transl. 1894. *Die Blenorrhöe der Sexualorgane und Ihre Complicationen.* Leipzig and Wien: Franz Deuticke. Translated by E. Finger. *Gonorrhoea and Its Complications.* 3rd rev. and enl. ed. New York: William Wood.

Finland, M. 1954. Treatment of bacterial endocarditis. *N. Engl. J. Med.* 250:372 and 419.

Finland, M., consulting ed. 1958. The basic and clinical research of the new antibiotic, kanamycin. A conference. Held July 10–11, 1958. *Ann. NY Acad Sci.* 76:17–408.

Finland, M., guest ed. 1969. International symposium on gentamicin. A new aminoglycoside antibiotic. Held October 30–31, 1968. *J. Infect. Dis.* 119:341.

Finland, M., and Barnes, M. W. 1970. Changing etiology of bacterial endocarditis in the antibacterial era. Experiences at Boston City Hospital 1933–1965. *Ann. Intern. Med.* 72:341.

Finland, M.; Brown, J. W.; and Rauh, A. E. 1938. Treatment of pneumococcic meningitis. A study of ten cases treated with sulfanilamide alone or in various combinations with specific antipneumococcic serum and complement, including six recoveries. *N. Engl. J. Med.* 218:1033.

Finland, M., and Kass, E. H., eds. 1973. Trimethoprim-sulfamethoxazole. Symposium. *J. Infect. Dis. Suppl.* 128:425 (November).

Finlay, A. C.; Hobby, G. L.; P'an, S. Y.; Regna, P. P.; Routien, J. B.; Seeley, D. B.; Shull, G. M.; Sobin, B. A.; Solomons, I. A.; Vinson, J. W.; and Kane, J. H. 1950. Terramycin, a new antibiotic. *Science* 111:85.

Finlay, C. J. 1937. The mosquito hypothetically considered as the agent of transmission of yellow fever. *Med. Class.* 2:590.

Fishbein, M., and Salmonsen, E. M., with Hektoen, L., eds. 1951. *A Bibliography of Infantile Paralysis 1789–1949.* 2nd ed. Philadelphia: J. B. Lippincott.

Flaum, A.; Malmros, H.; and Persson, E. 1926. Eine nosocomiale ikterus-epidemie. *Acta Med. Scand. Suppl.* No. 16:544.

Fleming, A. 1919. The action of chemical and physiological antiseptics in a septic wound. *Br. J. Surg.* 7:99.

Fleming, A. 1922. On a remarkable bacteriolytic element found in tissues and secretions. *Proc. R. Soc. Lond. (Biol.)* 93:306.

Fleming, A. 1924. A comparison of the activities of antiseptics on bacteria and on leucocytes. *Proc. R. Soc. Lond. (Biol.)* 96:171.

Fleming, A. 1929a. On the antibacterial action of cultures of a penicillium with special reference to their use in the isolation of *B. influenzae. Br. J. Exp. Pathol.* 10:226.

Fleming, A. 1929b. The staphylococci. In *A System of Bacteriology in Relation to Medicine* by Great Britain Medical Research Council. Vol. 2, p. 11. London: Her Majesty's Stationery Office.

Fleming, A. 1932. Lysozyme. President's Address given on October 18, 1932. *Proc. R. Soc. Med.* 26:71 (Pathology Sec.).

Fleming, A. 1947. Louis Pasteur. *Br. Med. J.* 1:517.

Fleming, J.; Bignall, J. R.; and Blades, A. N. 1947. Sand-fly fever. Review of 664 cases. *Lancet* 252:443.

Flexner, S. 1907. Concerning a serum-therapy for experimental infection with *Diplococcus intracellularis. J. Exp. Med.* 9:168.

Flexner, S. 1916. A note on the serum treatment of poliomyelitis (infantile paralysis). *JAMA* 67:583.

Flexner, S., and Jobling, J. W. 1908. Serum treatment of epidemic cerebro-spinal meningitis. *J. Exp. Med.* 10:141.

Flexner, S., and Lewis, P. A. 1910a. Experimental epidemic poliomyelitis in monkeys. *J. Exp. Med.* 12:227.

Flexner, S., and Lewis, P.A. 1910b. Experimental poliomyelitis in monkeys. Eighth note: Further contributions to the subjects of immunization and serum therapy. *JAMA* 55:662.

Flick, L. F. 1925. *Development of our Knowledge of Tuberculosis.* Philadelphia: Author, 738 Pine Street.

Florey, H. 1930. The relative amounts of lysozyme present in the tissues of some mammals. *Br. J. Exp. Pathol.* 11:251.

Florey, H. W., ed. 1954. *Lectures on General Pathology.* Philadelphia: W. B. Saunders.

Florey, H. W. 1955. Antibiotic products of a versatile fungus. *Ann. Intern. Med.* 43:480.

Florey, H. W. 1959. Penicillin in perspective. In *Antibiotics Annual 1958–1959*, edited by Henry Welch and Felix Marti-Ibanez. New York: Medical Encyclopedia.

Florey, H. W.; Chain, E.; Heatley, N. G.; Jennings, M. A.; Sanders, A. G.; Abraham, E. P.; and Florey, M. E. 1949. *Antibiotics. A Survey of Penicillin, Streptomycin, and other Antimicrobial Substances from Fungi, Actinomycetes, Bacteria, and Plants*. 2 vols. London: Oxford University Press.

Florey, M. E. 1952. *The Clinical Application of Antibiotics. Penicillin*. London: Oxford University Press.

Florey, M. E., and Florey, H. W. 1943. General and local administration of penicillin. *Lancet* 244:387.

Florio, L.; Stewart, M. O.; and Mugrage, E. R. 1946. The etiology of Colorado tick fever. *J. Exp. Med.* 83:1.

Flynn, E. H., ed. 1972. *Cephalosporins and Penicillins. Chemistry and Biology*. New York: Academic Press.

Foerster, R. 1933. Sepsis im Anschluß an ausgedehnte Periporitis. Heilung durch streptozon. *Zentbl. Haut- u. GeschlKrankh.* 45:549.

Ford, E. B. 1957. Polymorphism in plants, animals and man. *Nature* 180:1315.

Ford, J. 1971. *The Role of the Trypanosomiases in African Ecology: A Study of the Tsetse Fly Problem*. Oxford: Clarendon Press.

Ford, W. W. 1911. The distribution of haemolysins agglutinins and poisons in fungi, especially the Amanitas, the Entolomas, the Lactarius and the Inocybes. *J. Pharmacol. Exp. Ther.* 2:285.

Fosbinder, R. J., and Walter, L. A. 1939. Sulfanilamido derivatives of heterocyclic amines. *J. Am. Chem. Soc.* 61:2032.

Foster, W. D. 1965. *A History of Parasitology*. Edinburgh: E. & S. Livingstone.

Foster, W. D. 1970. *A History of Medical Bacteriology and Immunology*. London: Wm. Heinemann Medical Books.

Fothergill, J. 1751. *An Account of the Sore Throat Attended with Ulcers*. 3rd ed. London: C. Davis.

Fothergill, L. D.; Dingle, J. H.; Farber, S.; and Connerley, M. L. 1938. Human encephalitis caused by the virus of the eastern variety of equine encephalomyelitis. *N. Engl. J. Med.* 219:411.

Fothergill, L. D., and Wright, J. 1933. Influenzal meningitis. The relation of age incidence to the bactericidal power of blood against the causal organism. *J. Immunol.* 24:273.

Fox, H. 1923. *Disease in Captive Wild Mammals and Birds*. Philadelphia: J. B. Lippincott.

Fox, H. H. 1951. Synthetic tuberculostats show promise. *Chem. Engng. News* 29:3963.

Fox, H. H. 1953. The chemical attack on tuberculosis. *Trans. N Y Acad. Sci.* 15:234.

Fox, J. P.; Manso, C.; Penna, H. A.; and Para, M. 1942. Observations on the occurrence of icterus in Brazil following vaccination against yellow fever. *Am. J. Hyg.* 36:68.

Fracastoro, G. 1930. *De Contagione et Contagiosis Morbis et Eorum Curatione, Libri III.* Translated, with notes, by W. C. Wright. London: G. P. Putnam's Sons.

Fracastoro, G. 1934. *The Sinister Shepherd: A Translation by William Van Wyck of Girolamo Fracastoro's Syphilidis Sive De Morbo Gallico Libri Tres*. Los Angeles: The Primavera Press.

Fraenkel, A. 1886. Bakteriologische Mittheilungen. *Z. klin. Med.* 10:401.

Frame, J. D.; Baldwin, Jr., J. M.; Gocke, D. J.; and Troup, J. M. 1970. Lassa fever, a new virus disease of man from West Africa. I. Clinical description and pathological findings. *Am. J. Trop. Med. Hyg.* 19:670.

Francis, E. 1922. Tularaemia Francis 1921. A new disease of man. *U.S. Hyg. Lab. Bull.* No. 130.

Francis, E. 1925. Tularemia. *JAMA* 84:1243.

Francis, Jr., T. 1940. A new type of virus from epidemic influenza. *Science* 92 (N.S.):405.

Frazer, W. M. 1950. *A History of English Public Health*. London: Baillière, Tindall & Cox.

Frost, W. H. 1913. Epidemiologic studies of acute anterior poliomyelitis. *U.S. Hyg. Lab. Bull.* No. 90.

Frost, W. H.; Frobisher, Jr., M.; Van Volkenburgh, V. A.; and Levin, M. L. 1936. Diphtheria in Baltimore: A comparative study of morbidity carrier prevalence and antitoxic immunity in 1921–24 and 1933–36. *Am. J. Hyg.* 24:568.

Frothingham, Jr., C. 1906. A contribution to the knowledge of the lesions caused by *Trichina spiralis* in man. *J. Med. Res.* 15:483.

Frothingham, L. 1902. A tumor-like lesion in the lung of a horse caused by a blastomyces (Torula). *J. Med. Res.* 8:31.

Fuller, T. 1730. *Exanthematologia: Or, an Attempt to Give a Rational Account of Eruptive Fevers, Especially of the Measles and Small Pox.* London: Charles Rivington and Stephen Austen.

Furcolow, M. L., and Grayston, J. T. 1953. Occurrence of histoplasmosis in epidemics. Etiological studies. *Am. Rev. Tuberc.* 68:307.

Furman, B. 1973. *A Profile of the United States Public Health Service 1798–1948.* DHEW Publication No. NIH 73–369. Washington, D.C.: U.S. Government Printing Office.

Gaffky, G. 1884, transl. 1886. Zur Aetiologie des Abdominaltyphus. *Mitt. K. GesundhAmt.*, Berl. 2:372. Translated by J. J. Pringle. On the etiology of enteric fever. *New Sydenham Society* 115:205.

Gajdusek, D. C. 1962. Virus hemorrhagic fevers. Special reference to hemorrhagic fever with renal syndrome. (Epidemic hemorrhagic fever). *J. Pediatr.* 60:841.

Gajdusek, D. C., and Gibbs, Jr., C. J. 1973. Subacute and chronic diseases caused by atypical infections with unconventional viruses in aberrant hosts. In *Perspectives in Virology*, edited by M. Pollard, Vol. 8, p. 279. New York: Academic Press.

Gajdusek, D. C.; Gibbs, Jr., C. J.; and Alpers, M. 1966. Experimental transmission of a kuru-like syndrome to chimpanzees. *Nature* 209:794.

Garland, J. 1943. Varicella following exposure to herpes zoster. *N. Engl. J. Med.* 228:336.

Garnham, P. C. C. 1971. *Progress in Parasitology.* University of London Heath Clark Lecture 1968, delivered at the London School of Hygiene and Tropical Medicine. London: The Athlone Press.

Garrison, F. H. 1922a. *An Introduction to the History of Medicine with Medical Chronology, Suggestions for Study and Bibliographic Data.* 3rd ed. rev. Philadelphia: W. B. Saunders.

Garrison, F. H. 1922b. *Notes on the History of Military Medicine.* Washington, D.C.: Association of Military Surgeons.

Garrod, L. P.; James, D. G.; and Lewis, A. A. G., eds. 1969. The synergy of trimethoprim and sulphonomides, Symposium. Held at the Royal College of Physicians, London, on May 9, 1969. *Postgraduate Med. J. Suppl.* 45:3 (November).

Gay, F. P. 1918. *Typhoid Fever. Considered as a Problem of Scientific Medicine.* New York: Macmillan.

Geiling, E. M. K., and Cannon, P. R. 1938. Pathologic effects of elixir of sulfanilamide (diethylene glycol) poisoning. *JAMA* 111:919.

Gelmo, P. 1908. Über Sulfamide der p-Amidobenzolsulfonsäure. *J. prakt. Chem.* 77 (N.S.):369.

Gentles, J. C. 1958. Experimental ringworm in guinea pigs: Oral treatment with griseofulvin. *Nature* 182:476.

Gentles, J. C., ed. 1961. *Sabouraudia. Journal of the International Society for Human and Animal Mycology.* Vol. 1, Part 1. Edinburgh and London: E. & S. Livingstone.

Gerhard, W. W. 1833–34. Cerebral affections of children. *Am. J. Med. Sci.* 13:313 (1833) and 14:99 (1834).

Gerhard, W. W. 1836–37. On the typhus fever, which occurred at Philadelphia in the spring and summer of 1836; illustrated by clinical observations at the Philadelphia Hospital; showing the distinction between this form of disease and dothinenteritis or the typhoid fever with alteration of the follicles of the small intestine. *Am. J. Med. Sci.* 19:289 (1836) and 20:289 (1837).

Germany: Reichsgesundheitsamte 1935. Die Säuglingstuberkulose in Lübeck. *Arb. ReichsgesundhAmt.* 69:1.

Gersdorff, H., von. 1517. *Feldtbuch der Wundartzney.* Strassburg: J. Schott. Reprinted by Wissenschaftliche Buchgesellschaft, Darmstadt (Germany), 1967.

Gibbs, Jr., C. J., and Gajdusek, D. C. 1972. Transmission of scrapie to the Cynomolgus monkey (Macaca fascicularis). *Nature* 236:73.

Gibbs, Jr., C. J., and Gajdusek, D. C. 1974. Biology of kuru and Creutzfeldt-Jakob disease. In *Slow Virus Diseases*, edited by W. Zeman and E. H. Lennette, p. 39. Baltimore: Williams & Wilkins.

Gibbs, Jr., C. J.; Gajdusek, D. C.; Asher, D. M.; Alpers, M. P.; Beck, E.; Daniel, P. M.; and Matthews, W. B. 1968. Creutzfeldt-Jakob disease (spongiform encephalopathy): Transmission to the chimpanzee. *Science* 161:388.

Gibson, W. C. 1970. The bio-medical pursuits of Christopher Wren. *Med. Hist.* 14:331.

Gilchrist, T. C. 1896. A case of blastomycetic dermatitis in man. *Johns Hopkins Hosp. Rep.* 1:269.

Gilchrist, T. C., and Stokes, W. R. 1898. A case of pseudo-lupus vulgaris caused by a blastomyces. *J. Exp. Med.* 3:53.

Giles, J. P.; McCollum, R. W.; Berndtson, Jr., L. W.; and Krugman, S. 1969. Viral hepatitis. Relation of Australia/SH antigen to the Willowbrook MS-2 strain. *N. Engl. J. Med.* 281:119.

Gillett, J. D. 1973. The mosquito: Still man's worst enemy. *Am. Sci.* 61:430.

Gjestland, T. 1955. The Oslo study of untreated syphilis. *Acta Derm Venereol.* (Stockh) 35, *Supplement* No. 34.

Glade, P. R., ed. 1973. *Infectious Mononucleosis*. Proceedings of a symposium held in New York, N.Y. April 7, 1972. Philadelphia: J. B. Lippincott.

Glazier, W. C. W. 1881. *Report on Trichinae and Trichinosis*. U.S. Marine Hospital Service Treasury Dept. Document No. 84. Washington, D.C.: U.S. Government Printing Office.

Gley, P., and Girard, A. 1936. Un nourveau dérivé de la sulfamido-chrysoidine très actif contre l'infection streptococcique. *La Presse Medicale* 2:1775.

Gochenour, Jr., W. S.; Smadel, J. E.; Jackson, E. B.; Evans, L. B.; and Yager, R. H. 1952. Leptospiral etiology of Fort Bragg fever. *U.S. Public Health Rep.* 67:811.

Godlee, R. J. 1917. *Lord Lister*. London: Macmillan.

Goldblatt, L. A., ed. 1969. *Aflatoxin. Scientific Background, Control, and Implications*. New York: Academic Press.

Goldschmidt, R. 1933. Untersuchungen zur Ätiologie der Durchfallserkrankungen des Säuglings. *Jb. Kinderheilkunde* 139:318.

Goldschneider, I.; Gotschlich, E. C.; and Artenstein, M. S. 1969. Human immunity to the meningococcus. I. The role of humoral antibodies. II. Development of natural immunity. *J. Exp. Med.* 129:1307 and 1327.

Goldsworthy, N. E., and Florey, H. 1930. Some properties of mucus, with special reference to its antibacterial functions. *Br. J. Exp. Pathol.* 11:192.

Golgi, C. 1886. Sull'infezione malarica. *Arch. Sci. Med.* (Torino) 10:109.

Goodman, N. M. 1971. *International Health Organizations and Their Work*. 2d ed. Baltimore: Williams & Wilkins.

Goodpasture, E. W., and Talbot, F. B. 1921. Concerning the nature of "protozoan-like" cells in certain lesions of infancy. *Am. J. Dis. Child.* 21:415.

Gordon, A. 1795. *A Treatise on the Epidemic Puerperal Fever of Aberdeen*. London: G. G. & J. Robinson.

Gordon, J. E. 1948. Louse-borne typhus fever in the European Theater of Operations, U.S. Army, 1945. In *Rickettsial Diseases of Man*, edited by F. R. Moulton, p. 16. Washington, D.C.: American Association for the Advancement of Science.

Gordon, J. E. 1958. General considerations of modes of transmission. In *U.S. Army Medical Service: Preventive Medicine in World War II*. Vol. 4, p. 3. Washington, D.C.: Office of the Surgeon General, Department of the Army.

Gordon, M. H. 1915. Differentiation of meningococci. *Br. Med. J.* 2:942.

Gordon, M. H. 1920. *Cerebrospinal Fever: Studies in the Bacteriology, Preventive Control, and Specific Treatment of Cerebrospinal Fever among the Military Forces, 1915–19*. Great Britain Medical Research Council-Privy Council, Special Report Series No. 50. London: His Majesty's Stationery Office.

Gordon, M. H., and Murray, E. G. 1915. Identification of the meningococcus. *J. R. Army med Corps* 25:411.

Gotschlich, E. C.; Liu, T. Y.; and Artenstein, M. S. 1969. Human immunity to the meningococcus. III. Preparation and immunochemical properties of the group A, group B, and group C meningococcal polysaccharides. *J. Exp. Med.* 129:1349.

Gottlieb, D.; Bhattachryya, P. K.; Anderson, H. W.; and Carter, H. E. 1948. Some properties of an antibiotic obtained from a species of Streptomyces. *J. Bacteriol.* 55:409.

Gould, S. E., ed. 1970. *Trichinosis in Man and Animals.* Springfield: Chas. C Thomas.

Gram, C. 1884. Üeber die isolirte Färbung der Schizomyceten in Schnitt-und Trockenpräparaten. *Fortschr. Med.* 2:185.

Grassi, G. B. 1878. Intorno all'Anchilostomo duodenale (Dubini). *Gazz. med. ital. lomb.* 7 Ser. 5:193, 1878.

Grassi, G. B. 1899. Studii di uno zoologo sulla malaria. *Roma, R. Accad. Lincei Mem.* 3:299.

Graunt, J. 1665. *Natural and Political Observations Mentioned in a Following Index, and Made Upon the Bills of Mortality: With Reference to the Government, Religion, Trade, Growth, Air, Diseases and the Several Changes of the Said City.* Fourth impression. London: John Martyn, and James Allestry.

Graves, R. R. 1943. The story of John M. Buck's and Matilda's contribution to the cattle industry. *J. Am. Vet. Med. Assoc.* 102:193.

Great Britain, Local Government Board. 1859–70. *Great Britain Local Government Board: Report of the Medical Officer of the Privy Council, with Appendix, 1858–1870.* London: G. E. Eyre and W. Spottiswoode.

Great Britain Ministry of Health. 1920. *Report on the Pandemic of Influenza: 1918–1919.* Reports on Public Health and Medical Subjects No. 4. London: His Majesty's Stationery Office.

Great Britain Ministry of Health. 1938. Acute infective jaundice and administration of measles serum. In *On the State of the Public Health. Annual Report of the Chief Medical Officer of the Ministry of Health for the Year 1937*, p. 38. Chief Medical Officer: Sir Arthur S. MacNalty. London: His Majesty's Stationery Office.

Great Britain Ministry of Health. 1943. Homologous serum jaundice. Memorandum prepared by Medical Officers of the Ministry of Health. *Lancet* 244:83.

Great Britain Ministry of Health. 1959. *Staphylococcal Infections in Hospitals. Ministry of Health Central Services Council Standing Medical Advisory Committee. Report of the Sub-Committee on Staphylococcal Infections in Hospitals.* London: Her Majesty's Stationery Office.

Great Britain, Poor Law Commissioners. 1838. *Fourth Annual Report of the Poor Law Commissioners for England and Wales; Together with Appendices A.B. & C. Supplement No. 1 (pp. 103–129). Report on the Prevalence of certain Physical Causes of Fever in the Metropolis, which might be removed by proper Sanatory Measures. By Neil Arnott, M.D. & James Phillips Kay, M.D. Supplement No. 2 (pp. 129–139). Report on some of the Physical Causes of Sickness and Mortality to which the Poor are particularly exposed, and which are capable of removal by Sanatory Regulations; exemplified in the present condition of the Bethnal Green and Whitechapel Districts, as ascertained on a personal inspection.* By Southwood Smith, M.D., Physician to the London Fever Hospital. London: W. Clowes and Sons.

Great Britain, Poor Law Commissioners, 1839. *Fifth Annual Report of the Poor Law Commissioners for England and Wales; Together with Appendices A.B.C. & D. Supplement No. 2 (pp. 160–161). Report on the Prevalence of Fever in Twenty Metropolitan Unions or Parishes, during the Year ended the 20th March, 1838.* By Southwood Smith, M.D., Physician to the London Fever Hospital. London: W. Clowes and Sons.

Great Britain, Poor Law Commissioners. 1842 and 1965. *Report on the Sanitary Condition of the Labouring Population of Great Britain*, by Edwin Chadwick, Esq. London: W. Clowes and Sons (1842). Edinburgh: University Press (1965).

Great Britain, Royal Society of London. 1903 and 1905. *Reports of the Sleeping Sickness Commission of the Royal Society of London*. (No. I August 1903; No. II-III-IV November 1903; No. V July 1905; No. VI August 1905). London: Harrison and Sons.

Great Britain, Royal Society of London. Mediterranean Fever Commission Reports. 1905–1907. *Reports of the Commission for the Investigation of Mediterranean Fever. Parts I to VII*. London: Harrison and Sons.

Greenberg, M. 1948. Rickettsialpox in New York City. *Am. J. Med.* 4:866.

Greenberg, M.; Pellitteri, O.; and Barton, J. 1957. Frequency of defects in infants whose mothers had rubella during pregnancy. *JAMA* 165:675.

Greenwood, M. 1936. *The Medical Dictator, and Other Biographical Studies*. London: Williams & Norgate.

Gregg, N. M. 1941. Congenital cataract following German measles in the mother. *Trans. ophthalmol. Soc. Aust.* 3:35.

Gregory, J. E.; Golden, A.; and Haymaker, W. 1943. Mucormycosis of the central nervous system. A report of three cases. *Johns Hopkins Hosp. Bull.* 73:405.

Griffith, F. 1934. The serological classification of *Streptococcus pyogenes*. *J. Hyg.* (Camb.) 34:542.

Groman, N. B. 1961. Phage-host relationships in some genera of medical significance. *Annu. Rev. Microbiol.* 15:153.

Grönvold, C. 1884. *Leprosy in Minnesota*. Report to the State Board of Health of Minnesota. Chicago: A. G. Newell.

Gruber, M., and Durham, H. E. 1896. Eine neue Methode zur raschen Erkennung des Choleravibrio und des Typhusbacillus. *Münch. Med. Wochenschr.* 43:285.

Gruby, D. 1842. Sur une espèce de mentagre contagieuse résultant du developpement d'un nouveau cryptogame dans la racine des poils de la barbe de l'homme. *C. R. Acad. Sci.* (D) (Paris) 15:512.

Gruby, D. 1844. Recherches sur les cryptogames qui constituent la maladie contagieuse du cuir chevelu décrite sous le nom de Teigne tondante (Mahon), Herpes tonsurans (Cazenave). *C. R. Acad. Sci.* (D) (Paris) 18:583.

Grunberg, E., and Schnitzer, R. J. 1952. Studies on the activity of hydrazine derivatives of isonicotinic acid in the experimental tuberculosis of mice. *Q. Bull. Sea View Hosp.* 13:3.

Gsell, O. 1952. *Leptospirosen*. Bern: Hans Huber.

Guttmann, P., and Ehrlich, P. 1891, transl. 1960. Ueber die Wirkung des Methylenblau bei Malaria. *Berl. klin. Wschr.* 28:953. Translated by the editors. On the action of methylene blue on malaria. In *The Collected Papers of Paul Ehrlich*, compiled and edited by F. Himmelweit with the assistance of Martha Marquardt under the editorial direction of Sir Henry Dale. Vol. 3, p. 15. London: Pergamon Press.

Habel, K. 1942. Transmission of rubella to *Macacus mulatta* monkeys. *U.S. Public Health Rep.* 57:1126.

Habel, K. 1945. Cultivation of mumps virus in the developing chick embryo and its application to studies of immunity to mumps in man. *U.S. Public Health Rep.* 60:201.

Habel, K. 1946. Preparation of mumps vaccines and immunization of monkeys against experimental mumps infection. *U.S. Public Health Rep.* 61:1655.

Hackett, C. J. 1963. On the origin of the human treponematoses. *Bull. WHO* 29:7.

Hadlow, W. J. 1959. Scrapie and kuru. *Lancet* 2:289.

Haensell, P. 1881. Vorläufige Mittheilung über Versuche von Impfsyphilis der Iris und Cornea des Kaninchenauges. *Albrecht von Graefe's Arch. Klin. Ophthalmol.* 27:93.

Haffkine, W. M. 1897. Remarks on the plague prophylactic fluid. *Br. Med. J.* 1:1461.

Haggis, A. W. 1941. Fundamental errors in the early history of cinchona. Part 4. The fabulous story of the Countess of Chinchon. *Bull. Hist. Med.* 10:568.

Hahnemann, S. 1869. *Organon of Homoeopathic Medicine*. 4th American ed. Philadelphia: Wm. Radde.

Hall, M. C. 1921. The use of carbon tetrachlorid for the removal of hookworms. *JAMA* 77:1641.

Hall, M. W. 1928. Inflammatory diseases of the respiratory tract (bronchitis, influenza, bronchopneumonia, lobar pneumonia). In *The Medical Department of the United States Army in the World War* by the U.S. Surgeon-General's Office, Vol. 9, p. 61. Washington, D.C.: U.S. Government Printing Office.

Hall, W. H.; Alden, J.; Burt, G. M.; and Spink, W. W. 1946. The treatment of pneumococcic and staphylococcic meningitis with penicillin and sulfonamides: Report of 20 cases. *Minn. Med.* 29:553.

Hall, W. H., and Spink, W. W. 1947. In vitro sensitivity of Brucella to streptomycin: Development of resistance during streptomycin treatment. *Proc. Soc. Exp. Biol. Med.* 64:403.

Halstead, S. B. 1966. Mosquito-borne haemorrhagic fevers of south and south-east Asia. *Bull. WHO* 35:3.

Halstead, S. B. 1970. Observations related to pathogenesis of dengue hemorrhagic fever. VI. Hypotheses and discussion. *Yale J. Biol. Med.* 42:350.

Hambidge, G., ed. 1942. *Keeping Livestock Healthy. The Yearbook of Agriculture 1942.* Washington, D.C.: U.S. Dept. of Agriculture, U.S. Government Printing Office.

Hamilton, R. 1790. An account of a distemper, by the common people in England vulgarly called the mumps. *Trans. R. Soc. Edinb.* 2:59.

Hammon, W. McD., and Reeves, W. C. 1952. California encephalitis virus. A newly described agent. I. Evidence of natural infection in man and other animals. *Calif. Med.* 77:303.

Hansen, G. A. 1875. I. On the etiology of leprosy. English translation. *Br. and Foreign Med.-chir. Rev.* 55:459.

Hanshaw, J. B. 1970. Developmental abnormalities associated with congenital cytomegalovirus infection. In *Advances in Teratology*, edited by D. H. M. Woollam. Vol. 4, p. 64. New York: Academic Press.

Hanshaw, J. B., and Weller, T. H. 1961. Urinary excretion of cytomegaloviruses by children with generalized neoplastic disease. Correlation with clinical and histopathologic observations. *J. Pediatr.* 58:305.

Hanson, R. P., and Marsh, R. F. 1974. Biology of transmissible mink encephalopathy and scrapie. In *Slow Virus Diseases*, edited by W. Zeman and E. H. Lennette. Baltimore: Williams & Wilkins.

Hardy, A. V.; Jordan, C. F.; Borts, I. H.; and Hardy, G. C. 1931. Undulant fever: With special reference to a study of brucella infection in Iowa. *U.S. NIH Health Bull.* No. 158.

Hare, R. 1970. *The Birth of Penicillin and the Disarming of Microbes.* London: George Allen and Unwin.

Harned, B. K.; Cunningham, R. W.; Clark, M. C.; Cosgrove, R.; Hine, C. H.; McCauley, W. J.; Stokey, E.; Vessey, R. E.; Yuda, N. N.; and SubbaRow, Y. 1948. The pharmacology of duomycin. *Ann. NY Acad. Sci.* 51:182.

Hartsough, G. R., and Burger, D. 1965. Encephalopathy of mink. I. Epizootiologic and clinical observations. *J. Infect. Dis.* 115:387.

Haupt, E. W., and Rehaag, J. L. 1921. Durch Fledermäuse verbreitete seruchenhafte Tollwut unter Viehbeständen in Santa Catharina (Süd-Brasilien). *Z. InfektKrankh. parasit. Krankh. Hyg. Haustiere* 22:104.

Havens, Jr., W. P. 1968. Viral hepatitis. In *Internal Medicine in World War II* by Medical Department, U.S. Army, Vol. 3, p. 331. Washington, D.C.: Office of the Surgeon-General.

Hazen, E. L., and Brown, R. 1950. Two antifungal agents produced by a soil actinomycete. *Science* 112:423.

Heberden, W. 1768. On the chicken-pox. *Med. Trans. R. Coll. Phys. Lond.* 1:427.

Hebra, F. 1856–76. *Atlas der Hautkrankheiten.* 2 vols. in 10 parts. Wien: k. -k. Hof- & Staatsdr.

Hebra, F. 1874–76. *Lehrbuch der Hautkrankheiten.* 2 vols. Stuttgart: F. Enke. Reprinted from *Hanbuch der speciellen Pathologie und Therapie* by Rudolph Virchow. Vol. 3, 1854–1876. Stuttgart and Erlangen: F. Enke.

Hecker, J. F. C. 1844. *The Epidemics of the Middle Ages*. Translated by B. G. Babington. London: George Woodfall & Son.

Heffron, R. 1939. *Pneumonia; with Special Reference to Pneumococcus Lobar Pneumonia*. New York: Commonwealth Fund.

Heidelberger, M., and Jacobs, W. A. 1919. Syntheses in the cinchona series. III. Azo dyes derived from hydrocupreine and hydrocupreidine. *J. Am. Chem. Soc.* 41:2131.

Heine, J. 1840. *Beobachtungen über Lähmungszustände der untern Extremitäten und deren Behandlung*. Stuttgart: F. H. Köhler.

Hektoen, L. 1905. Experimental measles. *J. Infect. Dis.* 2:238.

Henderson, D. A. 1973. Eradication of smallpox: The critical year ahead. *Proc. R. Soc. Med.* 66:493.

Henle, F. G. J. 1840, transl. 1938. Von den Miasmen und Kontagien und von den Miasmatisch-Contagiösen Krankheiten. In *Pathologische Untersuchung*, p. 1. Berlin: A. Hirschwald. Translated by George Rosen. On miasmata and contagia. *Bull. Hist. Med.* 6:907.

Henle, G., and Deinhardt, F. 1955. Propagation and primary isolation of mumps virus in tissue culture. *Proc. Soc. Exp. Biol. Med.* 89:556.

Henle, G.; Henle, W.; and Diehl, V. 1968. Relation of Burkitt's tumor-associated herpes-type virus to infectious mononucleosis. *Proc. Natl. Acad. Sci. USA* 59:94.

Henrici, A. T. 1930. *Molds, Yeasts, and Actinomycetes. A Handbook for Students of Bacteriology*. New York: John Wiley & Sons.

Henrici, A. T., and Gardner, E. L. 1921. The acidfast actinomycetes. With a report of a case from which a new species was isolated. *J. Infect. Dis.* 28:232.

Hentsch, D., ed. 1971. *Toxoplasmosis*. Bern: Hans Huber.

Heracleitus. 1931. On the universe. Translated by W. H. S. Jones. In *Hippocrates*, p. 449. Vol. 4 of The Loeb Classical Library, edited by E. H. Warmington. Cambridge (Mass.): Harvard University Press.

Herrell, W. E.; Heilman, D. H.; and Williams, H. L. 1942. The clinical use of penicillin. *Proc. Staff Meet. Mayo Clin.* 17:609.

Hess, A. F. 1914. German measles (rubella): An experimental study. *Arch. Intern. Med.* 13:913.

Hill, J. 1943. Experimental infection with *Neisseria gonorrhoeae*. I. Human inoculations. *Am. J. Syph. Gonorrhea vener. Dis.* 27:733.

Hinshaw, H. C., and Feldman, W. H. 1945. Streptomycin in treatment of clinical tuberculosis: A preliminary report. *Proc. Staff Meet. Mayo Clin.* 20:313.

Hinsie, L. E., and Carpenter, C. M. 1931. Radiothermic treatment of general paralysis. *Psychiatr. Q.* 5:215.

Hippocrates. 1939. *The Genuine Works of Hippocrates*. Translation by Francis Adams. Baltimore: Williams & Wilkins.

Hiro, Y., and Tasaka, S. 1938. Die Röteln sind eine Viruskrankheit. *Monattschr. Kinderheilkd.* 76:328.

Hirsch, A. 1886. Meningitis cerebro-spinalis epidemica. In *Handbuch der Historisch-Geographischen Pathologie* by August Hirsch. 2nd ed. Vol. 3, p. 379. Stuttgart: F. Enke. Translation from the second German edition by Charles Creighton. *Epidemic Cerebrospinal Meningitis*. Vol. 117, p. 547. London: New Sydenham Society.

Hoagland, R. J. 1952. Infectious mononucleosis. *Am. J. Med.* 13:158.

Hoare, C. A. 1938. Early discoveries regarding the parasite of oriental sore: With an English translation of the memoir by P. F. Borovsky "On Sart Sore." 1898. *Trans. R. Soc. Trop. Med. Hyg.* 32:67.

Hobbs, B. C. 1969. Staphylococcal and *Clostridium welchii* food poisoning. In *Bacterial Food Poisoning*, edited by Joan Taylor, p. 67. London: Royal Society of Health.

Hobby, G. L.; Dougherty, N.; Lenert, T. F.; Hudders, E.; and Kiseluk, M. 1950. Antimicrobial action of terramycin *in vitro* and *in vivo*. *Proc. Soc. Exp. Biol. Med.* 73:503.

Hobby, G. L.; Meyer, K.; and Chaffee, E. 1942. Chemotherapeutic activity of penicillin. *Proc. Soc. Exp. Biol. Med.* 50:285.

Hodgkin, D. C., and Maslen, E. N. 1961. The x-ray analysis of the structure of cephalosporin C. *Biochem J.* 79:393.

Hoerlein, H. 1937. A new class of chemotherapeutic agents against streptococci. With special reference to prontosil and prontylin. *Int. Record Med., NY Med. J.* 146:11.

Hoffman, T. A.; Ruiz, C. J.; Counts, G. W.; Sachs, J. M.; and Nitzkin, J. L. 1975. Waterborne typhoid fever in Dade County, Florida: Clinical and therapeutic evaluation of 105 bacteremic patients. *Am. J. Med.* 59:481.

Holmes, O. W. 1843. The contagiousness of puerperal fever. Read before the Boston Society for Medical Improvement. *N. Engl. Q. J. Med. Surg.* 1:503.

Holmes, O. W. 1855. *Puerperal Fever, as a Private Pestilence*. Boston: Ticknor and Fields.

Holmes, W. H. 1940. *Bacillary and Rickettsial Infections, Acute and Chronic; A Textbook, Black Death to White Plague*. New York: Macmillan.

Home, F. 1759. *Medical Facts and Experiments*. London: A. Millar.

Hood, L.; Campbell, J. H.; and Elgin, S. C. R. 1975. The organization, expression, and evolution of antibody genes and other multigene families. In *Annual Review of Genetics*, edited by H. L. Roman, A. Campbell, and L. M. Sandler. Vol. 9, p. 305. Palo Alto (Calif.): Annual Reviews Inc.

Hopkins, J. G. 1927. The higher bacteria, molds and fungi. In *A Textbook of Bacteriology* by H. Zinsser. 6th ed., p. 819. New York: D. Appleton.

Hornibrook, J. W., and Nelson, K. R. 1940. An institutional outbreak of pneumonitis. I. Epidemiological and clinical studies. *U.S. Public Health Rep.* 55:1936.

Horta-Barbosa, L.; Fuccillo, D. A.; Sever, J. L.; and Zeman, W. 1969. Subacute sclerosing panencephalitis: Isolation of measles virus from a brain biopsy. *Nature* 221:974.

Horwitz, O.; Grünfeld, K.; Lysgaard-Hansen, B.; and Kjeldsen, K. 1974. The epidemiology and natural history of measles in Denmark. *Am. J. Epidemiol.* 100:136.

Hotchin, J. 1971. *Persistent and Slow Virus Infections*. New York: S. Karger.

Hotchkiss, R. D., and Dubos, R. J. 1940. Bactericidal fractions from an aerobic sporulating bacillus. *J. Biol. Chem.* 136:803.

Hotta, S. 1969. *Dengue and Related Hemorrhagic Diseases*. St. Louis: Warren H. Green.

Howard, J. 1791. *An Account of the Principal Lazarettos in Europe; with Various Papers Relative to the Plague: Together with Further Observations on Some Foreign Prisons and Hospitals; and Additional Remarks on the Present State of Those in Great Britain and Ireland*. 2nd. ed. London: J. Johnson, C. Dilly & T. Cadell.

Howard, J. 1792. *The State of the Prisons in England and Wales, with Preliminary Observations and an Account of Some Foreign Prisons and Hospitals*. 4th ed. London: J. Johnson, C. Dilly & T. Cadell.

Howard-Jones, N. 1975. *The Scientific Background of the International Sanitary Conferences 1851–1938*. Geneva: World Health Organization.

Howitt, B. 1938. Recovery of the virus of equine encephalomyelitis from the brain of a child. *Science* 88:455.

Hudson, E. H. 1963. Treponematosis and anthropology. *Ann. Intern. Med.* 58:1037.

Huebner, R. J.; Jellison, W. L.; and Pomerantz, C. 1946. Rickettsialpox — A newly recognized rickettsial disease. IV. Isolation of a Rickettsia apparently identical with the causative agent of rickettsialpox from *Allodermanyssus sanguineus*, a rodent mite. *U.S. Public Health Rep.* 61:1677.

Hughes, M. L. 1897. *Mediterranean, Malta or Undulant Fever*. London: Macmillan.

Hull, T. G., ed. 1955. *Diseases Transmitted from Animals to Man*. 4th ed. Springfield (Ill.): Chas. C Thomas.

Hunter, J. 1778. Of the heat, &c. of animals and vegetables. *Philos. Trans. R. Soc. Lond. (Biol. Sci.)* 68:7.

Hunter, J. 1835. A treatise on the venereal disease. In *The Works of John Hunter*, edited by James F. Palmer. Vol. 2. London: Longman, Rees, Orme, Brown, Green and Longman.

Hurst, E. W., and Pawan, J. L. 1931. An outbreak of rabies in Trinidad. *Lancet* 221:622.

Hurst, E. W., and Pawan, J. L. 1932. A further account of the Trinidad outbreak of acute rabic myelitis: Histology of the experimental disease. *J. Pathol. Bacteriol.* 35:301.

Hutchison, W. M. 1967. The nematode transmission of *Toxoplasma gondii*. *Trans. R. Soc. Trop. Med. Hyg.* 61:80.

Ido, Y.; Hoki, R.; Ito, H.; and Wani, H. 1917. The rat as a carrier of *Spirochaeta icterohaemorrhagiae*, the causative agent of Weil's disease (spirochaetosis icterohaemorrhagica). *J. Exp. Med.* 26:341.

Illinois State Agricultural Society, Commissioners of 1868. *Report on Texas or Spanish Fever*. Springfield (Ill.): Baker, Bailhache.

Imperato, P. J. 1974a. Leishmaniasis. In *The Treatment and Control of Infectious Diseases in Man*, p. 436. Springfield (Ill.): Chas. C Thomas.

Imperato, P. J. 1974b. The present status of diphtheria in New York City. *Bull. N Y Acad. Med.* 50:763.

Inada, R.; Ido, Y.; Hoki, R.; Kaneko, R.; and Ito, H. 1916. The etiology, mode of infection, and specific therapy of Weil's disease (spirochaetosis icterohaemorrhagica). *J. Exp. Med.* 23:377.

India. Plague Advisory Committee 1906–1917. Reports on plague investigations in India. *J. Hyg.* (Camb.) 6:421; 7:323, 693; 8:161; 10:313 (1906–1910). *J. Hygiene* (Camb.) *Plague Supplements* I–V, pp. 1–899 (1912–1917).

Ireland, Medical Research Council of. 1954. *Tuberculosis in Ireland. Report of the National Tuberculosis Survey 1950–53*. Dublin: Medical Research Council of Ireland.

Israël, J. 1878, transl. 1886. Neue Beobachtungen auf dem Gebiete der Mykosen des Menschen. *Virchow's Arch. Path. Anat.* 74:15. Translation abstracted by Thos. W. Hime. On actinomycosis in man. In *Bacteria in Relation to Disease*, edited by W. W. Cheyne. Vol. 115, p. 463. London: New Sydenham Society.

Ivanowski, D. 1942. Concerning the Mosaic disease of the tobacco plant. Translated by James Johnson. *Phytopathol. Classics* No. 7.

Jacobs, P. P. 1940. *The Control of Tuberculosis in the United States*. New York: National Tuberculosis Assn.

Jakob, A. 1921. Über eigenartige Erkrankungen des Zentralnervensystems mit bemerkenswertem anatomischen Befunde. *Z. ges. Neurol. Psychiat.* 64:147.

Janbon, M.; Bertrand, L.; and Combier, Ch. 1949. La traitment de la fièvre boutonneuse par la chloromycétine. *Presse med.* 57:1026.

Jellison, W. L.; Kohls, G. M.; Butler, W. J.; and Weaver, J. A. 1942. Epizootic tularemia in the beaver, *Castor Canadensis*, and the contamination of stream water with *Pasteurella tularensis*. *Am. J. Hyg.* 36:168.

Jenner, E. 1798. *An Inquiry into the Causes and Effects of the Variolae Vaccinae*. London: S. Low.

Jerne, N. K. 1955. The natural-selection theory of antibody formation. *Proc. Natl. Acad. Sci. USA* 41:849.

Jerne, N. K. 1973. The immune system. *Sci. Am.* 229:52 (July).

Jessen, O.; Rosendal, K.; Bülow, P.; Faber, V.; and Eriksen, K. R. 1969. Changing staphylococci and staphylococcal infections. A ten-year study of bacteria and cases of bacteremia. *N. Engl. J. Med.* 281:627.

Jobling, J. W., and Petersen, W. 1916. The nonspecific factors in the treatment of disease. *JAMA* 66:1753.

Jochmann, G. 1906. Versuche zur Serodiagnostik und Serotherapie der epidemischen Genickstarre. *Dtsch. med. Wochenschr.* 32:788.

Johnson, C. D., and Goodpasture, E. W. 1934. An investigation of the etiology of mumps. *J. Exp. Med.* 59:1.

Johnson, R. T. 1974. Slow virus infections: Virus-host relationships. In *Slow Virus Diseases*, edited by W. Zeman and E. H. Lennette, p. 1. Baltimore: Williams & Wilkins.

Jones, C. M., and Minot, G. R. 1923. Infectious (catarrhal) jaundice. An attempt to establish a clinical entity. Observations on the excretion and retention of the bile pigments, and on the blood. *Boston Med. Surg. J.* 189:531.

Jones, T. C.; Kean, B. H.; and Kimball, A. C. 1965. Toxoplasmic lymphadenitis. *JAMA* 192:87.

Jordan, E. O. 1927. *Epidemic Influenza: A Survey*. Chicago: American Medical Assn.

Jordan, E. O.; Whipple, G. C.; and Winslow, C-E. A. 1924. *A Pioneer of Public Health: William Thompson Sedgwick*. New Haven: Yale University Press.

Jukes, T. H. 1955. *Antibiotics in Nutrition*. Antibiotics Monographs No. 4. New York: Medical Encylcopedia.

Jukes, T. H. 1973. Public health significance of feeding low levels of antibiotics to animals. In *Advances in Applied Microbiology*, edited by D. Perlman. Vol. 16, p. 1. New York: Academic Press.

Kääriäinen, L.; Klemola, E.; and Paloheimo, J. 1966. Rise of cytomegalovirus antibodies in an infectious-mononucleosis-like syndrome after transfusion. *Br. Med. J.* 1:1270.

Kagan, I. G.; Osimani, J. J.; Varela, J. C.; and Allain, D. S. 1966. Evaluation of intradermal and serologic tests for the diagnosis of hydatid disease. *Am. J. Trop. Med. Hyg.* 15:172.

Kallmann, F. J., and Reisner, D. 1943. Twin studies on the significance of genetic factors in tuberculosis. *Am. Rev. Tuberc.* 47:549.

Kaneko, R., and Aoki, Y. 1928. Über die Encephalitis epidemica in Japan. *Ergeb. Inn. Med. Kinderheilkd.* 34:342.

Kanich, R. E., and Craighead, J. E. 1966. Cytomegalovirus infection and cytomegalic inclusion disease in renal homotransplant recipients. *Am. J. Med.* 40:874.

Kaplan, M. 1973. Science's role in the World Health Organization. *Science* 180:1028.

Kaplan, M. and Beveridge, W. I. B., eds. 1972. Influenza in animals. *Bull. WHO* 47:439–541.

Kaplan, M. M., and Webster, R. G. 1977. The epidemiology of influenza. *Sci. Am.* 237:88 (December).

Kaposi, M. 1875. Lepra. In *On Diseases of the Skin Including the Exanthemata* by F. Hebra and M. Kaposi. Vol. 64, p. 118. Translated by Waren Tay. London: New Sydenham Society.

Kayne, G. G. 1937. *The Control of Tuberculosis in England: Past and Present*. London: Oxford University Press.

Kean, B. H.; Kimball, A. C.; and Christenson, W. N. 1969. An epidemic of acute toxoplasmosis. *JAMA* 208:1002.

Keating, J. M. 1879. *A History of the Yellow Fever. The Yellow Fever Epidemic of 1878, in Memphis, Tenn.* Memphis (Tenn.): Howard Association.

Kedes, L. H.; Siemienski, J.; and Braude, A. I. 1964. The syndrome of the alcoholic rose gardener: Sporotrichosis of the radial tendon sheath. Report of a case cured with amphotericin B. *Ann. Intern. Med.* 61:1139.

Keefer, C. S. 1924. Report of a case of Malta fever originating in Baltimore, Maryland. *Johns Hopkins Hosp. Bull.* 35:6.

Keefer, C. S.; Blake, F. G.; Lockwood, J. S.; Long, P. H.; Marshall, Jr., E. K.; and Wood, Jr., W. B. 1946. Streptomycin in the treatment of infections: A report of one thousand cases. *JAMA* 132:4, 70.

Keefer, C. S.; Blake, F. G.; Marshall, Jr., E. K.; Lockwood, J. S.; and Wood, Jr., W. B. 1943. Penicillin in the treatment of infections. A report of 500 cases. Report by NRC Division of Medical Sciences Committee on Chemotherapeutic and Other Agents. *JAMA* 122:1217.

Keefer, C. S., and Hewitt, W. L. 1948. *The Therapeutic Value of Streptomycin. A Study of 3000 Cases*. Ann Arbor (Mich.): J. W. Edwards.

Keefer, C. S.; Ingelfinger, F. J.; and Spink, W. W. 1937. Significance of hemolytic streptococcic bacteremia. A study of two hundred and forty-six patients. *Arch. Intern. Med.* 60:1084.

Keefer, C. S., and Spink, W. W. 1936–37. Studies of hemolytic streptococcal infection. I. Factors influencing the outcome of erysipelas. *J. Clin. Invest.* 15:17 (1936). III. The characteristics of the hemolytic streptococci isolated from patients with erysipelas. *J. Clin. Invest.* 16:155 (1937).

Keefer, C. S., and Spink, W. W. 1937. Gonococcic arthritis: Pathogenesis, mechanism of recovery and treatment. *JAMA* 109:1448.

Keen, W. W. 1905. Surgical reminiscences of the Civil War. *Trans. Coll. Physicians Phila.* 27:95.

Kellaway, C. H.; MacCallum, P.; and Terbutt, A. H. 1928. *Report of the Commission to the Governor of the Commonwealth of Australia.* Melbourne.

Kelly, H. A. 1906. *Walter Reed and Yellow Fever.* New York: McClure, Phillips.

Khalil, M. B. 1931. *The Bibliography of Schistosomiasis (Bilharziasis). Zoological, Clinical and Prophylactic.* Published by the Egyptian University Faculty of Medicine, Publication No. 1. Cairo: Université Egyptienne Faculty of Med. Publ.

Khan, M. Y.; Zinneman, H. H.; and Hall, W. H. 1970. Vietnam malaria. Clinical experience with 50 patients. *Minn. Med.* 53:331 (March).

Kierman, Jr., F. A. 1959. The blood fluke that saved Formosa. *Harper's Magazine* (April) p. 45.

King, A. F. A. 1883. Insects and disease — mosquitoes and malaria. *Popular Sci. Monthly* 23:644 (September).

Kirby, W. M. M. 1944. Extraction of highly potent penicillin inactivator from penicillin resistant staphylococci. *Science* 99:452.

Kirchheimer, W. F., and Storrs, E. E. 1971. Attempts to establish the armadillo (*Dasypus novemcinctus* Linn.) as a model for the study of leprosy. I. Report of lepromatoid leprosy in an experimentally infected armadillo. *Int. J. Lepr.* 39:693.

Kirkes, W. S. 1852 and 1945. On some of the principle effects resulting from the detachment of fibrinous deposits from the interior of the heart, and their mixture with the circulating blood. *Trans. R. med-chir. Soc. London* 35:281 (1852). In *Classic Descriptions of Disease* by R. Major, 3rd ed., p. 464. Springfield (Ill.): Chas. C Thomas (1945).

Kitasato, S. 1889. Ueber den Tetanusbacillus. *Z. Hyg.* 7:225.

Kjellstrand, C. M.; Simmons, R. L.; Buselmeier, T. J.; and Najarian, J. S. 1972. Recipient selection, medical management and dialysis. In *Transplantation,* edited by J. S. Najarian and R. L. Simmons, p. 418. Philadelphia: Lea & Febiger.

Klebs, E. 1879. Das Contagium der Syphilis. Eine experimentelle Studie. *Arch. exp. Path. Pharmak.* 10:161.

Klee, P., and Römer, H. 1935. Prontosil bei Streptokokkenerkrankungen. *Dtsch. med. Wochenschr.* 61:253.

Klein, J. O., and Finland, M. 1963. The new penicillins. *N. Engl. J. Med.* 269:1019, 1074, and 1129.

Klemperer, G., and Klemperer, F. 1891. Versuche über Immunisirung und Heilung bei der Pneumokokkeninfection. *Berl. klin. Wschr.* 28:833.

Kneeland, Jr., Y. 1963a. Measles. In *Internal Medicine in World War II,* by Medical Department, U.S. Army, edited by J. B. Coates, Jr., and W. P. Havens, Jr. Vol. 2, p. 32. Washington, D.C.: Office of the Surgeon-General, Department of the Army.

Kneeland, Jr., Y. 1963b. Mumps. In *Internal Medicine in World War II* by Medical Department, U.S. Army, edited by J. B. Coates, Jr. and W. P. Havens, Jr. Vol. 2, p. 35. Washington, D.C.: Office of the Surgeon-General, Department of the Army.

Knyvett, A. F. 1966. The pulmonary lesions of chickenpox. *Q. J. Med.* 35:313.

Koch, R. 1877, transl. 1938. Untersuchungen über Bacterien. V. Die Aetiologie der Milzbrand-Krankheit, begründet auf die Entwicklungsgeschichte des Bacillus Anthracis. *Beitr. Biol. Pfl.* 2:277. Translation. Investigations of bacteria. The etiology of anthrax, based on the ontogeny of the anthrax bacillus. In *Medical Classics,* compiled by E. C. Kelly. Vol. 2, p. 787. Baltimore: Williams & Wilkins.

Koch, R. 1878, transl. 1880. *Untersuchungen über die Aetiologie der Wundinfectionskrankeiten.* Leipzig: F. C. W. Vogel. Translated by W. Watson Cheyne. *Investigations into the Etiology of Traumatic Infective Diseases* by R. Koch. Vol. 88, p. 1. London: New Sydenham Society.

Koch, R. 1882, transl. 1938. Die Aetiologie der Tuberculose. *Berl. klin. Wschr.* 19:221. Translated by W. de Rouville. The etiology of tuberculosis. In *Medical Classics,* compiled by E. C. Kelly. Vol. 2, p. 853. Baltimore: Williams & Wilkins.

Koch, R. 1886. Recent papers on disinfection by Robert Koch. Abstracted by B. Arthur Whitelegge. In *Recent Essays by Various Authors on Bacteria in Relation to Disease*, edited by W. Watson Cheyne. Vol. 115, p. 493. London: New Sydenham Society. Also in *Mitt. K. GesundhAmt., Berl.* Vol. 1, 1881.

Kock, R. 1890. Weittere Mittheilungen über ein Heilmittel gegen Tuberculose. *Dtsch. med. Wochenschr.* 16:1029.

Koch, R., and Carson, M. J. 1955. Management of *Hemophilus Influenzae*, type B meningitis: Analysis of 128 cases. *J. Pediatr.* 46:18.

Koen, J. S. 1919. A practical method for field diagnosis of swine diseases. *Am. J. vet Med.* 14:468.

Koenig, M. G.; Spickard, A.; Cardella, M. A.; and Rogers, D. E. 1964. Clinical and laboratory observations on type E botulism in man. *Medicine* 43:517.

Kohler, P. F. 1964. Hospital salmonellosis. *JAMA* 189:6.

Kolmer, J. A. 1935. Susceptibility and immunity in relation to vaccination in acute anterior poliomyelitis. *JAMA* 105:1956.

Krugman, S.; Giles, J. P.; and Hammond, J. 1967. Infectious hepatitis. Evidence for two distinctive clinical, epidemiological, and immunological types of infection. *JAMA* 200:365.

Krugman, S.; Giles, J. P.; and Hammond, J. 1971. Viral hepatitis, type B (MS-2 strain). Studies on active immunization. *JAMA* 217:41.

Krugman, S., and Ward, R. 1973a. Cytomegalovirus infections. In *Infectious Diseases of Children and Adults* by S. Krugman and R. Ward. 5th ed., p. 1. St. Louis: C. V. Mosby.

Krugman, S., and Ward, R. 1973b. Measles (rubeola). Ibid., p. 106.

Krugman, S., and Ward, R. 1973c. Rubella (German measles). Ibid., p. 236.

Krugman, S., and Ward, R. 1973d. Toxoplasmosis. Ibid., p. 336.

Kubes, V., and Ríos, F. A. 1939. The causative agent of infectious equine encephalomyelitis in Venezuela. *Science* 90:20.

Kuhn, T. S. 1962. *The Structure of Scientific Revolutions*. Chicago: University of Chicago Press.

Kützing, F. 1837. Microscopische Untersuchungen über die Hefe und Essigmutter, Nebst Mehreren Andern Dazu gehörigen Vegetablischen Gebilden. *J. prakt. Chem.* 11:385.

Laennec, R. T. H. 1819, transl. 1823. *De l'auscultation médiate, ou Traité du diagnostic des maladies des poumons et du coeur, fondé principalement sur ce nouveau moyen d'exploration*. 2 vols. Paris: J. -A. Brosson & J. -S. Chaude. Translated from 3rd French edition by John Forbes. *A Treatise on the Diseases of the Chest*. Philadelphia: J. Webster.

Lagrange, E. 1926. Concerning the discovery of the plague bacillus. *Am. J. Trop. Med. Hyg.* 29:299.

Lambert, R. 1963. *Sir John Simon: 1816–1904, and English Social Administration*. London: MacGibbon & Kee.

Lambert, S. M. 1941. *A Yankee Doctor in Paradise*. Boston: Little, Brown.

Lancefield, R. C. 1933. A serological differentiation of human and other groups of hemolytic streptococci. *J. Exp. Med.* 57:571.

Landsteiner, K. 1947. *The Specificity of Serological Reactions*. Rev. ed. with a chapter on Molecular Structure and Intermolecular Forces by Linus Pauling. Cambridge (Mass.): Harvard University Press.

Landsteiner, K., and Popper, E. 1909. Uebertragung der Poliomyelitis acuta auf Affen. *Z. Immunitätsforsch.* 2:377.

Lapeyssonnie, L. 1963. La méningite cérébro-spinale en Afrique. *Bull. WHO* Vol. 28 *Suppl.*

Laranja, F. S.; Dias, E.; Nobrega, G.; and Miranda, A. 1956. Chagas' disease: A clinical, epidemiologic, and pathologic study. *Circulation* 14:1035.

Latham, M. C. Nutrition and infection in national development. *Science* 188:561.

Laveran, A. 1880. Un nouveau parasite. Trouvé dans le sang de malades atteints de fiévre palustre. Origine Parasitaire des accidents de l'impaludisme. *Bull. Mém. Soc. méd. Hôp. Paris* 17 (II Series):158.

Laveran, A. 1893. *Paludism*. Translated by J. W. Martin. Vol. 146, p. 1. London: New Sydenham Society.

Lavinder, C. H.; Freeman, A. W.; and Frost, W. H. 1918. Epidemiologic Studies of Poliomyelitis in New York City and the Northeastern United States during the Year 1916. *USPHS Public Health Bull.* No. 91.

League of Nations. 1945. Bibliography of the technical work of the health organisation of the League of Nations, 1920–1945. *Bull. WHO* 11:1–235.

Leake, J. P. 1935. Poliomyelitis following vaccination against this disease. *JAMA* 105:2152.

Leidy, J. 1846. Remarks on *Trichina spiralis* in hogs. Minutes of meeting October 6, 1846. *Proc. Acad. nat. Sci. Philad.* 3:107.

Leiper, R. T. 1915–18. Report on the results of the Bilharzia Mission in Egypt, 1915. *J. R. Army med. Cps.* Part I, Transmission, 25:1 (1915); Part II, Prevention and eradication, 26:147 (1915); Part III, Development, 26:253 (1915); Part IV, Egyptian mollusca, 27:171 (1916); Part V, Adults and ova, 30:235 (1918).

Leishman,, W. B. 1903. On the possibility of the occurrence of trypanosomiasis in India. *Br. Med. J.* 1:1252.

Lennette, E. H., and Koprowski, H. 1943. Human infection with Venezuelan equine encephalomyelitis virus. A report of eight cases of infection acquired in the laboratory. *JAMA* 123:1088.

Leonard Wood Memorial Staff (American Leprosy Foundation) 1944. World wide distribution and prevalence of leprosy. *Int. J. Lepr. Suppl.* 12:1.

Lepper, M. H. 1956. *Aureomycin (Chlortetracycline)*. Antibiotics Monographs No. 7. New York: Medical Encyclopedia.

Lepper, M. H., and Spies, H. W. 1959. *Results of Treatment of Tuberculous Meningitis with Several Regimen. Transactions of the 18th Conference on the Chemotherapy of Tuberculosis, February 1959*. Vol. 18, p. 183. Washington, D.C.: V.A. Department of Medicine and Surgery.

Leslie, P. H., and Gardner, A. D. 1931. The phases of *Haemophilus pertussis. J. Hyg.* (Camb.) 31:423.

Leuckart, R. 1860. *Untersuchungen über Trichina spiralis*. Leipzig: C. F. Winter.

Levaditi, C., and Vaisman, A. 1935. Action curative et preventive du chlorhydrate de 4'-sulfamido-2, 4-diamino-azobenzene dans l'infection streptococcique experimentale. *C. R. Acad. Sci.* (D) (Paris) 200:1694.

Levinthal, W. 1930. Die Ätiologie der Psittakosis. *Klin. Wochenschr.* 9:654.

Lewis, T. R. 1872. On a haematozoon inhabiting human blood. Its relation to chyluria and other diseases. In: *Eighth Annual Report of the (Great Britain) Sanitary Commissioner with the Government of India, 1871*. Appendix E, p. 243. Calcutta: Office of the Superintendent of Government Printing.

Lewis, T. R. 1878. The microscopic organisms found in the blood of man and animals, and their relation to disease. In *Fourteenth Annual Report of the (Great Britain) Sanitary Commissioner with the Government of India for 1877*. Appendix B, p. 157. Calcutta: Office of the Superintendent of Government Printing.

Ley, Jr., H. L.; Woodward, T. E.; and Smadel, J. E. 1950. Chloramphenicol (chloromycetin) in the treatment of murine typhus. *JAMA* 143:217.

Lichtman, S. S., and Gross, L. 1932. Streptococci in the blood in rheumatic fever, rheumatoid arthritis and other diseases. Based on a study of 5, 233 consecutive blood cultures. *Arch. Intern. Med.* 49:1078.

Lien-Teh, W. 1926. *A Treatise on Pneumonic Plague*. Vol. 3, No. 13. Geneva: League of Nations.

Lien-Teh, W.; Chun, J. W. H.; Pollitzer, R.; and Wu, C. Y. 1936. *Plague. A Manual for Medical and Public Health Workers*. Shanghai Station (China): Weishengshu National Quarantine Service.

Lillie, R. D. 1930. Psittacosis: Rickettsia-like inclusions in man and in experimental animals. *U.S. Public Health Rep.* 45:773.

Lincoln, E. M., and Sewell, E. M. 1963. *Tuberculosis in Children*. New York: McGraw-Hill Book.

Lind, J. 1757a. *An Essay on the Most Effectual Means of Preserving the Health of Seamen, in the Royal Navy*. London: A. Millar.

Lind, J. 1757b. *A Treatise on the Scurvy*. 2nd ed. London: A. Millar.

Lind, J. 1771. *An Essay on Diseases Incidental to Europeans in Hot Climates. With the Method of Preventing their Fatal Consequences*. 2nd ed. London: T. Becket & P. A. DeHondt.

Link, V. B. 1955. A history of plague in the United States of America. *USPHS Publication* No. 392. *Public Health Monogr*. No. 26.

Linnemann, Jr., C. C. 1973. Measles vaccine: Immunity reinfection and revaccination. *Am. J. Epidemiol*. 97:365.

Lister, F. S. 1917. Prophylactic inoculation of man against pneumococcal infections, and more particularly against lobar pneumonia; including a report upon the results of the experimental inoculation, with a specific group vaccine, of the native mine labourers employed upon the Premier (diamond) mine and the Crown (gold) mines in the Transvaal and the De Beers (diamond) mines at Kimberley — covering the period from November 1, 1916 to October 31, 1917. Publication No. 10. *S. Afr. Inst. med. Res. Publ*. 1:303.

Lister, J. 1867. On a new method of treating compound fracture, abscess, etc., with observations on the conditions of suppuration. *Lancet* 1:326, 357, 387, 507 and 2:95.

Lister, J. 1870. On the effects of the antiseptic system of treatment upon the salubrity of a surgical hospital. *Lancet* 1:4 and 40.

Littauer, J., and Sørensen, K. 1965. The measles epidemic at Umanak in Greenland in 1962. *Dan. Med. Bull*. 12:43.

Littman, M. L.; Horowitz, P. L.; and Swadey, J. G. 1958. Coccidioidomycosis and its treatment with amphotericin B. *Am. J. Med*. 24:568.

Littman, M. L., and Zimmerman, L. E. 1956. *Cryptococcosis. Torulosis or European Blastomycosis*. New York: Grune & Stratton.

Livingstone, D. 1857. *Missionary Travels and Researches in South Africa*. London: John Murray.

Loder, B.; Newton, G. G. F.; and Abraham, E. P. 1961. The cephalosporin C nucelus (7-aminocephalosporanic acid) and some of its derivatives. *Biochem. J*. 79:408.

Loeffler, F. 1884. Untersuchungen über die Bedeutung der Mikroorganismen für die Entstehung der Diphtherie beim Menschen, bei der Taube und beim Kalbe. *Mitt. K. GesundhAmt., Berl*. 2:421.

Loeffler, F. 1908. The history of diphtheria. In: *The Bacteriology of Diphtheria*, edited by G. H. F. Nuttall and G. S. Graham-Smith, p. 1. Cambridge: University Press.

Loeffler, F., and Frosch, F. 1898. Berichte der Kommission zur Erforschung der Maul- und Klauenseuche bei dem Institut für Infectionskrankheiten in Berlin. *Zentbl. Bakt. ParasitKde. Hyg*. 23:371.

Long, E. R. 1961. Tuberculosis. *Encycloped. Brit*. 22:531.

Long, E. R. 1967. Forty years of leprosy research: History of the Leonard Wood Memorial (American Leprosy Foundation) 1928–1967. *Int. J. Lepr. (Suppl.)* 35 (Part 2):239.

Long, P. H., and Bliss, E. A. 1937. Para-amino-benzene-sulfonamide and its derivatives. Experimental and clinical observations on their use in the treatment of beta-hemolytic streptococcic infection: A preliminary report. *JAMA* 108:32.

Long, P. H., and Bliss, E. A. 1939. *The Clinical and Experimental Use of Sulfanilamide, Sulfapyridine and Allied Compounds*. New York: Macmillan.

Longcope, W. T. 1922. Infectious mononucleosis (glandular fever), with a report of ten cases. *Am. J. Med. Sci*. 164:781.

Looss, A. 1901. Ueber das Eindringen der Ankylostomalarven in die menschliche Haut. *Zentbl. Bakt. ParasitKde. Hyg. Abt*. 1, 29:733.

Lorber, J. 1954. The results of treatment of 549 cases of tuberculous meningitis. *Am. Rev. Tuberc*. 69:13.

Lord, F. T. 1928. The mycoses. In *A Textbook of Medicine*, edited by R. L. Cecil, p. 343. Philadelphia: W. B. Saunders.

Lord, F. T., and Heffron, R. 1938. *Pneumonia and Serum Therapy*. Rev. ed. of *Lobar Pneumonia and Serum Therapy*. New York: The Commonwealth Fund.

Lösch, F. 1875. Massenhafte Entwickelung von Amöben im Dickdarm. *Virchow's Arch. path. Anat. Physiol.* 65:196.

Lott, W. A., and Bergeim, F. H. 1939. 2 (p-aminobenzenesulfonamido)-thiazole: A new chemotherapeutic agent. *J. Am. Chem. Soc.* 61:3593.

Louis, P. Ch. A. 1836a. *Anatomical, Pathological and Therapeutic Researches Upon the Disease Known under the Name of Gastro-Enterite, Putrid, Adynamic, Ataxic, or Typhoid Fever, etc., Compared with the Most Common Acute Diseases.* 2 vols. Translated by H. I. Bowditch. Boston: I. R. Butts (Vol. 1), Hilliard Gray (Vol. 2).

Louis, P. Ch. A. 1836b. *Researches of the Effects of Bloodletting in Some Inflammatory Diseases, and on the Influence of Tartarized Antimony and Vesication in Pneumonitis.* Translated by C. G. Putnam. Boston: Hilliard Gray.

Louria, D. B. 1967. Deep-seated mycotic infections, allergy to fungi and mycotoxins. *N. Eng. J. Med.* 277:1065 and 1126.

Lovett, R. W. 1917. *The Treatment of Infantile Paralysis.* 2nd ed. Philadelphia: P. Blakiston's Sons.

Low, J. 1822. Cases of hydatids in the bladder and liver. *NY med. physical J.* 1:287.

Luby, J. P.; Sulkin S. E.; and Sanford, J. P. 1969. The epidemiology of St. Louis encephalitis: A review. *Annu. Rev. Med.* 20:329.

Lucas, C. T.; Chandler, Jr., F.; Martin, Jr., J. E.; and Schmale, J. D. 1971. Transfer of gonococcal urethritis from man to chimpanzee. *JAMA* 216:1612.

Lumsden, L. L. 1958. St. Louis encephalitis in 1933. Observations on epidemiological features. *U.S. Public Health Rep.* 73:340.

Lundström, R. 1962. Rubella during pregnancy. A follow-up study of children born after an epidemic of rubella in Sweden, 1951, with additional investigations on prophylaxis and treatment of maternal rubella. *Acta Paediatr.* (Uppsala) *Suppl.* 133, 51:1.

Lürman, A. 1885, transl. 1972. Eine Icterusepidemie. *Berl. klin. Wschr.* 22:20. Translated by Helene Smith. An epidemic of icterus. In *Heptatis-Associated Antigen and Viruses* by A. J. Zuckerman, p. 3. New York: Am. Elsevier Publ. Co.

Lutz, A. 1908. Uma mycose pseudococcidica localisada na bocca e observada no Brazil. Contribuicao ao conhecimento das hyphoblastomycoses americanas. *Brazil-med.* 22:121 and 141.

Lyons, C. 1943. Penicillin therapy of surgical infections in the U.S. Army. *JAMA* 123:1007.

MacArthur, W. 1955. An account of some of Sir David Bruce's researches, based on his own manuscript notes. *Trans. R. Soc. Trop. Med. Hyg.* 49:404.

MacCallum, F. O., and Bauer, D. J. 1944. Homologous serum jaundice. Transmission experiments with human volunteers. *Lancet* 246:622.

MacCallum, W. G. 1897. On the flagellated form of the malarial parasite. *Lancet* 2:1240.

Mackaness, G. B. 1971. Delayed hypersensitivity and the mechanism of cellular resistance to infection. In: *Progress in Immunology. First International Congress of Immunology*, edited by B. Amos, p. 413. New York: Academic Press.

Mackenzie, R. B.; Beye, H. K.; Valverde, L.; and Garrón, H. 1964. Epidemic hemorrhagic fever in Bolivia. I. A preliminary report of the epidemiologic and clinical findings in a new epidemic area in South America. *Am. J. Trop. Med. Hyg.* 13:620.

Mackerchar, E. 1949. *The Romance of Leprosy.* London: The Mission to Lepers.

Maclagan, T. 1876. The treatment of acute rheumatism by salicin. *Lancet* 1:342.

MacLeod, C. M.; Hodges, R. G.; Heidelberger, M.; and Bernhard, W. G. 1945. Prevention of pneumococcal pneumonia by immunization with specific capsular polysaccharides. *J. Exp. Med.* 82:445.

MacNevin, M. G., and Vaughan, H. S. 1930. *Mouth Infections and Their Relation to Systemic Diseases*. 2 vols. New York: Joseph Purcell Research Memorial.

Magath, T. B. 1937. Hydatid (Echinococcus) disease in Canada and the United States. *Am. J. Hyg.* 25:107.

Magoffin, R.; Anderson, D.; and Spink, W. W. 1949. Therapy of experimental brucella infection in the developing chick embryo. IV. Therapy with aureomycin. *J. Immunol.* 62:125.

Magoffin, R. L., and Spink, W. W. 1951. The protection of intracellular brucella against streptomycin alone and in combination with other antibiotics. *J. Lab. and Clin. Med.* 37:924.

Mahoney, J. F.; Arnold, R. C.; and Harris, A. D. 1943. Penicillin treatment of early syphilis: A preliminary report. *Am. J. Public Health* 33:1387.

Mahoney, J. F.; Van Slyke, C. J.; Cutler, J. C.; and Blum, H. L. 1946. Experimental gonococcic urethritis in human volunteers. *Am. J. Syph. Gonorrhea vener. Dis.* 30:1.

Maitland, H. B., and Maitland, M. C. 1928. Cultivation of vaccinia virus without tissue culture. *Lancet* 215:596.

Mann, C. H., consulting ed. 1966. Kanamycin: Appraisal after eight years of clinical application. A conference held Dec. 13–14, 1965. *Ann. NY Acad. Sci* 132:771.

Mann, C. H., consulting ed. 1967. Comparative assessment of the broad-spectrum penicillins and other antibiotics. *Ann. NY Acad. Sci.* 145:207–521.

Manson, P. 1877. Further observations on *Filaria sanguinis hominis*. *Med. Rep. China imp. marit. Customs* 14:1.

Manson, P. 1879. On the development of *Filaria sanguinis hominis*, and on the mosquito considered as a nurse. *J. Linn. Soc. London (Zoology)* 14:304.

Mantoux, C. 1910. L'intradermo-réaction à la tuberculine. Et son interprétation clinique. *Presse méd.* 18:10.

Marchiafava, E., and Bignami, A. 1894. *On Summer-Autumn Malarial Fevers*. Vol. 150, p. 1. Translated from the first Italian edition by J. Harry Thompson, M.D. London: New Sydenham Society.

Marquardt, M. 1951. *Paul Ehrlich*. New York: Henry Schuman.

Marsh, R. F.; Burger, D.; and Hanson, R. P. 1969. Transmissible mink encephalopathy: Behavior of the disease agent in mink. *Am. J. Vet. Res.* 30:1637.

Marshall, Jr., E. K. 1939. Bacterial chemotherapy: The pharmacology of sulfanilamide. *Physiol. Rev.* 19:240.

Marshall, Jr., E. K.; Emerson, Jr., K.; and Cutting, W. C. 1937. Para-aminobenzenesulfonamide. Absorption and excretion: Method of determination in urine and blood. *JAMA* 108:953.

Marten, B. 1720. *A New Theory of Consumptions: More Especially of a Phthisis, or Consumption of the Lungs*. London: R. Knaplock.

Martin, D. S., and Smith, D. T. 1939. Blastomycosis (American blastomycosis, Gilchrist's disease). I. A review of the literature. II. A report of thirteen new cases. *Am. Rev. Tuberc.* 39:275 and 488.

Martine, G. 1740. *Essays Medical and Philosophical*. London: A. Millar.

Massachusetts-Sanitary Commission of 1850, reprint 1948. *Report of the Sanitary Commission of Massachusetts, 1850 by Lemuel Shattuck and others, with a foreword by C-E. A. Winslow*. Part I, p. 109; Part II, p. 206. Boston: Dutton and Wentworth State Printers. Cambridge (Mass.): Harvard University Press (reprint).

Massachusetts State Board of Health. 1870. *First Annual Report of the State Board of Health of Massachusetts. January, 1870*. Boston: Wright & Potter.

Massachusetts State Board of Health. 1874. *Fifth Annual Report of the State Board of Health of Massachusetts. January, 1874*. Boston: Wright & Potter.

Mata, L. J. 1975. Malnutrition-infection interactions in the tropics. *Am. J. Trop. Med. Hyg.* 24:564.

Matsen, J. M. 1973. The sources of hospital infection. In *Infectious Disease*, edited by R. P. Gruninger and W. H. Hall, p. 271. Baltimore: Williams & Wilkins.

Matthey, A. 1806. Recherches sur une maladie particulière qui a régné à Genève en 1805. *J. Méd. Chir. Pharmacie* 11:243.

Maurois, A. 1959. *The Life of Sir Alexander Fleming. Discoverer of Penicillin*. Translated by Gerard Hopkins. London: Jonathan Cape.

Mauss, H., and Mietzsch, F. 1933. Atebrin, ein neues Heilmittel gegen Malaria. *Klin. Wochenschr*. 12:1276.

Maxcy, K. F. 1926. An epidemiological study of endemic typhus (Brill's disease) in the southeastern United States. With special reference to its mode of transmission. *U.S. Public Health Rep*. 41:2967.

Maxey, E. E. 1899. Some observations on the so-called spotted fever of Idaho. *Med. Sent*. 7:433.

Mayer, A. 1942. Concerning the mosaic disease of tobacco. Translated by James Johnson. *Phytopathol. Classics* No. 7.

Mays, T. J. 1904. Human slavery as a prevention of pulmonary consumption. *Trans. Am. Climatol. Assoc*. 20:192.

McCarty, M., ed. 1954. *Streptococcal Infections*. A Symposium of the Section on Microbiology, New York Academy of Medicine. Held February 25-26, 1953. New York: Columbia University Press.

McCoy, G. W. 1911. A plague-like disease of rodents. *USPHS Public Health Bull*. No. 43:53.

McCoy, G. W., and Chapin, C. W. 1912. Further observations on a plague-like disease of rodents with a preliminary note on the causative agent, *Bacterium tularense*. *J. Infect. Dis*. 10:61.

McCrumb, Jr., F. R.; Hall, H. E.; Imburg, J.; Merideth, A.; Helmhold, R.; Basora y Defillo, J.; and Woodward, T. E. 1951. Treatment of *Hemophilus influenzae* meningitis with chloramphenicol and other antibiotics. *JAMA* 145:469.

McDermott, W.; Muschenheim, C.; Clark, C.; Elmendorf, Jr., D.; and Cawthon, W. 1952. Isonicotinic acid hydrazide in tuberculosis in man. *Trans. Assoc. Am. Physicians* 55:191.

McDougall, J. B. 1949. *Tuberculosis. A Global Study in Social Pathology*. Edinburgh: E. & S. Livingstone.

McGowan, Jr., J. E.; Klein, J. O.; Bratton, L.; Barnes, M. W.; and Finland, M. 1974. Meningitis and bacteremia due to *Haemophilus influenzae*: Occurrence and mortality at Boston City Hospital in 12 selected years, 1935-1972. *J. Infect. Dis*. 130:119.

McGuinness, A. C. 1958. Diphtheria. In *Preventive Medicine in World War II* by U.S. Army Medical Service, Vol. 4, pp. 167-189. Washington, D.C.: Office of Surgeon-General, Department of the Army.

McGuire, J. M.; Bunch, R. L.; Anderson, R. C.; Boaz, H. E.; Flynn, E. H.; Powell, M. H.; and Smith, J. W. 1952. "Ilotycin," A new antibiotic. *Antibiot. Chemother*. 2:281.

McKinlay, C. A. 1935. Infectious mononucleosis. Part I. Clinical aspects. *JAMA* 105:761.

McNinch, J. H. 1955. Venereal disease problems, U.S. Army Forces, Far East 1950-1953. In *Recent Advances in Medicine and Surgery Based on Professional Medical Experiences in Japan and Korea 1950-1953*. Vol. 2, p. 144. Medical Science Publication No. 4. Washington, D.C.: U.S. Army Medical Service Graduate School — Walter Reed Army Medical Center.

M'Dowel, E. 1835. Observations on erysipelas. *Ir. J. Med. Sci*. 6:161.

Mead, R. 1720. *A Short Discourse Concerning Pestilential Contagion, and the Methods to be Used to Prevent It*. London: Sam Buckley and Ralph Smith.

Medin, O. 1890. En epidemi af infantil paralysi (An epidemic of infantile paralysis). *Hygiea* 52:657.

Melnick, J. L., and Paul, J. R. 1948. Experimental Fort Bragg fever (pretibial fever) in chimpanzees. *Proc. Soc. Exp. Biol. Med*. 67:263.

Melvin, A. D., Chief of Bureau 1914. Infectious abortion of cattle. In *Report of the Chief of the Bureau of Animal Industry, U.S. Department of Agriculture for Fiscal Year Ended June 30, 1914*. *Annu. Rep. Dept. Agric*., p. 30.

Menser, M. A., and Reye, R. D. K. 1974. The pathology of congenital rubella: A review written by request. *Pathology* (Aust.) 6:215 (July 6).

Metchnikoff, E. 1884. Ueber eine Sprosspilzkrankheit der Daphnien. Beitrag zur Lehre über den Kampf der Phagocyten gegen Krankheitserreger. *Virchow's Arch. path. Anat. Physiol.* 96:177.

Metchnikoff, E. 1892, transl. 1968. *Leçons sur la pathologie comparée de l'inflammation.* Paris: G. Masson. Translated by F. A. Starling and E. H. Starling. *Lectures on the Comparative Pathology of Inflammation.* New York: Dover Publications.

Metchnikoff, E. 1901, transl. 1905. *L'immunité dans les Maladies infectieuses.* Paris: G. Masson. Translated by Francis G. Binnie. *Immunity in Infective Diseases.* Cambridge: University Press.

Metchnikoff, E., and Roux, E. 1903–04. Études expérimentales sur la Syphilis. *Annls. Inst. Pasteur* 17:809 (1903), 18:1 (1904).

Metchnikoff, O. 1921. *Life of Elie Metchnikoff 1845–1916.* Boston: Houghton Mifflin.

Meyer, H. M., Jr.; Parkman, P. D.; and Panos, T. C. 1966. Attenuated rubella virus. II. Production of an experimental live-virus vaccine and clinical trial. *N. Engl. J. Med.* 275:575.

Meyer, K. F. 1942. The ecology of psittacosis and ornithosis. *Medicine* 21:175.

Meyer, K. F. 1956a. The status of botulism as a world health problem. *Bull. WHO* 15:281.

Meyer, K. F. 1956b. *The Zoonoses in their Relation to Rural Health.* Berkeley: University of California.

Meyer, K. F. 1958. Ornithosis: A public health problem. (62nd Annual) *Proc. U.S. Livestock Sanit. Assoc.,* p. 230 (November).

Meyer, K. F. 1959. Some general remarks and new observations on psittacosis and ornithosis. *Bull. WHO* 20:101.

Meyer, K. F., and Eddie, B. 1954–55. Chemotherapy of natural psittacosis and ornithosis; field trial of tetracycline (polyotic hydrochloride), chlortetracycline, and oxytetracycline. *Antibiot. Annu.* P. 544.

Meyer, K. F., and Eddie, B. 1965. *Sixty-Five Years of Human Botulism in the United States and Canada. Epidemiology and Tabulations of Reported Cases 1899 through 1964.* San Francisco: The George Williams Hooper Foundation, University of California-San Francisco Medical Center.

Meyer, K. F.; Eddie, B.; and Yanamura, H. Y. 1942. Ornithosis (psittacosis) in pigeons and its relation to human pneumonitis. *Proc. Soc. Exp. Biol. Med.* 49:609.

Meyer, K. F.; Haring, C. M.; and Howitt, B. 1931. The etiology of epizootic encephalomyelitis of horses in the San Joaquin Valley, 1930. *Science* 74:227.

Meyer, K. F.; Quan, S. F.; McCrumb, F. R.; and Larson, A. 1952. Effective treatment of plague. *Ann. NY Acad. Sci.* 55:1228.

Meyer, K. F.; Stewart-Anderson, B.; and Eddie, B. 1939. Canine leptospirosis in the United States. *J. Am. Vet. Med. Assoc.* 95:710.

Michie, H. C. 1928a. Encephalitis lethargica. In *The Medical Department of the United States Army in the World War* by the U.S. Surgeon-General's Office. Vol. 9, p. 473. Washington, D.C.: U.S. Government Printing Office.

Michie, H. C. 1928b. Mumps. Ibid., p. 451.

Michie, H. C. 1928c. The venereal diseases. Ibid., p. 263.

Michie, H. C., and Lull, G. E. 1928. Measles. In *The Medical Department of the United States Army in the World War* by the U.S. Surgeon-General's Office. Vol. 9, p. 409. Washington, D.C.: U.S. Government Printing Office.

Michigan Department of Health. 1945. Diphtheria increase in Michigan is due to failure to continue to immunize. *Mich. Public Health* 33:203.

Middleton, W. E. K. 1966. *A History of the Thermometer and Its Use in Meteorology.* Baltimore: The Johns Hopkins Press.

Middleton, W. E. K. 1971. *The Experimenters: A Study of the Accademia del Cimento.* Baltimore: Johns Hopkins Press.

Middleton, W. S. 1928. The yellow fever epidemic of 1793 in Philadelphia. *Ann. Med. Hist.* 10:434.

Miller, C. P., and Bohnhoff, M. 1946. Streptomycin resistance of gonococci and meningococci. *JAMA* 130:485.

Miller, C. P., and Bohnhoff, M. 1947. Two streptomycin-resistant variants of meningococcus. *J. Bacteriol.* 54:467.

Miller, E. B. 1961. *Medical Department, U.S. Army. United States Army Veterinary Service in World War II.* Washington, D.C.: Office of the Surgeon-General, Department of the Army.

Miller, G.; Niederman, J. C.; and Andrews, L-L. 1973. Prolonged oropharyngeal excretion of Epstein-Barr virus after infectious mononucleosis. *N. Engl. J. Med.* 288:229.

Miller, J. L., and Lusk, F. B. 1916. The treatment of arthritis by the intravenous injection of foreign protein. *JAMA* 66:1756.

Millous, M. 1936. Une épidémie de varicelle maligne au Cameroun. *Bull. Acad. Med.* 115 (Series 3):840.

Miner, R. W., ed. 1947. The relations of diseases in the lower animals to human welfare. Conference held by the Section of Biology on March 15–16, 1946 with a series of papers. *Ann. NY Acad. Sci.* 48:351.

Mitchell, J. K. 1849. *On the Cryptogamous Origin of Malarious and Epidemic Fevers.* Philadelphia: Lea and Blanchard.

Mitchell, R. S., and Bell, J. C. 1958. *Modern Chemotherapy of Tuberculosis.* Antibiotics Monographs No. 11. New York: Medical Encyclopedia.

Mitchell, S. W. 1892. The early history of instrumental precision in medicine. President's address. *Trans. Congr. Am. Physns. Surg.* 2:159.

Miyajima, M., and Okumura, T. 1917. On the life cycle of the "Akamushi," carrier of Nippon River fever. *Kitasato Arch. Exp. Med.* 1:1.

Monath, T. P. 1974. Lassa fever and Marburg virus disease. *WHO Chron.* 28:212.

Monath, T. P. C.; Nuckolls, J. G.; Berall, J.; Bauer, H.; Chappell, W. A.; and Coleman, P. H. 1970. Studies on California encephalitis in Minnesota. *Am. J. Epidemiol.* 92:40.

Moore, J. 1815. *The History of the Small Pox.* London: Longman, Hurst, Rees, Orme and Brown.

Moore, P. R.; Evenson, A.; Luckey, T. D.; McCoy, E.; Elvehjem, C. A.; and Hart, E. B. 1946. Use of sulfasuxidine, streptothricin, and streptomycin in nutritional studies with the chick. *J. Biol. Chem.* 165:437.

Mooser, H. 1928. Experiments relating to the pathology and the etiology of Mexican typhus (tabardillo). I. Clinical course and pathologic anatomy of tabardillo in guinea-pigs. *J. Infect. Dis.* 43:241.

Mooser, H.; Marti, H. R.; and Leemann, A. 1949. Beobachtungen an Füntagefieber. Hautläsionen nach kutaner und intrakutaner Inokulation mit Rickettsia quintana. *Schweiz. Z. Path. Bakt.* 12:476.

Morgagni, G. B. 1769 and 1960. *The Seats and Causes of Diseases Investigated by Anatomy; in Five Books, Containing a Great Variety of Dissections, with Remarks.* Translated by Benjamin Alexander, London, 1769. Published under auspices of the New York Academy of Medicine (1960). New York: Hafner Publishing Co.

Morgan, H. V., and Williamson, D. A. J. 1943. Jaundice following administration of human blood products. *Br. Med. J.* 1:750.

Morgenroth, J., and Levy, R. 1911. Chemotherapie der Pneumokokkeninfektion. *Berl. klin. Wschr.* 48:1979.

Morin, R. B.; Jackson, B. G.; Flynn, E. H.; and Roeske, R. W. 1962. Chemistry of cephalosporin antibiotics. I. 7-aminocephalosporanic acid from cephalosporin C. *J. Am. Chem. Soc.* 84:3400.

Morisset, R., and Spink, W. 1969. Epidemic canine brucellosis due to a new species, *Brucella canis. Lancet* 2:1000.

Morton, L. T. 1970. *A Medical Bibliography (Garrison and Morton).* 3rd ed. Philadelphia: J. P. Lippincott.

Most, H. 1968. Leishmaniasis. In *Internal Medicine in World War II* by U.S. Army Medical Department. Vol. 3. Infectious Diseases and General Medicine, p. 1. Washington, D.C.: Office of the Surgeon-General, Department of the Army.

Mostofi, F. K., ed. 1967. *Bilharziasis*. Berlin: Springer-Verlag.

Moulder, J. W. 1964. *The Psittacosis Group as Bacteria*. New York: John Wiley.

Moulton, F. R., ed. 1948. *Rickettsial Diseases of Man*. Washington, D.C.: American Association for the Advancement of Science.

Mowrey, F. H. 1963. Statistics of malaria. In *Internal Medicine in World War II* by U.S. Army Medical Department. Vol. 2, p. 449. Washington, D.C.: Office of the Surgeon-General, Department of the Army.

Muckenfuss, R. S.; Armstrong, C.; and McCordock, H. A. 1933. Encephalitis: Studies on experimental transmission. *U.S. Public Health Rep*. 48:1341.

Müller-Eberhard, H. J. 1972. The molecular basis of the biological activities of complement. In *The Harvey Lectures 1970–71*. Vol. 66, p. 75. New York: Academic Press.

Mulligan, H. W., ed. 1970. *The African Trypanosomiases*. London: George Allen and Unwin Ltd.

Murchison, C. 1862. *A Treatise on the Continued Fevers of Great Britain*. London: Parker, Son, & Bourn.

Murphy, J. B., and Rous, P. 1912. The behavior of chicken sarcoma implanted in the developing embryo. *J. Exp. Med*. 15:119.

Murray, E. S.; Baehr, G.; Schwartzman, G.; Mandelbaum, R. A.; Rosenthal, N.; Doane, J. C.; Weiss, L. B.; Cohen, S.; and Snyder, J. C. 1950. Brill's disease. I. Clinical and laboratory diagnosis. *JAMA* 142:1059.

Murray, E. S., and Snyder, J. C. 1951. Brill's disease. II. Etiology. *Am. J. Hyg*. 53:22.

Murray, M. J., and Murray, A. B. 1977. Starvation suppression and refeeding activation of infection. An ecological necessity? *Lancet* 1:123.

Musselman, M. M. 1956. *Terramycin (oxytetracycline)*. Antibiotics Monographs No. 6. New York: Medical Encyclopedia.

Mycotoxicoses 1973. Mycotoxicoses of domestic animals. Reports by several authors in single issue. *J. Am. Vet. Med. Assoc*. 163 (No. 11):1259.

Myers, J. A. 1944. *The Evolution of Tuberculosis: As Observed during Twenty Years at Lymanhurst, 1921 to 1941*. Minneapolis (Minn.): J-Lancet.

Myers, J. A. 1949. *Invited and Conquered. Historical Sketch of Tuberculosis in Minnesota*. St. Paul: Minnesota Public Health Association.

Myers, J. A., and Steele, J. H. 1969. *Bovine Tuberculosis Control in Man and Animals*. St. Louis: Warren H. Green.

Nadaždin, M., and Karlovac, K. 1977. Investigations on reactivity of sera in endemic syphilis from Bosnia 20 years after treatment. *Br. J. Vener. Dis*. 53:216.

Nahmias, A. J., and Eickhoff, T. C. 1961. Staphylococcal infections in hospitals. Recent developments in epidemiologic and laboratory investigation. *N. Engl. J. Med*. 265:74, 120, and 177.

Napier, L. E. 1946a. *The Principles and Practice of Tropical Medicine*. New York: Macmillan.

Napier, L. E. 1946b. Trypanosomiasis. In *The Principles and Practice of Tropical Medicine*, p. 197. New York: Macmillan.

National Academy of Sciences 1969. *The Use of Drugs in Animal Feeds. A Symposium*. Publication No. 1679. Washington, D.C.: National Academy of Sciences.

National Academy of Sciences-National Research Council. Agricultural Board 1956. *Proceedings First International Conference on the Use of Antibiotics in Agriculture* (Held October 19–21, 1955) Publication No. 397. Washington, D.C.: National Academy of Sciences, National Research Council (USA).

National Communicable Disease Center. 1968. Plague. *CDC Morbidity Mortality Weekly Rep*. No. 27 (July 6), 17:253 and No. 28 (July 13), 17:261.

National Communicable Disease Center. 1969. *Foodborne Outbreaks. Annual Summary*

1969 Center for Disease Control. Atlanta (Ga.): U.S. Department of Health, Education, and Welfare, Public Health Service.

National Communicable Disease Center. 1970. Outbreak of typhoid fever aboard ship. *CDC Morbidity Mortality Weekly Rep.* 19:13 (January 17).

National Research Council Committee on Viral Hepatitis. 1974. The public health implications of hepatitis B antigen in human blood. A revised statement. *CDC Morbidity and Mortality Statistics* 23:125 (April 6).

Neal, J. B. 1921. Influenzal meningitis. *Arch. Pediat.* 38:1.

Neal, J. B. et al. 1942. *Encephalitis. A Clinical Study.* New York: Grune & Stratton.

Neal, J. B.; Jackson, H. W.; and Appelbaum, E. 1934. Meningitis due to the influenza bacillus of Pfeiffer (*Hemophilus influenzae*). A study of 111 cases, with four recoveries. *JAMA* 102:513.

Negri, A. 1903. Beitrag zum Studium der Aetiologie der Tollwuth. *Z. Hyg. InfektKrankh.* 43:507.

Neisser, A. 1879. Ueber eine der Gonorrhoe eigentümliche Micrococcusform. *Zentbl. med. Wiss.* 17:497.

Nelson, E. R. 1960. Hemorrhagic fever in children in Thailand. Report of 69 cases. *J. Pediatr.* 56:101.

Neufeld, F. 1902. Ueber die Agglutination der Pneumokokken und über die Theorieen der Agglutination. *Z. Hyg. InfektKrankh.* 40:54.

Newman, R.; Doster, B. E.; Murray, F. J.; and Woolpert, S. F. 1974. Rifampin in initial treatment of pulmonary tuberculosis. *Am. Rev. Respir. Dis.* 109:216.

New York State Department of Health Joint Committee on Staphylococcal Infections 1958. *Control of Staphylococcal Infections in Hospitals.* Albany (N.Y.): New York State Department of Health.

Nichols, D. R., and Herrell, W. E. 1948. Penicillin in the treatment of actinomycosis. *J. Lab. Clin. Med.* 33:521.

Nicolle, C.; Comte, C.; and Conseil, E. 1909. Transmission experimentale du typhus exanthematique par le pou du corps. *C. R. Acad. Sci* (D) (Paris) 149:486.

Nicolle, C., and Manceaux, L. 1908. Sur une infection à corps de Leishman (ou organismes voisins) du gondi. *C. R. Acad. Sci.* (D) (Paris) 147:763.

Niederman, J. C. 1974. Infectious mononucleosis. In *Harrison's Principles of Internal Medicine* by T. R. Harrison and edited by M. M. Wintrobe, G. W. Thorn, R. D. Adams et al. 7th ed., p. 1063. New York: McGraw-Hill Book.

Niederman, J. C.; Evans, A. S.; Subrahmanyan, L.; and McCollum, R. W. 1970. Prevalence, incidence and persistence of EB virus antibody in young adults. *N. Engl. J. Med.* 282:361.

Niederman, J. C.; McCollum, R. W.; Henle, G.; and Henle, W. 1968. Infectious mononucleosis. Clinical manifestations in relation to EB virus antibodies. *JAMA* 203:205.

Nightingale, F. 1860. *Notes on Nursing: What It Is, and What It Is Not.* London: Harrison.

Nocard, E. 1888. Note sur la maladie des boeufs de Guadeloupe. *Annls. Inst. Pasteur* 2:293.

Nocard, E., and Roux, E. R. 1898. Le microbe de la pérepneumonie. *Annls. Inst. Pasteur* 12:240.

Noguchi, H. 1915. Pure cultivation in vivo of vaccine virus free from bacteria. *J. Exp. Med.* 21:539.

Noran, H. H., and Baker, A. B. 1945. Western equine encephalitis: The pathogenesis of the pathological lesions. *J. Neuropathol. Exp. Neurol.* 4:269.

North, E. 1811. *A Treatise on a Malignant Epidemic, Commonly Called Spotted Fever.* New York: T. & J. Swords.

Nott, J. C. 1848. Yellow fever contrasted with bilious fever — reasons for believing it a disease sui generis — its mode of propagation — remote cause — probable insect or animalcular origin. *New Orl. med. surg. J.* 4:563.

Nuttall, G. 1888. Experimente über die bacterienfeindlichen einflüsse des thierischen Körpers. *Z. Hyg.* 4:353.

Ochsner, A., and De Bakey, M. 1943. Amebic hepatitis and hepatic abscess. *Surgery* 13:460 and 612.

Ogata, M. 1897. Ueber die Pestepidemie in Formosa. *Zentbl. Bakt. ParasitKde. Hyg.*, Abt. 1, 21:769.

Ogata, N. 1931. Aetiologie der Tsutsugamushikrankheit: *Rickettsia tsutsugamushi. Zentbl. Bakt. ParasitKde. Hyg.*, Abt. I *Orig.*, 122:249.

Ogston, A. 1881. Report upon micro-organisms in surgical diseases. *Br. Med. J.* 1:369.

Ohara, H. 1930. Ueber Identitat von "Yato-Byo" (Ohara's Disease) and "Tularamie," sowie ihren Erreger. *Zentbl. Bakt. ParasitKde.* 117:440.

Opie, E. L.; Blake, F. G.; Small, J. C.; and Rivers, T. M. 1921. *Epidemic Respiratory Disease. The Pneumonias and Other Infections of the Respiratory Tract Accompanying Influenza and Measles.* St. Louis: C. V. Mosby.

Ordman, C. W.; Jennings, Jr., C. G.; and Janeway, C. A. 1944. Chemical, clinical, and immunological studies on the products of human plasma fractionation. XII. The use of concentrated normal human serum gamma globulin (human immune serum globulin) in the prevention and attenuation of measles. *J. Clin. Invest.* 23:541.

Ormerod, W. E. 1961. The epidemic spread of Rhodesian sleeping sickness 1908–1960. *Trans. R. Soc. Trop. Med. Hyg.* 55:525.

Orr, H. W. 1927. *The Treatment of Osteomyelitis and Other Infected Wounds by Drainage and Rest.* Reprinted from *Surgery, Gynecology and Obstetrics*, October 1927, p. 446. Chicago: The Surgical Publishing Co. of Chicago.

Osler, W. 1885. The Gulstonian lectures on malignant endocarditis. *Br. Med. J.* 1:467, 522, and 577.

Osler, W. 1901. *The Principles and Practice of Medicine, Designed for the Use of Practitioners and Students of Medicine.* 4th ed. New York: D. Appleton.

Osler, W. et al. 1891–1900. Report on typhoid fever. *Johns Hopkins Hosp. Rep.* 2:119 (1891); 4:1 (1894); 5:281 (1895); 8:155 (1900).

Owen, R. 1835. Description of a microscopic entozoon infesting the muscles of the human body. *Trans. zool. Soc. Lond.* 1:315.

Padjett, B. L.; Walker, D. L.; Zu Rhein, G. M.; and Eckroade, R. J. 1971. Cultivation of papova-like virus from human brain with progressive multifocal leucoencephalopathy. *Lancet* 1:1257.

Pagel, W.; Simmonds, F. A. H.; Macdonald, N.; and Nassau, E. 1964. *Pulmonary Tuberculosis.* 4th ed. London: Oxford University Press.

Paget, G. E. 1867. Note from Dr. Paget to the Editor of The Lancet: Memorandum on the nature and the mode of propagation of phthisis by William Budd, M. D. *Lancet* 2:451.

Paget, J. 1866. On the discovery of Trichina. *Lancet* 1:269.

Pankey, G. A. 1961. Subacute bacterial endocarditis at the University of Minnesota Hospital, 1939 through 1959. *Ann. Intern. Med.* 55:550.

Panum, P. L. 1939. Observations made during the epidemic of measles on the Faroe Islands in the year 1846. In *Medical Classics*, compiled by E. C. Kelly. Vol. 3, p. 829. Baltimore: Williams & Wilkins.

Parish, H. J., and Cannon, D. A. 1962. *Antisera, Toxoids, Vaccines and Tuberculins in Prophylaxis and Treatment.* 6th ed. Baltimore: Williams & Wilkins.

Park, W. H. 1906. A critical study of the results of serum therapy in the diseases of man. In *The Harvey Lectures 1905–06.* Vol. 1, p. 101. Philadelphia: J. B. Lippincott.

Park, W. H., and Bolduan, C. 1908. Mortality. In *The Bacteriology of Diphtheria*, edited by G. H. F. Nuttall and G. S. Graham-Smith. Cambridge: University Press.

Parker, Jr., F., and Nye, R. N. 1925a. Studies on filterable viruses. I. Cultivation of vaccine virus. *Am. J. Pathol.* 1:325.

Parker, Jr., F., and Nye, R. N. 1925b. Studies on filterable viruses. II. Cultivation of herpes virus. *Am. J. Pathol.* 1:337.

Parker, R. R. 1938. Rocky Mountain spotted fever. *JAMA* 110:1185 and 1273.

Parker, R. R., and Spencer, R. R. 1926. Rocky Mountain spotted fever. A study of the relationship between the presence of rickettsial-like organisms in tick smears and the infectiveness of the same ticks. *U.S. Public Health Rep.* 41:461.

Parkman, P. D.; Buescher, E. L.; and Artenstein, M. S. 1962. Recovery of rubella virus from army recruits. *Proc. Soc. Exp. Biol. Med.* 111:225.

Parodi, U. 1907. Ueber die Uebertragung der Syphilis auf den Hoden des Kaninchens. *Zentbl. Bakt. ParasitKde. Hyg.* 44:428.

Pasteur, L. 1870. *Études sur la maladie de vers à soie.* 2 vols. Paris: Gauthier-Villars.

Pasteur, L. 1880. Sur les maladies virulentes, et en particulier sur la maladie appelée vulgairement choléra des poules. *C. R. Acad. Sci.* (D) (Paris) 90:239.

Pasteur, L. 1881. Sur la rage. *C. R. Acad. Sci.* (D) (Paris) 92:1259.

Pasteur, L. 1922–1939. *Oeuvres de Pasteur* réunies par Pasteur Vallery-Radot. 7 vols. Paris: Masson et Cie.

Pasteur, L.; Chamberland; and Roux, E. 1881. De la possibilité de Rendre Les Moutons Réfractaires au Charbon par la méthode des inoculations préventives. *C. R. Acad. Sci.* (D) (Paris) 92:662.

Pasteur, L., and Joubert, J. 1877a. Charbon et Septicémie. *C. R. Acad. Sci.* (D) (Paris) 85:101.

Pasteur, L., and Joubert, J. 1877b. Étude sur la maladie charbonneuse. *C. R. Acad. Sci.* (D) (Paris) 84:900.

Paul, J. R. 1971. *A History of Poliomyelitis.* New Haven: Yale University Press.

Paul, J. R., and Bunnell, W. W. 1932. The presence of heterophile antibodies in infectious mononucleosis. *Am. J. Med. Sci.* 183:90.

Paul, J. R., and Gardner, H. T. 1960. Viral hepatitis. In *Preventive Medicine in World War II* by Medical Department, United States Army. Vol. 5, p. 411. Washington, D.C.: Office of the Surgeon-General, Department of the Army.

Pawan, J. L. 1936a. Rabies in the vampire bat of Trinidad, with special reference to the clinical course and the latency of infection. *Ann. Trop. Med. Parasitol.* 30:401.

Pawan, J. L. 1936b. The transmission of paralytic rabies in Trinidad by the vampire bat (*Desmodus Rotundus Murinus* Wagner, 1840). *Ann. Trop. Med. Parasitol.* 30:101.

Payne. F. E.; Baublis, J. V.; and Itabashi, H. H. 1969. Isolation of measles virus from cell cultures of brain from a patient with subacute sclerosing panencephalitis. *N. Engl. J. Med.* 281:585.

Peabody, F. W.; Draper, G.; and Dochez, A. R. 1912. *A Clinical Study of Acute Poliomyelitis.* Monograph No. 4. *Monogr. Rockefeller Inst. med. Res.* (June 24).

Pearse, R. A. 1911. Insect bites. *Northwest Med.* 3 (N.S.):81.

Pearson, R. T., and Hall, W. H. 1952. Canicola fever. Report of a human infection due to *Leptospira canicola* in Minnesota. *Minn. Med.* 35:1127.

Pejme, J. 1964. Infectious mononucleosis. A clinical and haematological study of patients and contacts, and a comparison with healthy subjects. *Acta Med. Scand. (Suppl)* 413.

Pelletier, J., and Caventou, J. B. 1820. Recherches Chimiques sur les Quinquinas. *Annls. Chim. Phys.* 15 (Second Series):289.

Penicillin, Special Issue. 1944. Penicillin in warfare. *Br. J. Surg. (Special Suppl.)* 32:108.

Pepper, D. S.; Flippin, H. F.; Schwartz, L.; and Lockwood, J. S. 1939. The results of sulfapyridine therapy in 400 cases of typed pneumococci pneumonia. *Am. J. Med. Sci.* 198:22.

Pepys, S. 1926. *The Diary: Vols. IV–VI, 1664–1667, Referring to the London Plague.* Transcribed by M. Bright with additions by H. B. Wheatley. New York: Harcourt Brace.

Petersen, W. F. 1922. *Protein Therapy and Nonspecific Resistance.* New York: Macmillan.

Pettenkofer, M. von, ed. 1869. *Das Kanal-oder Siel-System in München.* München: H. Manz.

Pfeiffer, E. 1889. Drüsenfieber. *Jb. Kinderheilkunde* 29:257.

Pfeiffer, R. 1892. Vorläufige Mittheilungen über die Erreger der Influenza. *Dtsch. med. Wochenschr.* 18:28.

Pfeiffer, R. 1894. Weitere Untersuchungen über das Wesen der Choleraimmunität und über specifisch baktericide Processe. *Z. Hyg. InfektKrankh.* 18:1.

Pfeiffer, R., and Issaeff (Dr.) 1894. Ueber die specifische Bedeutung der Choleraimmunität (bacteriolyse). *Z. Hyg. InfektKrankh.* 17:355.

Pfeiffer, R., and Kolle, W. 1896. Experimentelle untersuchungen zur Frage der Schutzimpfung des Menschen gegen Typhus abdominalis. *Dtsch. med. Wochenschr.* 22:735.

Philip, R. N.; Reinhard, K. R.; and Lackman, D. B. 1959. Observations on a mumps epidemic in a "virgin" population. *Am. J. Hyg.* 69:91.

Pickles, W. N. 1939. Epidemic catarrhal jaundice. In *Epidemiology in Country Practice* by W. N. Pickles p. 61. Bristol (England): John Wright & Sons.

Pincoffs, M. C.; Guy, E. G.; Lister, L. M.; Woodward, T. E.; and Smadel, J. E. 1948. The treatment of Rocky Mountain spotted fever with chloromycetin. *Ann. Intern. Med.* 29:656.

Pirquet, C. von. 1907. Der diagnostische Wert der kutanen Tuberkulinreaktion bei der Tuberkulose des Kindesalters auf Grund von 100 Sektionen. *Wien. Klin. Wochenschr.* 20:1123.

Pirquet, C. F. von and Schick, B. 1951. *Serum Sickness.* Translated by B. Schick. Baltimore: Williams & Wilkins.

Pittman, M. 1931. Variation and type specificity in the bacterial species *Hemophilus influenzae. J. Exp. Med.* 53:471.

Pollitzer, R. 1954. Plague. *WHO Monogr. Ser.* No. 22.

Pollock, M. R. 1962. Penicillinase. In *Resistance of Bacteria to the Penicillins*, edited by A. V. S. de Reuck and M. P. Cameron. Ciba Foundation Study Group No. 13, p. 56. Boston: Little, Brown.

Porter, R. R. 1967a. The structure of antibodies. *Sci. Am.* 217.81 (October).

Porter, R. R. 1967b. The structure of immunoglobulins. In *Essays in Biochemistry*, edited by P. N. Campbell and G. D. Greville. Vol. 3, p. 1. London: Academic Press.

Powell, G. M. 1954. Hemorrhagic fever: A study of 300 cases. *Medicine* 33:97.

Powell, J. H. 1949. *Bring Out Your Dead. The Great Plague of Yellow Fever in Philadelphia in 1793.* Philadelphia: University of Pennsylvania Press.

Pringle, J. 1810. *Observations on the Diseases of the Army.* First American edition with notes by Benjamin Rush. Philadelphia: Edward Earle.

Prowazek, S. von 1915. Ätiologische Untersuchungen über den Flecktyphus in Serbien 1913 und Hamburg 1914. *Beitr. Klin. InfektKrankh.* 4:5.

Pullan, B. 1971. *Rich and Poor in Renaissance Venice. The Social Institutions of a Catholic State, to 1620.* Oxford: Basil Blackwell.

Purvis, Jr., J. D., and Morris, G. C. 1946. Report of food-borne Streptococcus outbreak. *Nav. med. Bull.* 46:613.

Pusey, W. A. 1933a. *The History and Epidemiology of Syphilis.* Springfield (Ill.): Chas. C Thomas.

Pusey, W. A. 1933b. *The History of Dermatology.* Springfield (Ill.): Chas. C Thomas.

Quain, E. P. 1904. Report of six cases of tubercular ulcers and tubercular lymphangitis of the upper extremity. *St. Paul med. J.* 6:615.

Rabinovich, S.; Smith, I. M.; and January, L. E. 1968. The changing pattern of bacterial endocarditis. *Med. Clin. North Am.* 52:1091.

Raich, R.; Casey, F.; and Hall, W. H. 1961. Pulmonary and cutaneous nocardiosis. The significance of the laboratory isolation of Nocardia. *Am. Rev. Respir. Dis.* 83:505.

Rammelkamp, C. H., and Maxon, T. 1942. Resistance of *Staphylococcus aureus* to the action of penicillin. *Proc. Soc. Exp. Biol. Med.* 51:386.

Rammelkamp, Jr., C. H.; Weaver, R. S.; and Dingle, J. H. 1952. Significance of the epidemiological differences between acute nephritis and acute rheumatic fever. *Trans. Assoc. Am. Physicians* 65:168.

Rantz, L. A. 1958. Hemolytic streptococcal infections. In *Preventive Medicine in World War II* by Medical Department, United States Army. Vol. 4, p. 229. Washington, D.C.: Office of the Surgeon-General, Department of the Army.

Rantz, L. A.; Randall, E.; Spink, W. W.; and Boisvert, P. J. 1946. Sulfonamide and penicillin resistance of group A hemolytic streptococci. *Proc. Soc. Exp. Biol. Med.* 62:54.

Rantz, L. A.; Spink, W. W.; Boisvert, P.; and Coggeshall, H. 1945. The treatment of rheumatic fever with penicillin. *J. Pediatr.* 26:576.

Razzell, P. 1977. *Edward Jenner's Cowpox Vaccine: The History of a Medical Myth.* Sussex (England): Caliban Books.

Reed, D.; Brody, J.; Huntley, B.; and Overfield, T. 1966. An epidemic in an eskimo village due to group-B meningococcus. Part I. Epidemiology. *JAMA* 196:383.

Reed, D.; Brown, G.; Merrick, R.; Sever, J.; and Feltz, E. 1967. A mumps epidemic on St. George Island, Alaska. *JAMA* 199:967.

Reed, W.; Carroll, J.; and Agramonte, A. 1901. Experimental yellow fever. *Trans. Assoc. Am. Physicians* 16:45.

Reed, W.; Carroll, J.; Agramonte, A. A.; and Lazear, J. W. 1900. The etiology of yellow fever: A preliminary note. *Philad. Med. J.* 6:790.

Reed, W.; Vaughan, V. C.; and Shakespeare, O. E. 1900. *Abstract of Report on the Origin and Spread of Typhoid Fever in U.S. Military Camps during the Spanish War of 1898.* Washington, D.C.: U.S. Government Printing Office.

Reed, W. P.; Palmer, D. L.; Williams, Jr., R. C.; and Kisch, A. L. 1970. Bubonic plague in the southwestern United States. *Medicine* 49:465.

Regimen Sanitatis Salernitanum 1607 and 1922. *The School of Salernum; Regimen Sanitatis Salernitanum.* The English Version by Sir John Harington, first published in 1607. London: Oxford University Press.

Reimann, H. A. 1938. An acute infection of the respiratory tract with atypical pneumonia. A disease entity probably caused by a filtrable virus. *JAMA* 111:2377.

Reimann, H. A. 1954. *Pneumonia.* Springfield (Ill.): Chas. C Thomas.

Reinhart, A. S. 1931. Evolution of the clinical concept of rheumatic fever. *N. Engl. J. Med.* 204:1194.

Rennie, A. 1894. The plague in the East. *Br. Med. J.* 2:615.

Rénon, L. 1893. *Recherches Cliniques et Expérimentales sur la Pseudo-Tuberculose Aspergillaire.* Thése pour le Doctorat en Médecine (Faculté de médecine de Paris). Paris: G. Steinheil.

Reynolds, E. S.; Walls, K. W.; and Pfeiffer, R. I. 1966. Generalized toxoplasmosis following renal transplantation: Report of a case. *Arch. Intern. Med.* 118:401.

Rhazes. Transl. 1847 and 1939. *A Treatise on the Small-Pox and Measles.* Translated from Arabic by William Alexander Greenhill. Published in London for the Sydenham Society of England, 1847. In *Medical Classics,* compiled by E. C. Kelly. Vol. 4, p. 22. Baltimore: Williams & Wilkins.

Rich, A. R. 1930. The pathogenesis of the forms of jaundice. *Johns Hopkins Hosp. Bull.* 47:338.

Rich, A. R. 1944. *The Pathogenesis of Tuberculosis.* Springfield (Ill.): Chas. C Thomas.

Ricketts, H. T. 1911. *Contributions to Medical Science.* Chicago: University of Chicago Press.

Ricketts, H. T., and Wilder, R. M. 1910. The relation of typhus fever (tabardillo) to Rocky Mountain spotted fever. *Arch. Intern. Med.* 5:361.

Ricord, P. 1838, transl. 1848. *Traité Pratique des Maladies Vénériennes.* Paris: Librairie des Sciences Médicales De Just Rouvier et E. Le Bouvier. Translated by A. Sidney Doane. *A Practical Treatise on Venereal Disease; or, Critical and Experimental Researches on Inoculation, Applied to the Study of these Affections, with a Therapeutical Summary and Special Formulary.* 3rd ed. New York: J. S. Redfield.

Riley, W. A. 1933. Reservoirs of echinococcus in Minnesota. *Minn. Med.* 16:744.

Rippon, J. W. 1974. *Medical Mycology. The Pathogenic Fungi and the Pathogenic Actinomycetes.* Philadelphia: W. B. Saunders.

Rivers, T. M., and Scott, T. F. M. 1935. Meningitis in man caused by a filterable virus. *Science* 81:439.

Robbins, F. C. 1948. Q Fever, clinical features. In *The Rickettsial Diseases of Man*, edited by F. R. Moulton, p. 160. Washington, D.C.: American Association for the Advancement of Science.

Roberts, R. S. 1959. Botulism. In *Infectious Diseases of Animals; Diseases Due to Bacteria* by A. W. Stableforth and I. A. Galloway. Vol. 1, p. 209. New York: Academic Press.

Robitzek, E. H.; Selikoff, I. J.; and Ornstein, G. G. 1952. Chemotherapy of human tuberculosis with hydrazine derivatives of isonicotinic acid. *Q. Bull. Sea View Hosp.* 13:27.

Rocha-Lima, H. da 1916. Zur Aetiologie des Fleckfiebers. *Berliner klin. Wschr.* 53:567.

Rockefeller Foundation-International Health Board 1922. *Bibliography of Hookworm Disease*. Publication No. 11. New York: Rockefeller Foundation, International Health Board.

Roholm, K., and Iversen, P. 1939. Changes in the liver in acute epidemic hepatitis (catarrhal jaundice) based on 38 aspiration biopsies. *Acta Pathol. Microbiol. Scand.* 16:427.

Rolleston, J. D. 1937. *The History of the Acute Exanthemata*. The Fitzpatrick Lectures 1935–1936 delivered before the Royal College of Physicians of London. London: Wm. Heinemann.

Romano, M. N.; Brunetti, O. A.; Schwabe, C. W.; and Rosen, M. N. 1974. Probable transmission of *Echinococcus granulosus* between deer and coyotes in California. *J. Wildl. Dis.* 10:225.

Rosen, G. 1958. *A History of Public Health*. New York: M D Publications.

Rosenau, M. J. 1902. Laboratory course in pathology and bacteriology. *U.S. Hyg. Lab. Bull.* No. 8.

Rosenau, M. J. 1913. *Preventive Medicine and Hygiene*. New York: D. Appleton.

Rosenbach, F. J. 1884, transl. 1886. *Mikro-organismen bei den Wund-infections-krankheiten des Menschen*. Weisbaden: J. F. Bergmann. Translated and abstracted by W. W. Cheyne. *Recent researches on micro-organisms in relation to suppuration and septic diseases. I. Micro-organisms in human traumatic infective diseases*. In *Recent Essays by Various Authors on Bacteria in Relation to Disease*, selected and edited by W. Watson Cheyne. Vol. 115, p. 397. London: New Sydenham Society.

Rosenberg, C. E. 1962. *The Cholera Years, the United States in 1832, 1849, and 1866*. Chicago: University of Chicago Press.

Rosenkrantz, B. G. 1972. *Public Health and the State: Changing Views in Massachusetts, 1842–1936*. Cambridge (Mass.): Harvard University Press.

Rosenow, E. C. 1914. The newer bacteriology of various infections as determined by special methods. *JAMA* 63:903.

Rosenow, E. C. 1917. The treatment of epidemic poliomyelitis with immune horse serum: Preliminary report. *JAMA* 69:1074.

Rosenow, E. C. 1949. Bacteriologic studies by new methods of a major epidemic of poliomyelitis, 1947. *J-Lancet* 69:47.

Rosenow, E. C.; Towne, E. B.; and Wheeler, G. W. 1916. The etiology of epidemic poliomyelitis: Preliminary note. *JAMA* 67:1202.

Rosenthal, T. 1932. David Gruby (1810–1898). *Ann. Med. Hist.* 4 (N.S.):339.

Ross, R. 1897. On some peculiar pigmented cells found in two mosquitos fed on malarial blood. With note by Surgeon-Major Smyth, M.D. *Br. Med. J.* 2:1786.

Ross, R. 1898. Report on the cultivation of Proteosoma, *Labbé* in grey mosquitoes. *Indian med. Gaz.* 33:401.

Ross, R. 1923. *Memoirs. With a Full Account of the Great Malaria Problem and Its Solution*. London: John Murray.

Ross, R. 1930. *Memories of Sir Patrick Manson*. London: Harrison and Sons.

Rosselet, J. P.; Marquez, J.; Meseck, E.; Murawski, A.; Hamdan, A.; Joyner, C.; Schmidt, R.; Migliore, D.; and Herzog, H. L. 1964. Isolation, purification and characterization of gentamicin. In *Antimicrobial Agents and Chemotherapy 1963*, edited by J. C. Sylvester, p. 14. Ann Arbor (Mich.): American Society for Microbiology.

Rothstein, W. G. 1972. *American Physicians in the Nineteenth Century: From Sects to Science*. Baltimore: Johns Hopkins University Press.

Roueché, B. 1954. The alerting of Mr. Pomerantz. In *Eleven Blue Men* by B. Roueché, p. 48. Boston: Little, Brown.

Rountree, P. M., and Thomson, E. F. 1949. Incidence of penicillin-resistant and streptomycin-resistant staphylococci in a hospital. *Lancet* 2:501.

Rous, P. 1911. Transmission of a malignant new growth by means of a cell-free filtrate. *JAMA* 56:198.

Roux, E., and Yersin, A. 1888–1890. Contribution à l'étude de la diphthérie. *Annls. Inst. Pasteur* 2:629 (1888); 3:273 (1889); 4:385 (1890).

Rowse, A. L. 1972. Nature and medicine. In *The Elizabethan Renaissance*. Vol. 2, p. 247. London: Macmillan.

Ruediger, G. F. 1912. Sporotrichosis in the United States. *J. Infect. Dis.* 11:193.

Rush, B. 1794. *An Account of the Bilious Remitting Yellow Fever as it Appeared in the City of Philadelphia in the Year 1793*. Philadelphia: Thomas Dobson.

Russell, A. 1756. *The Natural History of Aleppo*. London: A. Millar.

Sabin, A. B. 1947. Epidemic encephalitis in military personnel. Isolation of Japanese B virus on Okinawa in 1945, serologic diagnosis, clinical manifestations, epidemiologic aspects and use of mouse brain vaccine. *JAMA* 133:281.

Sabin, A. B. 1952. Research on dengue during World War II. *Am. J. Trop. Med. Hyg.* 1:30.

Sabin, A. B. 1965. Oral poliovirus vaccine: History of its development and prospects for eradication of poliomyelitis. *JAMA* 194:872.

Sabin, A. B., and Feldman, H. A. 1948. Dyes as microchemical indicators of a new immunity phenomenon affecting a protozoan parasite (toxoplasma). *Science* 108:660.

Sabin, A. B.; Hennessen, W. A.; and Winsser, J. 1954. Studies on variants of poliomyelitis virus: I. Experimental segregation and properties of avirulent variants of 3 immunologic types. *J. Exp. Med.* 99:551.

Sabin, A. B., and Olitsky, P. K. 1936. Cultivation of poliomyelitis virus *in vitro* in human embryonic nervous tissue. *Proc. Soc. Exp. Biol. Med.* 34:357.

Sabin, A. B., and Olitsky, P. K. 1937. Toxoplasma and obligate intracellular parasitism. *Science* 85:336.

Sabin, A. B.; Philip, C. B.; and Paul, J. R. 1944. Phlebotomus (pappataci or sandfly) fever. A disease of military importance. *JAMA* 125:603 and 693.

Sabouraud, R. 1894a. *La Teigne Trichophytique et la Teigne Spéciale de Grüby*. Paris: Rueff et Cie.

Sabouraud, R. 1894b. *Les Trichophyties Humaines*. Paris: Rueff & Cie.

Sabouraud, R. 1910. *Maladies du Cuir Chevelu. III. Les Maladies Cryptogamiques: Les Teignes*. Paris: Masson et Cie.

Salk, J. E. 1953. Studies in human subjects on active immunization against poliomyelitis. I. A preliminary report of experiments in progress. *JAMA* 151:1081.

Salmon, D. E. 1886. Report on swine plague. In *U.S. Department of Agriculture: Second Annual Report of the Bureau of Animal Industry for the Year 1885*, p. 184. Washington, D.C.: U.S. Government Printing Office.

Salmon, D. E., and Smith, T. 1886. On a new method of producing immunity from contagious diseases. *Proc. biol. Soc. Wash.* 3:29.

Sanford, J. P. 1974. Arbovirus and arenovirus infections. In *Harrison's Principles of Internal Medicine* by T. R. Harrison. Edited by M. M. Wintrobe, R. D. Thorn, R. D. Adams et al. 7th ed., p. 990. New York: McGraw-Hill.

Sarot, I. A.; Weber, D.; and Schecter, D. C. 1970. Cardiac surgery in active, primary infective endocarditis. *Chest* 57:58.

Sawyer, R. N.; Evans, A. S.; Niederman, J. C.; and McCollum, R. W. 1971. Prospective studies of a group of Yale University freshmen. I. Occurrence of infectious mononucleosis. *J. Infect. Dis.* 123:263.

Sawyer, W. A. 1947. Achievements of UNRRA as an international health organization. *Am. J. Public Health* 37:41.

Schaeffer, M. 1951. Leptospiral meningitis: Investigation of a water-borne epidemic due to *L. pomona*. Abstract. *J. Clin. Invest.* 30:670.

Schamberg, J. F. 1908. *Diseases of the Skin and the Eruptive Fevers*. Philadelphia: W. B. Saunders.

Schatz, A.; Bugie, E.; and Waksman, S. A. 1944. Streptomycin, a substance exhibiting antibiotic activity against gram-positive and gram-negative bacteria. *Proc. Soc. Exp. Biol. Med.* 55:66.

Schatz, A., and Waksman, S. A. 1944. Effect of streptomycin and other antibiotic substances upon *Mycobacterium tuberculosis* and related organisms. *Proc. Soc. Exp. Biol. Med.* 57:244.

Schaudinn, F., and Hoffmann, E. 1905. Vorläufiger Bericht über das Vorkommen von Spirochaeten in syphilitischen Krankheitsprodukten und bei Papillomen. *Arb. K. GesundhAmt.* 22:527.

Schenck, B. R. 1898. On refractory subcutaneous abscesses caused by a fungus possibly related to the sporotricha. *Johns Hopkins Hosp. Bull.* 9:286.

Schick, B. 1908. Kutanreaktion bei impfung mit Diphtherietoxin. *Münch. Med. Wochenschr.* 55:504.

Schneider, H. A. 1955. Recapitulation and prospects. In *Nutrition in Infections. A Conference*, edited by W. A. Wright. *Ann. NY Acad. Sci.* 63:314.

Schoenlein, J. L. 1839, transl. 1933. Zur Pathogenie der Impetigines. *Arch. Anat. Physiol. wiss. Med.* p. 82. Translated by W. A. Pusey in *The History of Dermatology* by W. A. Pusey, p. 93. Springfield (Ill.): Chas. C Thomas.

Schottmüller, H. 1903. Die Artunterscheidung der für den Menschen pathogenen Streptokokken durch Blutagar. *Münch. Med. Wochenschr.* 50:849.

Schottmüller, H. 1910. Endocarditis lenta. *Münch. Med. Wochenschr.* 12:617 and 697.

Schreus, H. Th. 1935. Chemotherapie des Erysipels und anderer Infektionen mit Prontosil. *Dtsch. med. Wochenschr.* 61:255.

Schüffner, W. 1934. Recent work on leptospirosis. *Trans. R. Soc. Trop. Med. Hyg.* 28:7.

Schulemann, W. 1932. Synthetic anti-malarial preparations. *Proc. R. Soc. Med.* 25:897.

Schultz, W., and Charlton, W. 1918. Serologische Beobachtungen am Scharlachexanthem. *Z. Kinderheilkd.* 17:328.

Schwabe, C. W. 1969. *Veterinary Medicine and Human Health*. 2nd ed. Baltimore: Williams & Wilkins.

Schwabe, C. W.; Ruppanner, R.; Miller, C. W.; Fontaine, R. E.; and Kagan, I. G. 1972. Hydatid disease is endemic in California. *Calif. Med.* 117:13 (November).

Schwann, Th. 1837. Vorläufige Mittheilung, betreffend Versuche über die Weingährung und Fäulniss. *Annln. Phys. Chem.* 41:184.

Schwentker, F. F.; Gelman, S.; and Long, P. H. 1937. The treatment of meningococcic meningitis with sulfanilamide. *JAMA* 108:1407.

Scott, H. H. 1939a. Chagas. In *A History of Tropical Medicine* by H. H. Scott. Vol. 1, p. 532. London: Edward Arnold.

Scott, H. H. 1939b. Human trypanosomiasis. Ibid., p. 454.

Scott, H. H. 1939c. Leishmaniasis. Ibid., p. 548.

Scoville, A. B., Jr. 1948. Epidemic typhus fever in Japan and Korea. In *Rickettsial Diseases of Man*, edited by F. R. Moulton, p. 28. Washington, D.C.: American Association for the Advancement of Science.

Scrimshaw, N. S.; Taylor, C. E.; and Gordon, J. E. 1968. Interactions of nutrition and infection. *WHO Monogr. Ser.* No. 57.

Sedgwick, W. T. 1902. *Principles of Sanitary Science and the Public Health with Special Reference to the Causation and Prevention of Infectious Diseases*. New York: Macmillan.

Seegal, D., and Earle, Jr., D. P. 1941. A consideration of certain biological differences between glomerulonephritis and rheumatic fever. *Am. J. Med. Sci.* 201:528.

Semmelweis, I. P. 1861, transl. 1941. *Die aetiologie, der Begriff, und die Prophylaxis des Kindbettfiebers*. Pest: C. A. Hartleben. Translated by F. P. Murphy. *The etiology, the concept and the prophylaxis of childbed fever*. In *Medical Classics*, compiled by E. C. Kelly. Vol. 5, p. 350. Baltimore: Williams & Wilkins.

Sexton, Jr., R. C.; Eyles, D. E.; and Dillman, R. E. 1953. Adult toxoplasmosis. *Am. J. Med.* 14:366.

Shaffer, J. M.; Kucera, C. J.; and Spink, W. W. 1953a. Evaluation of prolonged antibiotic therapy in mice with chronic brucella infection due to *Brucella melitensis J. Immunol.* 70:31.

Shaffer, J. M.; Kucera, C. J.; and Spink, W. W. 1953b. The protection of intracellular brucella against therapeutic agents and the bactericidal action of serum. *J. Exp. Med.* 97:77.

Shaffer, J. M., and Spink, W. W. 1948. Therapy of experimental brucella infection in the developing chick embryo. III. The synergistic action of streptomycin and sulfadiazine. *J. Immunol.* 60:405.

Shankman, B. 1946. Report on an outbreak of endemic febrile illness, not yet identified, occurring in New York City. *NY State J. Med.* 46:2156.

Shelley, W. B., and Crissey, J. T. 1953. *Classics in Clinical Dermatology*. Springfield (Ill.): Chas. C Thomas.

Shepard, C. C. 1971. The first decade in experimental leprosy. *Bull. WHO* 44:821.

Shiga, K. 1898. Ueber den Dysenteriebacillus *(Bacillus dysenteriae)*. *Zentbl. Bakt. ParasitKde. Hyg., Abt.* 1, 24:817 and 870.

Shope, R. E. 1931. Swine influenza. III. Filtration experiments and etiology. *J. Exp. Med.* 54:373.

Shope, R. E. 1944. Old, intermediate, and contemporary contributions to our knowledge of pandemic influenza. *Medicine* 23:415.

Shortt, H. E.; Smith, R. O. A.; Swaminath, C. S.; and Krishnan, K. V. 1931. Transmission of Indian kala-azar by the bite of *Phlebotomus argentipes*. *Indian J. Med. Res.* 18:1373.

Sigurdsson, B. 1954a. Maedi, a slow progressive pneumonia of sheep: An epizoological and a pathological study. *Br. Vet. J.* 110:255.

Sigurdsson, B. 1954b. Rida, a chronic encephalitis of sheep. With general remarks on infections which develop slowly and some of their special characteristics. Ibid., p. 341.

Sigurdsson, B., and Pálsson, P. A. 1958. Visna of sheep. A slow, demyelinating infection. *Br. J. Exp. Pathol.* 39:519.

Siim, J. C. 1961. *Toxoplasmosis Acquisita Lymphonodosa*. Copenhagen: Munksgaard.

Siler, J. F.; Hall, M. W.; and Hitchens, A. P. 1926. *Dengue. Its History, Epidemiology, Mechanism of Transmission, Etiology, Clinical Manifestations, Immunity, and Prevention*. Monograph No. 20. Manila: Government of Philippine Islands, Department of Agriculture and Natural Resources, Bureau of Science.

Silverman, M. 1943. *Magic in a Bottle*. New York: Macmillan.

Simmons, J. S., and Michie, H. C. 1928. Cerebrospinal meningitis. In *The Medical Department of the United States Army in the World War* by the U.S. Surgeon-General's Office. Vol. 9, p. 203. Washington, D.C.: U.S. Government Printing Office.

Simmons, J. S.; St. John, J. H.; and Reynolds, F. H. K. 1926. *Experimental Studies of Dengue*. Manila: Government of Philippine Islands, Department of Agriculture and Natural Resources, Bureau of Science.

Simon, J. 1887. *Public Health Reports*, edited for The Sanitary Institute of Great Britain by Edward Seaton. Vol. 1. London: Offices of the Sanitary Institute. (Note: Indexed in British Museum General Catalog of Printed Books to 1955, Vol. 15, p. 980, column 1730 under "London-Royal Society for the Promotion of Health.")

Simpson, J. Y. 1847. On a new anaesthetic agent, more efficient than sulfuric ether. *Lancet* 2:549.

Simpson, W. J. 1905. *A Treatise on Plague Dealing with the Historical, Epidemiological, Clinical, Therapeutic and Preventive Aspects of the Disease.* Cambridge: Cambridge University Press.

Skinner, D., and Keefer, C. S. 1941. Significance of bacteremia caused by *Staphylococcus aureus*. A study of one hundred and twenty-two cases and a review of the literature concerned with experimental infection in animals. *Arch. Intern. Med.* 68:851.

Slawyk. 1899. Ein Fall von Allgemeininfection mit Influenzabacillen. *Z. Hyg. Infekt-Krankh.* 32:443.

Smadel, J. E. 1949. Chloramphenicol (chloromycetin) in the treatment of infectious diseases. *Am. J. Med.* 7:671.

Smadel, J. E.; Bailey, C. A.; and Lewthwaite, R. 1950. Synthetic and fermentative type chloramphenicol (chloromycetin) in typhoid fever: Prevention of relapses by adequate treatment. *Ann. Intern. Med.* 33:1.

Smadel, J. E., and Jackson, E. B. 1947. Chloromycetin. An antibiotic with chemotherapeutic activity in experimental rickettsial and viral infections. *Science* 106:418.

Smadel, J. E.; Jackson, E. B.; Ley, Jr., H. L.; and Lewthwaite, R. 1949. Comparison of synthetic and fermentation chloramphenicol (chloromycetin) in rickettsial and viral infections. *Proc. Soc. Exp. Biol. Med.* 70:191.

Smadel, J. E.; León, A. P.; Ley, Jr., H. L.; and Varela, G. 1948. Chloromycetin in the treatment of patients with typhus fever. *Proc. Soc. Exper. Biol. Med.* 68:12.

Smadel, J. E.; Ley, Jr., H. L.; and Diercks, F. H. 1951. Treatment of typhoid fever. I. Combined therapy with cortisone and chloramphenicol. *Ann. Intern. Med.* 34:1.

Smadel, J. E.; Woodward, T. E.; Ley, Jr., H. L.; and Lewthwaite, R. 1949. Chloramphenicol (chloromycetin) in the treatment of tsutsugamushi disease (scrub typhus). *J. Clin. Invest.* 28:1196.

Smallpox Editorial 1974. Smallpox target zero? *Lancet* 1:295.

Smith, C. E. 1943. Coccidioidomycosis. *Med. Clin. North Am.* 27:790.

Smith, C. E. G.; Simpson, D. I. H.; Bowen, E. T. W.; and Zlotnik, I. 1967. Fatal human disease from vervet monkeys. *Lancet* 2:1119.

Smith, C. H. 1944. Acute infectious lymphocytosis: A specific infection. Report of our cases showing its communicability. *JAMA* 125:342.

Smith, H. F. 1921. Epidemic encephalitis (encephalitis lethargica, Nona). Report of studies conducted in the United States. *U.S. Public Health Rep.* 36:207.

Smith, L. D. 1916. The value of anaphylaxis in the treatment of gonorrheal complications. Allergy, a therapeutic agent? *JAMA* 66:1758.

Smith, M. G. 1954. Propagation of salivary gland virus of the mouse in tissue cultures. *Proc. Soc. Exp. Biol. Med.* 86:435.

Smith, M. G. 1956. Propagation in tissue cultures of a cytopathogenic virus from human salivary gland virus (SGV) disease. *Proc. Soc. Exp. Biol. Med.* 92:424.

Smith, N. 1824. *A Practical Essay on Typhous Fever.* New York: E. Bless and E. White.

Smith, S. 1835. *A Treatise on Fever.* 3rd American ed. (first published in 1829). Philadelphia: Carey, Lea and Blanchard.

Smith, S. 1911. *The City That Was.* New York: Frank Allaben.

Smith, T. 1898. A comparative study of bovine tubercle bacilli and of human bacilli from sputum. *J. Exp. Med.* 3:451.

Smith, T. 1934. *Parasitism and Disease.* Princeton (N.J.): Princeton University Press.

Smith, T., and Kilborne, F. L. 1893. Investigations into the nature, causation, and prevention of Southern Cattle Fever. In *Eighth and Ninth Annual Reports of the Bureau of Animal Industry for the Years 1891 and 1892*, p. 177. Washington, D.C.: United States Government Printing Office.

Smith, W.; Andrewes, C. H.; and Laidlaw, P. P. 1933. A virus obtained from influenza patients. *Lancet* 225:66.

Smorodintsev, A. A.; Kazbintsev, L. I.; and Chudakov, V. G. 1964. *Virus Hemorrhagic Fevers.* Washington, D.C.: Office Tech. Services, U.S. Department of Commerce.

Snow, J. 1853 and 1855, reproduced in 1936. *Snow on Cholera,* being a reprint of two papers by John Snow, M.D. 1. On the mode of communication of cholera. 1st ed. (1849), 2nd ed. (1855). 2. On continuous molecular changes, more particularly in their relation to epidemic diseases (1853). New York: Commonwealth Fund.

Soper, F. L., and Smith, H. H. 1938. Yellow fever vaccination with cultivated virus and immune and hyperimmune serum. *Am. J. Trop. Med.* 18:111.

Soper, F. L., and Wilson, D. B. 1943. *Anopheles gambiae in Brazil: 1930 to 1940.* New York: Rockefeller Foundation.

Soper, G. A. 1919. Typhoid Mary. *Milit. Surg.* 45:1.

Souza de Morais, J.; Munford, R. S.; Risi, J. B.; Antezana, E.; and Feldman, R. A. 1974. Epidemic disease due to serogroup C *Neisseria meningitidis* in Sao Paulo, Brazil. *J. Infect. Dis.* 129:568.

Spink, W. W. 1934. Effects of vaccines and bacterial and parasitic infections on eosinophilia in trichinous animals. *Arch. Intern. Med.* 54:805.

Spink, W. W. 1937. Pathogenesis of erythema nodosum. With special reference to tuberculosis, streptococcic infection and rheumatic fever. *Arch. Intern. Med.* 59:65.

Spink, W. W. 1939a. The bactericidal effect of sulfanilamide upon pathogenic and nonpathogenic staphylococci. *J. Immunol.* 37:345.

Spink, W. W. 1939b. The pathogenesis of gonococcal infection. In *The Gonococcus and Gonococcal Infection,* p. 23. Publication No. 11 of the American Association for the Advancement of Science. Lancaster (Pa.): Science Press.

Spink, W. W. 1941a. Rocky Mountain spotted fever in Minnesota. *Proc. Sixth Pacif. Sci. Congr.* 5:585.

Spink, W. W. 1941b. *Sulfanilamide and Related Compounds in General Practice.* Chicago: Year Book Publishers.

Spink, W. W. 1941c. The pathogenesis and treatment of staphylococcal infections. *New Int. Clins.* 4:237.

Spink, W. W. 1943. Atypical pneumonia. *Minn. Med.* 26:337.

Spink, W. W. 1951. Clinical and biologic significance of penicillin-resistant staphylococci, including observations with streptomycin, aureomycin, chloramphenicol, and terramycin. *J. Lab. and Clin. Med.* 37:278.

Spink, W. W. 1952a. Human leptospirosis due to *Leptospira pomona.* Report of first case in Minnesota. *Minn. Med.* 35:525.

Spink, W. W. 1952b. Some biologic and clinical problems related to intracellular parasitism in brucellosis. *N. Engl. J. Med.* 247:603.

Spink, W. W. 1956. *The Nature of Brucellosis.* Minneapolis: University of Minnesota Press.

Spink, W. W. 1958. From endotoxin to snake venom. *Yale J. Biol. Med.* 30:355.

Spink, W. W. 1960. Brucellosis as a model for metabolic studies on bacterial shock and inflammation. In *The Biochemical Response to Injury,* edited by H. B. Stoner, p. 361. Oxford: Blackwell Scientific Publications.

Spink, W. W. 1962. Pathogenesis and therapy of shock due to infection: Experimental and clinical studies. In *Shock: Pathogenesis and Therapy. An International Symposium,* edited by K. D. Bock, p. 225. Berlin: Springer-Verlag Publishers.

Spink, W. W. 1965. *The Dilemma of Bacterial Shock: With Special Reference to Endotoxin Shock.* The Freeland Barbour Fellowship Lecture delivered on March 3, 1964 at the Royal College of Physicians of Edinburgh. Publication No. 29, Royal College of Physicians of Edinburgh.

Spink, W. W., and Anderson, D. 1951. Studies relating to the differential diagnosis of brucellosis and infectious mononucleosis: Clinical, hematologic, and serologic observations. *Trans. Assoc. Am. Physicians* 64:428.

Spink, W. W., and Augustine, D. L. 1935a. The diagnosis of trichinosis with especial reference to skin and precipitin tests. *JAMA* 104:1801.

Spink, W. W., and Augustine, D. L. 1935b. Trichinosis in Boston. *N. Engl. J. Med.* 213:527.

Spink, W. W., and Bradley, G. M. 1960. Persistent parasitism in experimental brucellosis: Attempts to eliminate brucellae with long-term tetracycline therapy. *J. Lab. Clin. Med.* 55:535.

Spink, W. W.; Braude, A. I.; Castaneda, M. R.; and Goytia, R. S. 1948. Aureomycin therapy in human brucellosis due to *Brucella melitensis. JAMA* 138:1145.

Spink, W. W., and Crago, F. H. 1939. Evaluation of sulfanilamide in the treatment of patients with subacute bacterial endocarditis. *Arch. Intern. Med.* 64:228.

Spink, W. W., and Ferris, V. 1945a. Penicillin inhibitor from staphylococci which have developed resistance to penicillin in the human body. *Proc. Soc. Exp. Biol. Med.* 59:188.

Spink, W. W., and Ferris, V. 1945b. Quantitative action of penicillin inhibitor from penicillin-resistant strains of staphylococci. *Science* 102:221.

Spink, W. W., and Ferris, V. 1947. Penicillin-resistant staphylococci: Mechanisms involved in the development of resistance. *J. Clin. Invest.* 26:379.

Spink, W. W.; Ferris, V.; and Vivino, J. J. 1944. Comparative in vitro resistance of staphylococci to penicillin and to sodium sulfathiazole. *Proc. Soc. Exp. Biol. Med.* 55:207.

Spink, W. W.; Hall III, J. W.; Finstad, J.; and Mallet, E. 1962. Immunization with viable Brucella organisms. Results of a safety test in humans. *Bull. WHO* 26:409.

Spink, W. W., and Hall, W. H. 1945. Penicillin therapy at the University of Minnesota Hospitals 1942–1944. *Ann. Intern. Med.* 22:510.

Spink, W. W., and Hall, W. H. 1952. The influence of cortisone and adrenocorticotrophic hormone on brucellosis. II. Adrenocorticotrophic hormone (ACTH) in acute and chronic human brucellosis. *J. Clin Invest.* 31:958.

Spink, W. W.; Hall, W. H.; and Ferris, V. 1945. Clinical significance of staphylococci. With natural or acquired resistance to the sulfonamides and to penicillin. *JAMA* 128:555.

Spink, W. W.; Hall, W. H.; Shaffer, J. M.; and Braude, A. I. 1948. Human brucellosis: Its specific treatment with a combination of streptomycin and sulfadiazine. *JAMA* 136:382.

Spink, W. W., and Hansen, A. E. 1940. Sulfathiazole: Clinical evaluation. *JAMA* 115:840.

Spink, W. W.; Hansen, A. E.; and Paine, J. R. 1941. Staphylococcic bacteremia. Treatment with sulfapyridine and sulfathiazole. *Arch. Intern. Med.* 67:25.

Spink, W. W., and Jermsta, J. 1941. Effects of sulfonamide compounds upon growth of staphylococci in presence and absence of p-aminobenzoic acid. *Proc. Soc. Exp. Biol. Med.* 47:395.

Spink, W. W., and Paine, J. R. 1940. The bactericidal power of blood from patients and normal controls for staphylococci. *J. Immunol.* 38:383.

Spink, W. W.; Rantz, L. A.; Boisvert, P. J.; and Coggeshall, H. 1946. Sulfadiazine and penicillin for hemolytic streptococcus infections of the upper respiratory tract. An evaluation in tonsillitis, nasopharyngitis and scarlet fever. *Arch. Intern. Med.* 77:260.

Spink, W. W., and Thompson, H. 1953. Human brucellosis caused by *Brucella abortus*, strain 19. *JAMA* 153:1162.

Spink, W. W., and Vivino, J. J. 1942. The coagulase test for staphylococci and its correlation with the resistance of organisms to the bactericidal action of human blood. *J. Clin Invest.* 21:353.

Spink, W. W.; Wright, L. D.; Vivino, J. J.; and Skeggs, H. R. 1944. Para-aminobenzoic acid production by staphylococci. *J. Exp. Med.* 79:331.

Splendore, A. 1908. Un nouvo protozoa parassita dei conigli. Incontrato nelle lesioni anatomiche d'una malattia che ricorda in molti punti il Kala azar dell'uomo. *Revta. Soc. scient. S. Paulo* 3:109.

Splendore, A. 1909. Sobre um Novo Caso de Blastomycose Generalizada. *Revta. Soc. scient. S. Paulo* 4:52.

Sprunt, T. P., and Evans, F. A. 1920. Mononuclear leucocytosis in reaction to acute infections ("infectious mononucleosis"). *Johns Hopkins Hosp. Bull.* 31:410.

Stableforth. A. W. 1959. Brucellosis. In *Diseases Due to Bacteria* edited by A. W. Stableforth and I. A. Galloway. Vol. 1, p. 53. New York: Academic Press.

Stavitsky, A. B., and Green, R. G. 1945. A survey of leptospirosis (Weil's disease) in Minnesota. *Minn. Med.* 28:549.

Stearn, E. Wagner, and Stearn, A. E. 1945. *The Effect of Smallpox on the Destiny of the Amerindian.* Boston: Bruce Humphries.

Steele, J. H. 1973. A bookshelf on veterinary public health. *Am. J. Public Health* 63:291.

Steenken, Jr., W., and Wolinsky, E. 1952. Antituberculous properties of hydrazines of isonicotinic acid (Rimifon, Marsilid). *Am. Rev. Tuberc.* 65:365.

Stefferud, A., ed. 1956. *Animal Diseases. The Yearbook of Agriculture 1956.* Washington, D.C.: U.S. Department of Agriculture, U.S. Government Printing Office.

Sterling, C. 1972. Superdams: The perils of progress. *Atlantic* (Boston) 229:35 (June).

Sternberg, G. M. 1884. *Malaria and Malarial Diseases.* New York: William Wood.

Stiles, C. W. 1903. Report upon the prevalence and geographical distribution of hookworm disease (uncinariasis or anchylostomiasis) in the United States. *U.S. Marine Hospital Service Hygienic Laboratory Bulletin* No. 10 *(U.S. Hyg. Lab. Bull.).*

Stillé, A. 1867. *Epidemic Meningitis, or Cerebro-Spinal Meningitis.* Philadelphia: Lindsay and Blakiston.

Stoddard, J. L., and Cutler, E. C. 1916. Torula infection in man. A group of cases, characterized by chronic lesions of the central nervous system, with clinical symptoms suggestive of cerebral tumor, produced by an organism belonging to the Torula group *(Torula histolytica*, N. Sp.). *Stud. Rockefeller Inst. med. Res.* 25:1.

Stokes, J. H., and Ruedemann, Jr., R. 1920. Epidemic infectious jaundice and its relation to the therapy of syphilis. *Arch. Intern. Med.* 26:521.

Stookey, P. F.; Ferris, C. R.; Parker, H. M.; Scarpellino, L. A.; and English, K. E. 1934. Necrotizing ulcers complicating erysipelas. *JAMA* 103:903.

Strode, G. K., ed. 1951. *Yellow Fever.* New York: McGraw-Hill.

Strom, R. L.; Hall, W. H.; and Casey, F. 1964. Coccidioidomycosis. A Minnesota experience. *Minn. Med.* 47:1189.

Strong, R. P. 1938. Onchocerciasis in Africa and Central America. *Am. J. Trop. Med. (Suppl.)* 18:1.

Strong, R. P.; Sandground, J. H.; Bequaert, J. C.; and Ochoa, M. M. 1934. *Onchocerciasis, with Special Reference to the Central American Form of the Disease.* Four parts. Cambridge (Mass.): Harvard University Press.

Strong, R. P.; Shattuck, G. C.; Zinsser, H.; Sellards, A. W.; and Hopkins, J. G. 1920. *Typhus Fever with Particular Reference to the Serbian Epidemic.* Cambridge (Mass.): Harvard University Press.

Stuart-Harris, C. H. 1961. Twenty years of influenza epidemics. In *International Conference on Asian Influenza.* Held February 17–19, 1960. *Am. Rev. Respir. Dis.* 83 (No. 2, Part 2):54.

Stuart-Harris, C. H.; Andrewes, C. H.; and Smith, W. 1938. *A Study of Epidemic Influenza: With Special Reference to the 1936–7 Epidemic.* Great Britain Medical Research Council Special Report Series No. 228. London: His Majesty's Stationery Office.

Sturdee, E. L., and Scott, W. M. 1930. *A Disease of Parrots Communicable to Man (Psittacosis).* Reports on Public Health and Medical Subjects No. 61, Ministry of Health. London: His Majesty's Stationery Office.

Sundman, O. 1970. *The Flight of the Eagle.* Translated by Mary Sandbach. New York: Pantheon Books.

Svedberg, T. 1937. The ultra-centrifuge and the study of high-molecular compounds. *Nature (Suppl.)* 139:1051.

Svedberg, T.; Boestad, G.; and Eriksson-Quensel, I. -B. 1934. Possibility of sedimentation measurements in intense centrifugal fields. *Nature* 134:98.

Swift, H. F. 1927. Rheumatic fever. In *A Textbook of Medicine,* edited by R. L. Cecil, p. 77. Philadelphia: W. B. Saunders.

Swift, H. W. 1921. Trench fever. In *Harvey Lectures 1919–20,* Series 15, p. 58. Philadelphia: J. B. Lippincott.

Sydenham, T. 1848 and 1850. *The Works of Thomas Sydenham.* 2 vols. (Vol. 1, 1848; Vol. 2, 1850). Translated from the Latin edition of Dr. Greenhill with a life of the author by R. G. Latham. London: Sydenham Society.

Sydenham, T. 1939. Of epidemic diseases: Of the measles of 1670. In *Medical Classics,* compiled by E. C. Kelly. Vol. 4, p. 313. Baltimore: Williams & Wilkins.

Talbott, J. H. 1970. Sir Ronald Ross (1857–1932). In *A Biographical History of Medicine* by John H. Talbott, p. 770. New York: Grune & Stratton.

Taniguchi, T.; Hosokawa, M.; and Kuga, S. 1936. A virus isolated in 1935 epidemic of summer encephalitis of Japan. *Jap. J. Exp. Med.* 14:185.

Tasker, A. N. 1928. Infectious jaundice; typhus fever; trench fever. In *The Medical Department of the United States Army in the World War* by the U.S. Surgeon-General's Office. Vol. 9, p. 483. Washington, D.C.: U.S. Government Printing Office.

Tassel, D., and Madoff, M. A. 1968. Treatment of Candida sepsis and Cryptococcus meningitis with 5-fluorocytosine. A new antifungal agent. *JAMA* 206:830.

Tatlock, H. 1947. Studies on a virus from a patient with Fort Bragg fever (pretibial fever). *J. Clin. Invest.* 26:287.

Taylor, J. 1960. The diarrhoeal diseases in England and Wales: With special reference to those caused by *Salmonella, Escherichia* and *Shigella. Bull. WHO* 23:763.

Taylor, R. M.; Lisbonne, M.; Vidal, L. F.; and Hazemann, R. H. 1938. Investigations on undulant fever in France. *Bull. Hlth. Org.* 7:503.

Terramycin 1950. Conference on terramycin with several authors. Held June 16–17, 1950. *Ann. NY Acad. Sci.* 53:221 (September 15).

Thacher, J. 1812. *Observations on Hydrophobia. Produced by the Bite of a Mad Dog, or Other Rabid Animal.* Plymouth (Mass.): Joseph Avery.

Thatcher, R. W., and Pettit, T. H. 1971. Gonorrheal conjunctivitis. *JAMA* 215:1494.

Thayer, W. S. 1926. Studies on bacterial (infective) endocarditis. *Johns Hopkins Hosp. Rep.* 22:1.

Theiler, A. 1919. Acute liver-atrophy and parenchymatous hepatitis in horses. In *Union of South Africa Department of Agriculture, Fifth Report of the Director of Veterinary Research, April 1918,* p. 7. Pretoria (South Africa): Government Printing and Stationery Office.

Theiler, M. 1930. Studies on the action of yellow fever virus in mice. *Ann. Trop. Med. Parasitol.* 24:249.

Theiler, M. 1933. A yellow fever protection test in mice by intracerebral injection. *Ann. Trop. Med. Parasitol.* 27:57.

Theiler, M. 1934. Spontaneous encephalomyelitis of mice — a new virus disease. *Science* 80:122.

Theiler, M. 1937. Spontaneous encephalomyelitis of mice. A new virus disease. *J. Exp. Med.* 65:705.

Theiler, M. 1941. Studies on poliomyelitis. *Medicine* 20:443.

Theiler, M., and Smith, H. H. 1937. The use of yellow fever virus modified by an in vitro cultivation for human immunization. *J. Exp. Med.* 65:787.

Theologides, A.; Osterberg, K.; and Kennedy, B. J. 1966. Cerebral toxoplasmosis in multiple myeloma. *Ann. Intern. Med.* 64:1071.

Thomas, H. E. 1947. *A Study of Leprosy Colony Policies.* New York: American Mission to Lepers, Inc.

Thomas, L., ed. 1952. *Rheumatic Fever.* A symposium held at the University of Minnesota on November 29, 30 and December 1, 1951 under the sponsorship of the Minnesota Heart Association. Minneapolis: University of Minnesota Press.

Thompson, T. 1852. *Annals of Influenza or Epidemic Catarrhal Fever in Great Britain from 1510 to 1837.* Vol. 21, p. 1. London: The Sydenham Society.

Thompson, W. H., and Inhorn, S. L. 1967. Arthropodborne California group viral encephalitis in Wisconsin. *Wis. Med. J.* 66:250.

Thompson, W. H.; Kalfayan, B.; and Anslow, R. O. 1965. Isolation of California encephalitis group virus from a fatal human illness. *Am. J. Epidemiol.* 81:245.

Thompson, W. H.; Trainer, D. O.; Allen, V.; and Hale, J. B. 1963. The exposure of wildlife workers in Wisconsin to ten zoonotic diseases. *Trans. N. Am. Wildl. Nat. Resources Conf.* 28:215.

Thomson, D., and Thomson, R. 1928. An historical survey of researches on the role of the streptococci in acute articular rheumatism or rheumatic fever. *Ann. Pickett-Thomson Res. Lab. Monograph* 1. Vol. 4, p. 1.

Thomson, D., and Thomson, R. 1928–29. The pathogenic streptococci. An historical survey of their role in human and animal disease. *Ann. Pickett-Thomson Res. Lab.* Part I. *Monographs* 1–4. Vol. 4, p. 1 (1928); Part II. *Monographs* 5–7. Vol. 4, p. 251 (1929).

Thomson, D., and Thomson, R. 1932. The common cold. With special reference to the part played by streptococci, pneumococci, and other organisms. *Ann. Pickett-Thomson Res. Lab. Monograph* 15. Vol. 8, p. 1.

Thomson, D., and Thomson, R. 1933–34. Influenza. *Ann. Pickett-Thomson Res. Lab.* Part I. *Monograph* 16. Vol. 9, p. 1 (1933); Part II. *Monograph* 16, Vol. 10, p. 641 (1934).

Thormar, H., and Pálsson, P. A. 1967. Visna and Maedi — Two slow infections of sheep and their etiological agents. In *Perspectives in Virology*, edited by M. Pollard. Vol. 5, p. 291. New York: Academic Press.

Thucydides 1954. *The Peloponnesian War.* Translated with an introduction by Rex Warner. London: Cassell.

Tileston, W. 1928. Focal infections. In *A Textbook of Medicine*, edited by R. L. Cecil, p. 75. Philadelphia: W. B. Saunders.

Transvaal Mine Medical Officers' Association, Proceedings 1947. *Sporotrichosis Infection on Mine of the Witwatersrand. A Symposium.* Johannesburg (South Africa): Transvaal Chamber of Mines.

Traub, E. 1935. A filterable virus recovered from white mice. *Science* 81:298.

Tréfouël, J.: Tréfouël, Mme. J.; Nitti, F.; and Bovet, D. 1935. Activité du p-aminophénylsulfamide sur les infections streptococciques expérimentales de la souris et du lapin. *C. R. Séanc. Soc. Biol.* 120:756.

Troup, J. M.; White, H. A.; Fom, A. L. M. D.; and Carey, D. E. 1970. An outbreak of Lassa fever on the Jos Plateau, Nigeria, in January–February 1970. A preliminary report. *Am. J. Trop. Med. Hyg.* 19:695.

Trousseau, A. 1861. *Clinique médicale de l'Hôtel-Dieu de Paris.* Vol. 1, p. 1. Paris: J. -B. Baillière & fils.

Trudeau, E. L. 1916. *An Autobiography.* Garden City (N.Y.): Doubleday Page.

Trueta, J. 1943. *The Principles and Practice of War Surgery. With Reference to the Biological Method of the Treatment of War Wounds and Fractures.* St. Louis: C. V. Mosby.

Trumbull, M. L., and Greiner, D. J. 1951. Homologous serum jaundice. An occupational hazard to medical personnel. *JAMA* 145:965.

Tulloch, W. J. 1955. Sir David Bruce: An appreciation. *J. R. Army med. Cps.* 101:81.

Turk, D. C., and May, J. R. 1967. *Haemophilus influenzae. Its Clinical Importance.* London: The English Universities Press Ltd.

Turner, L. H. 1974. Genus V. Leptospira. In *Bergey's Manual of Determinative Bacteriology*, edited by R. E. Buchanan and N. E. Gibbons. 8th ed., p. 190. Baltimore: Williams & Wilkins.

Twort, F. W. 1915. An investigation on the nature of ultra-microscopic viruses. *Lancet* 189:1241.

Tyndall, J. 1882. *Essays on the Floating-Matter of the Air in Relation to Putrefaction and Infection.* New York: D. Appleton.

Typhoid Panel, UK Department of Technical Co-operation 1964. A controlled field trial of acetone-dried and inactivated and heat-phenol-inactivated typhoid vaccines in British Guiana. *Bull. WHO* 30:631.

Tyrrell, D. A. 1965. *Common Colds and Related Diseases*. Baltimore: Williams & Wilkins.

Tyzzer, E. E. 1906. The histology of the skin lesions in varicella. *J. Med. Res.* 14:361.

Uhr, J. W., ed. 1964. *The Streptococcus, Rheumatic Fever and Glomerulonephritis*. A symposium held at New York University School of Medicine November 27–28, 1962. Baltimore: Williams & Wilkins.

Underwood, M. 1795. Debility of the lower extremities. In *A Treatise on the Diseases of Children, with General Directions for the Management of Infants from the Birth* by M. Underwood. Vol. 2, p. 54. London: J. Mathews.

United States Army Medical Service-Graduate School, 1953. *Symposium on the Leptospiroses*. Held at the Walter Reed Army Medical Center December 11–12, 1952. Medical Science Publication No. 1. Washington, D.C.: Government Printing Office.

United States Bureau of Animal Industry. 1913. *U.S. Bureau of Animal Industry: Twenty-eighth Annual Report for the Year 1911*. Washington, D.C.: U.S. Government Printing Office.

United States Department of Health, Education and Welfare. 1958. *On Hospital-Acquired Staphylococcal Disease*. Proceedings of the National Conference held at Atlanta, Georgia September 15–17, 1958. Atlanta: Communicable Disease Center.

United States Department of Health, Education and Welfare. 1974. Cattle tuberculosis epizootic — Georgia. CDC Vet. Public Health Notes (September).

United States Department of Health, Education and Welfare, National Institutes of Health. 1976. *NIH Research Advances-1976*. DHEW Publication No. (NIH) 76-3.

United States Public Health Service. 1936. Epidemic amebic dysentery. The Chicago outbreak of 1933. *U.S. NIH Health Bull.* No. 166, pp. 1–187.

United States Public Health Service, Report to the Surgeon-General. 1964. Oral poliomyelitis vaccines: Report of special advisory committee on oral poliomyelitis vaccines to the Surgeon General of the Public Health Service. *JAMA* 190:49.

United States Surgeon-General's Office. 1888. Jaundice. In *The Medical and Surgical History of the War of the Rebellion, Medical History*. Prepared under the direction of the Surgeon General, U.S. Army, by Charles Smart, Major and Surgeon, U.S. Army. Vol. 1, Part III, p. 874. Washington, D.C.: Government Printing Office.

Unna, P. G. 1896. *The Histopathology of the Diseases of the Skin*. Translated by Norman Walker from the 1894 German edition. New York: Macmillan.

Vallery-Radot, R. [1923]. *The Life of Pasteur*. Translated by Mrs. R. L. Devonshire. Garden City (N.Y.): Garden City Publishing.

Vandeputte, J.; Wachtel, J. L.; and Stiller, E. T. 1956. Amphotericins A and B, antifungal antibiotics produced by a streptomycete. II. The isolation and properties of the crystalline amphotericins. In *Antibiotics Annual 1955–56*, edited by Henry Welch and Felix Marti-Ibanez. New York: Medical Encyclopedia.

Van Ermengem, E. 1897. Contribution à l'étude des intoxications alimentaires. Recherches sur des accidents à caractères botuliniques provoqués par du jambon. *Archs. Pharmacodyn.* 3:213.

Van Oye, E., ed. 1964. *The World Problem of Salmonellosis*. The Hague: Dr. W. Junk Publishers.

Veale, H. 1866. History of an epidemic of Rötheln, with observations on its pathology. *Edinb. med. J.* 12:404.

Venters, H. D.; Hoffert, W. R.; Scatterday, J. E.; and Hardy, A. V. 1954. Rabies in bats in Florida. *Am. J. Public Health* 44:182.

Vickery, H. F., and Richardson, O. 1904. Three cases of probable psittacosis. *Med. News* 85:780.

Vieusseux, M. 1806. Mémoire sur la maladie qui a régné a Genève au printemps de 1805. *J. Méd. Chir. Pharmacie* 11:163.

Villemin, J. -A. 1868. *Etudes sur La Tuberculose*. Paris: J. B. Baillière et Fils.

Viral Hepatitis: Symposium 1976. Viral hepatitis: Present status of basic clinical and laboratory studies. Tenth annual ASCP research symposium. *Am. J. Clin. Pathol.* 65:No. 5 *(Suppl.)*.

Virchow, R. 1855. Infectionen durch contagiose thiergifte (Zoonosen). In *Handbuch der Speciellen Pathologie und Therapie*, p. 337. Erlangen: Rud. Virchow.

Virchow, R. 1856. Beiträge zur Lehre von den beim Menschen vorkommenden pflanzlichen Parasiten. *Virchow's Arch. path. Anat. Physiol.* 9:557.

Virchow, R. 1858. Ueber die Nature der constitutionell-syphilitischen Affectionen. *Virchow's Arch. path. Anat. Physiol.* 15:217.

Virchow, R. 1864. *Darstellung der Lehre von den Trichinen.* Berlin: G. Reimer.

Virchow, R. 1868, transl. 1868. *Ueber den Hungertyphus und einige verwandte Krankheitsformen.* Berlin: August Hirschwald. Translation. *On Famine Fever and Some of the Other Cognate Forms of Typhus.* London: Williams & Norgate.

Volkert, M. 1965. Studies on immunologic tolerance to LCM virus. In *Perspectives in Virology*, edited by Morris Pollard. Vol. 4, p. 269. New York: Hoeber Medical Division-Harper & Row.

Wagner-Jauregg, J. 1921. Die Behandlung der progressiven Paralyse und Tabes. *Wien. Med. Wochenschr.* 71:1106 and 1210.

Wahdan, M. H.; Rizk, F.; El-Akkad, A. M.; El Ghoroury, A. A.; Hablas, R.; Girgis, N. I.; Amer, A.; Boctar, W.; Sippel, J. E.; Gotschlich, E. C.; Triau, R.; Sanborn, W. R.; Cvjetanovic, B. 1973. A controlled field trial of a serogroup A meningococcal polysaccharide vaccine. *Bull. WHO* 48:667.

Waksman, S. A. 1945. *Microbial Antagonisms and Antibiotic Substances.* New York: The Commonwealth Fund.

Waksman, S. A. 1948. *The Literature on Streptomycin 1944–1948.* New Brunswick (N.J.): Rutgers University Press.

Waksman, S. A. 1949. *Streptomycin. Its Nature and Practical Application.* Baltimore: Williams & Wilkins.

Waksman, S. A. 1954. *My Life with the Microbes.* New York: Simon and Schuster.

Waksman, S. A., ed 1958. *Neomycin. Its Nature and Practical Application.* Baltimore: Williams & Wilkins.

Waksman, S. A., and Henrici, A. T. 1943. The nomenclature and classification of the actinomycetes. *J. Bacteriol.* 46:337.

Wallgren, A. 1925. Une nouvelle maladie infectieuse du système nerveux central? *Acta Paediatr.* 4:158.

Walsh, G. P.; Storrs, E. E.; Burchfield, H. P.; Cottrell, E. H.; Vidrine, M. F.; and Binford, C. H. 1975. Leprosy-like disease occurring naturally in armadillos. *J. Reticuloendothel. Soc.* 18:347.

Wangensteen, O. H. 1936. The role of surgery in the treatment of actinomycosis. *Ann. Surg.* 104:752.

Wangensteen, O. H. 1970. Nineteenth century wound management of the parturient uterus and compound fracture: The Semmelweis-Lister priority controversy. *Bull. NY Acad. Med.* 46:565.

Wangensteen, O. H.; Wangensteen, S. D.; and Klinger, C. F. 1973. Some pre-Listerian and post-Listerian antiseptic wound practices and the emergence of asepsis. *Surg. Gynecol. Obstet.* 137:677.

Wannamaker, L. W., and Matsen, J. M., eds. 1972. *Streptococci and Streptococcal Diseases.* New York: Academic Press.

Waring, J. J.; Neubuerger, K.; and Geever, E. F. 1942. Severe forms of chickenpox in adults. With autopsy observations in a case with associated pneumonia and encephalitis. *Arch. Intern. Med.* 69:384.

Warren, S. L.; Scott, W. W.; and Carpenter, C. M. 1937. Artificially induced fever for the treatment of gonococcic infections in the male. *JAMA* 109:1430.

Washburn, W. L. 1950. Leprosy among Scandinavian settlers in the upper Mississippi Valley, 1864–1932. *Bull. Hist. Med.* 24:123.

Wassermann, A. 1907. Ueber die bisherigen Erfahrungen mit dem Meningococcen-Heilserum bei Genickstarrekranken. *Dtsch. med. Wochenschr.* 33:1585.

Wassermann, A.; Neisser, A.; and Bruck, C. 1906. Eine serodiagnostische Reaktion bei Syphilis. *Dtsch. med. Wochenschr.* 32:745.

Watson, C. J., and Riley, W. A. 1926. A case of Darling's histoplasmosis originating in Minnesota. *Arch. Pathol. Lab. Med.* 1:662.

Watson, T. 1853a. Catarrh. In *Lectures on the Principles and Practice of Physic* by T. Watson, p. 532. Philadelphia: Blanchard & Lea.

Watson, T. 1853b. Hooping-Cough. Ibid., p. 552.

Watt, R. 1813. *Treatise on the History, Nature, and Treatment of Chincough. Including a Variety of Cases and Dissections*. Glasgow: John Smith & Son.

Webb, G. B. 1936. *Tuberculosis*. New York: P. B. Hoeber.

Webster, L. T., and Fite, G. L. 1933. A virus encountered in the study of material from cases of encephalitis in the St. Louis and Kansas City epidemics of 1933. *Science* 78:463.

Weed, L. A.; Andersen, H. A.; Good, C. A.; and Baggenstoss, A. H. 1955. Nocardiosis: Clinical, bacteriologic and pathological aspects. *N. Engl. J. Med.* 253:1137.

Weichselbaum, A. 1887a. Ueber die Aetiologie der Akuten Meningitis Cerebro-spinalis. *Fortschr. Med.* 5:573 and 620.

Weichselbaum, A. 1887b. Zusammenfassender historischer Bericht über die Aetiologie der acuten Lungen-und Rippenfellentzündungen. *Zentbl. Bakt. ParasitKde* 1:553.

Weil, A. 1886. Ueber eine eigenthümliche, mit Milztumor, Icterus und Nephritis einhergehende, acute Infectionskrankheit. *Dtschs. Arch. klin. Med.* 39:209.

Weiner, L. P.; Herndon, R. M.; Narayan, O.; Johnson, R. T.; Shah, K.; Rubinstein, L. J.; Preziosi, T. J.; and Conley, F. K. 1972. Isolation of virus related to SV40 from patients with progressive multifocal leukoencephalopathy. *N. Engl. J. Med.* 286:385.

Weinstein, L. 1975a. Rifampin. In *The Pharmacological Basis of Therapeutics*, edited by L. S. Goodman and A. Gilman. 5th ed., p. 1208. New York: Macmillan.

Weinstein, L. 1975b. Sulfonamides and trimethoprim-sulfamethoxazole. Ibid., p. 1113.

Weinstein, L., and Ehrenkranz, N. J. 1958. *Streptomycin and Dihydrostreptomycin*. Antibiotics Monograph No. 10. New York: Medical Encyclopedia.

Weinstein, L., and Kaplan, K. 1970. The cephalosporins. A review of microbiological, chemical, and pharmacological properties and use in chemotherapy of infection. *Ann. Intern. Med.* 72:729.

Weinstein, M. J.; Luedemann, G. M.; Oden, E. M.; and Wagman, G. H. 1964. Gentamicin, a new broad-spectrum antibiotic complex. In *Antimicrobial Agents and Chemotherapy-1963*, edited by J. C. Sylvester, p. 1. Ann Arbor (Mich.): American Society for Microbiology.

Welch, W. H. 1888. The Cartwright Lectures on the general pathology of fever. *Med. News* 52:365 (Lecture I); 393 (Lect. I contd.); 397 (Lect. II); 539 (Lect. III); 565 (Lect. III contd.).

Weller, T. H. 1953. Serial propagation *in vitro* of agents producing inclusion bodies derived from varicella and herpes zoster. *Proc. Soc. Exp. Biol. Med.* 83:340.

Weller, T. H. 1971. The cytomegaloviruses: Ubiquitous agents with protean clinical manifestations. *N. Engl. J. Med.* 285:203 and 267.

Weller, T. H.; Macauley, J. C.; Craig, J. M.; and Wirth, P. 1957. Isolation of intranuclear inclusion producing agents from infants with illnesses resembling cytomegalic inclusion disease. *Proc. Soc. Exp. Biol. Med.* 94:4.

Weller, T. H., and Neva, F. A. 1962. Propagation in tissue culture of cytopathic agents from patients with rubella-like illness. *Proc. Soc. Exp. Biol. Med.* 111:215.

Wesselhoeft, C. 1947. Rubella (German measles.) *N. Engl. J. Med.* 236:943 and 948.

Wesselhoeft, C.; Smith, E. C.; and Branch, C. F. 1938. Human encephalitis: Eight fatal cases, with four due to the virus of equine encephalomyelitis. *JAMA* 111:1735.

West, J. P. 1896. An epidemic of glandular fever. *Arch. Pediat.* 13:889.

Wherry, W. B., and Lamb, B. H. 1914. Infection of man with *Bacterium tularense*. *J. Infect. Dis.* 15:331.

Whipple, G. C. 1908. *Typhoid Fever: Its Causation, Transmission and Prevention.* New York: John Wiley and Sons.

Whitby, L. E. H. 1938. Chemotherapy of pneumococcal and other infections with 2-(p-aminobenzenesulphonamido) pyridine. *Lancet* 234:1210.

White, B. 1924. *Smallpox and Vaccination.* Cambridge (Mass.): Harvard University Press.

White, B. 1938. *The Biology of Pneumococcus. The Bactericidal, Biochemical, and Immunological Characters and Activities of Diplococcus pneumoniae.* New York: Commonwealth Fund.

White, C. 1773. *A Treatise on the Management of Pregnant and Lying-in Women and the Means of Curing, but More Especially of Preventing the Principle Disorders to Which They Are Liable.* London: E. & C. Dilly.

Whitehair, C. K. 1956. Antibiotics in growth promotion of livestock. In *Symposium on Medicated Feeds,* edited by H. Welch and F. Marti-Ibanez, p. 38. New York: Medical Encyclopedia.

Whytt, R. 1768. *Observations on the Dropsy in the Brain.* Edinburgh: Balfour, Auld & Smellie.

Wickman, I. 1913. *Acute Poliomyelitis (Heine-Medin's Disease).* Translated by J. W. Maloney. *Nervous and Mental Disease Monograph Series* No. 16. New York: Journal of Nervous and Mental Disease Publishing Co.

Widal, F. 1896. Sérodiagnostic de la fièvre typhoide. *Bull. Mem. Soc. méd. Hôp. Paris.* 13 (Third Series): 561.

Wilensky, A. O. 1934. *Osteomyelitis. Its Pathogenesis, Symptomatology and Treatment.* New York: Macmillan.

Wilks, S. 1868. Pyaemia as a result of endocarditis. *Br. Med. J.* 1:297.

Willan, R. 1809. *On Cutaneous Diseases.* Vol. 1. Philadelphia: Kimber and Conrad.

Williams, J. H., Consulting ed. 1948. Aureomycin — A new antibiotic. A conference. Held July 21, 1948. *Ann. NY Acad. Sci.* 51:175–342.

Williams, J. T. 1936. Epidemic puerperal sepsis. *N. Engl. J. Med.* 215:1022.

Williams, R. C. 1951. *The United States Public Health Service, 1798–1950.* Washington, D.C.: Commissioned Officers Association of the U.S. Public Health Service.

Willis, T. 1684. *Dr. Willis's Practice of Physick; Being the Whole Works of that Renowned and Famous Physician.* London: T. Dring, C. Harper and J. Leigh.

Wilson, G. S., and Miles, A. A. 1964a. Staphylococcus and Micrococcus. In *Topley and Wilson's Principles of Bacteriology and Immunity,* revised by G. S. Wilson and A. A. Miles. 5th ed. Vol. 1, p. 746. Baltimore: Williams & Wilkins.

Wilson, G. S., and Miles, A. A. 1964b. Tetanus. Ibid., p. 2095.

Wilson, G. S., and Miles, A. A. 1964c. *Topley and Wilson's Principles of Bacteriology and Immunity,* revised by G. S. Wilson and A. A. Miles. 5th ed. 2 vols. Baltimore: Williams & Wilkins.

Wilson, G. S., and Miles, A. A. 1964d. Tuberculosis. Ibid., p. 1588.

Wilson, G. S., and Miles, A. A. 1975. The streptococci. In *Topley and Wilson's Principles of Bacteriology, Virology and Immunity,* by G. S. Wilson and A. A. Miles. 6th ed. Vol. 1, p. 712. Baltimore: Williams & Wilkins.

Wilson, J. F.; Diddams, A. C.; and Rausch, R. L. 1968. Cystic hydatid disease in Alaska. A review of 101 autochthonous cases of *Echinococcus granulosus* infection. *Am. Rev. Respir. Dis.* 98:1.

Wiltshire, H. W., and MacGillycuddy, A.R.N. 1915. Experiences in the treatment of typhoid fever by stock typhoid vaccine. *Lancet* 189:685.

Winge, E.F.H. 1945. Mycosis endocardii (1869). In *Classic Description of Disease* by R. Major. 3rd ed., p. 471. Springfield (Ill.): Chas. C Thomas.

Winslow, C-E. A. 1920. The untilled fields of public health. *Science* 51(N.S.):23.

Winslow, C-E. A. 1929. The contribution of Herman Biggs to public health. *Am. Rev. Tuberc.* 20:1.

Winslow, C-E. A., and Herrington, L. P. 1949. *Temperature and Human Life.* Princeton (N.J.): Princeton University Press.

Winterbottom, T. M. 1803. *An Account of the Native Africans in the Neighborhood of Sierra Leoni*. Vol. 2. London: C. Wittingham.

Winternitz, M. C.; Wason, I. M.; and McNamara, F. P. 1920. *The Pathology of Influenza*. New Haven (Conn.): Yale University Press.

Wise, R. I. 1965. The staphylococcus — approach to therapy. *Med. Clin. North Am.* 49:1403.

Wise, R. I. 1973. Modern management of severe staphylococcal disease. *Medicine* 52:295.

Wise, R. I.; Cranny, C.; and Spink, W. W. 1956. Epidemiologic studies on antibiotic-resistant strains of *Micrococcus pyogenes*. *Am. J. Med.* 20:176.

Wogan, G. N., ed. 1965. *Mycotoxins in Foodstuffs*. International symposium held in Cambridge, Massachusetts, 1964. Cambridge (Mass.): The M.I.T. Press.

Wolbach, S. B. 1919. Studies on Rocky Mountain spotted fever. *J. Med. Res.* 41:1.

Wolbach, S. B.; Todd, J. L.; and Palfrey, F. W. 1922. *The Etiology and Pathology of Typhus*. Cambridge (Mass.): Harvard University Press.

Wolf, A., and Cowen, D. 1937. Granulomatous encephalomyelitis due to an encephalitozoan (encephalitozoic encephalomyelitis). A new Protozoan disease of man. *Bull. neurol. Inst. NY* 6:306.

Wollenman, Jr., O. J., and Finland, M. 1943. Pathology of staphylococcal pneumonia complicating clinical pneumonia. *Am. J. Pathol.* 19:23.

Wollstein, M. 1911a. Influenzal meningitis and its experimental production. *Am. J. Dis Child.* 1:42.

Wollstein, M. 1911b. Serum treatment of influenzal meningitis. *J. Exp. Med.* 14:73.

Wood, H. C. 1881. Fever: A study in morbid and normal physiology. *Smithson. Contr. Knowl.* 23:Article VI (No. 357) p. 1.

Woodhead, G. S., and Varrier-Jones, P. C. 1916. Investigations on clinical thermometry: Continuous and quasi-continuous temperature records in man and animals in health and disease. *Lancet* 190: 173, 281, 338, 450, and 495.

Woodruff, A. M., and Goodpasture, E. W. 1931. The susceptibility of the chorio-allantoic membrane of chick embryos to infection with the fowl-pox virus. *Am. J. Pathol.* 7:209.

Woods, D. D. 1940. The relation of p-aminobenzoic acid to the mechanism of the action of sulphanilamide. *Br. J. Exp. Pathol.* 21:74.

Woodward, T. E. 1974. The rickettsioses. In *Harrison's Principles of Internal Medicine*, edited by M. M. Wintrobe et al. 7th ed., p. 909. New York: McGraw-Hill.

Woodward, T. E.; Hall, H. E.; Dias-Rivera, R.; Hightower, J. A.; Martinez, E.; and Parker, R. T. 1951. Treatment of typhoid fever. II. Control of clinical manifestations with cortisone. *Ann. Intern. Med.* 34:10.

Woodward, T. E.; Smadel, J. E.; Ley, Jr., H. L.; Green, R.; and Mankikar, D. S. 1948. Preliminary report on the beneficial effect of chloromycetin in the treatment of typhoid fever. *Ann. Intern. Med.* 29:131.

Woodward, T. E., and Wisseman, Jr., C. L. 1958. *Chloromycetin (Chloramphenicol)*. Antibiotics Monographs No. 8. New York: Medical Encyclopedia.

Woodworth, J. M. 1875. *Cholera Epidemic of 1873 in the United States: The Introduction of Epidemic Cholera through the Agency of the Mercantile Marine: Suggestions of Measures of Prevention*. Washington, D.C.: U.S. Government Printing Office.

World Health Organization. 1947. Constitution of the World Health Organization. *WHO Chron.* 1:29.

World Health Organization. 1955. Eighth World Health Assembly. *Off. Rec. Wld. Hlth. Org.* No. 63.

World Health Organization. 1958a. Eleventh World Health Assembly. *WHO Chron.* 12:224.

World Health Organization. 1958b. *The First Ten Years of the World Health Organization*. Geneva: World Health Organization.

World Health Organization. 1959. Hydatidosis. In *Joint WHO/FAO Expert Committee on Zoonoses. Second Report. WHO Tech Rep Ser.* No. 169, p. 44.

World Health Organization. 1960. *Bibliography on Bilharziasis 1949–1958.* Geneva: World Health Organization.

World Health Organization. 1965. *Bibliography of Hookworm Disease (Ancylostomiasis) 1920–1962.* Geneva: World Health Organization.

World Health Organization. 1967a. Arboviruses and human disease. Report of a scientific group. *WHO Tech. Rep. Ser.* No. 369.

World Health Organization. 1967b. Chemotherapy of malaria. Report of a WHO scientific group. *WHO Tech. Rep. Ser.* No. 375.

World Health Organization. 1967c. Echinococcosis control in Iceland and New Zealand. In *Joint FAO/WHO Expert Committee on Zoonoses. Third Report. WHO Tech. Rep. Ser.* No. 378, p. 124.

World Health Organization. 1968a. Echinococcosis (hydatidosis): Symposium. *Bull. WHO* 39:1–36.

World Health Organization. 1968b. *The Second Ten Years of the World Health Organization 1958–1967.* Geneva: World Health Organization.

World Health Organization. 1969a. African trypanosomiasis: Report of Joint FAO/WHO Expert Committee. *WHO Tech Rep. Ser.* No. 434.

World Health Organization. 1969b. Cerebrospinal meningitis in Africa. *WHO Chron.* 23:54.

World Health Organization. 1969c. Comparative studies of American and African trypanosomiasis. Report of a WHO scientific group. *WHO Tech. Rep. Ser.* No. 411.

World Health Organization. 1970. Principles and practice of cholera control. *Publ. Hlth Pap. WHO* No. 40.

World Health Organization. 1971a. *International Health Regulations, 1969.* Adopted by the twenty-second World Health Assembly. 1st annotated ed. Geneva: World Health Organization.

World Health Organization. 1971b. Leishmaniasis. *Bull. WHO* 44 *(Suppl.)* No. 4:471–584.

World Health Organization. 1971c. Morbidity statistics: Trachoma, 1955–1969. *WHO Stat. Rep.* 24:274.

World Health Organization. 1972a. Reports on malaria in the WHO Technical Series: An evaluation. *WHO Chron.* 26:496.

World Health Organization. 1972b. Trypanosomiasis. *Bull. WHO* 47 *(Suppl.)* No. 6:685–820.

World Health Organization. 1973. Chemotherapy of malaria and resistance to antimalarials: Report of WHO scientific group. *WHO Tech. Rep. Ser.* No. 529.

World Health Organization. 1974a. Communicable diseases and vector control in 1973: Leprosy. *WHO Chron.* 28:318.

World Health Organization. 1974b. Communicable diseases and vector control in 1973: Onchocerciasis. *WHO Chron.* 28:322.

World Health Organization. 1974c. Communicable diseases and vector control in 1973: Tuberculosis. *WHO Chron.* 28:317.

World Health Organization. 1974d. WHO Expert Committee on Tuberculosis. Ninth Report. *WHO Tech. Rep. Ser.* No. 552.

World Health Organization. 1974e. *World Health Organization Publications: 1947–1973. A Catalogue.* Geneva: World Health Organization.

World Health Organization. 1976. Resistance of vectors and reservoirs of disease to pesticides. 22nd report of the WHO Expert Committee on Insecticides. *WHO Tech. Rep. Ser.* No. 585.

World Health Organization, Director General. 1972. Malaria eradication in 1971. *WHO Chron.* 26:485.

World Health Organization, Director General. 1974. Trachoma. In *The Work of WHO*

1973: Annual Report of the Director-General to the World Health Assembly and to the United Nations. Off. Rec. Wld. Hlth. Org. No. 213, p. 12.

World Health Organization Expert Committee on Filariasis. 1974. WHO Expert Committee on Filariasis. Third Report. *WHO Tech. Rep. Ser.* No. 542.

World Health Organization Expert Committee on Plague. 1970. WHO Expert Committee on Plague. Fourth Report. *WHO Tech. Rep. Ser.* No. 447.

World Health Organization Expert Committee on Poliomyelitis. 1958. Expert Committee on Poliomyelitis. Second Report. *WHO Tech. Rep. Ser.* No. 145.

World Health Organization Expert Committee on Rabies. 1966. WHO Expert Committee on Rabies. Fifth Report. *WHO Tech. Rep. Ser.* No. 321.

World Health Organization Expert Committee on Streptococcal and Staphylococcal Infections. 1968. Streptococcal and Staphylococcal Infections: Report of a WHO Expert Committee. *WHO Tech. Rep. Ser.* No. 394.

World Health Organization Expert Committee on Trachoma. 1962. Expert Committee on Trachoma. Third Report. *WHO Tech. Rep. Ser.* No. 234.

World Health Organization Expert Committee on Zoonoses. 1951; 1959; 1967. Joint FAO/WHO Expert Committee on Zoonoses. First Report *WHO Tech. Rep. Ser.* No. 40 (1951); Second Report *WHO Tech. Rep. Ser.* No. 169 (1959); Third Report *WHO Tech. Rep. Ser.* No. 378 (1967).

World Health Organization Expert Panel on Brucellosis. 1951; 1953; 1958; 1964; 1971. Joint FAO/WHO Expert Panel on Brucellosis. First Report *WHO Tech. Rep. Ser.* No. 37 (1951); Second Report *WHO Tech. Rep. Ser.* No. 67 (1953); Third Report *WHO Tech. Rep. Ser.* No. 148 (1958); Fourth Report *WHO Tech. Rep. Ser.* No. 289 (1964); Fifth Report *WHO Tech. Rep. Ser.* No. 464 (1971).

World Health Organization Report of a WHO Expert Group. 1967. Current problems in leptospirosis research. *WHO Tech. Rep. Ser.* No. 380.

Wright, A. E. 1908. The principles of vaccine therapy. In *The Harvey Lectures 1906–07.* Vol. 2, p. 17. Philadelphia: J. B. Lippincott.

Wright, A. E. 1915. A lecture on wound infections and their treatment. *Br. Med. J.* 2:629.

Wright, A. E. 1919. A lecture on the lessons of the war and on some new prospects in the field of therapeutic immunisation. *Lancet* 196:489.

Wright, A. E.; Fleming, A.; and Colebrook, L. 1918. The conditions under which the sterilisation of wounds by physiological agency can be obtained. *Lancet* 194:831.

Wright, A. E.; Morgan, W. P.; Cantab, M. B.; Colebrook, L.; and Dodgson, M. D. 1914. Observations on prophylactic inoculation against pneumococcus infections, and on the results which have been achieved by it. *Lancet* 186:1 and 87.

Wright, A. E., and Semple, D. 1897. Remarks on vaccination against typhoid fever. *Br. Med. J.* 1:256.

Wucherer, O. 1868. Noticia preliminar sobre vermes de uma especie ainda não descripta, encontrados na urina de doentes de hematuria intertropical no Brazil. *Gazeta med. Bahia* 3:97.

Wunderlich, C. A. 1871. *On the Temperature in Diseases: A Manual of Medical Thermometry.* Translated by W. Bathurst Woodman from the second German edition. Vol. 49, p. 1. London: New Sydenham Society.

Wunderlich, C. A., and Seguin, E. 1871. *Medical Thermometry, and Human Temperature.* New York: William Wood.

Yersin 1894. La peste bubonique à Hong-Kong. *Annls. Inst. Pasteur* 8:662.

Youmans, G. P.; Williston, E. H.; Feldman, W. H.; and Hinshaw, H. C. 1946. Increase in resistance of tubercle bacilli to streptomycin: A preliminary report. *Proc. Staff Meet. Mayo Clin.* 21:126.

Young, H. H.; White, E. C.; and Swartz, E. O. 1919. A new germicide for use in the genito-urinary tract: "Mercurochrome-220." *JAMA* 73:1483.

Young, J. H. 1976. Botulism and the ripe olive scare of 1919–1920. *Bull. Hist. Med.* 50:372.

Young, L. S.; Bicknell, D. S.; Archer, B. G.; Clinton, J. M.; Leavens, L. J.; Feeley, J. C.;

and Brachman, P. S. 1969. Tularemia epidemic: Vermont, 1968. Forty-seven cases linked to contact with muskrats. *N. Engl. J. Med.* 280:1253.

Yow, E. M., and Spink, W. W. 1949. Experimental studies of the action of streptomycin, aureomycin, and chloromycetin on brucella. *J. Clin. Invest.* 28:871.

Yugoslav Typhoid Commission 1964. A controlled field trial of the effectiveness of acetone-dried and inactivated and heat-phenol-inactivated typhoid vaccines in Yugoslavia. *Bull. WHO* 30:623.

Zarafonetis, C.J.D. 1949. Infectious mononucleosis. *J.-Lancet* 69:364.

Zarafonetis, C.J.D., and Baker, M. P. 1963. Scrub typhus. In *Internal Medicine in World War II* by U.S. Army Medical Service. Vol. 2, p. 111. Washington, D.C.: Office of the Surgeon-General, Department of the Army.

Zenker, F. A. 1866. Beiträge zur Lehre von der Trichinenkrankheit. *Dtschs. Arch. klin. Med.* 1:90.

Zinsser, H. 1922. The etiology and epidemiology of influenza. *Medicine* 1:213.

Zinsser, H. 1927. *A Textbook of Bacteriology.* 6th ed. New York: D. Appleton.

Zinsser, H. 1934. Varieties of typhus virus and the epidemiology of the American form of European typhus fever (Brill's disease). *Am. J. Hyg.* 20:513.

Zinsser, H. 1935. *Rats, Lice and History.* Boston: Little, Brown.

Zuckerman, A. J. 1972. *Hepatitis-Associated Antigen and Viruses.* New York: American Elsevier Publishing Co.

INDEXES

Name Index

Subject Index

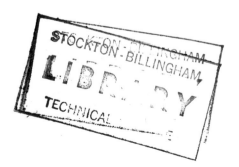